Clinical Pathways in Neuro-Ophthalmology

An Evidence-Based Approach

Clinical Pathways in Neuro-Ophthalmology
An Evidence-Based Approach

Andrew G. Lee, M.D.
Assistant Professor
Departments of Ophthalmology, Neurology, and Neurosurgery
Baylor College of Medicine
Department of Neurosurgery
M.D. Anderson Cancer Center
The University of Texas
Houston, Texas

Paul W. Brazis, M.D.
Associate Professor of Neurology
Mayo School of Medicine
Consultant in Neurology and Neuro-Ophthalmology
Mayo Clinic Jacksonville
Jacksonville, Florida

1998
Thieme
New York • Stuttgart

Thieme New York
333 Seventh Avenue
New York, NY 10001

Clinical Pathways in Neuro-Ophthalmology
Andrew G. Lee, M.D.
Paul W. Brazis, M.D.

Lee, Andrew G.
Clinical pathways in neuro-ophthalmology / Andrew G. Lee, Paul Brazis.
p. cm.
Includes bibliographical references and index.
ISBN 0-86577-755-1. — ISBN 3-13-108641-6 (German)
1. Neuroophthalmology. 2. Medical protocols. I. Brazis, Paul W.
II. Title.
[DNLM: 1. Eye Diseases. 2. Optic Nerve Diseases. 3. Critical
Pathways. 4. Neurologic Manifestations. WW 460 L477c 1998]
RE725.L44 1998
617.7—dc21
DNLM/DLC
for Library of Congress 97-51525
CIP

Printed in the United States of America
Composition by V&M Graphics, Inc.; Printed by Hamilton Printing Company

5 4 3 2 1

TNY ISBN 0-86577-755-1
GTV ISBN 3-13-108641-6

To our wives, Hilary and Liz

and

to our parents, Alberto C. Lee, M.D.,
and Rosalind G. Lee, M.D., and
Dr. and Mrs. Peter T. Brazis

Contents

Foreword

Never in the history of medicine have physicians had so many ways to both diagnose and treat disease and never have physicians had so many bureaucratic barriers to performing these activities. This paradox has necessitated a return to the days when clinical judgment was at least as important as diagnostic testing. The challenge to all of us who care for patients is thus to understand the signs and symptoms that distinguish among many different local and systemic disorders so that we can perform the most logical, expeditious, safe, and economic assessment.

Andrew Lee is an ophthalmologist and head of the neuro-ophthalmology service at the Cullen Eye Institute of the Baylor College of Medicine in Houston, Texas. Paul Brazis is a neurologist and head of the neuro-ophthalmology service at the Mayo Clinic in Jacksonville, Florida. Both of these authors have extensive training and experience in the field of neuro-ophthalmology, and both have contributed singly and together to the field of neuro-ophthalmology with numerous articles, chapters, and textbooks. In this book, these authors provide the reader with a triumverate of information. First, they describe the symptoms and signs of a variety of neuro-opthalmologic disorders, such as anterior and retrobulbar optic neuropathies, ocular motor nerve pareses and other disorders of ocular motility and alignment, and anisocoria. Second, they provide algorithms for differentiating, both in the office and using laboratory and neuroimaging studies, among conditions that often have overlapping clinical manifestations. Finally, they provide a basic set of references about each subject that the reader can use to expand his or her knowledge.

By providing basic, clinically relevant information regarding various disorders, their diagnosis, and treatment, this book teaches the reader how to approach a patient with a known or presumed neuro-ophthalmologic problem in a logical, straight-forward, and cost-effective manner. As such, it is a welcome addition to the neuro-opthalmologic repertoire.

Neil R. Miller
Baltimore, MD

Preface

In this textbook, we present an evidence-based critical literature review of the most important clinical problems in neuro-ophthalmology. In preparing to write this volume, we have reviewed all of the pertinent English language literature (MEDLINE 1966 to 1996) concerning each topic and have attempted to summarize a large body of knowledge into useful decision making points. Many of these literature reviews are summarized in table form and extensive reference lists are provided. We have strived to consolidate the clinical data into simple and user friendly, practical decision-making diagnosis-specific algorithms. These algorithms are not intended to be extensive and cover all possibilities, but are used as an outline approach to the text and a general guide to the decision-making involved in various neuro-ophthalmologic problems.

As several excellent texts on neuro-ophthalmology already exist, we have not endeavored to write an all-inclusive general neuro-ophthalmology textbook and will not, in this volume, discuss extensively the basic anatomy, physiology, and pharmacology of the afferent and efferent visual systems. Instead, we assume that the clinician has a basic understanding of neurologic and ophthalmologic principles and wants to know "what to do" with the neuro-ophthalmologic patient in the clinical setting. The reader is referred to the existing excellent review texts mentioned above for the details of the neuro-ophthalmology exam, pathophysiology, etc. In addition, this text is intended mainly as a guide in the evaluation of the adult neuro-ophthalmologic patient. The text is specifically aimed at "front-line" clinicians, that is, physicians in ophthalmology, neurology, and neurosurgery, especially residents and fellows, who are daily evaluating and treating neuro-ophthalmologic problems.

We would especially like to thank our mentor, colleague, and friend, Dr. Neil R. Miller, for his scholarship, advice, and example. We would also like to thank the following individuals for their support: Dr. Dan Jones, Dr. Robert Grossman, Dr. Stanley Appel, Dr. James Corbett, and Dr. Jonathan Trobe. Ms. Jackie Nichols was invaluable in providing secretarial assistance. We also appreciate the excellent counsel and encouragement of our editor, Ms. Andrea Seils, of Thieme New York. Finally, we wish to thank the faculty, residents, and staff of the Departments of Ophthalmology, Neurology, and Neurosurgery at Baylor College of Medicine, the Department of Neurosurgery at the University of Texas, M.D. Anderson Cancer Center, and the Mayo Clinic Jacksonville and Rochester for their interest and academic stimulation.

Andrew G. Lee, M.D.
Paul W. Brazis, M.D.

Clinical Pathways in Neuro-Ophthalmology

An Evidence-Based Approach

1

The Diagnosis of Optic Neuropathies

The diagnosis of an optic neuropathy is usually made on clinical grounds alone. Several excellent references discuss in detail the anatomy of the optic nerve as well as examination techniques (Burde, 1992; Chisholm, 1969; Glaser, 1976, 1978; Griffin, 1978; Hoyt, 1976; Johnson, 1988; Levin, 1983; Miller, 1982; Sanders, 1976; Smith, 1977; Sunga, 1970; Thompson, 1976, 1982; Younge, 1980). The clinical features of optic neuropathies are summarized in Table 1–1.

Other more sophisticated (and time consuming) tests for optic neuropathy, such as visual-evoked potentials, formal color vision testing, or contrast sensitivity (Lorance, 1987; Rubin, 1988), are not presented. An extensive discussion of the objective and subjective testing of visual function and the neuro-ophthalmologic exam is beyond the scope of this text and is contained in many excellent reviews (Burde, 1992; Chisholm, 1969; Glaser, 1976, 1978; Miller, 1982; Smith, 1977; Sunga, 1970; Younge, 1980).

Once the diagnosis of optic neuropathy has been made, it is important to consider a wide differential diagnosis of possible etiologies, including hereditary, inflammatory, infiltrative, ischemic, demyelinating (optic neuritis), and compressive optic neuropathies. We refer the reader to the specific chapter on each type of optic neuropathy for further details.

Table 1–1. Clinical Features of an Optic Neuropathy

Clinical Features
Decreased visual acuity
Decreased color vision
Visual field defect
Ipsilateral relative afferent pupillary defect in unilateral or bilateral, asymmetric cases
Light-near dissociation of the pupils in bilateral and symmetric cases
Optic disc edema or disc atrophy (although the optic nerve may appear normal in retrobulbar optic neuropathy)

Source: Burde, 1992; Chisholm, 1969; Glaser, 1976, 1978; Griffin, 1978; Hoyt, 1976; Levin, 1983; Miller, 1982; Sanders, 1976; Smith, 1977; Sunga, 1970; Thompson, 1976; Younge, 1980.

Can the Appearance of the Optic Nerve Differentiate Etiology?

In general, the appearance of the optic nerve (e.g., normal, swollen, or pale) is not specific and cannot differentiate among the various possible etiologies for optic neuropathy. Trobe et al. reviewed 163 color fundus photographs of several entities resulting in optic atrophy, including glaucoma, central retinal artery occlusion (CRAO), ischemic optic neuropathy (ION), optic neuritis (ON), hereditary optic neuropathy (Leber's and non-Leber's types), compressive optic neuropathy (CON), and traumatic optic neuropathy (TON) (Trobe, 1980). These photographs were reviewed by five ophthalmologists as "unknowns." Glaucoma, CRAO, and ION were correctly identified as the etiology by at least one of five observers with an accuracy above 80%, but the remaining etiologies were correctly identified in less than 50% of cases! Helpful features in differentiating the entities included:

1. The presence of retinal arteriolar attenuation and sheathing in ischemic lesions (e.g., CRAO or ION).
2. Temporal pallor in entities selectively involving central vision and central visual field with sparing of peripheral visual field (e.g., optic neuritis and toxic optic neuropathies).
3. Superior or inferior (sector) optic disc pallor in ION.

Although optic disc cupping was often identified in glaucoma, it was also seen in 20% of cases not associated with glaucoma. Optic disc cupping in glaucoma cases, however, was more profound than in nonglaucomatous cases and greater neuroretinal rim pallor occurred in the nonglaucomatous cases. Interestingly, only 11% of these cases with a known history of papillitis or ION had sufficient clues to identify previous disc swelling (Trobe, 1980).

In addition, numerous authors have stressed the localizing value to the optic chiasm or optic tract of a special type of optic disc atrophy caused by specific involvement of the nerve fiber layer of the nasal and temporal retina, respectively. Involvement of these fibers results in atrophy of the nasal and temporal optic disc with sparing of the inferior and superior poles ("band" or "bowtie" atrophy). Band atrophy occurs in the eye contralateral to the involved optic tract and may be unilateral or bilateral with lesions of the optic chiasm.

Neither the pattern (e.g., central scotoma, arcuate, altitudinal) of ipsilateral visual field impairment nor the severity of visual loss is not pathognomonic for a specific optic neuropathy (Harms, 1976; Trobe and Glaser, 1978) and virtually any visual field defect may occur with any optic neuropathy (Gutman, 1984; Slavin, 1986). In their report on 35 eyes in 20 patients with CON and 70 eyes in 54 patients with ON, Trobe and Glaser found central scotomas in 33% of cases of CON (vs. 75% in ON) and felt that a central scotoma could not be used as a differentiating feature between the two entities (Trobe and Glaser, 1978).

The following sections describe the evaluation of optic neuropathy; this approach is summarized in Figure 1–1. We begin with an age-based differential diagnosis of an acute optic neuropathy.

Two of the most common causes of acute optic neuropathy are anterior ischemic optic neuropathy (AION) and ON. Although there is considerable overlap in their clinical presentation, age can be used as an initial differentiating feature in many cases (Rizzo, 1991). In younger patients (< 40 years old) with acute unilateral optic disc edema and evidence for an optic neuropathy, ON is more likely than AION. Conversely, in the older patient with acute optic disc edema and visual loss, AION is more common.

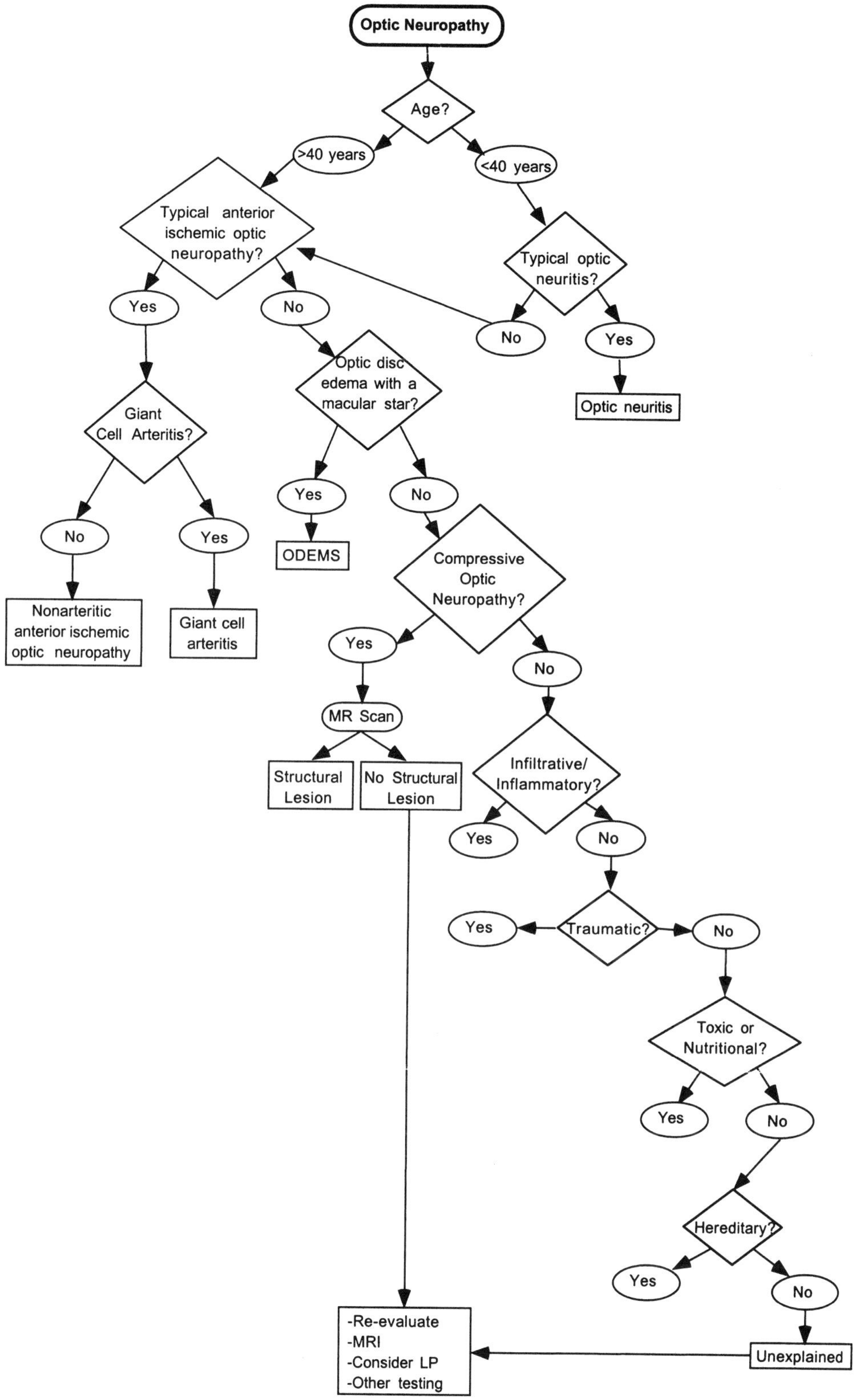

Figure 1–1. Evaluation of an optic neuropathy.

Is the Clinical Presentation Typical for Anterior Ischemic Optic Neuropathy?

The features of typical AION are discussed in Chapter 4. If these features are present, the patient should undergo an evaluation for underlying vasculopathic risk factors and giant cell arteritis.

Is the Clinical Presentation Typical for Optic Neuritis?

The features and evaluation of typical ON are described in Chapter 2. The evaluation of optic disc edema with a macular star is outlined in Chapter 3.

Is the Clinical Presentation Consistent with Optic Disc Edema with a Macular Star (ODEMS)?

Is a Compressive Optic Neuropathy Present?

Optic nerve compression (CON) usually causes painless, progressive, gradual loss of visual function (visual acuity, visual field, and color vision), a relative afferent pupillary defect (in unilateral or asymmetric cases), and optic disc edema or atrophy (but the optic disc may initially appear normal) (Burde, 1992; Clifford-Jones, 1985; Cruysberg, 1982; Frisen, 1980; Glaser and Trobe, 1979; Knight, 1972; Miller, 1982; Trobe, 1978). Unfortunately, CON may also present acutely or be steroid responsive and may masquerade as an inflammatory or demyelinating optic neuropathy (Hirst, 1980; Kamin, 1972; Kennerdell, 1974; Senelick, 1974; Spoor, 1982).

CON that is due to orbital or intracanalicular lesions may result in ipsilateral optic disc edema followed by optic atrophy; it may be associated with the development of abnormal blood vessels on the disc head called optociliary shunt vessels. These vessels probably represent collateral circulation between the retinal and choroidal venous circulation that allows venous blood to bypass the compression at the level of the optic nerve. The presence of an unexplained relative afferent pupillary defect or unexplained optic atrophy should prompt appropriate neuroimaging studies (usually magnetic resonance imaging of the involved optic nerve) (Guy, 1990). Orbital signs such as proptosis, chemosis, or conjunctival injection should direct the imaging studies to the orbit. Table 1–2 lists some possible causes of CON.

Table 1–2. Lesions Causing Compressive Optic Neuropathy

Intracranial or intraorbital benign and malignant tumors
Meningioma
Glioma
Craniopharyngioma
Pituitary adenoma
Lymphoma
Metastasis

Inflammatory or infectious sinus disease (e.g., mucoceles)
Primary bone disease (e.g., osteopetrosis, fibrous dysplasia)
Vascular etiologies
  Orbital hemorrhage
  Carotid artery aneurysm
  Dolichoectasia of the carotid artery
  Arteriovascular malformations
Hydrocephalus
Iatrogenic
  Intranasal balloon catheter
  Intracranial oxidized cellulose hemostat
Thyroid ophthalmopathy

Source: Aasved, 1970; Alper, 1976; Anderson, 1970; Arseni, 1970; Berson, 1966; Brazis, 1995; Burde, 1978, 1992; Burnbaum, 1978; Colapinto, 1996; Calderon, 1969; Calogero, 1971; Carlin, 1981; Carrion, 1979; Crivelli, 1970; Decker, 1979; Durston, 1970; Dutton, 1983; Ginsberg, 1970; Glaser, 1971; Golnik, 1996; Goodman, 1975; Goodwin, 1978; Gregorius, 1975; Guidetti, 1970; Hakuba, 1975; Hoyt, 1966; Imachi, 1981; Johnson, 1986; Kattah, 1993; Katz, 1991; Kazim, 1992; Kirkham, 1977; Kline, 1984; Kodsi, 1993; Kollarits, 1976; Kothandaram, 1971; Krohel, 1979; Long, 1985; Manz, 1979; Matsuo, 1980; McCarthy, 1972; Michelson, 1975; Miller, 1975, 1995; Newton, 1989; Nugent, 1970; Peiris, 1980; Puliafito, 1981; Raitta, 1968; Raymond, 1978; Reese, 1971; Ridgeway, 1976; Rutka, 1985; Savy, 1996; Senelick, 1974; Sengupta, 1976; Shields, 1986; Simpson, 1988; Slavin, 1986; Spoor, 1980; Stern, 1973; Susac, 1973; Trobe, 1978; Weiter, 1979; Yee, 1977; Zimmerman, 1975.

Is There Clinical Evidence for an Infiltrative or Inflammatory Optic Neuropathy?

Infiltrative or inflammatory optic neuropathy may present with the typical features of an optic neuropathy discussed above. As described in Chapter 2, the clinical profile of typical ON (e.g., pain with eye movement, typical age of onset, etc.) should be differentiated from atypical ON (e.g., lack of pain, atypical age of onset, anterior or posterior segment inflammation, etc.). Atypical cases should undergo an evaluation for infiltrative or inflammatory etiologies as listed in Table 1–3.

Table 1–3. Infiltrative or Inflammatory Optic Neuropathies

Neoplastic
  Plasmacytoma (Kamin, 1972) and multiple myeloma (Gudas, 1971)
  Carcinomatous meningitis (Altrocchi, 1972; Appen, 1978; Cantillo, 1979; Katz, 1991; Little, 1974; Susac, 1973)
  Leukemia (Currie, 1988; Nikaido, 1988; Phanthumchinda, 1988)
  Lymphoma (Bullock, 1979; Guyer, 1990; Kansu, 1980; Kattah, 1980; Kay, 1986; Miller, 1975; Purvin, 1984; Yen, 1985)
Paraneoplastic disease (Bennett, 1986; Boghen, 1988; Coppeto, 1988; Hoogenraad, 1989; Oohira, 1991; Pillay, 1984; Rudge, 1973; Waterston, 1986)
Infectious etiologies
  Cryptococcal meningitis (Kupfer, 1974)
  Aspergillus
  Lyme disease (Halperin, 1989; Pachner, 1989; Schecter, 1986)
  Tuberculosis
  Syphilis (Weinstein, 1981)

(continued)

Table 1–3. *(continued)*

Inflammatory diseases (Fleet, 1986)
Churg-Strauss (Acheson, 1993)
Contiguous sinus disease
Sarcoidosis (Delaney, 1977; Graham, 1986; Gelwan, 1988; Stern, 1985)
Systemic lupus erythematosus (Ahmadieh, 1994; Deutsch, 1988; Jabs, 1986; Kenik, 1987; Oppenheimer, 1986; Rosenbaum, 1997)
Sjogren's syndrome (Wise, 1988)
Relapsing polychondritis (Killian, 1978)
Polyarteritis nodosa (Kimbrell, 1967)
Inflammatory bowel disease

Source: Acheson, 1993; Achiron, 1995; Allen, 1961; Altrocchi, 1972; Appen, 1978; Barr, 1975; Belden, 1993; Brown, 1992, 1994; Bullock, 1979; Burde, 1992; Cacciatori, 1996; Cohen, 1993; Colvard, 1977; Delaney, 1977; Ellis, 1973; Freilich, 1995; Goldberg, 1989; Golnik, 1994; Graham, 1986; Gudas, 1971; Gudeman, 1982; Ing, 1996; Jabs, 1986; Jampol, 1972; Kansu, 1979, 1989; Kattah, 1980; Kay, 1986; Kinkaid, 1983; Kline, 1984; Kraus, 1963; Kupfer, 1974; Lesser, 1990; Litvak, 1964; Miller and Iliff, 1975; Nikaido, 1988; Olson, 1974; Purvin, 1984; Ridgway, 1976; Rosenthal, 1975, 1983; Rothstein, 1984; Rubinfeld, 1988; Rush, 1980; Schwartz, 1989; Sedwick, 1984; Siatkowski, 1992; Spoor, 1982; Stern, 1985; Susac, 1973; Teare, 1991; Weaver, 1986; Weinstein, 1989; Winward, 1989; Wise, 1988; Zaidman, 1986.

Patients with inflammatory autoimmune optic neuropathy often have a progressive or recurrent steroid responsive or steroid dependent clinical course (Dutton, 1982; Kupersmith, 1988). A more detailed discussion of the evaluation of atypical ON and these alternative etiologies is found in Chapter 2.

In patients with a possible inflammatory or infiltrative optic neuropathy, a lumbar puncture and additional laboratory studies (e.g., complete blood count, syphilis serology, antinuclear antibody, Lyme titer, chest radiograph, etc.) should be considered. The appropriate specific laboratory studies should be directed by pertinent history and examination findings. Table 1–9 reviews the evaluation of an atypical or unexplained optic neuropathy.

Is There Evidence for Traumatic Optic Neuropathy?

The features and evaluation of TON are discussed in Chapter 5.

Is There Evidence for a Toxic or Nutritional Optic Neuropathy?

Patients with toxic optic neuropathies usually present with painless, bilaterally symmetric, and slowly progressive visual loss. The visual field defect is typically bilateral central or cecocentral scotomas. The optic nerves may appear normal until late in the course of the disease when optic atrophy (often temporal pallor) usually develops. A number of medications and toxins may result in optic neuropathy (Ainley, 1970; Benton, 1952; Bronte-Stewart, 1976; Carroll, 1935, 1944, 1947, 1966, 1971; Chisholm, 1967, 1970, 1978; Crew, 1970; Dreyfus, 1965; Krumsiek, 1985; Leibold, 1971; Potts, 1973; Rucker, 1960; Samples, 1981; Sedwick, 1991, 1992; Sharpe, 1982; Smiddy, 1987). These are summarized in Table 1–4. Most of these etiologies can be excluded by a careful and detailed exposure and occupational history.

Table 1–4. Etiologies for Toxic Optic Neuropathy

Common Etiologies

Ethambutol (Addington, 1979; Barron, 1974; Campbell, 1988; Carr, 1962; Chatterjee, 1986; Citron, 1969, 1986; DePalma, 1989; DeVita, 1987; Harcombe, 1991; Jimenez-Lucho, 1987; Kahana, 1987, 1988; Kakisu, 1988; Karmon, 1979; Karnik, 1985; Kumar, 1993; Kuming, 1979; Leibold, 1966, 1971; Leppert, 1988; Miller, 1982; Nasemann, 1989; Polak, 1985; Roberts, 1974; Roussos, 1970; Russo, 1994; Salmon, 1987; Schild, 1991; Seth, 1991; Smith, 1987; Thomas, 1994; Walker, 1968; Yiannikas, 1983).

Ethanol and tobacco (tobacco alcohol amblyopia) (Ainley, 1958; Benton, 1952; Bronte-Stewart, 1976; Carroll, 1935, 1944, 1947, 1966, 1971; Chisholm, 1967, 1970, 1978; Crew, 1970; Dreyfuss, 1965; Krumsiek, 1985; Leibold, 1971; Potts, 1973; Rucker, 1960; Samples, 1981; Sedwick, 1991, 1992; Sharpe, 1982; Smiddy, 1987)

Chloramphenicol (Cocke, 1967; Cogan, 1973; Charache, 1977; Godel, 1980; Harley, 1970; Lamba, 1968; Snavely, 1984; Thomas, 1994)

Less Common Etiologies

Amantadine

Amiodarone (Feiner, 1987; Garrett, 1988; Gittinger, 1987; Nazarian, 1988; Sedwick, 1992)

Amoproxan

Aniline dyes

Aspidium (male fern)

Barbiturates

Cafergot (Gupta, 1972)

Caramifen (Panparnit)

Cabromal

Carbon disulfide

Carbon tetrachloride

Cephaloridine (Ballingall, 1967)

Chlorodinitrobenzene

Chlorpromazine (Rab, 1969)

Chlorpropamide (Diabenese) (Wymore, 1982)

Cobalt chloride (Licht, 1972)

Corticosteroids (Teus, 1991)

Cyanide intoxication (dietary) (Tuboku-Metzger, 1969)

Dichlorodiphenyltrichloroethane (DDT)

Digitalis

Dinitrobenzene

Dinitrotoluene

Disulfuram (Antabuse) (Norton, 1972)

D-penicillamine

Elcatonin (Kimura, 1996)

Emetine

Ethylchlorvinol (Placidyl, Serenesil) (Brown, 1969)

Ethylene glycol (Ahmed, 1971; Berger, 1981)

5-Fluoruracil (Adams, 1984)

Glue sniffing (Ehyai, 1983)

Halogenated hydroxyquinolone (Behrens, 1974; Berggren, 1968; Billson, 1972; Fleisher, 1974; Kjaersgaard, 1971; Oakley, 1973; Osterman, 1971; Pittman, 1974; Selby, 1972; Spillane, 1971, 1972; van Balen, 1971)

- Boxyquinoline (Colipar)
- Chlorquinadol (Steroxin)
- Clioquinol

(continued)

Table 1–4. *(continued)*

Cliquinol
Diiodohydroxyquin (Diodoquin)
Iodochlorhydroxyquin (Entero-Vioform)
Vioform
Heavy metals (e.g., arsenic, lead, mercury)
Hexachlorophene (PhisoHex) (Goutieres, 1977; Martinez, 1974; Slamovits, 1980)
Iodoform
Iodopyracet (Diodrast)
Isoniazid (Hughes, 1977; Jimenez-Lucho, 1987; Karmon, 1979; Kiyosawa, 1981; Snavely, 1984; Thomas, 1994)
Lead (Baghdassarian, 1968; Tennekoon, 1979)
Lysol
Methanol (Baumbach, 1977; Benton, 1976; Roe, 1943; Sharpe, 1982)
Methotrexate (Johansson, 1992)
Methyl acetate
Methyl bromide (Chavez, 1985)
Octamoxin
Organic arsenicals
Organophosphate pesticides (Uga, 1977)
Penicillamine (Goldstein, 1966)
Phenazone (Antipyrene)
Pheniprazine (Catron)
Plasmocid
Quinine
Sodium fluoride
Streptomycin
Styrene (vinyl benzyl)
Sulfonamides
Thallium
Thioglycolates
Tolubutamide (Orinase)
Trichloroethylene
Tricresyl phosphate
Vincristine (Norton, 1979; Sanderson, 1976; Sandler, 1969)

Source: Modified from Miller, 1982.

Ethambutol is a prominent etiology of toxic optic neuropathy. The mechanism of ethambutol toxicity is poorly understood but may be related to zinc depletion (Kahana, 1987; Schild, 1991). The incidence of toxicity is dose and duration dependent (Addington, 1979; Barron, 1974; Campbell, 1988; Carr, 1962; Chatterjee, 1986; Citron, 1969, 1986; DePalma, 1989; DeVita, 1987; Harcombe, 1991; Jimenez-Lucho, 1987; Kahana, 1987, 1988; Kakisu, 1988; Karmon, 1979; Karnik, 1985; Kumar, 1993; Kuming, 1979; Leibold, 1966; Leppert, 1988; Miller, 1982; Nasemann, 1989; Polak, 1985; Roberts, 1974; Roussos, 1970; Russo, 1994; Salmon, 1987; Schild, 1991; Seth, 1991; Smith, 1987; Thomas, 1994; Walker, 1968; Yiannikas, 1983). It is felt that the incidence of optic neuropathy may be as high as 6% at doses of 25 mg/kg/day. Doses less than 15 mg/kg/day are felt to be relatively safe (Citron, 1969). Barron et al. reported ethambutol optic neuropathy in 3 of 304 (1.03%)

patients treated with ethambutol at 25 mg/kg/day for 60 days followed by 15 mg/kg/day (Barron, 1974). Leibold described two types of visual loss due to ethambutol toxicity, a central toxicity (e.g., decreased visual acuity, central scotomas, and impaired color perception) and a periaxial toxicity (e.g., normal or almost normal visual acuity, normal color perception, and peripheral quadrantic scotomas or constriction) (Leibold, 1966). There was a 20% incidence of central toxicity and an 11% incidence of peripheral toxicity in 35 patients receiving doses higher than 35 mg/kg/day for a minimum of 185 days. A 5.3% incidence of periaxial toxicity occurred in the 38 patients receiving less than 35 mg/kg/day (Leibold, 1966). Although many authors feel that doses of 25 mg/kg/day for less than 2 months followed by maintenance doses of 15 mg/kg/day are safe, there are cases of visual loss even at these "safe" doses (Addington, 1979; Alvarez, 1993; Chatterjee, 1986; Karnik, 1985; Thomas, 1994). Bronte-Stewart et al. reported five patients with severe visual loss after 25 mg/kg/day for 2 months followed by 15 mg/kg/day (Bronte-Stewart, 1976). Three of these five patients had renal disease that may have increased drug levels because 70% of the ethambutol dose is excreted by the kidneys (Citron, 1986). Isoniazid (especially in combination with ethambutol) has also been reported to cause a toxic optic neuropathy and isoniazid toxicity should be suspected as the etiology in cases of persistent visual loss despite discontinuation of ethambutol (Jimenez-Lucho, 1987). Visual-evoked potential studies may be useful in evaluating patients with early ethambutol toxicity (Kakisu, 1988; Kumar, 1993).

Nutritional deficiencies may result in optic neuropathy (Dang, 1981; Lerman, 1961; Obal, 1951; Rodger, 1952, 1953, 1954). Some vitamin and nutrient deficiencies causing an optic neuropathy are listed in Table 1–5.

Pernicious anemia or dietary deficiency (e.g., vegetarian) may result in a vitamin B_{12} deficiency optic neuropathy (Lerman, 1961; Smith, 1962; Stambolian, 1977). The pathophysiology of "alcohol amblyopia" is also probably related to a deficiency (nutritional amblyopia) of vitamin B_{12} and/or folate (rather than a direct toxic effect of alcohol). The ability of tobacco alone to cause toxic optic neuropathy has been asserted by several authors (Harrington, 1977; Samples and Younge, 1981). Samples and Younge, for example, state that central and cecocentral scotomas may occur in association with smoking alone (especially cigar smoking) (Samples and Younge, 1981). A toxic effect of cyanide may be the basis for tobacco optic neuropathy (Bronte-Stewart, 1976; Jestico, 1984; Lessell, 1971). Smoking may also impair intestinal vitamin B_{12} absorption (Watson-Williams, 1969).

Patients suspected of harboring a toxic or nutritional optic neuropathy should be screened for nutritional deficiencies and treated with appropriate supplementation. These patients should be urged to discontinue alcohol and tobacco use (Enoksson, 1960; Foulds, 1969a, 1969b; Friedman, 1970; Frisen, 1983; Harrington, 1962; Heaton, 1958; Hind, 1970; Hoyt, 1977; King, 1955; Kupersmith, 1983; Phillips, 1970; Potts, 1973; Victor, 1965, 1980; Watson-Williams, 1969). Both serum and erythrocyte folate levels should be checked

Table 1–5. Etiology of Nutritional Optic Neuropathy

B_6 deficiency (Phillipsen, 1970)
B_{12} deficiency (Troncoso, 1979)
Folate deficiency (Golnik, 1994)
Niacin
Riboflavin
Thiamine (B_1) deficiency (Dreyfus, 1965; Hoyt, 1977, 1979)

Table 1–6. Evaluation of Painless Progressive Bilateral Optic Neuropathy (Presumed Toxic or Nutritional Optic Neuropathy)

Magnetic resonance imaging of the optic nerves (exclude CON)
Vitamin B_{12} level (serum)
Folate level (serum and erythrocyte)
Complete blood count with differential
Urine heavy metal screen (mercury, lead, arsenic) if history suggestive of exposure
Syphilis serology
Leber's hereditary optic neuropathy mutational analysis

because there may be variability in the serum folate level alone (especially related to recent meals) (Golnik, 1994; Knox, 1982).

Toxic or nutritional optic neuropathies are often painless, subacute in onset, and bilateral, and usually involve central visual acuity and visual fields (e.g., central or cecocentral scotomas), but their clinical presentation may be variable. Unfortunately, CON may mimic the clinical presentation of toxic optic neuropathy and neuroimaging is recommended. The determination of presumed toxic or nutritional optic neuropathy should include a complete evaluation to exclude other etiologies of bilateral, painless, and progressive optic neuropathies (e.g., hereditary optic neuropathy, bilateral compressive optic neuropathy, etc.). The evaluation of presumed toxic optic neuropathy is outlined in Table 1–6.

Is There Clinical Evidence for a Hereditary Optic Neuropathy?

Miller has divided the hereditary optic neuropathies into three groups:

1. Those without associated neurologic signs or symptoms.
2. Those with neurologic signs or symptoms.
3. Those in which the optic neuropathy is secondary to the underlying systemic disease (Miller, 1982).

The hereditary optic neuropathies may have an isolated, dominant, recessive, or mitochondrial (Leber's hereditary optic neuropathy) inheritance pattern. We will not discuss these forms in detail (Caldwell, 1971; Harding, 1979; Hoyt, 1980; Johnston, 1979; Kline, 1979; Kok-van Alphen, 1970; Krill, 1970; Miller, 1982; Smith, 1972a, 1972b).

Leber's hereditary optic neuropathy (LHON) usually occurs in young males (up to 80 to 90% of the cases in the United States), although it may rarely occur in females and develop at any age. The clinical features of LHON are summarized in Table 1–7 (Carroll, 1979; deWeerdt, 1971; Dorfman, 1977; Erikson, 1972; Fine, 1977; Foulds, 1968; Livingstone, 1980; Nikoskelainen, 1977; Smith, 1973; Wallace, 1970; Wilson, 1965).

Some patients thought to have tobacco-alcohol amblyopia may actually harbor a LHON mutation (Cullom, 1993) and testing for LHON mutations may therefore be indicated in patients with presumed toxic or nutritional optic neuropathy. Although the diagnosis of LHON can be confirmed by serological testing for the known LHON mutations, little consensus exists regarding the treatment of LHON. Some authors have recommended reducing metabolic stress on the optic nerve (e.g., discontinue smoking, known optic nerve

Table 1–7. Clinical Features of Leber's Hereditary Optic Neuropathy

- Visual acuity loss
  - Usually acute, rapid, unremitting, and painless
  - Ultimately 20/200 to hand motions (20/20 to NLP range)
- Visual field loss (central or cecocentral scotomas)
- Sequential bilateral involvement (second eye days to weeks to months later with 40–50% simultaneous onset)
- Fundus findings at the time of visual loss
  - Triad of the "suspect fundus"
    - Telangiectatic microangiopathy
    - Apparent swelling of nerve fiber layer around disc ("pseudoedema")
    - Fluorescein angiogram often shows "pseudoedema" but may rarely see disc leakage
- Fundus appearance after visual loss
  - Attenuated arterioles
  - Nerve fiber layer loss especially papillomacular bundle
  - Optic nerve pallor (temporally)
  - May develop nonglaucomatous cupping
- Usually systemically normal but may have some associated findings
  - Occasional cardiac conduction defects
  - Dystonia and other minor neurological deficits
  - Multiple sclerosis-like clinical pattern
- "Primary" mitochondrial DNA mutation (e.g., 11778, 3460, 14484)

toxins, trauma). Medical therapy also remains unproven, but some authors suggest supplementation with multivitamins, folate, vitamin B_{12}, ibedinone and other coenzyme Q10 analogs, and thiamine.

Other hereditary optic neuropathy syndromes are listed in Table 1–8.

Table 1–8. Hereditary Optic Atrophy (OA) Associated with Other Neurologic or Systemic Signs

- Dominant OA with congenital deafness (Konigsmark, 1974; Kollarits, 1976)
- Dominant OA with progressive hearing loss and ataxia
- Recessive OA with progressive hearing loss, spastic quadriplegia, mental deterioration, and death
- Recessive OA with juvenile diabetes mellitus, diabetes insipidus, and hearing loss ("DIDMOAD" or Wolfram's syndrome) (Gunn, 1976; Lessell, 1977; Marquardt, 1974; Richardson, 1978)
- Hereditary OA with progressive hearing loss and polyneuropathy (Iwashita, 1970; Rosenberg, 1967)
- Hereditary infantile OA with pyramidal tract signs, ataxia, mental retardation, urinary incontinence, and pes cavus (Behr's syndrome) (Dunn, 1972; Francois, 1968; Horoupian, 1979; Landrigan, 1973; Monaco, 1979)
- OA with hereditary ataxias (Friedreich's ataxia, Marie's ataxia) (Carroll, 1980; Geoffrey, 1976; Livingstone, 1981)
- Dominant OA with ataxia and pes cavus (Lundberg, 1967)
- OA with Charcot-Marie-Tooth disease (hereditary sensorimotor neuropathy)

Source: Miller, 1982.

Table 1–9. Evaluation of an Atypical or Unexplained Optic Neuropathy

First line testing
Magnetic resonance imaging of the optic nerve(s)
Erythrocyte sedimentation rate
Complete blood count with differential
Syphilis serology
Antinuclear antibody
Chest radiograph
Angiotensin converting enzyme
Lumbar puncture
Second line testing
Gallium scan if sarcoidosis suspected
Purified protein derivative (ppd) skin testing if tuberculosis suspected
Antidouble-stranded DNA, complement levels, etc. if systemic lupus erythematosus or other collagen vascular disease suspected
Leber's hereditary optic neuropathy mutation blood test
Heavy metal screen
Serum vitamin B_{12} and folate levels
Lyme titer if endemic area or exposure history

Is this an Atypical or Unexplained Optic Neuropathy?

A number of patients with optic neuropathy do not fit into the categories listed in our approach. For patients with an unexplained or atypical optic neuropathy a suggested evaluation is listed in Table 1–9.

References

Aasved H. (1970). Osteopetrosis from the ophthalmological point of view. *Acta Ophthalmol 48:*771–778.

Acheson JF, Cockerell OC, Bentley CR, Sanders MD. (1993). Churg-Strauss vasculitis presenting with severe visual loss due to bilateral sequential optic neuropathy. *Br J Ophthalmol 77:*118–119.

Achiron L, Stominger M, Witkin N, Primo S. (1995). Sarcoid optic neuropathy: A case report. *J Am Optometr Assoc 66:*646–651.

Adams JW, Bofenkamp TM, Tobrin J, et al. (1984). Recurrent acute toxic optic neuropathy secondary to 5-FU. *Cancer Treat Rep 68:*565–566.

Addington WV. (1979). The side effects and interactions of antituberculous drugs. *Chest 76* (Supp):782–784.

Ahmadieh H, Roodpeyma S, Azarmina M, Soheilian M, Sajjadi SH. (1994) Bilateral simultaneous optic neuritis in childhood systemic lupus erythematosus. A case report. *J Neuro-ophthalmol 14:*84–86.

Ahmed MM. (1971). Ocular effects of antifreeze poisoning. *Br J Ophthalmol 55:*854–855.

Ainley RG. (1970). The Farnsworth-Munsell 100 Hue test in tobacco amblyopia. *Trans Ophthalmol Soc UK 90:*765–772.

Allen RA, Straatsma BR. (1961). Ocular involvement in leukemia and allied disorders. *Arch Ophthalmol 66:*490–508.

Alper MG. (1976). Mucoceles of the sphenoid sinus. Neuro-ophthalmic manifestations. *Trans Am Ophthalmol Soc 74:*53–81.

Altrocchi PA, Reinhardt PH, Eckman PB. (1972). Blindness and meningeal carcinomatosis. *Arch Ophthalmol 88:*508–512.

Alvarez KL, Krop LC. (1993). Ethambutol-induced ocular toxicity revisited. *Ann Pharmacother 27:*102–103.

Anderson DR, Spencer WH. (1970). Ultrastructural and histochemical observations of optic nerve gliomas. *Arch Ophthalmol 83:*324–335.

Appen RE, de Venecia G, Selliken JH, Giles LT. (1978). Meningeal carcinomatosis with blindness. *Am J Ophthalmol 86:*661–665.

Arseni C, Ghitescu M, Cristescu A, Mihaila G. (1970). Intrasellar aneurysms simulating hypophyseal tumors. *Eur Neurol 3:*321–329.
Baghdassarian SA. (1968). Optic neuropathy due to lead poisoning. *Arch Ophthalmol 80:*721–723.
Ballingall DK, Turpie AG. (1967). Cephaloridine toxicity. *Lancet 2:*835–836.
Barr CC, Green WR, Payne JW, et al. (1975). Intraocular reticulum cell sarcoma: Clinicopathological study of four cases and review of the literature. *Surv Ophthalmol 19:*224–239.
Barron CJ, Tepper L, Ioving E. (1974). Ocular toxicity from ethambutol. *Am J Ophthalmol 77:*256–266.
Baumbach GL, Cancilla PA, Martin-Amat G, et al. (1977). Methyl alcohol poisoning IV. Alterations of the morphological findings of the retina and optic nerve. *Arch Ophthalmol 95:*1859–1865.
Behrens MM. (1974). Optic atrophy in children after diiodohydroxyquin therapy. *JAMA 228:*693–694.
Belden CJ, Hamed LM, Mancuso AA. (1993). Bilateral isolated retrobulbar optic neuropathy in limited Wegener's granulomatosis. *J Clin Neuro-ophthalmol 13 (2):*119–123.
Bennett WM. (1986). Bronchial carcinoma presenting with non-metastatic bilateral papillitis. *Br J Dis Chest 80:*189–190.
Benton CD, Jr., Calhoun FP, Jr. (1976). The ocular effects of methyl alcohol poisoning: Report of a catastrophe involving three hundred and twenty persons. *Trans Am Acad Ophthalmol Otolaryngol 56:*875–885.
Berger JR, Ayyar DR. (1981). Neurological complications of ethylene glycol intoxication. Report of a case. *Arch Neurol 38:*724–726.
Berggren L, Hansson O. (1968). Absorption of intestinal antiseptics derived from 8-hydroxyquinolines. *Clin Pharmacol Ther 9:*67–70.
Berson EL, Freeman MI, Gay AJ. (1966). Visual field defects in giant suprasellar aneurysms of internal carotid. *Arch Ophthalmol 76:*52–58.
Billson FH, Reich J, Hopkins IH. (1972). Visual failure in a patient with ulcerative colitis treated by clioquinol. *Lancet 1:*1015–1016.
Bjorkenheim B. (1966). Optic neuropathy caused by vitamin B12 deficiency in carriers of the fish tapeworm, Diphyllobothrium latum. *Lancet 1:*688–690.
Boghen D, Debag M, Michaud J. (1988). Paraneoplastic optic neuritis and encephalomyelitis, report of a case. *Arch Neurol 45:*353–356.
Brazis PW, Menke DM, McLeish et al. (1995). Angiocentric T-cell lymphoma presenting with multiple cranial nerve palsies and retrobulbar optic neuropathy. *J Neuro-ophthalmol 15 (3):*152–157.
Bronte-Stewart J, Pettigrew AR, Foulds WS. (1976). Toxic optic neuropathy and its experimental production. *Trans Ophthalmol Soc UK 96:*355–358.
Brown DM, Kimura AE, Ossinig KC, Weiner GJ. (1992). Acute promyelocytic infiltration of the optic nerve treated by oral trans-retinoic acid. *Ophthalmology 99:*1463–1467.
Brown E, Meyer GG. (1969). Toxic amblyopia and peripheral neuropathy with ethchlorvynol abuse. *Am J Psychiatr 126:*882–884.
Brown et al. (1992) Mitochondrial DNA complex I and III mutations associated with Leber's hereditary optic neuropathy. *Genetics 103:*163.
Brown GC, Shields JA, Augsburger JT, et al. (1981). Leukemic optic neuropathy. *Int Ophthalmol 8:*111–116.
Brown P, Demaerel P, McNaught A, et al. (1994). Neuro-ophthalmological presentation of non-invasive Aspergillus sinus disease in the non-immunocompromised host. *J Neurol Neurosurg Psychiatr 57:*234–237.
Bullock JD, Yanner B, Kelly M, et al. (1979). Non-Hodgkins lymphoma involving the optic nerve. *Ann Ophthalmol 11:*1477–1480.
Burde RM, Gittinger J, Keltner JL, Miller NR. (1978). Neuro-ophthalmologic dilemma. Chronic optic neuritis? *Surv Ophthalmol 23:*173–176.
Burde RM, Savino PJ, Trobe JD. (1992). *Clinical Decisions in Neuro-ophthalmology.* St. Louis, Mosby Year Book, pp. 56–57.
Burnbaum MD, Harbison JW, Selhorst JB, Young HF. (1978). Blue-domed cyst with optic nerve compression. *J Neurol Neurosurg Psychiatr 41:*987–991.
Cacciatori M, Ling CS, Dhillon B. (1996). Retrobulbar neuritis in a patient with acquired immune deficiency syndrome. *Acta Ophthalmol Scand 74:*194–196.
Calderon M, Brady HR. (1969). Fibrous dysplasia of bone. *Am J Ophthalmol 68:*513–515.
Caldwell JBH, Howard RO, Riggs LA. (1971). Dominant juvenile optic atrophy: A study of two families and review of the hereditary disease in childhood. *Arch Ophthalmol 85:*133–147.
Calogero JA, Alexander E, Jr. (1971). Unilateral amaurosis in a hydrocephalic child with an obstructed shunt. *J Neurosurg 34:*236–240.
Campbell IA, Ormerod LP. (1988). Ethambutol and the eye. *Lancet ii:*113–114.
Cantillo R, Jain J, Singhakowinta A, et al. (1979). Blindness as initial manifestation of meningeal carcinomatosis in breast cancer. *Cancer 44:*755–757.
Carlin L, Biller J, Laster W, O'Toole JF. (1981). Monocular blindness in nasopharyngeal cancer. *Arch Neurol 38:*600.
Carr RE, Henkind P. (1962). Ocular manifestations of ethambutol. *Arch Ophthalmol 67:*566–571.
Carrion LT, Edwards WC, Perry LD. (1979). Spontaneous subperiosteal orbital hematoma. *Ann Ophthalmol 11:*1754–1757.
Carroll FD. (1935). Analysis of fifty-five cases of tobacco-alcohol amblyopia. *Arch Ophthalmol 14:*421–434.

Carroll FD. (1944). The etiology and treatment of tobacco-alcohol amblyopia. Parts I and II. *Am J Ophthalmol 27*:713–725, 847–863.
Carroll FD. (1947). Nutritional retrobulbar neuritis. *Am J Ophthalmol 30*:172–176.
Carroll FD. (1966). Nutritional amblyopia. *Arch Ophthalmol 76*:406–411.
Carroll FD. (1971). Jamaican optic neuropathy in immigrants to the United States. *Am J Ophthalmol 71*:261–265.
Carroll WM, Kriss A, Baraitser M, Barrett G, Halliday AM. (1980). The incidence and nature of visual pathway involvement in Friedreich's ataxia: A clinical and visual evoked potential study of 22 patients. *Brain 103*:413–434.
Carroll WM, Mastaglia FL. (1979). Leber's optic neuropathy: A clinical and visual evoked potential study of affected and asymptomatic members of a six generation family. *Brain 102*:559–580.
Chalfin AI, Nash BM, Goldstein JH. (1973). Optic nerve head involvement in lymphocytic leukemia. *J Pediatr Ophthalmol 10*:39–43.
Charache S, Finkelstein D, Lietman PS, Scott J. (1977). Peripheral and optic neuritis in a patient with hemoglobin SC disease during treatment of Salmonella osteomyelitis with chloramphenicol. *Johns Hopkins Med J 140*:121–124.
Chatterjee VK, Buchanan DR, Friedmann AI, Green M. (1986). Ocular toxicity following ethambutol in standard dosage. *Br J Dis Chest 80*:288–291.
Chavez CT, Hepler RS, Straatsma BR. (1985). Methyl bromide optic atrophy. *Am J Ophthalmol 99*:715.
Chisholm IA. (1969). An evaluation of the Farnsworth-Munsell 100 Hue test as a clinical tool in investigation and management of ocular neurological deficit. *Trans Ophthalmol Soc UK 89*:243–250.
Chisholm IA. (1978). Serum cobalamin and folate in the optic neuropathy associated with tobacco smoking. *Can J Ophthalmol 13*:105–109.
Chisholm IA, Bronte-Stewart J, Foulds WS. (1967). Hydroxycobalamin versus cyanocobalamin in the treatment of tobacco amblyopia. *Lancet 2*:450–451.
Chisholm IA, Pettigrew AR. (1970). Biochemical observations in toxic optic neuropathy. *Trans Ophthalmol Soc UK 90*:827–838.
Citron KM. (1969). Ethambutol. A review with special reference to ocular toxicity. *Tubercle 50*:32–36.
Citron KM, Thomas GO. (1986). Ocular toxicity from ethambutol. *Thorax 41*:737–739.
Clifford-Jones RE, McDonald WI, Landon DN. (1985). Chronic optic nerve compression: An experimental study. *Brain 108*:241–262.
Cocke JG. (1967). Chloramphenicol optic neuritis. *Am J Dis Child 114*:424–426.
Cogan DG, Truman JT, Smith TR. (1973). Optic neuropathy, chloramphenicol and infantile genetic agranulocytosis. *Invest Ophthalmol 12*:534–537.
Cohen SB, Glasgow BJ. (1993). Bilateral optic nerve cryptocooccosis in sudden blindness in patients with acquired immune deficiency syndrome. *Ophthalmology 100*:1689–1694.
Colapinto EV, Cabeen MA, Johnson LN. (1996). Optic nerve compression by a dolichoectatic internal carotid artery: Case report. *Neurosurgery 39*:604–606.
Colvard DM, Robertson DM, O'Duffy JD. (1977). The ocular manifestations of Behcet's disease. *Arch Ophthalmol 95*:1813–1817.
Coppetto JR, Monteiro MLR, Cannarozzi DB. (1988). Optic neuropathy associated with chronic lymphomatous meningitis. *J Clin Neuro-ophthalmol 8*:39–43.
Crew SJ, James B, Masters JB, West RH. (1970). Drug and nutritional factors in optic neuropathy. *Trans Ophthalmol Soc UK 90*:773–794.
Crivelli G, Riviera LC. (1970). Unilateral blindness from aspergilloma at the right optic foramen. *J Neurosurg 33*:207–211.
Cruysberg JRM, Pinckers A. (1982). Acquired color vision defects in compressive optic neuropathy. *Neuro-ophthalmology 2*:169–181.
Cullen JF, Haining WM, Crombie AL. (1966). Cerebral aneurysms presenting with visual field defects. *Br J Ophthalmol 50*:251–256.
Cullom ME, Heher KL, Miller NR, et al. (1993). Leber's hereditary optic neuropathy masquerading as tobacco-alcohol amblyopia. *Arch Ophthalmol 111*:1482.
Currie JN, Lessell S, Lessell IM, Weiss JS, Albert DM, Benson EM. (1988). Optic neuropathy in chronic lymphocytic leukemia. *Arch Ophthalmol 106*:654–660.
Dang CV. (1981). Tobacco-alcohol amblyopia: A proposed biochemical basis for pathogenesis. *Med Hypoth 7*:1317–1328.
Decker RF, Mardayat M, Marc J, Rasool A. (1979). Neurosarcoidosis with computerized tomographic visualization and transphenoidal excision of a supra- and intrasellar granuloma. *J Neurosurg 50*:814–816.
Delaney P. (1977). Neurologic manifestations in sarcoidosis: Review of the literature with report of 23 cases. *Ann Intern Med 87*:336–345.
DePalma P, Franco F, Bragliani G, et al. (1989). The incidence of optic neuropathy in 84 patients treated with ethambutol. *Met Ped Syst Ophthalmol 12*:80–82.
Deutsch TA, Corwin HL. (1988). Lupus optic neuritis with negative serology. *Ann Ophthalmol 20*:383–384.
DeVita EG, Miao M, Sadun AA. (1987). Optic neuropathy in ethambutol-treated renal tuberculosis. *J Clin Neuro-ophthalmol 7*:77–83.
deWeerdt CJ, Went LN. (1971). Neurological studies in families with Leber's optic atrophy. *Acta Neurol Scand 47*:541–545.

Dorfman LF, Nikoskelainen E, Rosenthal AR, Sogg RL. (1977). Visual evoked potentials in Leber's hereditary optic neuropathy. *Ann Neurol 1*:565–568.
Dreyfus PM. (1965). Blood transketolase levels in tobacco-alcohol amblyopia. *Arch Ophthalmol 74*:617–620.
Dunn HG, Dolman CL. (1972). Necrotizing encephalomyelopathy: Report of a case with manifestations resembling Behr's syndrome. *Eur Neurol 7*:34–55.
Durston JHJ, Parsons-Smith BG. (1970). Blindness due to aneurysm of anterior communicating artery. *Br J Ophthalmol 54*:170–176.
Dutton JJ, Tse DT, Anderson RL. (1983). Compressive optic neuropathy following use of intracranial oxidized cellulose hemostat. *Ophthalmic Surg 14*:487–490.
Ehyai A, Freenib FR. (1983). Progressive optic neuropathy and sensorineural hearing loss due to chronic glue sniffing. *J Neurol Neurosurg Psychiatr 46*:349–351.
Ellis W, Little HL. (1973). Leukemic infiltration of the optic nerve head. *Am J Ophthalmol 75*:867–871.
Enoksson P, Norden A. (1960). Vitamin B-12 deficiency affecting the optic nerve. *Acta Med Scand 167*:199–208.
Erikson RP. (1972). Leber's optic atrophy: A possible example of maternal inheritance. *Am J Hum Genet 24*:348–349.
Etheridge JE, Jr., Stewart GT. (1966). Treating acrodermatitis enteropathica. *Lancet 1*:261–262.
Feiner LA, Younge BR, Kazmier FJ, et al. (1987). Optic neuropathy and amiodarone therapy. *Mayo Clin Proc 62*:702–717.
Fine PEM. (1977). Analysis of family history data for evidence of non-Mendelian inheritance resulting from vertical transmission. *J Med Genet 14*:399–407.
Fleet WS, Watson RT. (1986). Autoimmune optic neuritis: A potentially treatable form of visual loss. *Ann Ophthalmol 18*:144–146.
Fleisher DI, Hepler RS, Landau JW. (1974). Blindness during diiodohydroxyquin (Diodoquin) therapy. A case report. *Pediatrics 54*:1106–1108.
Foulds WS, Cant JS, Chisholm IA, Bronte-Stewart J, Wilson J. (1968). Hydroxycobalamin in the treatment of Leber's hereditary optic atrophy. *Lancet 1*:896–897.
Foulds WS, Chisholm IA, Bronte-Stewart J, Reid HCR. (1970). The investigation and therapy of the toxic optic amblyopias. *Trans Ophthalmol Soc UK 90*:739–763.
Foulds WS, Chisholm IA, Bronte-Stewart J, Wilson TM. (1960). Vitamin B-12 absorption in tobacco amblyopia. *Br J Ophthalmol 53*:393–397.
Foulds WS, Chisholm IA, Bronte-Stewart J, Wilson TM. (1969). The optic neuropathy of pernicious anemia. *Arch Ophthalmol 82*:427–432.
Francois J. (1968). Hereditary degeneration of the optic nerve (hereditary optic atrophy). *Int Ophthalmol Clin 8*:999–1054.
Freilich RJ, Krol G, DeAngelis LM. (1995). Neuroimaging and cerebrospinal fluid cytology in the diagnosis of leptomeningeal metastasis. *Ann Neurol 38*:51–57.
Friedman AI. (1970). Visual field examination in the toxic and nutritional optic neuropathies. *Trans Ophthalmol Soc UK 90*:795–808.
Frisen L. (1980) The neurology of visual acuity. *Brain 103*:639–670.
Frisen L. (1983). Fundus changes in acute malnutritional optic neuropathy. *Arch Ophthalmol 101*:577–579.
Frisen L, Hoyt WF, Tengroth BM. (1973). Optociliary veins, disc pallor and visual loss. *Acta Ophthalmologica 51*:241–249.
Garrett SN, Kearney JL, Schiffman JS. (1988). Amiodarone optic neuropathy. *J Clin Neuro-ophthalmol 8*:105–110.
Gelwan MJ, Kellen RI, Burde RM, et al. (1988). Sarcoidosis of the anterior visual pathway: Successes and failures. *J Neurol Neurosurg Psychiatr 51*:1473–1480.
Geoffrey FH, Barbeau A, Breton G, Lemieux B, Aube M, Leger C, Bouchard JP. (1976). Clinical description and roetgenologic evaluation of patients with Friedrich's ataxia. *Can J Neurol Sci 3*:279–286.
Gillum WN, Anderson RL. (1981). Reversible visual loss in subperiosteal hematoma of the orbit. *Ophthalmic Surg 12*:203–209.
Ginsberg J, Freemond AS, Calhoun JB. (1970). Optic nerve involvement in metastatic tumors. *Ann Ophthalmol 2*:604–617.
Gittinger JW, Jr., Asdourian GK. (1987). Papillopathy caused by amiodarone. *Arch Ophthalmol 105*:349–351.
Glaser JS. (1976). Clinical evaluation of optic nerve function. *Trans Ophthalmol Soc UK 96*:359–362.
Glaser JS. (1978). *Neuro-ophthalmology*, pp 5–24. Hagerstown, MD, Harper and Row.
Glaser JS, Hoyt WF, Corbett J. (1971). Visual morbidity with chiasmal glioma: Long term studies of visual fields in treated and untreated cases. *Arch Ophthalmol 85*:3–12.
Glaser JS, Trobe JD. (1979). Perspective on perimetry. *Arch Ophthalmol 97*:775–780.
Gleeson MH, Graves PS. (1974). Complications of dietary deficiency of vitamin B12 in young caucasians. *Postgrad Med J 50*:462–464.
Godel V, Nemet P, Lazar M. (1980). Chloramphenicol optic neuropathy. *Arch Ophthalmol 98*:1417–1421.
Goldberg RA, Weisman JS, McFarland JE, Krauss HR, Hepler RS, Shorr N. (1989). Orbital inflammation and optic neuropathies associated with chronic sinusitis of intranasal cocaine abuse. Possible contiguous inflammation. *Arch Ophthalmol 107*:831–835.
Goldstein NP, Hollenhorst RW, Randall RV, Gross JB. (1966). Possible relationship of optic neuritis, Wilson's disease, and DL-penicillamine therapy. *JAMA 196*:734–735.

Golnik KC, Schaible ER. (1994). Folate-responsive optic neuropathy. *J Neuro-ophthalmol 14:*163–169.

Golnik KC, Hund PW, Stroman GA, Stewart WC. (1996). Magnetic resonance imaging in patients with unexplained optic neuropathy. *Ophthalmology 103:*515–520.

Golnik KC, Marotto ME, Fanous MM, Heitter D, King LP, Halpern JI, Holley PH, Jr. (1994). Ophthalmic manifestations of Rochalimaea species. *Am J Ophthalmol 118:*145–151.

Goodwin JA, Glaser JS. (1978). Chiasmal syndrome in sphenoid sinus mucocoele. *Ann Neurol 4:*440–444.

Goutieres F, Aicardi J. (1977). Accidental percutaneous hexachlorophene intoxication in children. *Br Med J 2:*663–667.

Graham EM, Ellis CJK, Sanders MD, et al. (1986). Optic neuropathy in sarcoidosis. *J Neurol Neurosurg Psychiatr 49:*756–763.

Gregorius FK, Hepler RS, Stern WE. (1975). Loss and recovery of vision with suprasellar meningiomas. *J Neurosurg 42:*69–75.

Griffin JF, Wray SH. (1978). Acquired color vision defects in retrobulbar neuritis. *Am J Ophthalmol 86:*193–201.

Gudas PP, Jr. (1971). Optic nerve myeloma. *Am J Ophthalmol 71:*1085–1089.

Gudeman SK, Selhorst JB, Susac JO, Waybright EA. (1982). Sarcoid optic neuropathy. *Neurology 32:*597–603.

Guidetti B, LaTorre E. (1970). Carotid ophthalmic aneurysms. *Acta Neurchir 22:*289–304.

Gunn T, et al. (1976). Juvenile diabetes mellitus, optic atrophy, sensory nerve deafness and diabetes insipidus-a syndrome. *J Pediatr 89:*565–570.

Gupta DR, Strobos RJ. (1972). Bilateral papillitis associated with cafergot therapy. *Neurology 22:*793–797.

Gutman I, Behrens M, Odel J. (1984). Bilateral central and centocaecal scotomata due to mass lesions. *Br J Ophthalmol 68:*336–342.

Guy J, Mancuso A, Quisling RG, Beck R, Moster M. (1990). Gadolinium-DTPA-enhanced magnetic resonance imaging in optic neuropathies. *Ophthalmology 97 (5):*592–600.

Guyer DR, Green WR, Schachat AP, Bastacky S, Miller NR. (1990). Bilateral ischemic optic neuropathy and retinal vascular occlusions associated with lymphoma and sepsis. *Ophthalmology 97:*882–888.

Hakuba A, Katsuyama J, Matsuoka Y, Shim JH, Nishimura S. (1975). Sphenoid sinus mucocoeles: report of two cases. *J Neurosurg 43:*368–373.

Halperin JJ, Luft BJ, Anand AK, et al. (1989). Lyme neuroborreliosis: Central nervous system manifestations. *Neurology 39:*753–759.

Harcombe A, Kinnear W, Britton J, Macfarlane J. (1991). Ocular toxicity of ethambutol. *Resp Med 85:*151–153.

Harding GFA, Crews SJ, Pitts SM. (1979). Psychophysical and visual evoked potential findings in hereditary optic atrophy. *Trans Ophthalmol Soc UK 99:*96–102.

Harley RD, Huang NN, Macri CH, Green WR. (1970). Optic neuritis and optic atrophy following chloramphenicol in cystic fibrosis patients. *Trans Am Acad Ophthalmol Otolaryngol 74:*1011–1031.

Harms H. (1976). Role of perimetry in assessment of optic nerve dysfunction. *Trans Ophthalmol Soc UK 96:*363–367.

Harrington DO. (1962). Amblyopia due to tobacco, alcohol and nutritional deficiency. *Am J Ophthalmol 53:*967–972.

Harrington DO. (1977). What is the etiology of alcohol and tobacco amblyopia? In Brockhurst RJ, Boruchoff SA, Hutchinson BT, Lessell S (eds). *Controversy in Ophthalmology.* Philadelphia, W.B. Saunders, pp. 866–872.

Heaton JM, McCormick AJA, Freeman AG. (1958). Tobacco amblyopia: A clinical manifestation of vitamin B-12 deficiency. *Lancet 2:*286–290.

Hedges TR. (1995). Two brothers with bilateral optic neuropathy. *Surv Ophthalmol 39:*417.

Hedges TR, Leung LE. (1976). Parasellar and orbital apex syndrome caused by aspergillosis. *Neurology 26:*117.

Hind VMD. (1970). Degeneration in the peripheral visual pathway of vitamin B-12 deficient monkeys. *Trans Ophthalmol Soc UK 90:*839–846.

Hirst LW, Miller NR, Kumar AJ, Udvarhelyi GB. (1980). Medulloblastoma causing a corticosteroid responsive optic neuropathy. *Am J Ophthalmol 89:*437–442.

Hoogenraad TU, Sanders EACM, Tan KEWP. (1989). Paraneoplastic optic neuropathy with histopathological verification of absence of meningeal metastases. *Neuro-ophthalmology 9:*247–250.

Hoover DL, Smith LEH, Turner SJ, Gelber RD, Sallan SE. (1988). Ophthalmic evaluation of survivors of acute lymphoblastic leukemia. *Ophthalmology 95:*151–155.

Horoupian DS, Zucker SK, Moshe S, Peterson de C. (1979). Behr syndrome: A clinico-pathologic report. *Neurology 29:*323–327.

Howell et al. (1993). Leber's hereditary optic neuropathy. The etiological role of a mutation in the mitochondrial cyochrome b gene. *Genet 133;*133.

Hoyt CS III. (1980). Autosomal dominant optic atrophy: A spectrum of disability. *Ophthalmology 87:*245–251.

Hoyt CS III, Billson FA. (1977). Low-carbohydrate diet optic neuropathy. *Med J Aust 1:*65–66.

Hoyt CS III, Billson FA. (1979). Optic neuropathy in ketogenic diet. *Br J Ophthalmol 63:*191–194.

Hoyt WF. (1976). Fundoscopic changes in the retinal nerve-fiber layer in chronic and acute optic neuropathies. *Trans Ophthalmol Soc UK 96:*368–371.

Hoyt WF, Beeston D. (1966). *The Ocular Fundus in Neurologic Disease.* St. Louis, C.V. Mosby.

Hughes RAC, Mair WGP. (1977). Acute necrotic myelopathy with pulmonary tuberculosis. *Brain 100:*223–238.

Huopenen et al. (1991). A new mtDNA mutation associated with Leber's hereditary optic neuroretinopathy. *Am J Hum Genet 48:*1147.

Imachi J, Tajino M, Okamoto N, Nakajima T, Shiraki K. (1981). Rhinogenous retrobulbar optic neuritis: Pathogenetic problems and case reports. *Neuro-ophthalmology 1:*273–280.

Ing EB, Augburger JJ, Eagle RC. (1996). Lung cancer with visual loss. *Surv Ophthalmol 40:*505–510.

Iwashita H, Inoue N, Araki S, Kuroiwa Y. (1970). Optic atrophy, neural deafness and distal neurogenic amyotrophy. *Arch Neurol 22:*357–363.

Jabs DA, Miller NR, Newman SA, Johnson MA, Stevens MB. (1986). Optic neuropathy in systemic lupus erythematosus. *Arch Ophthalmol 104:*564–568.

Jampol LM, Woodfin W, McLean EB. (1972). Optic nerve sarcoidosis: report of a case. *Arch Ophthalmol 87:*355–360.

Jestico JV, O'Brien MD, Teoh R, et al. (1984). Whole blood cyanide levels in patients with tobacco amblyopia. *J Neurol Neurosurg Psychiatr 47:*573–578.

Jimenez-Lucho VE, Del Bustro R, Odel J. (1987). Isoniazid and ethambutol as a cause of optic neuropathy. *Eur J Resp Dis 71:*42–45.

Johansson BA. (1992). Visual field defects during low-dose methotrexate therapy. *Doc Ophthalmol 79:*91.

Johns DR and Neufeld MJ. (1993). Cytochrome c oxidase mutations in Leber's hereditary optic neuropathy. *Biochem Biophy Res Comm 196:*810–815.

Johns DR, Smith KH, Miller NR. (1992). Leber's hereditary optic neuropathy. Clinical manifestations of the 3460 mutation. *Arch Ophthalmol 110:*1577–1581.

Johns DR et al. (1993). Leber's hereditary optic neuropathy. Clinical manifestations of the 15257 mutation. *Ophthalmol 100:*981.

Johns DR, Heher KL, Miller NR, Smith KH. (1993). LHON: clinical manifestations of the 14484 mutation. *Arch Ophthalmol 111:*495–498.

Johnson LN, Hepler RS, Yee RD, Batzdorf U. (1986). Sphenoid sinus mucocele mimicking diabetic ophthalmoplegia and retrobulbar neuritis. *Am J Ophthalmol 102:*111–115.

Johnson LN, Hill RA, Bartholomew MJ. (1988). Correlation of afferent pupillary defect with visual loss on automated perimetry. *Ophthalmology 95:*1649–1655.

Johnston PB, Gaster RN, Smith VC, Tripathi RC. (1979). A clinicopathologic study of autosomal dominant optic atrophy. *Am J Ophthalmol 88:*868–875.

Kahana LM. (1987). Toxic ocular effects of ethambutol. *Can Med Assoc J 137:*213–216.

Kahana LM. (1988). Ethambutol and the eye. *Lancet ii:*627.

Kakisu Y, Adach-Usani E, Mizota A. (1988). Pattern electroretinogram and visual evoked potential in ethambutol optic neuropathy. *Doc Ophthalmol 67:*327–334.

Kamin DF, Hepler RS. (1972). Solitary intracranial plasmacytoma mistaken for retrobulbar neuritis. *Am J Ophthalmol 73:*584.

Kansu T, Kirkali P, Kansu E, Zileli T. (1989). Optic neuropathy in Behcet's disease. *J Clin Neuro-ophthalmol 9:*277–280.

Kansu T, Orr LS, Savino PJ, Schatz NJ, Corbett JJ. (1979). Optic neuropathy as initial manifestation of lymphoreticular diseases: A report of five cases. In Smith JL (ed). *Neuro-ophthalmology Focus.* New York, Masson, pp. 125–136.

Karmon G, Savir H, Zevin D, Levi J. (1979). Bilateral optic neuropathy due to combined ethambutol and isoniazid treatment. *Ann Ophthalmol 11:*1013–1017.

Karnik AM, Al-Shamali MA, Fewech FF. (1985). A case of ocular toxicity to ethambutol—an idiosyncratic reaction. *Postgrad Med J 61:*811–813.

Kattah JC, Chrousos GC, Roberts J, Kolsky M, Zimmerman L, Manz H. (1993). Metastatic prostate cancer to the optic canal. *Ophthalmol 100:*1711–1715.

Kattah JC, Suski ET, Killen JY, et al. (1980). Optic neuritis and systemic lymphoma. *Am J Ophthalmol 89:*431–436.

Katz B. (1991). Disc edema, transient obscurations of vision, and a temporal fossa mass. *Surv Ophthalmol 36:*133–139.

Kay MC. (1986). Optic neuropathy secondary to lymphoma. *J Clin Neuro-ophthalmol 61:*31–34.

Kayan A, Earl CJ. (1975). Compressive lesions of the optic nerve and chiasm. *Brain 98:*13–28.

Kazim M, Kennerdell JS, Rothfus W, Marquardt M. (1992). Orbital lymphangioma. Correlation of magnetic resonance images and intraoperative findings. *Ophthalmol 99:*1588–1594.

Kenik JG, Krohn K, Kelly RB, Bierman M, Hammeke MD, Hurley JA. (1987). Transverse myelitis and optic neuritis in systemic lupus erythematosus: A case report with magnetic resonance imaging findings. *Arthrit Rheum 31:*1105–1110.

Kennerdell JS, Janetta PJ, Johnson BNL. (1974). A steroid-sensitive solitary intracranial plasmacytoma. *Arch Ophthalmol 92:*393.

Kerrison JB, Howell N, Miller NR, et al. (1995). Leber hereditary optic neuropathy: Electron microscopy and molecular genetic analysis of a case. *Ophthalmology 102:*1509–1516.

Killian PJ, Susac J, Lawless OJ. (1978) Optic neuropathy in relapsing polychondritis. *JAMA 239:*49–50.

Kimbrell OC, Wheliss JA. (1967). Polyarteritis nodosa complicated by bilateral optic neuropathy. *JAMA 201:*139–140.

Kimura H, Masai H, Kashii S. (1996). Optic neuropathy following elcatonin therapy. *J Neuro-ophthalmol 16:*134–136.

King JH, Jr., Passmore JW. (1955). Nutritional amblyopia: A study of American prisoners of war in Korea. *Am J Ophthalmol 39:*173–186.

Kinkaid MC, Green WR. (1983). Ocular and orbital involvement in leukemia. *Surv Ophthalmol 27:*211–232.
Kirkham TH. (1977). Optic atrophy in the bobble-head doll syndrome. *J Pediatr Ophthalmol 14:*299–301.
Kiyosawa M, Ishikawa S. (1981). A case of isoniazid-induced optic neuropathy. *Neuro-ophthalmol 2:*67–70.
Kjaersgaard K. (1971). Amnesia after clioquinol. *Lancet 2:*1086.
Kline LB, Garcia JH, Harsh GR. (1984). Lymphomatous optic neuropathy. *Arch Ophthalmol 102:*1655–1657.
Kline LB, Glaser JS. (1979). Dominant optic atrophy: The clinical profile. *Arch Ophthalmol 97:*1680–1686.
Knight CL, Hoyt WF, Wilson CB. (1972). Syndrome of incipient prechiasmal optic nerve compression, progress towards early diagnosis and surgical management. *Arch Ophthalmol 87:*1–11.
Knox DL, Chen MF, Guilarte TR, et al. (1982). Nutritional amblyopia: Folic acid, vitamin B-12, and other vitamins. *Retina 2:*288–293.
Kodsi SR, Younge BR, Leavitt JA, Campbell RJ, Scheithauer BW. (1993). Intracranial plasma cell granuloma presenting as an optic neuropathy. *Surv Ophthalmol 38:*70–74.
Kok-van Alphen CC. (1970). Four families with the dominant infantile form of optic nerve atrophy. *Acta Ophthalmol 48:*905–916.
Kollarits CR, Lubow M, Johnson JC. (1976). Visual loss and perioptic vascular malformations in the eye and orbit. *Am J Ophthalmol 82:*237–240.
Kollarits CR, Pinheiro ML, Swann ER, Marcus DF, Corrie WS. (1979). The autosomal dominant syndrome of progressive optic atrophy and congenital deafness. *Am J Ophthalmol 87:*789–792.
Konigsmark BW, Knox DL, Hussels IE, Moses H. (1974). Dominant congenital deafness and progressive optic nerve atrophy: Occurrence in four generations of a family. *Arch Ophthalmol 91:*99–103.
Kothandaram P, Dawson BH, Kruyt R. (1971). Carotid-ophthalmic aneurysms. *J Neurosurg 34:*544–548.
Kraus AM, O'Rourke JO. (1963). Lymphomatous optic neuritis. *Arch Ophthalmol 70:*173–175.
Krill AE, Smith VC, Pokorny J. (1970). Similarities between congenital tritan defects and dominant optic nerve atrophy: Coincidence or identity? *J Opt Soc Am 60:*1132–1139.
Krohel GB, Wright JE. (1979). Orbital hemorrhage. *Am J Ophthalmol 88:*254–258.
Krumsiek J, Kruger C, Patzold U. (1985). Tobacco-alcohol amblyopia neuro-ophthalmological findings and clinical course. *Acta Neurol Scand 72:*180–187.
Kumar A, Sandramouli S, Verma L, Tewari HK, Khosla PK. (1993). Ocular ethambutol toxicity: Is it reversible? *J Clin Neuro-ophthalmol 13:*15–17.
Kuming BS, Braude L. (1979). Anterior optic neuritis caused by ethambutol toxicity. *S Afr Med J 55:*4.
Kupersmith MJ, Weiss PA, Carr RE. (1983). The visual-evoked potential in tobacco-alcohol and nutritional amblyopia. *Am J Ophthalmol 95:*307–314.
Kupfer C, McCrane E. (1974). A possible cause of decreased vision in cryptococcal meningitis. *Invest Ophthalmol 13:*801–804.
Lamba PA, Sood NN, Moorthy SS. (1968). Retinopathy due to chloramphenicol. *Scott Med J 13:*166–169.
Landrigan PJ, Berenberg W, Bresnan M. (1973). Behr's syndrome: Familial optic atrophy, spastic diplegia, and ataxia. *Dev Med Child Neurol 15:*41–47.
Leibold JE. (1966). The ocular toxicity of ethambutol and its relationship to dose. *Ann NY Acad Sci 135:*904–909.
Leibold JE. (1971). Drugs having a toxic effect on the optic nerve. *Int Ophthalmol Clin 11:*137–157.
Leppert D, Waespe W. (1988). Neurotoxicity of antituberculosis drugs in a patient without active tuberculosis. *Neuro-Ophthalmol 8:*95–99.
Lerman S, Feldmahn AL. (1961). Cecocentral scomatata as the presenting sign in pernicious anemia. *Arch Ophthalmol 65:*381–385.
Lessell S. (1971). Experimental cyanide optic neuropathy. *Arch Ophthalmol 86:*194–220.
Lessell S, Rosman NP. (1977). Juvenile diabetes mellitus and optic atrophy. *Arch Neurol 34:*759–765.
Lesser RL, Kornmehl EW, Pachner AR, et al. (1990). Neuro-ophthalmologic manifestations of Lyme disease. *Ophthalmology 97:*699–706.
Levin PS, Newman SA, Quigley HA, Miller NR. (1983). A clinicopathologic study of optic neuropathies associated with intracranial mass lesions with quantification of remaining axons. *Am J Ophthalmol 95:*295–306.
Licht A, Oliver M, Rachmilewitz WA. (1972). Optic atrophy following treatment with cobalt chloride in a patient with pancytopenia and hypercellular marrow. *Isr J Med Sci 8:*61–66.
Little JR, Dale AJD, Okazaki H. (1974). Meningeal carcinomatosis: Clinical manifestations. *Arch Neurol 30:*138.
Litvak J, Leder MM, Kauvar AJ. (1964). Hodgkin's disease involving optic nerve and brain. *J Neurosurg 21:*798–801.
Livingstone IR, Mastaglia FL, Edis R, Howe JW. (1981). Visual involvement in Friedrich's ataxia and hereditary spastic ataxia: A clinical and visual evoked response study. *Arch Neurol 38:*75–79.
Livingstone IR, Mastaglia FL, Howe JW, Aherne GES. (1980). Leber's optic neuropathy: Clinical and visual evoked response studies in asymptomatic and symptomatic members of a 4-generation family. *Br J Ophthalmol 64:*751–757.
Long DM. (1985). Neurosurgical involvement in tumors of the orbit. *Clin Neurosurg 32:*514–523.
Lorance RW, Kaufman D, Wray SH, et al. (1987). Contrast visual testing in neurovisual diagnosis. *Neurology 37:*923–929.
Lorber J, Zachary RB. (1968). Primary congenital hydrocephalus: Long term results of controlled therapeutic trial. *Arch Dis Child 43:*516–527.
Lundberg PO, Wranne I, Brun A. (1967). Family with optic atrophy and neurological symptoms. *Acta Neurol Scand 43:*87–105.

Mackey DA, Buttery RD. (1992). LHON in Australia. *Aust NZ J Ophthalmol 20:*179.

Manor RS, Ouaknine GE, Matz S, Shalit MN. (1980). Nasal visual field loss with intracranial lesions of the optic nerve pathways. *Am J Ophthalmol 90:*1–10.

Manz HJ, Klein LH, Fermaglich J, Kattah J, Lussenhop AJ. (1979). Cavernous hemangioma of optic chiasm, optic nerves, and right optic tract. *Virchows Arch (Pathol Anat) 383:*225–231.

Markovits AS. (1977). Evacuation of orbital hematoma by continuous suction. *Ann Ophthalmol 9:*1255–1258.

Marquardt JL, Loriaux DL. (1974). Diabetes mellitus and optic atrophy—with associated findings of diabetes insipidus and neurosensory hearing loss in two siblings. *Arch Int Med 134:*32–37.

Martinez AJ, Boehm R, Hadfield MG. (1974). Acute hexachlorophene encephalopathy: Clinical neuropathological correlation. *Acta Neuropathol 28:*93–101.

Mashima et al. (1995). Lack of differences among mitochondrial DNA in family members with LHON and differing visual outcomes. *J Neuro-ophthalmol 15:*15.

Mashima Y, Hiida Y, Oguchi Y. (1992). Remission of LHON with idebedone. *Lancet 340:*368–369.

Matsuo K, Kobayashi S, Sugita K. (1980). Bitemporal hemianopsia associated with sclerosis of the intracranial internal carotid arteries. *J Neurosurg 53:*566–569.

Mattson RH, Peterson EW. (1966). Glioblastome multiforme of the optic nerve. *JAMA 196:*799–800.

McCarthy WL, Jr., Frenkel M, Busse BJ. (1972). Visual loss as the only symptom of sphenoid sinus mucocoele. *Am J Ophthalmol 74:*1134–1140.

McEwan LM. (1971). Neuropathy after clioquinol. *Br Med J 3:*169–170.

McEwan LM, Constantinopoulos P. (1970). The use of dietary and antibacterial regime in the management of intrinsic allergy. *Ann Allergy 28:*256–266.

McLennan R, Taylor HR. (1978). Optic neuroretinitis in association with BCNU and procarbazine therapy. *Med Pediatr Oncol 4:*43–48.

Melon O, Weinberg PE, Kim KS, Hemmati M, Siqeria EB. (1980). Fibrous dysplasia of bone with acute visual loss. *Ann Ophthalmol 12:*734–739.

Michelson JB, Shields JA, Leonard BC, et al. (1975). Periorbital chloroma and proptosis in a two-year-old child with acute myelogenous leukemia. *J Pediatr Ophthalmol 12:*255–258.

Miller NR. (1982). *Walsh and Hoyt's Clinical Neuro-ophthalmology.* 4th edition. Baltimore, Maryland, Williams and Wilkins, vol. 1, pp. 108–111.

Miller NR, Green WR. (1975). Arachnoid cysts involving a portion of the intraorbital optic nerve. *Arch Ophthalmol 93:*1117–1121.

Miller NR, Iliff WJ. (1975). Visual loss as the initial symptom in Hodgkin's disease. *Arch Ophthalmol 93:*1158–1161.

Miller NR, Savino PJ, Schneider T. (1995). Rapid growth of an intracranial aneurysm causing apparent retrobulbar optic neuritis. *J Neuro-ophthalmol 15 (4):*212–218.

Monaco F, Pirisi A, Sechi GP, Mutani R. (1979). Complicated optic atrophy (Behr's disease) associated with epilepsy and amino acid imbalance. *Eur Neurol 18:*101–105.

Murray KH, Paolino F, Goldman JM, et al. (1977). Ocular involvement in leukemia: Report of three cases. *Lancet 1:*829–831.

Nakae K, Yamamoto S, Shigematsu I, Kono R. (1973). Relation between subacute myelo-optic neuropathy (SMON) and clioquinol: Nationwide survey. *Lancet 1:*171–173.

Nasemann J, Zrenner E, Riedel KG. (1989). Recovery after severe ethambutol intoxication: Psychophysical and electrophysical correlations. *Doc Ophthalmol 71:*179–192.

Nazarian SM, Jay WM. (1988). Bilateral optic neuropathy associated with amiodarone therapy. *J Clin Neuro-ophthalmol 8:*25–28.

Newman NJ. (1993). Leber's hereditary optic neuropathy: New genetic considerations. *Arch Neurol 50:*540–548.

Newman NJ, Lott MT, Wallace DC. (1991). The clinical characteristics of pedigrees of Leber's hereditary optic neuropathy with the 11778 mutation. *Am J Ophthalmol 111:*750.

Newton N, Jr., Baratham G, Sinniah R, Lim A. (1989). Bilateral compressive optic neuropathy secondary to bilateral sphenoethmoidal mucoceles. *Ophthalmologica 198:*13–19.

Nikaido H, Mishima H, Ono H, et al. (1988). Leukemic involvement of the optic nerve. *Am J Ophthalmol 105:*294–298.

Nikoskelainen E, Sogg RL, Rosenthal AR, Friberg TR, Dorfman LJ. (1977). The early phase in Leber's hereditary optic atrophy. *Arch Ophthalmol 96:*969–978.

Nikoskelainen E, et al. (1983). Ophthalmoscopic findings in Leber's hereditary optic neuropathy. II. The fundus findings in the affected family members. *Arch Ophthalmol 101:*1059.

Norton AL, Walsh FB. (1972). Disulfiram-induced optic neuritis. *Trans Am Acad Ophthalmol Otolaryngol 76:*1263–1265.

Nugent GR, Sprinkle P, Bloor BM. (1970). Sphenoid sinus mucocoeles. *J Neurosurg 32:*443–451.

Oakley GP, Jr. (1973). The neurotoxicity of the halogenated hydroxyquinolines. *JAMA 225:*395–397.

Obal A. (1951). Nutritional amblyopia. *Am J Ophthalmol 34:*857–865.

Olson ME, Chernik NL, Posner JB. (1974). Infiltration of the leptomeninges by systemic cancer. *Arch Neurol 30:*122–137.

Oohira A, Inoue T, Fukuda N, Uchida K-I. (1991). A case with paraneoplastic optic neuropathy presenting bitemporal hemianopsia. *Neuro-ophthalmology 11:*325–328.

Oppenheimer S, Hoffbrand BI. (1986). Optic neuritis and myelopathy in systemic lupus erythematosus. *Can J Neurol Sci 13:*129–132.
Osterman PO. (1971). Myelopathy after Clioquinol treatment. *Lancet 2:*544.
Pachner AP, Duray P, Steere AC. (1989). Central nervous manifestations of Lyme disease. *Arch Neurol 46:*790–795.
Pearlman JT, Kadish AH, Ramseyer JC. (1977). Vision loss associated with amantadine hydrochloride use. *JAMA 237:*1200.
Peiris JB, Ross Russell RW. (1980). Giant aneurysms of the carotid system presenting as visual field defect. *J Neurol Neurosurg Psychiatr 43:*1053–1064.
Phanthumchinda K, Intragumtornchai T, Kasantikul V. (1988). Guillain-Barre syndrome and optic neuropathy in acute leukemia. *Neurology 38:*1324–1326.
Phillips CI, Wang MK, Van Peborgh PF. (1970). Some observations on the mechanism of tobacco amblyopia and its treatment with sodium thiosulphate. *Trans Ophthalmol Soc UK 90:*809–826.
Philipsen WM, Hommes OR. (1970). Atrophy of the optic nerve and vitamin B6 deficiency. *Ophthalmologica 160:*103–104.
Pillay N, Gilbert JJ, Ebers GC, Brown JD. (1984). Internuclear ophthalmoplegia and "optic neuritis": Paraneoplastic effects of bronchial carcinoma. *Neurology 34:*788–791.
Pittman FE, Westphal MC. (1974). Optic atrophy following treatment with diiodohydroxyquin. *Pediatrics 54:*81–83.
Polak BCP, Leys M, van Lith GHM. (1985). Blue-yellow colour vision changes as early symptoms of ethambutol oculotoxicity. *Ophthalmologica 191:*223–226.
Potts AM. (1973). Tobacco amblyopia. *Surv Ophthalmol 17:*313–339.
Pruett RC, Wepsic JG. (1979). Delayed diagnosis of chiasmal compression. *Am J Ophthalmol 76:*229–236.
Puliafito CA, Wray SH, Murray JE, Boger WP, III. (1981). Optic atrophy and visual loss in craniometaphyseal dysplasia. *Am J Ophthalmol 92:*696–701.
Purvin V, Van Dyck HJL. (1984). Primary reticulum cell sarcoma of the brain presenting as steroid-responsive optic neuropathy. *J Clin Neuro-ophthalmol 4:*15–23.
Pyle MM. (1966). Ethambutol in the retreatment and primary treatment of tuberculosis: A four-year clinical investigation. *Ann NY Acad Sci 135:*835–845.
Rab SM, Alam MN, Sadequzzaman MD. (1969). Optic atrophy during chlorpromazine therapy. *Br J Ophthalmol 53:*208–209.
Raitta C. (1968). Ophthalmic artery aneurysm. *Br J Ophthalmol 52:*707–709.
Raymond LA, Tew J. (1978). Large suprasellar aneurysms imitating pituitary tumour. *J Neurol Neurosurg Psychiatr 41:*83–87.
Reese AB. (1971). Expanding lesions of the orbit. *Trans Ophthalmol Soc UK 91:*85–104.
Reich JA, Billson FA. (1973). Toxic optic neuritis: Clioquinol ingestion in a child. *Med J Aust 2:*593–595.
Repka MX, Miller NR. (1988). Optic atrophy in children. *Am J Ophthalmol 106:*191–193.
Richardson JE, Hamilton W. (1978). Diabetes insipidus, diabetes mellitus, optic atrophy and deafness: Three cases of DIDMOAD syndrome. *Arch Dis Child 52:*796–798.
Ridgeway EW, Jaffe N, Walton DS. (1976). Leukemic ophthalmopathy in children. *Cancer 38:*1744–1749.
Rizzo JF III, Lessell S. (1991). Optic neuritis and ischemic optic neuropathy: Overlapping clinical profiles. *Arch Ophthalmol 109:*1668–1672.
Rizzo JF III, Lessell S. (1993). Tobacco amblyopia. *Am J Ophthalmol 116:*84–88.
Roberts SM. (1974). A review of the patterns on the ocular toxicity of ethambutol hydrochloride (Myambutol) on anti-tuberculosis drug. *Am J Optom Physiol Opt 51:*982–987.
Robertson DM, Hollenhorst RW, Callahan JA. (1966a). Ocular manifestations of digitalis toxicity. *Arch Ophthalmol 76:*640–645.
Robertson DM, Hollenhorst RW, Callahan JA. (1966b). Receptor function in digitalis therapy. *Arch Ophthalmol 76:*852–857.
Rodger FC. (1952). Nutritional amblyopia. A statistical report of the course and progress in two hundred thirty-eight cases. *Arch Ophthalmol 47:*570–583.
Rodger FC. (1953). Experimental thiamin deficiency as a cause of degeneration in the visual pathway of the rat. *Br J Ophthalmol 37:*11–29.
Rodger FC. (1954). Degenerative changes in the rat visual pathway when thiamin and riboflavin deficiencies are combined. *Br J Ophthalmol 38:*144–155.
Roe O. (1943). Clinical investigations of methyl alcohol poisoning with special reference to the pathogenesis and treatment of amblyopia. *Acta Med Scand 113:*558–608.
Rosenbaum JT, Simpson J, Neuwelt CM. (1997). Successful treatment of optic neuropathy in association with systemic lupus erythematosus using intravenous cyclophosphamide. *Br J Ophthalmol 81:*130–132.
Rosenberg RN, Chutorian A. (1967). Familial opticacoustic nerve degeneration and polyneuropathy. *Neurology 17:*827–832.
Rosenthal AR. (1983). Ocular manifestations of leukemia: A review. *Ophthalmology 90:*899–905.
Rosenthal AR, Egbert PR, Wilbur JR, Probert JC. (1975). Leukemic involvement of the optic nerve. *J Ped Ophthalmol 12:*84–93.
Rothstein J, Maisel RH, Berlinger NT, Wirtschafter JD. (1984). Relationship of optic neuritis to disease of the paranasal sinuses. *Laryngoscope 94:*1501–1508.

Roussos T, Tsolkas A. (1970). The toxicity of Myambutol on the human eye. *Ann Ophthalmol 2:*577–580.
Rubin GS. (1988). Reliability and sensitivity of clinical contrast sensitivity tests. *Clin Vis Sci 2:*169–177.
Rubinfeld RS, Gootenberg JE, Chavis RM, Zimmerman LE. (1988). Early onset acute orbital involvement in childhood acute lymphoblastic leukemia. *Ophthalmol 95:*116–120.
Rubinstein MK, Wilson G, Levin DC. (1968). Intraorbital aneurysms of the ophthalmic artery. *Arch Ophthalmol 80:*42–44.
Rucker CW. (1960). Tobacco amblyopia. *Proc Staff Meet Mayo Clin 35:*344–348.
Rudge P. (1973). Optic neuritis as a complication of carcinoma of the breast. *Proc R Soc Med 66:*1106–1107.
Rush JA. (1980). Retrobulbar optic neuropathy in sarcoidosis. *Ann Ophthalmol 12:*390–394.
Russo PA, Changlasian MA. (1994). Toxic optic neuropathy associated with ethambutol: Implications for current therapy. *J Am Optom Assoc 65:*332–338.
Rutka JD, Sharpe JA, Resch L, Fleming JF. (1985). Compressive optic neuropathy and ependymoma of the third ventricle. *J Clin Neuro-ophthalmol 5:*194–198.
Sadowsky AE, Leavenworth N, Wirtschafter JD. (1985). Compressive optic neuropathy induced by intranasal balloon catheter. *Am J Ophthalmol 99:*487–489.
Salmon JF, Carmichael TR, Welsh NH. (1987). Use of contrast sensitivity measurement in the detection of subclinical ethambutol toxic optic neuropathy. *Br J Ophthalmol 71:*192–196.
Samples JR, Younge BR. (1981). Tobacco-alcohol amblyopia. *J Clin Neuro-ophthalmol 11:*213–218.
Sanders MD. (1976). Diagnostic difficulties in optic nerve disease and in papilloedema and disc oedema. *Trans Ophthalm Soc UK 96:*386–394.
Sanderson PA, Kuwabara T, Cogan DG. (1976). Optic neuropathy presumably caused by vincristine therapy. *Am J Ophthalmol 81:*146–150.
Sandler SGH, Tobin W, Henderson ES. (1969). Vincristine-induced neuropathy. *Neurology 19:*367–372.
Savy LE, Moseley IF. (1996). Intracranial arterial calcification and ectasia in visual failure. *Br J Radiology 69:*394–401.
Schecter SL. (1986). Lyme disease associated with optic neuropathy. *Am J Med 81:*143–145.
Schild HS, Fox BC. (1991). Rapid-onset reversible ocular toxicity from ethambutol therapy. *Am J Med 90:*404–406.
Schwartz CL, Miller NR, Wharam MD, Leventhal BG. (1989). The optic nerve as the site of initial relapse in childhood lymphoblastic leukemia. *Cancer 63:*1616–1620.
Sedwick LA. (1991). The perils of Pauline: Visual loss in a tippler. *Surv Ophthalmol 35:*454–462.
Sedwick LA. (1992). Getting to the heart of visual loss: When cardiac medication may be dangerous to the optic nerves. *Surv Ophthalmol 36:*366–372.
Sedwick LA, Klingele TG, Burde RM, Behrens MM. (1984). Optic neuritis in inflammatory bowel disease. *J Clin Neuro-ophthalmol 4:*3–6.
Selby G. (1972). Subacute myelo-optic neuropathy in Australia. *Lancet 1:*123–125.
Senelick RC, Van Dyk HJL. (1974). Chromophobe adenoma masquerading as corticosteroid-responsive optic neuritis. *Am J Ophthalmol 78:*485–488.
Sengupta RP, Gryspeerdt GL, Hankinson J. (1976). Carotid ophthalmic aneurysms. *J Neurol Neurosurg Psychiatr 39:*837–853.
Seth B, Khosla PK, Semwal OP, D'Monty V. (1991). Visual evoked responses in tuberculous children on ethambutol therapy. *Indian Ped 28:*713–717.
Sharpe JA, Hostovsky M, Bilbao JM, Rewcastle NB. (1982). Methanol optic neuropathy: A histopathological study. *Neurology 32:*1093–1100.
Shields JA, Bakewell B, Augsburger JJ, et al. (1986). Space-occupying orbital masses in children: A review of 250 consecutive biopsies. *Ophthalmol 93:*379–384.
Shoffner JM, Brown MD, Stugard C, et al. (1995). Leber's hereditary optic neuropathy plus dystonia is caused by a mitochondrial DNA point mutation. *Ann Neurol 38:*163–169.
Siatkowski RM, Lam BL, Schatz NJ, Glaser JS, Byrne SF, Hughes JR. (1992). Optic neuropathy in Hodgkin's disease. *Am J Ophthalmol 114:*625–629.
Simpson DE, Moser LA. (1988). Compressive optic neuropathy secondary to chronic sinusitis. *Am J Optometry Physiol Optics 65:*757–762.
Singh et al. (1989). A mitochondrial DNA mutation as a cause of Leber's hereditary optic neuropathy. *NEJM 320:*1300.
Slamovits TL, Burde RM, Klingele TG. (1980). Bilateral optic atrophy caused by chronic oral ingestion and topical application of hexachlorophene. *Am J Ophthalmol 89:*676–679.
Slavin ML. (1986). Acute, severe, symmetric visual loss with cecocentral scotomas due to olfactory groove meningioma. *J Clin Neuro-ophthalmol 6:*224–227.
Smiddy WE, Green WR. (1987). Nutritional amblyopia. A histopathologic study with retrospective clinical correlation. *Graefe's Arch Clin Exp Ophthalmol 225:*321–324.
Smith ADM. (1961). Retrobulbar neuritis in Addisonian pernicious anaemia. *Lancet 1:*1001–1002.
Smith ADM. (1962). Veganism: A clinical survey with observations on vitamin B-12 metabolism. *Br Med J 1:* 1655–1658.
Smith DP. (1972a). Diagnostic criteria in dominantly inherited juvenile optic atrophy. A report of three new families. *Am J Optom Physiol Opt 49:*183–200.

Smith DP. (1972b). The assessment of acquired dyschromatopsia and clinical investigation of the acquired tritan defect in dominantly inherited juvenile atrophy. *Am J Optom Physiol Opt 49:*574–588.

Smith JL. (1977). The optic nerve work-up. *Trans Am Acad Ophthalmol Otolaryngol 83:*778–785.

Smith JL. (1987). Should ethambutol be barred? *J Clin Neuro-ophthalmol 7:*84–86.

Smith JL, Hoyt WF, Susac JO. (1973). Ocular fundus in acute Leber optic neuropathy. *Arch Ophthalmol 90:*349–354.

Snavely SR, Hodges GR. (1984). The neurotoxicity of antibacterial agents. *Ann Int Med 101:*92–104.

Spillane JD. (1971). SMON. *Lancet 2:*1371–1372.

Spillane JD. (1972). SMON. *Lancet 1:*154.

Spoor TC, Hartel WC, Harding S, Kocher G. (1982). Aspergillosis presenting as a corticosteroid responsive optic neuropathy. *J Clin Neuro-ophthalmol 2:*103–107.

Spoor TC, Kennerdell JS, Martinez AJ, Zorub D. (1980). Malignant gliomas of the optic nerve pathways. *Am J Ophthalmol 89:*284–292.

Stambolian D, Behrens M. (1977). Optic neuropathy associated with vitamin B-12 deficiency. *Am J Ophthalmol 83:*465–468.

Stern B, Krumholz A, Johns C, et al. (1985). Sarcoidosis and its neurological manifestations. *Arch Neurol 42:*909–917.

Stern WE. (1973). Meningiomas in the cranio-orbital junction. *J Neurosurg 38:*428–437.

Stern WE, Ernest JT. (1975). Intracranial ophthalmic artery aneurysm. *Am J Ophthalmol 80:*203–206.

Stone et al. (1992).Visual recovery in patients with Leber's hereditary optic neuropathy and the 11778 mutation. *J Clin Neuro-ophthalmol 12 (1):*10.

Strandvik B, Zetterstrom R. (1968). Amaurosis after broxyquinoline. *Lancet 1:*922–923.

Sunga RN, Enoch JM. (1970). Further perimetric analysis of patients with lesions of the visual pathways. *Am J Ophthalmol 70:*403–422.

Susac JO, Smith JL, Powell JO. (1973). Carcinomatous optic neuropathy. *Am J Ophthalmol 76:*672–679.

Susac JO, Smith JL, Walsh FB. (1977). The impossible meningioma. *Arch Neurol 34:*36–38.

Teare JP, Whitehad M, Rake MO, Coker RJ. (1991). Rapid onset of blindness due to meningeal carcinomatosis from an oesophageal adenocarcinoma. *Postgrad Med J 67:*909–911.

Tennekoon G, Aitchison CS, Frangia J, Price DL, Goldberg AM. (1979). Chronic lead intoxication: effects on developing optic nerve. *Ann Neurol 5:*558–564.

Teus MA, Teruel JL, Pascual J, et al. (1991). Corticosteroid induced toxic optic neuropathy. *Am J Ophthalmol 112:*605.

Thomas RJ. (1994). Neurotoxicity of antibacterial therapy. *South Med J 87:*869–874.

Thompson HS. (1976). Pupillary signs in the diagnosis of optic nerve disease. *Trans Ophthalmol Soc UK 96:*377–381.

Thompson HS, Montague P, Cox TA, et al. (1982). The relationship between visual acuity, pupillary defect, and visual field loss. *Am J Ophthalmol 93:*681–686.

Trobe JD, Glaser JS. (1978). Quantitative perimetry in compressive optic neuropathy and optic neuritis. *Arch Ophthalmol 96:*1210–1216.

Trobe JD, Glaser JS, Cassady JC. (1980). Optic atrophy: Differential diagnosis by fundus observation alone. *Arch Ophthalmol 98:*1040–1045.

Trobe JD, Glaser JS, Post JD, Page LK. (1978). Bilateral optic canal meningiomas. A case report. *Neurosurgery 3:*68–74.

Troncoso J, Mancall EL, Schatz NJ. (1979). Visual evoked responses in pernicious anemia. *Arch Neurol 36:*168–169.

Tsubaki T, Honma Y, Hoshi M. (1971). Neurological syndrome associated with Clioquinol. *Lancet 1:*696–697.

Tuboku-Metzger AF. (1969). Diet and neuropathy. *Br Med J 4:*239.

Uga S, Ishikawa S, Mukuno K. (1977). Histopathological study of canine optic nerve and retina treated by organophosphate pesticide. *Invest Ophthalmol Vis Sci 16:*877–881.

van Balen ATM. (1971). Toxic damage to the optic nerve caused by iodochlorhydroxyquinoline (Entero-Vioform). *Ophthalmologica 163:*8–9.

Victor M. (1970). Neuro-ophthalmic disorders due to alcoholism and malnutrition, in Smith JL (ed). *Neuro-Ophthalmology Symposium of the University of Miami and the Bascom Palmer Eye Institute.* Hallandale FL, Huffman Publishing Company.

Victor M, Dreyfus PM. (1965). Tobacco-alcohol amblyopia. Further comments on its pathology. *Arch Ophthalmol 74:*649–657.

Victor M, Mancall EL, Dreyfus PM. (1960). Deficiency amblyopia in the alcoholic patient. *Arch Ophthalmol 64:*1–33.

Waldman AL, Merrell R, Daroff RB, Geltzer A. (1967). Mucocele of the sphenoid sinus: A benign imitator. *Br J Ophthalmol 51:*674–678.

Walker CB. (1968). Visual screener for ethambutol toxicity. *Lancet 1:*493–494.

Wallace DC. (1970). A new manifestation of Leber's disease and a new explanation for the agency responsible for its unusual pattern of inheritance. *Brain 93:*121–132.

Wallace DC, et al. (1988). Mitochondrial DNA mutation associated with Leber's hereditary optic neuropathy. *Science 242:*1427.

Waterston JA, Gilligan BS. (1986). Parneoplastic optic neuritis and external ophthalmoplegia. *Aust NZ J Med 16:*703–704.

Watson-Williams EJ, Bottomley AC, Ainley RG, Phillips CI. (1969). Absorption of vitamin B-12 in tobacco amblyopia. *Br J Ophthalmol 53:*549–552.

Weaver RG, Jr., Chauvenet AR, Smith TJ, Schwartz AC. (1986). Ophthalmic evaluation of long-term survivors of childhood acute lymphoblastic leukemia. *Cancer 58:*963–968.
Weinstein JM, Lexow SS, Ho P, et al. (1989). Acute syphilitic optic neuritis. *Arch Ophthalmol 99:*1392–1395.
Weinstein JM, Morris GL, ZuRhein GM, Gentry LR. (1989). Posterior ischemic optic neuropathy due to Aspergillus fumigatus. *J Clin Neuro-ophthalmol 9:*7–13.
Weiter JJ. (1979). Retinociliary vein associated with a craniopharyngioma. *Ann Ophthalmol 11:*751–754.
Weleber RG, Shults WT. (1981). Digoxin retinal toxicity: Clinical and electrophysiolic evaluation of a cone dysfunction syndrome. *Arch Ophthalmol 99:*1568–1572.
White DW. (1972). Progressive visual loss. *Am J Ophthalmol 74:*752.
Wilson J. (1965). Skeletal manifestations in Leber's optic atrophy: A possible disorder of cyanide metabolism. *Ann Phys Med 44:*91–95.
Winward KW, Hamed LM, Glaser JS. (1989). The spectrum of optic nerve disease in human immunodeficiency virus infection. *Am J Ophthalmol 107:*373–380.
Wise CM, Agudelo CA. (1988). Optic neuropathy as an initial manifestation of Sjogren's syndrome. *J Rheumatol 15:*799–802.
Wymore J, Carter JE. (1982). Chlorpropamide-induced optic neuropathy. *Arch Intern Med 142:*381.
Yee RD, Cogan DG, Thorp TR, Schut L. (1977). Optic nerve compression due to aneurysmal bone cyst. *Arch Ophthalmol 95:*2176–2179.
Yen M-Y, Liu J-H. (1985). Malignant lymphoma involving the optic nerve and retina. *Ann Ophthalmol 17:*697–700.
Yiannikas C, Walsh JC, McLeod JG. (1983). Visual evoked potentials in the detection of subclinical optic toxic effect secondary to ethambutol. *Arch Neurol 40:*645–648.
Younge BR, Trautmann JC. (1980). Computer-assisted perimetry in neuro-ophthalmic disease. *Mayo Clin Proc 55:*207–222.
Zaidman GW. (1986). Neurosyphilis and retrobulbar neuritis in a patient with AIDS. *Ann Ophthalmol 18:*260.
Zimmerman LE, Font RL. (1975). Ophthalmologic manifestations of granulocytic sarcoma (myeloid sarcoma or chloroma). *Am J Ophthalmol 80:*975–990.
Zimmerman LE, Thoreson HT. (1964). Sudden loss of vision in acute leukemia: A clinicopathological report of two cases. *Surv Ophthalmol 9:*467–473.

◆ 2 ◆

Optic Neuritis

Optic neuritis (ON) is a general term for an optic neuropathy resulting from an idiopathic, inflammatory, infectious, or demyelinating etiology. If the optic nerve is swollen on ophthalmoscopy, then the terms *papillitis* or *anterior ON* are used. If the optic nerve is normal on ophthalmoscopy, then it is called *retrobulbar ON.*

What Are the Features of Typical Optic Neuritis?

Patients with idiopathic or demyelinating ON usually present with a "typical" clinical profile shown in Table 2–1 (Beck, 1992, 1993a, 1993b, 1993c, 1993d, 1994; Bradley, 1967; Burde, 1975, 1978, 1981; Cleary, 1993; Cox, 1981; Earl, 1967; Optic Neuritis Study Group, 1991; Fleischman, 1987; Frederiksen, 1991; Griffin, 1978; Keltner, 1993a, 1993b; Kupersmith, 1983; Kurtzke, 1985; Nikoskelainen, 1975; Sanders, 1986; Slamovits, 1991).

Table 2–1. Features of Typical Optic Neuritis (ON)

- Acute, usually, unilateral loss of visual acuity and/or visual field
- A relative afferent pupillary defect in unilateral or bilateral but asymmetric cases
- Periocular pain (90%), especially with eye movement
- Normal (65%) or swollen (35%) optic nerve head
- A young adult patient (< 40 years) but ON may occur at any age
- Eventual visual improvement
  - Improvement over several weeks in most patients (90%) to normal or near normal visual acuity
  - Visual recovery may continue for months
  - Patients may complain of residual deficits in contrast sensitivity, color vision, stereopsis, light-brightness, visual acuity, or visual field (Cleary, 1993; Fleishman, 1987)

Table 2–2. Features of Atypical Optic Neuritis (ON)

Bilateral simultaneous onset of ON in an adult patient
Lack of pain
Ocular findings suggestive of an inflammatory process
Anterior uveitis
Posterior chamber inflammation more than trace
Macular exudate or star figure
Retinal infiltrate or retinal inflammation
Lack of significant improvement of visual function or worsening of visual function after 30 days
Lack of at least one line of visual acuity improvement within the first 3 weeks after onset of symptoms
Age greater than 50 years
Diagnosis or evidence of other systemic conditions (e.g., inflammatory or infectious diseases [including human immunodeficiency virus infection]) other than multiple sclerosis that might cause optic neuropathy
Exquisitely steroid sensitive or steroid dependent optic neuropathy

What Are the Features of Atypical Optic Neuritis?

Patients who meet the criteria in Table 2–1 are considered to have *typical* ON. Conversely, patients with the features listed in Table 2–2 have an *atypical* ON (Ashworth, 1967, 1987; Beck, 1993a–d, 1994; Burde, 1978; Griffin, 1978; Moschos, 1990; Optic Neuritis Study Group, 1991; Parkin, 1984; Roseman, 1981; Sergott, 1988).

What Disorders May Be Associated with Optic Neuritis?

Table 2–3 lists a number of disorders that may be associated with typical or atypical ON. The presence of one of these disorders is usually suggested by the historical or examination findings.

What Is the Evaluation of Optic Neuritis?

In atypical cases, consideration should be made for a lumbar puncture and additional laboratory studies (e.g., in the Optic Neuritis Treatment Trial [ONTT] the following tests were performed: syphilis serology, antinuclear antibody, and chest radiograph). The required evaluation depends on the history and examination, with specific attention to infectious or inflammatory etiologies as listed in Table 2–3. In addition, patients with inflammatory autoimmune ON often have progressive or recurrent, steroid responsive, or steroid dependent optic neuropathy (Beck, 1994; Dutton, 1982; Kupersmith, 1988).

The ONTT was developed to evaluate the efficacy of corticosteroid treatment for acute ON and to investigate the relationship between ON and multiple sclerosis (MS) (Beck, 1992, 1993a–d, 1995). The ONTT was sponsored by the National Eye Institute as a randomized, controlled clinical trial that enrolled 457 patients at 15 clinical centers in the United States between the years 1988 and 1991. The ONTT entry criteria included patients

Table 2–3. Disorders Associated with Optic Neuritis

Guillain-Barré syndrome
Infections
Bacteria (e.g., syphilis, Lyme disease, cat scratch disease, meningitis, mycoplasma, Whipple's disease, tuberculosis)
Viruses (e.g., adenovirus, rubella, chicken pox, herpes zoster, human immunodeficiency virus, infectious mononucleosis, measles, mumps, influenza)
Protozoa (e.g., toxoplasmosis)
Fungi (e.g., Aspergillus, Histoplasmosis)
Parasites (e.g., intraocular nematodes)
Post-vaccination (e.g., smallpox, tetanus, rabies, influenza and Bacille Calmette-Guérin [BCG])
Focal infection or inflammation (e.g., paranasal sinusitis or mucocoele, beesting)
Systemic inflammation
Behçet's disease
Inflammatory bowel disease
Reiter's syndrome
Sarcoid
Systemic lupus erythematosus

Source: Abd Elrazak, 1991; Ahmadieh, 1994; Alexander, 1986; Beardsley, 1984; Beck, 1984; Berrios, 1994; Bienfang, 1977; Bird, 1970, 1976; Brazis, 1986; Breen, 1983; Cangemi, 1980; Carter, 1987; Cinefro, 1978; Confavreux, 1985; Connolly, 1975; Consul, 1968; Cox, 1983; Deane, 1995; Dutton, 1982; Farris, 1988, 1990; Finkel, 1988; Fleet, 1986; Folk, 1983, 1984; Frey, 1973; Frohman, 1997; Galetta, 1989; Gressel, 1983; Grossniklaus, 1987; Gunduz, 1994; Hackett, 1974; Harbison, 1984; Hart, 1979; Husted, 1975; Jabs, 1986; Jacobson, 1991; Johnson, 1986; Kazarian, 1978; Kupersmith, 1988; Lesser, 1990; Lew, 1983; Lustgarten, 1983; MacDonald, 1987; Macoul, 1982; McKibbin, 1995; McLeish, 1990; Molk, 1982; Nikoskelainen, et al., 1972, 1975; Openheimer, 1986; Pal, 1987; Perry, 1979; Pickens, 1975; Riffenburgh, 1961; Robinson, 1986; Rothstein, 1984; Schecter, 1986; Schuil, 1985; Sedwick, 1984; Shimo-Oku, 1989; Sombrono, 1987; Strong, 1974; Tarkkannen, 1971; van de Geijn, 1994; Winward, 1989; Wu, 1986; Yau, 1996; Yen, 1991; Zaidman, 1986.

who were between the ages of 18 and 46 years; presented with a relative afferent pupillary defect as well as a visual field defect in the affected eye; and examined within 8 days of the onset of visual symptoms of a first attack of acute unilateral ON. Patients were excluded if they had previous episodes of ON in the affected eye; previous corticosteroid treatment for ON or MS; or systemic disease other than MS that might be a cause for the ON (Beck, 1992, 1993a–d, 1995).

In the ONTT, all patients underwent testing for collagen vascular disease (antinuclear antibody [ANA]), serologic testing for syphilis (FTA-ABS), and a chest radiograph for sarcoidosis. A lumbar puncture was optional. An ANA antibody test was positive in a titer less than 1:320 in 13% of patients, and 1:320 or greater in 3% of them. Only one patient was eventually diagnosed with a collagen vascular disease. Visual and neurologic outcomes in these patients were no different from those of the other ONTT patients. The FTA-ABS was positive in six patients (1.3%) but none had syphilis. A chest radiograph did not reveal sarcoidosis in any patient. However, in a separate report Jacobson et al. described four of 20 patients with isolated ON with positive serology for Lyme disease. These authors recommended serologic testing for Lyme disease in patients with ON with or without the typical rash of erythema migrans, who live in or have visited Lyme endemic areas. Cerebrospinal fluid (CSF) analysis was recommended for patients with positive serology and intravenous (IV) antibiotic therapy for unexplained pleocytosis (Jacobson, 1991). We do not order Lyme titers for patients with ON from nonendemic regions.

The evaluation recommendations of the ONTT study group for patients with typical acute ON are listed in Table 2–4.

Table 2–4. Modified Evaluation Recommendations of the Optic Neuritis Treatment Trial (ONTT) for Optic Neuritis (ON)

Laboratory testing
Chest radiograph, laboratory tests (e.g., syphilis serology, collagen vascular disease, serum chemistries, complete blood counts, etc.), and lumbar puncture are not necessary for typical ON (see Table 2–1) but should not be considered in atypical cases (see Table 2–2).
Neuroimaging (MRI)
Neuroimaging studies in the ONTT disclosed an alternative etiology for visual loss in only one patient with a pituitary adenoma; a second patient had an ophthalmic artery aneurysm that was not detected on the initial magnetic resonance (MR) scan. The ONTT authors concluded that neuroimaging was of limited value in establishing the diagnosis of ON. MR imaging of the brain was felt to be a powerful predictor of multiple sclerosis (MS) and should be considered to assess risk of future neurologic events of MS and for treatment decision making.

What Are the Neuroimaging Findings in Optic Neuritis?

Periventricular white matter signal abnormalities on magnetic resonance imaging (MRI) consistent with MS (Baumhefner, 1990; Gebarski, 1985; Jacobs, 1986a,b, 1991; Johnson, 1983; Kinkel, 1984; Lukes, 1983; Scotti, 1986; Young, 1981) have been reported in 40 to 70% of cases of isolated ON (Christiansen, 1992; Feinstein, 1992; Francis, 1995; Friedrickson, 1989, 1991; Gebarski, 1985; Jacobs, 1986a,b, 1991; Jackson, 1985; Johns, 1986; Kinnunen, 1987; Miller, 1988a, 1988b; Morrissey, 1993; Moulin, 1983; Ormerod, 1986, 1987; Paty, 1988; Rudick, 1986; Shabas, 1987; Staedt, 1989). MRI with gadolinium may show enhancing lesions in 26 to 37% of patients with isolated ON (Christiansen, 1992; Merandi, 1991) and may increase the detection of disease activity (Guy, 1990; Merandi, 1991b; Miller, 1988; Thompson, 1990).

Although computed tomography (CT) scan of the head may also show abnormalities in MS and ON (Cala, 1976; Harding, 1978; Osher, 1980), CT has been relatively insensitive to the detection of MS plaques compared with MRI (Jacobs, 1986a, 1986b; Paty, 1988). MRI is a very sensitive test for detecting lesions consistent with MS (Baumhefner, 1990; Paty, 1988; Uhlenbrock, 1988). Paty reported 19 cases of clinically definite MS out of 200 consecutive patients with suspected MS comparing the predictive value of MR scanning with CT scanning, evoked potentials (EP), and CSF analysis for oligoclonal bands (Paty, 1988). Eighteen of these 19 (95%) patients had MR scans that were "strongly suggestive of MS" at first evaluation, compared to 14 of 19 (74%) patients with positive oligoclonal bands, 10 of 19 (53%) patients with abnormal somatosensory EPs, 9 of 19 (47%) patients with abnormal visual EP (VEP), and 9 of 19 (47%) patients with abnormal CT scans. Combining multiple reports, the risk of developing MS within 1 to 4 years is about 30% (range 23–35%) in patients with isolated ON and an abnormal MR scan (Beck, 1993; Frederiksen, 1992; Jacobs, 1986a,b; Miller, 1988a). Morrissey et al. reported 89 patients (44 with ON, 17 brainstem involvement, and 28 spinal cord involvement) with an acute demyelinating attack (Morrissey, 1993). Of these 89 patients, 57 (65%) had one or more MR scan abnormalities and 32 had no MR scan abnormalities. Only 1 of the 32 patients with a normal MR scan developed MS, versus development of MS in 37 of 57 patients (65%) with an abnormal MR scan. Of the three isolated clinical syndromes (optic nerve, brainstem, spinal cord), ON with an abnormal MR scan had the highest rate of progression to MS of 82%. Jacobs et al. reported 42 patients with isolated monosymptomatic optic neuritis (Jacobs, 1991). During 5.6 years of follow-up, 21 patients developed MS. Of these 21 patients, 16 (76%) had abnormal MR scans and 5 had normal MR scans (Jacobs, 1991). It should be emphasized, however, that MS is a clinical diagnosis that cannot be made on the basis of MR scan abnormalities alone (Guy, 1994; Paty, 1993) and the absence of MR scan abnormalities does not protect against the future development of MS (Beck, 1993c; Jacobs, 1991).

Should a Lumbar Puncture be Performed in Patients with Optic Neuritis?

Patients with ON may show abnormalities in CSF analysis consistent with those seen in MS such as increased cell count (> 5 cells per cubic mm), increased total protein, increased CSF-immunoglobulin G (IgG) concentration, oligoclonal bands, antibodies to myelin basic protein (MBP) and proteolipid protein (PLP), and increased CSF myelin basic protein (MBP) levels (Corridori, 1987; Ebers, 1980; Fredericksen, 1992; Frick, 1980; Hume, 1988; Link, 1971; McDonald, 1977; Moulin, 1983; Nikoskelainen, 1975a,b, 1981; Paty, 1988; Rudick, 1986; Schenck, 1969; Schwartz, 1970; Sellebjerg, 1994, 1995; Soderstrom, 1993; Sola, 1987; Stendal-Brodin, 1983; Warren, 1988, 1994). Lumbar puncture (LP), however, did not produce any additional unsuspected diagnoses in the 141 patients in the ONTT undergoing CSF analysis. In addition, a normal initial CSF after ON did not preclude the eventual development of MS (Sandberg-Wollheim, 1975). Although several authors have reported that abnormal CSF results may be predictive of eventual MS (Anmarkrud, 1989; Corridori, 1987; Ebers, 1985; Feasby, 1982; Fredericksen, 1992; Kinnunen, 1987; McDonald, 1977; Moulin, 1983; Nikoskelainen, 1981; Paty, 1988; Sandberg-Wollheim, 1990; Stendahl-Brodin, 1983), others have not found CSF abnormalities to have predictive value (Sandberg-Wollheim, 1975). We follow the recommendations of the ONTT and reserve LP for patients with atypical ON and do not routinely perform LP for typical ON.

Should Visual Evoked Potentials Be Performed on Patients with Optic Neuritis?

Although the VEP is often abnormal in patients with ON (Ashworth, 1994; Asselman, 1975; Bobak, 1987; Fujimoto, 1988; Ghezzi, 1986; Hoeppner, 1978; Honan, 1990; Kakisu, 1987; Kinnunen, 1987; MacFadyen, 1988), an abnormal VEP in the setting of a clinically diagnosed ON does not alter the diagnostic or treatment plan nor does the VEP provide additional prognostic information for visual recovery or the development of MS (Heinrichs, 1988; Kirkham, 1981). Nevertheless, although we do not feel that the routine use of VEP in typical ON is justified, VEP may be helpful in identifying a second site of neurologic involvement (previous ON) to strengthen the clinical diagnosis of MS in patients with no history or examination findings of an optic neuropathy (Asselman, 1975; Blumhardt, 1982; Celesia, 1990; Diener, 1980; Eisen, 1983; Ellenberger, 1977; Feinsod, 1975; Halliday, 1972; Hennerici, 1977; Kinnunen, 1987; Kupersmith, 1983; Matthews, 1977; Nilsson, 1978; Ormerod, 1987; Paty, 1988; Regan, 1976; Sola, 1987; Zeese, 1977).

What Is the Treatment of Optic Neuritis?

Although corticosteroids have been used for acute ON (Bowden, 1974; Gould, 1977; Lessell, 1992; Rawson, 1966, 1969; Silderberg, 1993; Spoor, 1988; Smith, 1986) and have been shown to improve symptoms in MS (Compston, 1987; Milligan, 1987), well-controlled data to support the treatment efficacy of steroids in ON have been lacking until recently (Beck, 1992; Durelli, 1986). IV methylprednisolone (MP) treatment has been reported to decrease CSF, anti-MBP, intrathecal IgG synthesis, and oligoclonal bands; to decrease gadolinium enhancement of MS plaques (and presumably blood-brain barrier disruption) on MRI; and to improve clinical disability. The clinical effect of treatment might be due to reduction of inflammation and myelin breakdown (Barkhof, 1991, 1992; Compston, 1987; Durelli, 1986; Warren, 1994).

Rawson et al. reported a more rapid visual recovery, but no difference in visual outcome after one year, in a double-blind, placebo-controlled, prospective study of 50 patients with ON treated with adrenocorticotrophic hormone (ACTH) (Rawson, 1966). Rose et al. observed similar more rapid improvement in patients with ON treated with ACTH versus placebo (Rose, 1970). Bowden et al., however, reported no benefit from ACTH compared with placebo in 54 patients with ON (Bowden, 1974). Gould et al. reported a prospective, single-blinded, controlled, randomized clinical trial of 74 patients with ON who experienced more rapid improvement with a retrobulbar injection of triamcinolone, but patients had no difference in outcome after 6 months (Gould, 1977).

In the ONTT, the patients were randomly assigned to one of three treatment arms in the study:

1. IV methylprednisolone sodium succinate (250 mg every 6 hours for 3 days) followed by oral prednisone (1 mg/kg per day for 11 days).
2. Oral prednisone (1 mg/kg per day for 14 days).
3. Oral placebo for 14 days followed by a short oral taper.

The major conclusions of the ONTT related to treatment are summarized in Table 2–5.

Based on the ONTT results, it is recommended that treatment with oral prednisone in standard doses be avoided in ON. Treatment with IV MP should be considered in patients with abnormal MRI of the brain or a particular need (e.g., monocular patient or occupational requirement) to recover visual function more rapidly. Beck, et al. felt that, although brain MRI may not be necessary for the diagnosis of ON, imaging was valuable for prognostic purposes (Beck, 1992, 1993a–d). In the ONTT, patients with multiple signal abnormalities on MRI most clearly benefited from IV corticosteroid therapy in terms of the development of MS. The rate of development of MS was too low in the patients with normal MRI to assess treatment benefit in this group. Although ON patients in the ONTT had MRI within 9 days of the onset of visual loss, some authors

Table 2–5. Treatment Summary of the ONTT

High-dose intravenous (IV) steroids followed by oral corticosteroids accelerated visual recovery (particularly with visual field defects; $p = 0.0001$) but provided no long-term benefit to vision
"Standard dose" oral prednisone alone did not improve the visual outcome, and was associated with an increased rate of new attacks of ON
IV followed by oral corticosteroids reduced the rate of development of clinically definite multiple sclerosis (MS) during the first 2 years, particularly in patients with magnetic resonance (MR) signal abnormalities, but by 3 years the treatment effect had subsided (Beck, 1993, 1995). Beck et al. reported that of 150 patients with two or more MR imaging lesions, 36% developed clinically definite MS within 2 years, versus only 5% of 202 patients with normal or minimal abnormalities on MR imaging.
Treatment was well tolerated with few major side effects.

have suggested that patients presenting later than this interval with an abnormal MR scan may still benefit from treatment with IV MP within a treatment window of about 2 months (Guy, 1994).

Finally, even though the ONTT was a large, well-designed study, several criticisms have been raised including:

1. The lack of an intravenous control group.
2. Incomplete masking of the patients (i.e., in-hospital IV treated patients knew they had received IV MP).
3. Data regarding treatment effect of IV MP on the development of MS were obtained from a retrospective analysis of a study that was primarily designed for a different purpose (to evaluate the treatment effect).
4. The role of retrobulbar steroids was not assessed.
5. The role of higher doses of MP, such as the 30 mg per kg dose suggested for the treatment of acute spinal cord injury, was not determined.
6. The efficacy of oral prednisone at higher doses was not assessed.
7. The need or lack of need for the oral tapering doses of corticosteroids following IV MP was not addressed.

Despite these concerns, the ONTT is the only well-controlled prospective clinical trial available in the literature to date on the treatment and evaluation of ON. We follow the evaluation and the treatment recommendations of the ONTT.

Are There Treatments Other than Steroids for Optic Neuritis?

Intravenous immunoglobulin (IVIg) has also been reported to improve visual acuity in an uncontrolled study of five patients with definite MS and unilateral or bilateral but stable demyelinating optic neuritis (van Engelen, 1992). These results must be replicated on a larger scale before any recommendation on the use of IVIg can be made.

What Is the Risk of Developing Multiple Sclerosis following Optic Neuritis?

The risk for the eventual development of MS following ON is quite variable in the literature, with reports ranging from 8 to 85% (Alter, 1973; Anmarkund, 1989; Bradley, 1968; Cohen, 1979; Collis, 1965; Ebers, 1981, 1985; Francis, 1987; Hely, 1986; Hutchison, 1976; Hyllested, 1961; Kinnunen, 1983; Kurland, 1966; Kuroiwa, 1973, 1975; Kurtzke, 1985; Miller, 1988; Nikoskelainen, 1974, 1981; Percy, 1972; Rizzo, 1988; Rodriguez, 1995; Sandberg-Wollheim, 1976; Sanders, 1986; Stendahl-Brodin, 1983; Wikstrom, 1980). Most studies indicate a 25 to 35% risk of patients with ON developing MS. This variability is probably related to differences in patient populations (e.g., clinic or hospital versus population based); sample sizes; study design (retrospective versus prospective); duration of follow-up (longer interval studies tend to report higher incidence rates); differences in selection criteria and diagnostic evaluation of ON cases; and different study diagnostic criteria for both ON and MS. Rodriguez, et al. found a cumulative probability of developing clinically definite MS of 24% after 5 years and 39% after 10 years (Rodriguez, 1995). Rizzo and Lessell studied 60 patients with ON, with a mean follow-up of 14.9 years

(Rizzo, 1988). Life table analysis indicated that 74% of the women and 34% of the men developed MS 15 years after their attack of ON, and 91.3% of the women and 44.8% of the men would develop MS after 20 years. As previously discussed, MR scan abnormalities may be the best predictor for the eventual development of MS after ON. Increased risk of MS has also been reported in patients with HLA-DR2 and HLA-B7 tissue types, but we do not recommend routine HLA screening for ON (Aranson, 1974; Hely, 1986; Kinnunen, 1987; Morrissey, 1993; Sandberg-Wollheim, 1975; Stendahl-Brodin, 1978).

Our approach to ON is summarized in Figure 2–1.

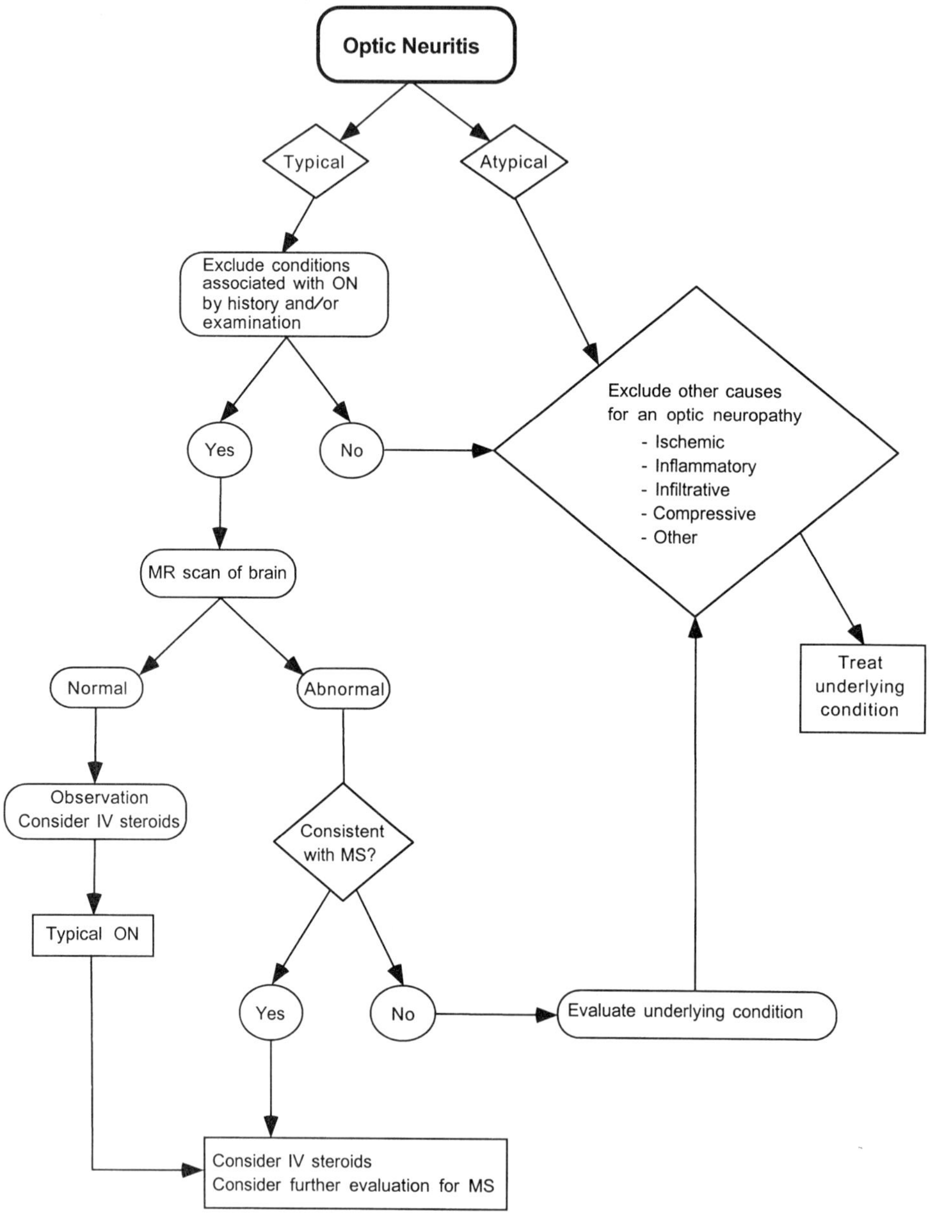

Figure 2–1. Evaluation of optic neuritis.

References

Abd Elrazak M. (1991). Brucella optic neuritis. *Arch Intern Med 151:*776-778.

Ahmadieh H, Roodpeyma S, Azarmina M, Soheilian M, Sajjadi SH. (1994). Bilateral simultaneous optic neuritis in childhood systemic lupus erythematosus. A case report. *J Neuro-ophthalmol 14:*84–86.

Alexander EL, Malinow K, Lejewski JE, et al. (1986). Primary Sjogren's syndrome with central nervous system disease mimicking multiple sclerosis. *Ann Intern Med 104:*323–330.

Alter M, Good J, Okihiro M. (1973). Optic neuritis in orientals and caucasians. *Neurology 23:*631–639.

Anmarkrud N, Slettnes ON. (1989). Uncomplicated retrobulbar neuritis and the development of multiple sclerosis. *Acta Ophthalmol 67:*306–309.

Aranson BGW, Fuller TC, Lehrich FR, et al. (1974). Histocompatibility types and measles antibodies in multiple sclerosis and optic neuritis. *J Neurol Sci 22:*419–428.

Ashworth B. (1967). Chronic retrobulbar and chiasmal neuritis. *Br J Ophthalmol 51:*698–702.

Ashworth B. (1987). Chronic demyelinating optic neuritis. *Neuro-ophthalmology 7:*75–79.

Ashworth B, Aspinall PA, Mitchell JD. (1994). Visual function in multiple sclerosis. *Doc Ophthalmol 73:*209–224.

Assleman P, Chadwick DW, Marsden CD. (1975). Visual evoked responses in the diagnosis and management of patients suspected of multiple sclerosis. *Brain 98:*261–282.

Barkhoff F, Frequin STFM, Hommes OR, et al. (1992). A correlative triad of gadolinium-DTPA MRI, EDSS, and CSF-MBP in relapsing multiple sclerosis patients treated with high-dose intravenous methylprednisolone. *Neurology 42:*63–67.

Barkhoff F, Hommes OR, Lamers KJB, et al. (1991). High dose intravenous methylprednisolone in multiple sclerosis. *Neurology 41:*1219–1222.

Baumhefner RO, Tourtellotte WW, Syndulko K, et al. (1990). Quantitative multiple sclerosis plaque assessment with magnetic resonance imaging: Its correlation with clinical parameters, evoked potentials, and intra-blood-barrier IgG synthesis. *Arch Neurol 47:*19–26.

Beardsley TL, Brown SVL, Syndnor CF, Grimson BS, Klintworth GK. (1984). Eleven cases of sarcoidosis of the optic nerve. *Am J Ophthalmol 97:*62–77.

Beck RW. (1992). Corticosteroid treatment of optic neuritis. *Neurology 42:*1133–1135.

Beck RW. (1995). The optic neuritis treatment trial: Three year follow-up results. *Arch Ophthalmol 113:*136–137.

Beck RW, Arrington J, Murtagh FR, Cleary PA, Kaufman DI. (1993a). Brain magnetic resonance imaging in acute optic neuritis experience of the optic neuritis study group. *Arch Neurol 50:*841–846.

Beck RW, Cleary PA. (1993a). Recovery from severe visual loss in optic neuritis. *Arch Ophthalmol 111:*300.

Beck RW, Cleary PA. (1993b). Optic neuritis treatment trial: One year follow-up results. *Arch Ophthalmol 111:773–775.*

Beck RW, Cleary PA, Anderson MA, et al. (1992). A randomized, controlled trial of corticosteroids in the treatment of acute optic neuritis. *N Engl J Med 326:*581–588.

Beck RW, Cleary PA, Backlund JC. (1994). The course of visual recovery after optic neuritis. *Ophthalmology 101:*1771–1778.

Beck RW, Cleary PA, Trobe JD, et al. (1993c). The effect of corticosteroids for acute optic neuritis on the subsequent development of multiple sclerosis. *N Engl J Med 329:*1764–1769.

Beck RW, Kupersmith MJ, Cleary PA, Katz B. (1993d). Fellow eye abnormalities in acute unilateral optic neuritis. *Ophthalmology 100:*691–698.

Beck RW, Sergott RC, Barr CC, Annesley WH. (1984). Optic disc edema in the presumed ocular histoplasmosis syndrome. *Ophthalmology 91:*183–185.

Beck RW, Trobe J. (1995). What we have learned from the optic neuritis treatment trial. *Ophthalmology 102:*1504–1508.

Behan PO, Lessell S, Roche M. (1976). Optic neuritis in the Landry-Guillain-Barre-Strohl syndrome. *Br J Ophthalmol 60:*58–59.

Berrios RR, Serrano LA. (1994). Bilateral optic neuritis after a bee sting. *Am J Ophthalmol 117:*677–678.

Bienfang DC, Kantrowitz FG, Noble JL, Raynor AM. (1977). Ocular abnormalities after influenza immunization. *Arch Ophthalmol 95:*1649.

Bird AC, Smith JL, Curtin VT. (1970). Nematode optic neuritis. *Am J Ophthalmol 69:*72–77.

Bird AC. (1976). Treatment of acute optic neuritis. *Trans Ophthalmol Soc UK 96:*412–414.

Blumhardt LD, Barrett G, Halliday AM. (1982). The pattern visual evoked potential in the clinical assessment of undiagnosed spinal cord disease. *Adv in Neurol 32:*463–471.

Bobak P. (1987). The visual evoked potential contrast response function in recovering optic neuritis. *Curr Eye Res 6:*981.

Bowden AN, Bowden PMA, Friedmann AI, et al. (1974). A trial of corticotrophin gelatin injection in acute optic neuritis. *J Neurol Neurosurg Psychiatr 37:*869–873.

Bradley WG, Whitty CWM. (1967). Acute optic neuritis: Its clinical features and their relation to prognosis for recovery of vision. *J Neurol Neurosurg Psychiatr 30:*531–538.

Bradley WG, Whitty CWM. (1968). Acute optic neuritis: Prognosis for the development of multiple sclerosis. *J Neurol Neurosurg Psychiatr 31:*1010–1018.

Brazis PW, Stokes HR, Ervin FR. (1986). Optic neuritis in cat scratch disease. *J Clin Neuro-ophthalmol 6:*172–174.

Breen LA, Burde RM, Mendelsohn GE. (1983). Beesting papillitis. *J Clin Neuro-ophthalmol 3:*97–100.

Brodsky MC, Beck RW. (1994). The changing role of MR imaging in the evaluation of acute optic neuritis. *Radiology 192:*22–23.

Buckley C, Kennard C, Swash M. (1982). Treatment of acute exacerbations of multiple sclerosis with intravenous methylprednisolone. *J Neurol Neurosurg Psychiatr 45:*179–186.

Burde RM, Gallin PF. (1975). Visual parameters associated with recovered retrobulbar optic neuritis. *Am J Ophthalmol 79:*1034–1037.

Burde RM, Gittinger J, Keltner JL, Miller NR. (1978). Neuro-ophthalmologic dilemma: Chronic optic neuritis? *Surv Ophthalmol 23:*173–176.

Burde RM, Keltner JL, Miller NR, Gittinger JW. (1981). Central visual dysfunction with disc swelling. *Surv Ophthalmol 26:*43–48.

Bynke H, Rosen I, Sandberg-Wolheim M. (1980). Correlation of visual evoked potentials, ophthalmological and neurological findings after unilateral optic neuritis. *Acta Ophthalmol 58:*673–687.

Cala LA, Mastaglia FL, Black JL. (1978). Computerized tomography of brain and optic nerve in multiple sclerosis. *J Neurol Sci 36:*411–426.

Cangemi FE, Bergen RL. (1980). Optic atrophy following swine flu vaccination. *Ann Ophthalmol 12:*857–863.

Carter JB, Hamill RJ, Matoba AY. (1987). Bilateral syphilitic optic neuritis in a patient with a positive test for HIV. *Arch Ophthalmol 105:*1485–1486.

Celesia GG, Kaufman DI, Brigell M, et al. (1990). Optic neuritis: A prospective study. *Neurology 40:*919–923.

Christiansen P, Frederiksen JL, Henriksen O, et al. (1992). Gd-DTPA-enhanced lesions in the brain of patients with acute optic neuritis. *Acta Neurol Scand 85:*141–146.

Cinefro RJ, Frenkel M. (1978). Systemic lupus erythematosus presenting as optic neuritis. *Ann Ophthalmol 10:*559–563.

Cleary PA, Beck RW, Anderson MM, et al. (1993). Design, methods and conduct of the Optic Neuritis Treatment Trial. *Controlled Clin Trials 14:*123–142.

Cohen M, Lessell S, Wolf P. (1979). A prospective study of the risk of developing multiple sclerosis in uncomplicated optic neuritis. *Neurology 29:*208–213.

Collins DWK, Black JL, Mastaglia FL. (1978). Pattern-reversal visual evoked potential. *J Neurol Sci 36:*83–95.

Collis WJ. (1965). Acute unilateral retrobulbar neuritis. *Arch Neurol 13:*409–412.

Compston DAS, Batchelor JR, Earl CH, McDonald WI. (1978). Factors influencing the risk of multiple sclerosis developing in patients with optic neuritis. *Brain 101:*495–511.

Compston DAS, Milligan NM, Hughes PJ, Gibbs J, McBroom V, Morgan BP, Campbell AK. (1987). A double-blind controlled clinical trial of high-dose methylprednisolone in patients with multiple sclerosis. 2. Laboratory results. *J Neurol Neurosurg Psych 50:*517–522.

Confavreux C, Girard-Madoux P, Moulin T. (1985). Acute acquired toxoplasmosis causing neuroptico-meningoencephalitis in an immunocompetent boy. *J Neurol Neurosurg Psychiatr 48:*715–716.

Connolly JH, Hutchinson WM, Allen IV, et al. (1975). Carotid artery thrombosis, encephalitis, myelitis and optic neuritis associated with rubella virus infections. *Brain 98:*583–594.

Consul BN, Purohit GK, Chhabra H. (1968). Antirabic vaccine optic neuritis. *Indian J Med Sci 22:*630–632.

Corridori F, Salmaggi A, Bortolami C, et al. (1987). Prognostic value of cerebrospinal fluid electrophoresis in optic neuritis and suspected multiple sclerosis. *Ital J Neurol Sci (supp) 6:*77–80.

Cox TA, Haskins GE, Gangitano JL, Antonson DL. (1983). Bilateral toxocara optic neuropathy. *J Clin Neuro-ophthalmol 3:*267–274.

Cox TA, Thompson HS, Corbett JJ. (1981). Relative afferent pupillary defects in optic neuritis. *Am J Ophthalmol 92:*685–690.

Cox TA, Woolson RF. (1981). Steroid treatment of optic neuritis. *Arch Ophthalmol 99:*336.

Deane JS, Bibby K. (1995). Bilateral optic neuritis following herpes zoster ophthalmicus. *Arch Ophthalmol 113:*972–973.

Diener CH, Scheibler H. (1980). Follow-up studies of visual potentials in multiple sclerosis evoked by checkerboard and foveal stimulation. *Electroencephal Clin Neurophys 49:*490–496.

Durelli L, Cocito D, Riccio A, et al. (1986). High-dose intravenous methylprednisolone in the treatment of multiple sclerosis: clinical-immunologic correlations. *Neurology 36:*238–243.

Dutton JJ, Anderson RL. (1985). Idiopathic inflammatory perioptic neuritis simulating optic nerve sheath meningioma. *Am J Ophthalmol 100:*424–430.

Dutton JJ, Burde RM, Klingele TG. (1982). Autoimmune retrobulbar optic neuritis. *Am J Ophthalmol 94:*11–17.

Earl CJ, Martin B. (1967). Prognosis in optic neuritis related to age. *Lancet 1:*74.

Ebers GC. (1985). Optic neuritis and multiple sclerosis. *Arch Neurol 42:*702–704.

Ebers GC, Cousin HK, Feasby TE, Paty DW. (1981). Optic neuritis and familial multiple sclerosis. *Neurology 31:*1138–1142.

Ebers GC, Paty DW. (1980). CSF electrophoresis in one thousand patients. *Can J Neurol Sci 7:*275–280.

Eisen A, Cracco RQ. (1983). Overuse of evoked potentials. Caution. *Neurology 33:*618–621.

Ellenberger C, Ziegler SB. (1977). Visual evoked potentials and quantitative perimetry in multiple sclerosis. *Ann Neurol 1:*561–564.

Farlow MR, Markand ON, Edwards MK, Stevens JC, Kolar OJ. (1986). Multiple sclerosis: Magnetic resonance imaging, evoked responses, and spinal fluid electrophoresis. *Neurology 36:*828–831.

Farris BK, Pickard DJ. (1990). Bilateral postinfectious optic neuritis and intravenous steroid therapy in children. *Ophthalmology 97:*339–345.

Farris BK, Webb RM. (1988). Lyme disease and optic neuritis. *J Clin Neuro-ophthalmol 8:*73–78.
Feasby TE, Ebers GC. (1982). Risk of multiple sclerosis in isolated optic neuritis (abstract). *Can J Neurol Sci 9:*269.
Feinsod M, Hoyt WF. (1975). Subclinical optic neuropathy in multiple sclerosis. *J Neurol Neurosurg Psychiatr 38:*1109–1114.
Feinstein A, Youl B, Ron M. (1992). Acute optic neuritis. *Brain 115:*1403–1415.
Finkel MF. (1988). Lyme disease and its neurologic complications. *Arch Neurol 45:*99–104.
Fleet WS, Watson RT. (1986). Autoimmune optic neuritis. A potentially treatable form of visual loss. *Ann Ophthalmol 18:*144–146.
Fleishman JA, Beck RW, Linares OA, Klein JW. (1987). Deficits in visual function after resolution of optic neuritis. *Ophthalmology 94:*1029–1035.
Folk JC, Lobes LA. (1984). Presumed toxoplasmic papillitis. *Ophthalmology 92:*64–67.
Folk JC, Weingesist TA, Corbett JJ, et al. (1983). Syphilitic neuroretinitis. *Am J Ophthalmol 95:*480–486.
Francis DA, Compston DAS, Batchelor JR, McDonald WI. (1987). A reassessment of the risk of multiple sclerosis developing in patients with optic neuritis after extended follow-up. *J Neurol Neurosurg Psych 50:*758–765.
Francis GS, Evans AC, Arnold DL. (1995). Neuroimaging in multiple sclerosis. *Neurologic Clinics 13:*147–170.
Fredericksen JL, Larsson HBW, Henriksen O, Olesen J. (1989). Magnetic resonance imaging of the brain in patients with acute monosymptomatic optic neuritis. *Acta Neurol Scand 80:*512–517.
Fredericksen JL, Larsson HBW, Olesen J. (1992). Correlation of magnetic resonance imaging and CSF findings in patients with acute monosymptomatic optic neuritis. *Acta Neurol Scand 86:*317–322.
Fredericksen JL, Larsson HBW, Olesen J, Stigsby B. (1991a). MR, VEP, SEP, and biotesiometry suggest monosymptomatic acute optic neuritis to be a first manifestation of multiple sclerosis. *Acta Neurol Scand 83:*343–350.
Fredericksen JL, Larsson HBW, Ottovay E, Stigsby B, Olesen J. (1991b). Acute optic neuritis with normal visual acuity. *Acta Ophthalmol 69:*357–366.
Frey T. (1973). Optic neuritis in children. Infectious mononucleosis as an etiology. *Doc Ophthalmol 34:*183–188.
Frick E, Stickl H. (1980). Optic neuritis and multiple sclerosis: An immunological study. *Eur Neurol 19:*185–191.
Frohman L, Wolansky L. (1997). Magnetic resonance imaging of syphilitic optic neuritis/perineuritis. *J Neuro-ophthalmol 17:*57–59.
Fujimoto N, Adachi-Usami E. (1988). Comparison of automated perimetry and pattern visually evoked cortical potentials in optic neuritis. *Doc Ophthalmol 69:*263–269.
Galetta S, Schatz N, Glaser JS. (1989). Acute sarcoid optic neuropathy with spontaneous recovery. *J Clin Neuro-ophthalmol 9:*27–32.
Gebarski SS, Gabrielsen TO, Gilman S, Knake JE, Latack JT, Aisen AM. (1985). The initial diagnosis of multiple sclerosis: Clinical impact of magnetic resonance imaging. *Ann Neurol 13:*592–601.
Ghezzi A, Zaffaroni M, Caputo D, et al. (1986). Evaluation of evoked potentials and lymphocyte subsets as possible markers of multiple sclerosis: One year follow up of 30 patients. *J Neurol Neurosurg Psych 49:*913–919.
Gould ES, Bird AC, Leaver PK, McDonald WI. (1977). Treatment of optic neuritis by retrobulbar injection of triamcinolone. *Br Med J 1:*1495–1497.
Gressel MG, Tomsak RL. (1983). Recurrent bilateral optic neuropathy in mixed connective tissue disease. *J Clin Neuro-ophthalmol 3:*101–104.
Griffin JF, Wray SH. (1978). Acquired color vision deficits in retrobulbar neuritis. *Am J Ophthalmol 86:*193.
Grossman RI, Gonzalez-Scarano F, Atlas SW, Galetta S, Silberberg SH. (1986). Multiple sclerosis: Gadolinium enhancement in MR imaging. *Radiology 161:*721–725.
Grossniklaus HE, Frank KE, Tomsak RL. (1987). Cytomegalovirus retinitis and optic neuritis in acquired immunodeficiency syndrome: Report of a case. *Ophthalmology 94:*1601–1604.
Gunduz K, Ozdermir O. (1994). Bilateral retrobulbar neuritis following unilateral herpes zoster ophthamicus. *Ophthalmologica 208:*61–64.
Guy JR, Mancuso AA, Quisling R. (1994). The role of magnetic resonance imaging in optic neuritis. *Ophthalmol Clin No Amer 7(3):*449–458.
Guy J, Mancuso A, Quisling R, Beck R, Moster M. (1990). Gadolinium-DTPA enhanced magnetic resonance imaging in optic neuropathies. *Ophthalmology 97:*592–599.
Hackett ER, Martinez RD, Larson PF, Paddison RM. (1974). Optic neuritis in systemic lupus erythematosus. *Arch Neurol 31:*9–11.
Halliday AM, McDonald WI, Mushin J. (1972). Delayed visual evoked response in optic neuritis. *Lancet 1:*982–985.
Halliday AM, McDonald WI, Mushin J. (1973a). Visual evoked response in diagnosis of multiple sclerosis. *Brit Med J 4:*661–664.
Halliday AM, McDonald WI, Mushin J. (1973b). Delayed pattern evoked responses in optic neuritis in relation to visual acuity. *Trans Ophthalmol Soc UK 93:*315–324.
Hammond SR, Yiannikkas C. (1986). Contribution of pattern reversal foveal and half field stimulation to analysis of VEP abnormalities in multiple sclerosis. *Electroencephal Clin Neurophys 64:*101–118.
Harbison JW, Lessell S, Selhorst JB. (1984). Neuro-ophthalmology of sphenoid sinus carcinoma. *Brain 107:*855–870.
Harding AE, Radae EW, Whitely AM. (1978). Contrast enhanced lesions on computerized tomography in multiple sclerosis. *J Neurol Neurosurg Psych 41:*754–758.
Hart WM, Jr., Burde RM. (1979). Optic disk edema in sarcoidosis. *Am J Ophthalmol 88:*769–771.

Heinrichs IH, McLean DR. (1988). Evolution of visual evoked potentials in optic neuritis. *Can J Neurolog Sci 15:*394–396.
Hely MA, McManis PG, Doran TJ, Walsh JC, McLeod JG. (1986). Acute optic neuritis: A prospective study of risk factors for multiple sclerosis. *J Neurol Neurosurg Psychiatr 49:*1125–1130.
Hennerici M, Wenzel D, Freund HJ. (1977). The comparison of small-size rectangle and checkerboard stimulation for the evaluation of delayed visual evoked responses in patients suspected of multiple sclerosis. *Brain 100:*119–136.
Herishanu YO, Badarna S, Sarov B, et al. (1989). A possible harmful late effect of methylprednisolone therapy on a time cluster of optic neuritis. *Acta Neurologica Scand 80:*569–574.
Hoeppner T, Lolas F. (1978). Visual evoked responses and visual symptoms in multiple sclerosis. *J Neurol Neurosurg Psych 41:*493–498.
Honan WP, Heron JR, Foster DH, et al. (1990). Visual loss in multiple sclerosis and its relation to previous optic neuritis, disease duration, and clinical classification. *Brain 113:*975–987.
Hume AL, Waxman SG. (1988). Evoked potentials in suspected multiple sclerosis: Diagnostic value and prediction of clinical course. *J Neurol Sci 83:*180–185.
Husted RC, Shock JP. (1975). Acute presumed histoplasmosis of the optic nerve head. *Br J Ophthalmol 59:*409–412.
Hutchinson WM. (1976). Acute optic neuritis and the prognosis for multiple sclerosis. *J Neurol Neurosurg Psych 39:*283–289.
Hyllested K, Moller PM. (1961). Follow-up on patients with a history of optic neuritis. *Acta Ophthalmol 39:*655–662.
Jabs DA, Johns CJ. (1986). Ocular involvement in chronic sarcoidosis. *Am J Ophthalmol 102:*297–301.
Jabs DA, Miller NR, Neman SA, Johnson MA, Stevens MB. (1986). Optic neuropathy in systemic lupus erythematosus. *Arch Ophthalmol 104:*564–568.
Jackson JA, Leake DR, Schneiders NJ, Rolak LA, Kelley GR, Ford JJ, Appeal SH, Bryan RN. (1985). Magnetic resonance imaging in multiple sclerosis: Results in 32 cases. *Am J Neuroradiol 6:*171–176.
Jacobs L, Kinkel PR, Kinkel WR. (1986a). Silent brain lesions in patients with isolated idiopathic optic neuritis. *Arch Neurol 43:*452–455.
Jacobs L, Kinkel WR, Polachini I, Kinel PR. (1986b). Correlations of nuclear magnetic resonance imaging, computerized tomography and clinical profiles in multiple sclerosis. *Neurology 36:*27–34.
Jacobs L, Munschauer FE, Kaba SE. (1991). Clinical and magnetic resonance imaging in optic neuritis. *Neurology 41:*15–19.
Jacobson DM, Marx JJ, Dlesk A. (1991). Frequency and clinical significance of Lyme seropositivity in patients with isolated optic neuritis. *Neurol 41:*706–711.
Johns K, Lavin P, Elliot JH, Partain GL. (1986). Magnetic resonance imaging of the brain in isolated optic neuritis. *Arch Ophthalmol 104:*1486–1488.
Johnson LN, Hepler RS, Yee RD, et al. (1986). Sphenoid sinus mucocoele (anterior clinoid variant) mimicking diabetic ophthalmoplegia and retrobulbar neuritis. *Am J Ophthalmol 102:*111–115.
Kahana E, Alter M, Feldman S. (1976). Optic neuritis in relation to multiple sclerosis. *J Neurol 213:*87–95.
Kahana E, Liebowitz U, Fishback N, Alter M. (1973). Slowly progressive visual impairment in multiple sclerosis. *Neurology 23:*729–733.
Kakisu Y, Adachi-Usami E, Fujimoto N. (1991). Pattern visually evoked cortical potential and magnetic resonance imaging in optic neuritis. *J Clin Neuro-ophthalmol 11:*205–212.
Kakisu Y, Adachi-Usami E, Mizota E. (1987). Pattern VECPs in optic neuritis caused by multiple sclerosis (abstract). *Acta Soc Ophthalmol Jpn 91:*230–234.
Kazarian E, Gager W. (1978). Optic neuritis complicating measles, mumps, and rubella vaccination. *Am J Ophthalmol 86:*544–547.
Keltner JL, Johnson CA, Beck RW, Cleary PA, Spurr JO and the Optic Neuritis Study Group. (1993a). Quality control functions of the visual field reading center (VFRC) for the optic neuritis treatment trial (ONTT). *Controlled Clin Trials 14:*143–159.
Keltner JL, Johnson CA, Spurr JO, Beck RW. (1993b). Baseline visual field profile of optic neuritis: The experience of the Optic Neuritis Treatment Trial. *Arch Ophthalmol 111:*231–234.
Kinnunen E. (1983). The incidence of optic neuritis and its prognosis for multiple sclerosis. *Acta Neurologica Scand 68:*371–377.
Kinnunen E, Larsen A, Ketonen L, Koskimies S, Sandstrom A. (1987). Evaluation of central nervous system involvement in uncomplicated optic neuritis after prolonged follow-up. *Acta Neurol Scand 76:*147–151.
Kirkham TH, Coupland SG. (1981). Multiple regression analysis of diagnostic predictors in optic nerve disease. *Can J Neurologic Sci 8:*67–72.
Kupersmith MJ, Burde RM, Warren FA, Klingele TG, Frohman L, Mitnick H. (1988). Autoimmune optic neuropathy: Evaluation and treatment. *J Neurol Neurosurg Psychiatr 51:*1381–1386.
Kupersmith MJ, Nelson JI, Seiple WH, Carr RE, Weiss PA. (1983). The 20/20 eye in multiple sclerosis. *Neurology 33:*1015–1020.
Kurland LT, Beebe GW, Kurzke JF, Nagler B, Auth EL, Lessell S, Nefzenger MD. (1966). Studies on the natural history of multiple sclerosis. 2. The progression of optic neuritis to multiple sclerosis. *Acta Neurolog Scand 42 (suppl. 19):*157–176.
Kuroiwa Y, Igata A, Itahara K, et al. (1975). Nationwide survey of multiple sclerosis in Japan. Clinical analysis of 1084 cases. *Neurology 25:*845–851.

Kuroiwa Y, Shibasaki H. (1973). Clinical studies of multiple sclerosis in Japan. A current appraisal of 83 cases. *Neurology 23:*609–617.

Kurtzke, JF. (1985). Optic neuritis and multiple sclerosis. *Arch Neurol 42:*702–704.

Landy PJ. (1983). A prospective study of the risk of developing multiple sclerosis in optic neuritis in a tropical and subtropical area. *J Neurol Neurosurg Psych 46:*659–661.

Lessell S. (1992). Corticosteroid treatment of acute optic neuritis. *N Engl J Med 326:*634–635.

Lesser RL, Kornmehl EW, Pachner WR, et al. (1990). Neuro-ophthalmologic manifestations of Lyme disease. *Ophthalmology 97:*699–706.

Lew D, Sothwick FS, Montgomery WW, et al. (1983). Sphenoid sinusitis. *N Engl J Med 309:*1149–1154.

Link H, Muller R. (1971). Immunoglobulins in multiple sclerosis and infections of the nervous system. *Arch Neurol 25:*326–344.

Lowitzsch K, Kuhnt U, Sakmann C, et al. (1976). Visual pattern evoked responses and blink reflexes in assessment of MS diagnosis. *J Neurol 213:*17–32.

Lukes SA, Crooks LE, Aminoff MJ, Kaufman L, Panitch HS, Mills C, Norman D. (1983). Nuclear magnetic resonance imaging in multiple sclerosis. *Ann Neurol 13:*592–601.

Lustgarten JS, Mindel JS, Yablonski ME, Friedman AH. (1983). An unusual presentation of isolated optic nerve sarcoidosis. *J Clin Neuro-ophthalmol 3:*13–18.

MacDonald AB. (1987). Lyme disease: A neuro-ophthalmologic view. *J Clin Neuro-ophthalmol 7:*185–190.

MacFadyen DJ, Drance SM, Douglas GR, et al. (1988). The retinal nerve fiber layer, neuroretinal rim area and visual evoked potentials in MS. *Neurology 38:*1353–1358.

Macoul KL. (1982). Bilateral optic nerve atrophy and blindness following swine influenza vaccination. *Ann Ophthalmol 14:*398–399.

Matthews WB, Small DG, Small M, Pountney E. (1977). Pattern reversed evoked potential in the diagnosis of multiple sclerosis. *J Neurol Neurosurg Psych 40:*1009–1014.

Matthews WB, Small DG. (1979). Serial recording of visual and somatosensory evoked potentials in multiple sclerosis. *J Neurol Sci 40:*11–21.

McDonald WI, Halliday AM. (1977). Diagnosis and classification of MS. *Br Med Bull 33:*4–9.

McDonald WI. (1983). The significance of optic neuritis. *Trans Ophthalmol Soc UK 103:*230–236.

McKibbin M, Cleland PG, Morgan SJ. (1995). Bilateral optic neuritis after hepatitis A. *J Neurol Neurosurg Psychiatr 58:*508.

McLeish WM, Pulido JS, Holland S, Culbertson WW, Winward K. (1990). The ocular manifestations of syphilis in the human immunodeficiency virus type 1-infected host. *Ophthalmology 97:*196–203.

Merandi SF, Kudryk BT, Murtagh FR, Arrington JA. (1991). Contrast-enhanced MR imaging of optic nerve lesions in patients with acute optic neuritis. *AJNR 12:*923–926.

Miller DH, Omerod IEC, McDonald WI, et al. (1988a). The early risk of multiple sclerosis after optic neuritis. *J Neurol Neurosurg Psychiatr 51:*1569–1571.

Miller DH, Johnson G, McDonald WI, et al. (1986). Detection of optic nerve lesions in optic neuritis with magnetic resonance imaging. *Lancet 1:*1490–1491.

Miller DH, Newton MR, Van der Poel JC, et al. (1988b). Magnetic resonance imaging of the optic nerve and optic neuritis. *Neurology 38:*175–179.

Molk R. (1982). Treatment of toxocaral optic neuritis. *J Clin Neuro-ophthalmol 2:*109–112.

Morrissey SP, Miller DH, Kendall BE, et al. (1993). The significance of brain magnetic resonance imaging abnormalities at presentation with clinically isolated syndromes suggestive of multiple sclerosis. A 5-year follow-up study. *Brain 116:*135–146.

Moschos M. (1990). Acute bilateral optic neuritis. *Doc Ophthalmol 73:*225–230.

Moulin D, Paty DW, Ebers GC. (1983). The predictive value of cerebrospinal fluid electrophoresis in "possible" multiple sclerosis. *Brain 106:*809–816.

Mulligan NM, Newcombe R, Compston DAS. (1987). A double-blind controlled trial of high dose methylprednisolone in patients with multiple sclerosis: I clinical effects. *J Neurol Neurosurg Psychiatr 50:*511–516.

Newman NJ, Lessell S, Winterkorn JS. (1991). Optic chiasmal neuritis. *Neurology 41:*1203–1210.

Nikoskelainen E, Frey H, Salmi A. (1981). Prognosis of optic neuritis with special reference to cerebrospinal fluid immunoglobulins and measles virus antibodies. *Ann Neurol 9:*545–550.

Nikoskelainen E, Irjala K, Salmi TT. (1975a). Cerebrospinal fluid findings in patients with optic neuritis. *Acta Ophthalmol 53:*105–119.

Nikoskelainen E, Nikoskelainen J, Salmi AA, Halonen PE. (1975b). Virus antibody levels in serum specimens from patients with optic neuritis and from matched controls. *Acta Neurol Scand 51:*333–346.

Nikoskelainen E, Riekkinen P. (1974). Optic neuritis—A sign of multiple sclerosis or other diseases of the central nervous system. A retrospective analysis of 116 patients. *Acta Neurol Scand 50:*690–718.

Nilsson BY. (1978). Visual evoked responses in multiple sclerosis: Comparison of two methods of pattern reversal. *J Neurol Neurosurg Psychiatr 41:*499–504.

Openheimer S, Hoffbrand BI. (1986). Optic neuritis and myelopathy in systemic lupus erythematosus. *Can J Neurol Sci 13:*129–132.

Optic Neuritis Study Group. (1991). The clinical profile of optic neuritis: Experience of the Optic Neuritis Treatment Trial. *Arch Ophthalmol 109:*1673–1678.

Ormerod IEC, McDonald WI. (1984). Multiple sclerosis presenting with progressive visual failure. *J Neurol Neurosurg Psychiatr 47:*943–946.

Ormerod IEC, McDonald WI, DuBoulay GH, Kendall BE, Moseley IF, Halliday AM, Kakigi R, Kreiss A, Peringer E. (1986). Disseminated lesions at presentation in patients with optic neuritis. *J Neurol Neurosurg Psychiatr 49:*124–127.
Ormerod IEC, Miller DH, McDonald WI, DuBoulay GH, Rudge P, Kendall BE, Moseley IF, Johnson G, Tofts PS, Halliday AM, Bronstein AM, Scaravilli F, Harding AE, Barnes D, Zisha KJ. (1987). The role of MNR imaging in the assessment of multiple sclerosis and isolated neurological lesions. A quantitative study. *Brain 110:*1579–1616.
Osher RH, Tomsak RL. (1980). Computed tomographic features in optic neuritis. *Am J Ophthalmol 89:*699–702.
Pal HD, Williams AC. (1987). Subacute polyradiculopathy with optic and auditory nerve involvement. *Arch Neurol 44:*885–887.
Parkin PJ, Hierons R, McDonald WI. (1984). Bilateral optic neuritis. *Brain 107:*951–964.
Paty DW. (1988). Magnetic resonance imaging in the assessment of disease activity in multiple sclerosis. *Can J Neurol Sci 15:*266–272.
Paty DW, Li DKB, the UBC MS/MRI Study Group, et al. (1993). Interferon beta-1b is effective in relapsing-remitting multiple sclerosis, II: MRI analysis results of a multicenter, randomized, double-blind, placebo-controlled trial. *Neurology 43:*662–667.
Paty DW, Oger JJF, Kastrukoff LF, Hashimoto SA, Hooge JP, Eisen AA, Eisen KA, Purves SJ, Low MD, Brandejs V, Robertson WD, Li DKB. (1988). MRI in the diagnosis of MS: A prospective study with comparison of clinical evaluation, evoked potentials, oligoclonal banding and CT. *Neurology 38:*180–185.
Percy AK, Norbrega FT, Kurland LT. (1972). Optic neuritis and multiple sclerosis. *Arch Ophthalmol 87:*135–139.
Perry HD, Mallen FJ, Grodin RW, Cossari AJ. (1979). Reversible blindness in optic neuritis associated with influenza vaccination. *Ann Ophthalmol 11:*545–550.
Pickens S, Sangster G. (1975). Retrobulbar neuritis and infectious mononucleosis. *Br Med J 4:*729.
Quinn JR, Wolfson WQ. (1952). Improved results from individualized intensive hormonal treatment in certain eye diseases reported to respond poorly to ACTH or cortisone. *Univ Mich Med Bull 18:*1–21.
Rawson MD, Liversedge LA. (1969). Treatment of retrobulbar neuritis with corticotrophin. *Lancet 2:*222.
Rawson MD, Liversedge LA, Goldfarb G. (1966). Treatment of acute retrobulbar neuritis with corticotrophin. *Lancet 2:*1044–1046.
Regan D, Milner BA, Heron JR. (1976). Delayed visual perception and delayed visual evoked potentials in the spinal form of multiple sclerosis and in retrobulbar neuritis. *Brain 99:*43–66.
Riffenburgh RS. (1961). Ocular manifestations of mumps. *Arch Ophthalmol 66:*155–159.
Rizzo JF, Lessell S. (1988). Risk of developing multiple sclerosis after uncomplicated optic neuritis: A long term prospective study. *Neurology 38:*185–190.
Robertson WD, Li DKB, Mayo JR, Fache JS, Paty DW. (1987). Assessment of multiple sclerosis by magnetic resonance imaging. *J Can Assoc Radiol 38:*177–182.
Robinson MR, Streeten BW, Hampton GR, et al. (1986). Treatment of cytomegalovirus optic neuritis with dihydroxy propoxymethyl guanine. *Am J Ophthalmol 101:*95–101.
Rodriguez M, Siva A, Cross SA, et al. (1995). Optic neuritis: A population based study in Olmsted County, Minnesota. *Neurology 45:*244–250.
Rose AS, Kuzma JW, Kurtzke JF, et al. (1970). Cooperative study in the evaluation of therapy in multiple sclerosis. ACTH vs. placebo-final report. *Neurology 20:*1–59.
Roseman R, Ellenberger C. (1982). Slowly progressive optic neuritis. *Neuro-ophthalmol 2:*183–194.
Rothstein J, Maisel RH, Berlinger NT, Wirtschafter JD. (1984). Relationship of optic neuritis to disease of the paranasal sinuses. *Laryngoscope 94:*1501–1508.
Rudick RA, Jacobs L, Kinkel PR, Kinkel WR. (1986). Isolated idiopathic optic neuritis. Analysis of free kappa-light chains in cerebrospinal fluid and correlation with nuclear magnetic resonance findings. *Arch Neuro 43:*456–458.
Sandberg M, Bynke H. (1973). Cerebrospinal fluid in 25 cases of optic neuritis. *Acta Neurol Scand 49:*443–452.
Sandberg-Wollheim M. (1975). Optic neuritis: Studies on the cerebrospinal fluid in relation to clinical course in 61 patients. *Acta Neurol Scand 52:*167–178.
Sandberg-Wollheim M, Bynke H, Cronqvist S, Holtas S, Platz P, Ryder LP. (1990). A long-term prospective study of optic neuritis: Evaluation of risk factors. *Ann Neurol 27:*386–393.
Sandberg-Wollheim M, Platz P, Ryder LP, et al. (1975). HLA-Histocompatibility antigens in optic neuritis. *Acta Neurol Scand 52:*161–166.
Sanders EACM, Billen ELEC, van der Velde EA. (1986). Presenting signs and symptoms in multiple sclerosis. *Acta Neurol Scand 73:*269–272.
Sanders EACM, Reulen JPH, Hogenuis LAH. (1984). Central nervous system involvement in optic neuritis. *J Neurol Neurosurg Psychiatr 47:*241–249.
Sanders EACM, Van Lith GHM. (1989). Optic neuritis, confirmed by visual evoked response, and the risk for multiple sclerosis: A prospective survey. *J Neurol Neurosurg Psych 52:*799–810.
Sanders EACM, Volkers ACW, Van der Poel JC, Van Lith GHM. (1986). Estimation of visual function after optic neuritis: A comparison of clinical tests. *Br J Ophthalmol 70:*918–924.
Schecter SL. (1986). Lyme disease associated with optic neuropathy. *Am J Med 81:*143–145.
Schenck SA, Claman HN. (1969). CSF immunoglobulins in multiple sclerosis and other neurologic diseases. Measurement by electroimmunodiffusion. *Arch Neurol 20:*132–139.
Schmidt D. (1983). Treatment of optic neuritis. *Bull Soc Belge Ophthalmol 208:*493–500.

Schuil J, Richardus JH, Baarsma GS, Schaap GJP. (1985). Q fever as a possible cause of bilateral optic neuritis. *Br J Ophthalmol 69:*580–583.

Schwartz S, Rieder HP, Wutrich R. (1970). The protein fractions in cerebrospinal fluid in the various states of multiple sclerosis. *Europ Neurol 4:*267–282.

Scotti G, Scialfa G, Biondi A, Landoni L, Caputo D, Cazzullo CL. (1986). Magnetic resonance in multiple sclerosis. *Neuroradiology 28:*319–323.

Sedwick LA. (1991). Optic neuritis. *Neurologic Clinics 9:*97–112.

Sedwick LA, Klingele TG, Burde RM, Behrens MM. (1984). Optic neuritis in inflammatory bowel disease. *J Clin Neuro-ophthalmol 4:*3–6.

Sellebjerg FT, Frederkisen JT, Olsson T. (1994). Anti-myelin basic protein and anti-proteolipid protein antibody-secreting cells in the cerebrospinal fluid of patients with acute optic neuritis. *Arch Neurol 51:*1032–1036.

Seelebjerg F, Madsen HO, Frederiksen JL, et al. (1995). Acute optic neuritis: Myelin basic protein and proteolipid protein antibodies, affinity and the HLA system. *Ann Neurol 38:*943–950.

Sergott RC, Brown MJ. (1988). Current concepts of the pathogenesis of optic neuritis associated with multiple sclerosis. *Surv Ophthalmol 33:*108–116.

Shabas D, Gerard G, Slavin M. (1987). MRI in optic neuritis. *Neuro-ophthalmol 7:*267–272.

Shimo-Oku M, Miyazaki S, Shiraki K, Sugimoto T, Sotani H. (1989). Optic nerve involvement in posterior paranasal sinus diseases. *Neuro-ophthalmology 9:*147–155.

Silberberg DH. (1993). Corticosteroids and optic neuritis. *N Engl J Med 329:*1808–1810.

Slamovits TL, Macklin R. (1991). What to tell the patient with optic neuritis about multiple sclerosis. *Surv Ophthalmol 36:*47–50.

Slamovits TL, Rosen CE, Cheng KP, Striph GG. (1991). Visual recovery in patients with optic neuritis and visual loss to no light perception. *Am J Ophthalmol 111:*209–214.

Smith T, Zeeberg I, Sjo O. (1986). Evoked potentials in multiple sclerosis before and after high-dose methylprednisolone infusion. *Eur Neurol 25:*67–73.

Soderstrom M, Link H, Sun J-B, et al. (1994). Autoimmune T cell repertoire in optic neuritis and multiple sclerosis: T cells recognizing multiple myelin proteins are accumulated in cerebrospinal fluid. *J Neurol Neurosurg Psychiatr 57:*544–551.

Soderstrom M, Link H, Xu Z, Fredriksson S. (1993). Optic neuritis and multiple sclerosis: Anti-MBP and anti-MBP peptide antibody-secreting cells are accumulated in CSF. *Neurology 43:*1215–1222.

Sola P, Merelli E, Schoenhuber R, et al. (1987). Neurophysiological and CSF immunological study of 19 patients affected by acute idiopathic optic neuritis. *Acta Neurol Scand 75:*140–144.

Sombrono WGM, Smith JL. (1987). Acute syphilitic blindness in AIDS. *J Clin Neuro-ophthalmol 7:*1–5.

Spoor TC. (1986). Treatment of optic neuritis with megadose corticosteroids. *J Clin Neuro-ophthalmol 6:*137–143.

Spoor TC, Rockwell DL. (1988). Treatment of optic neuritis with intravenous megadose corticosteroids: A consecutive series. *Ophthalmology 95:*131–134.

Staedt D, Kappos L, Rohrbach E, Heun R. (1989). Contributions of magnetic resonance imaging to the diagnosis of MS in isolated optic neuritis. *Psych Res 29:*295–296.

Staedt D, Kappos L, Rohrbach E, Heun R, Ratzka M. (1990). Occurrence of MRI abnormalities in patients with isolated optic neuritis. *Eur Neurol 30:*305–309.

Stendahl-Brodin L, Link H. (1983). Optic neuritis: Oligoclonal bands increase the risk of multiple sclerosis. *Acta Neurol Scand 67:*301–304.

Stendahl-Brodin L, Link H, Moller E, et al. (1978). Optic neuritis and distribution of genetic markers of the HLA system. *Acta Neurol Scand 57:*418–443.

Stewart JM, Houser OW, Baker HL, Jr., et al. (1987). Magnetic resonance imaging and clinical relationships in multiple sclerosis. *Mayo Clin Proc 62:*174–184.

Strong LE, Henderson JW, Gangitano JL. (1974). Bilateral retrobulbar neuritis secondary to mumps. *Am J Ophthalmol 78:*331–332.

Tarkkanen J, Tarkkanen A. (1971). Otorhinolaryngological pathology in patients presenting as optic neuritis. *Acta Ophthalmologica 49:*649–657.

Thompson AJ, Kermode A, MacManus DG, et al. (1990). Patterns of disease activity in multiple sclerosis; clinical and magnetic resonance imaging study. *BMJ 300:*631–634.

Thompson AJ, Miller D, Youl B, et al. (1992). Serial gadolinium-enhanced MRI in relapsing/remitting multiple sclerosis of varying disease duration. *Neurology 42:*60–63.

Trobe JD. (1994). High-dose corticosteroid regimen retards development of multiple sclerosis in optic neuritis treatment trial. *Arch Ophthalmol 112:*35–36.

Trotter JL, Garvey WF. (1980). Prolonged effects of large-dose methylprednisolone infusion in multiple sclerosis. *Neurology 30:*702–708.

Uhlenbrock D, Seidel D, Gehlen W, et al. (1988). MR imaging in multiple sclerosis: Comparison with clinical, CSF, and visual evoked potentials. *AJNR 9:*59–67.

van de Geijn EJ, Tukkie R, van Phillips LA, Punt H. (1994). Bilateral optic neuritis with branch retinal artery occlusion associated with vaccination. *Doc Ophthalmology 86:*403–408.

van Engelen BGM, Hommes OR, Pinckers A, Cruysberg JRM, Barkhof F, Rodriguez M. (1992). Improved vision after intravenous immunoglobulin in stable demyelinating optic neuritis. *Ann Neurology 32:*834.

Warren KG, Catz I, Bauer C. (1988). Cerebrospinal fluid antibodies to myelin basic protein in acute idiopathic optic neuritis. *Ann Neurol 23:*297–299.

Warren KG, Catz I, Jeffrey VM, Carroll D. (1986). Effect of methylprednisolone on CSF IgG parameters, myelin basic protein, and antimyelin basic protein in multiple sclerosis exacerbations. *Can J Neurol Sci 13*:25–30.
Warren KG, Catz I, Johnson E, Mielke B. (1994). Anti-myelin basic protein and anti-proteolipid protein specific forms of multiple sclerosis. *Ann Neurol 35*:280–289.
Warren KG, Catz I, McPherson TA. (1983). CSF myelin basic protein levels in acute optic neuritis and multiple sclerosis. *Can J Neurol Sci 10*:235–238.
Weintraub MI. (1988). Optic neuritis and MS [letter]. *Neurology 38*:1660–1661.
Wikstrom J, Poser S, Ritter G. (1980). Optic neuritis as an initial symptom in multiple sclerosis. *Acta Neurol Scand 61*:178–185.
Winward KE, Hamed LM, Glaser JS. (1989). The spectrum of optic nerve disease in human immunodeficiency virus infection. *Am J Ophthalmol 107*:373.
Wu G, Lincoff H, Ellsworth RM, Haik BG. (1986). Optic disc edema and Lyme disease. *Ann Ophthalmol 18*:252–255.
Yau TH, Rivera-Velasquez PM, Mark AS, et al. (1996). Unilateral optic neuritis caused by Histoplasma capsulatum in a patient with acquired immunodeficiency syndrome. *Am J Ophthalmol 121*:324–326.
Yen MY, Liu JH. (1991). Bilateral optic neuritis following bacille Calmette-Guerin (BCG) vaccination. *J Clin Neuro-ophthalmol 11*:246–249.
Zaidman GW. (1987). Neurosyphilis and retrobulbar neuritis in a patient with AIDS. *Ann Ophthalmol 18*:260–261.
Zeese JA. (1977). Pattern evoked responses in multiple sclerosis. *Arch Neurol 34*:314–316.

◆ 3 ◆

Optic Disc Edema with a Macular Star and Neuroretinitis

Optic disc edema with a macular star (ODEMS) is a descriptive term encompassing a heterogeneous group of disorders. In 1916 Leber described patients with idiopathic unilateral visual loss, optic disc edema, and macular exudate (Leber, 1916). He incorrectly theorized that the pathologic process was primarily retinal and called the condition *stellate retinopathy.* The condition was subsequently called *Leber's stellate maculopathy, Leber's idiopathic stellate neuroretinitis,* or simply *neuroretinitis.* In 1977 Gass suggested that this syndrome was caused by a prelaminar disc vasculitis that results in leakage of disc capillaries and concluded that this entity was not a retinal vasculopathy but a primary optic neuropathy and termed it *neuroretinitis* (Gass, 1977). This syndrome is characterized by swelling of the optic disc, peripapillary and macular hard exudates that often occur in a star pattern, and, often, vitreous cells (Dreyer, 1984; Maitland, 1984; Ricci, 1961). Because the macular exudate likely results from primary optic nerve disease and not a retinitis, we prefer the term *idiopathic optic disc edema with a macular star* (ODEMS) for idiopathic cases and use the term *neuroretinitis* when optic disc swelling and a macular star are associated with retinitis, especially if an infectious cause is documented (Brazis, 1996).

What Are the Clinical Features of ODEMS and Neuroretinitis?

The clinical features of ODEMS have been described by a number of authors (Brazis, 1996; Carroll, 1982; Dreyer, 1984; Francois, 1969; Grehn, 1984; Hamard, 1994; King, 1991; Maitland, 1984; Papastratigakis, 1981; Parmley, 1987; Ricci, 1961) and are summarized in Table 3–1. Patients are usually children or young adults, with the average age of onset between 20 and 40 years. Men and women are affected equally. Most cases are unilateral, but bilateral involvement has been noted in up to a third of the cases in some series. Most patients present with acute unilateral loss of vision. The condition is often painless, but retrobulbar pain, pain on eye movement, or associated headache may occur. A nonspecific "viral" illness precedes or accompanies the visual loss in approximately half the cases.

Table 3–1. Clinical Characteristics of Optic Disc Edema with Macular Star (ODEMS)

Age at onset	Childhood to young adult (6–50 years)
Gender	Men = women
Bilateral involvement	5–33%
Pain	Occasional
Antecedent viral illness	Approximately 50%
Initial visual acuity	Variable (20/20 to light perception)
Dyschromatopsia	Often prominent
Fields	Central, cecocentral, arcuate, or altitudinal defects; possible generalized constriction
Relative afferent pupil defect	Present; may be absent if bilateral involvement
Optic disc swelling	Present; occasional subsequent optic atrophy
Macular star	Present but may take 1–2 weeks to develop
Vitreous cells	Common (90%)

Visual acuity with ODEMS may range from 20/20 to light perception, but most cases are in the 20/40 to 20/200 range. Dyschromatopsia is often present. Perimetry most often reveals a central or cecocentral scotoma, but other "optic nerve-type" field abnormalities may occur, including arcuate and altitudinal defects or generalized constriction. Most patients have a relative afferent pupillary defect unless involvement is bilateral and relatively symmetric.

Optic disc edema is the earliest sign of ODEMS and may be severe. The disc edema tends to resolve over 2 weeks to 2 months, but in some patients optic atrophy ensues. Optic disc edema is associated with leakage of disc capillaries, with the fluid spreading from the disc through the outer plexiform layer of the retina. The serous component of the fluid accumulation in Henle's layer is resorbed, and the lipid precipitate forms a macular star. This macular star may be present at the onset of visual loss or only noted after 1 to 2 weeks following development of the disc edema. The macular star may even be observed only after the disc swelling is starting to resolve. Patients with acute disc swelling with a normal macula should thus be reexamined within 2 weeks to investigate for the presence of a macular star, especially because it is of prognostic importance for the patient's subsequent risk of developing multiple sclerosis (see below).

ODEMS is often associated with cells in the vitreous. Other occasional findings include cells in the anterior chamber (Dreyer, 1984), chorioretinitis (Carroll, 1982; Dreyer, 1984; Gass, 1977; Grehn, 1984; Maitland, 1984), inflammatory sheathing of the peripapillary veins (Dreyer, 1984), scleritis and uveitis (Grehn, 1984) and (rarely) central or branch retinal artery occlusions (May, 1995). The association of ODEMS with these latter findings suggests a more diffuse vasculitis or an infectious cause.

What Is the Etiology and Differential of ODEMS and Neuroretinitis?

Most cases of ODEMS are "idiopathic" and thought to be the result of a nonspecific viral infection or some immune mediated process. In general, ODEMS is usually a benign, self-limited inflammatory process. However, a number of infectious agents and inflammatory diseases have been reported to cause ODEMS and neuroretinitis. These include viruses (hepatitis B, herpes simplex, herpes zoster, Epstein-Barr, influenza A, mumps, and coxsackie B) (Audry-Chaboud, 1981; Carroll, 1982; Farthing, 1986; Foster, 1990; Francois, 1969; Frey, 1973; Glaser, 1978; Jensen, 1948; Johnson, 1977; Knapp, 1916; Koch, 1939; Maitland, 1984; Margolis, 1988; Monroe, 1979; Riffenburgh, 1961; Spalton, 1989), bacteria (cat-scratch disease, tuberculosis, and salmonella) (Bar, 1990; Chrousos, 1990; Dreyer, 1984; Duke-Elder, 1967; Fish, 1992; Fusco, 1986; Gass, 1977; Golnik, 1994; King, 1991; McCrary, 1994; Perkin, 1979; Sweeney, 1970; Ulrich, 1992; Zhao, 1991), spirochetes (Lyme disease, syphilis, and leptospirosis) (Arruga, 1985; Bialasiewicz, 1989, 1992; Dreyer, 1984; Fewell, 1932; Folk, 1983; Graveson, 1950; Halperin, 1992; Lesser, 1990; McCleish, 1990; Miller, 1995; Ninomiya, 1990; Schönherr, 1990, 1991; Smith, 1968; Veldman, 1986), fungi (histoplasmosis) (Beck, 1984), parasites and protozoa (toxoplasmosis and toxocara) (Brown, 1981; Cox, 1983; Fish, 1993; Margo, 1986; Molk, 1982; Moreno, 1992; Roach, 1985), and sarcoidosis (Miller, 1995). Some of these infectious agents have been implicated in single case reports, but it appears that syphilis, cat-scratch disease, Lyme disease, and perhaps toxoplasmosis are the most common causes of ODEMS and neuroretinitis in cases where an etiological agent can be identified. Infectious agents should be aggressively sought in cases of ODEMS and neuroretinitis because appropriate antibiotic treatment is then indicated.

ODEMS or neuroretinitis may occur as part of syphilitic meningitis (usually bilateral) or as an isolated entity in patients with secondary syphilis, in which case it may be associated with unilateral or bilateral uveitis (Arruga, 1985; Fewell, 1932; Folk, 1983; Graveson, 1950; Halperin, 1992; McCleish, 1990; Ninomiya, 1990; Smith, 1968; Veldman, 1986). ODEMS or neuroretinitis is a not uncommon manifestation of cat-scratch disease (Bar, 1990; Chrousos, 1990; Dreyer, 1984; Fish, 1992; Gass, 1977; Golnik, 1994; Grehn, 1984; McCrary, 1994; Perkin, 1979; Sweeney, 1970; Ulrich, 1992; Zhao, 1991), and, in fact, optic neuritis (papillitis) without a macular star has only rarely been reported with this disease (Brazis, 1986; Golnik, 1994). Cat-scratch disease may cause ODEMS or a neuroretinitis with chorioretinitis that at times is associated with uveitis, cells in the anterior chamber, and even branch or central retinal artery occlusions (Fish, 1992; Golnik, 1994; May, 1995; Ulrich, 1992; Zhao, 1991). This disease may also cause a multifocal retinitis with optic disc edema (without macular star), branch retinal artery occlusion, and vitritis (Cohen, 1995). Cat-scratch disease should, therefore, be considered in any patient who presents with ODEMS or neuroretinitis, especially if there is associated lymphadenopathy or retinal artery occlusion. ODEMS may also occur with stage II Lyme disease (Bialasiewicz, 1989, 1992; Lesser, 1990; Miller, 1995; Schönherr, 1990, 1991). Toxoplasmosis may also cause ODEMS or neuroretinitis (Fish, 1993; Moreno, 1992; Roach, 1985). Two features that often occur with toxoplasmosis neuroretinitis, but are uncommon with idiopathic ODEMS, are a prominent anterior chamber inflammation along with toxoplasmosis chorioretinal scars. Toxoplasmosis neuroretinitis is perhaps more likely to cause recurrent episodes of ODEMS or neuroretinitis compared to the usual monophasic course of idiopathic ODEMS.

ODEMS and neuroretinitis must be differentiated from other entities in which optic disc swelling is associated with macular star formation, including vascular causes (anterior ischemic optic neuropathy, branch or central retinal artery occlusion, hypertension, diabetes, polyarteritis nodosa, and Eales' disease), papilledema from increased intracranial pressure, optic nerve tumors or infiltrative processes, diffuse unilateral subacute neuroretinitis (DUSN), and the acute neuroretinopathy that may occur with progressive facial hemiatrophy (Parry-Romberg syndrome) (Dreyer, 1984; Garcia-Arumi, 1994; Gass, 1991; Maitland, 1984; Matsuda, 1994; Parmley, 1987; Verm, 1997). With many of these etiologies macular stars are rarely seen and usually the differential diagnosis is not difficult on clinical grounds. A suggested work-up for patients with optic disc edema with macular star is outlined in Figure 3–1.

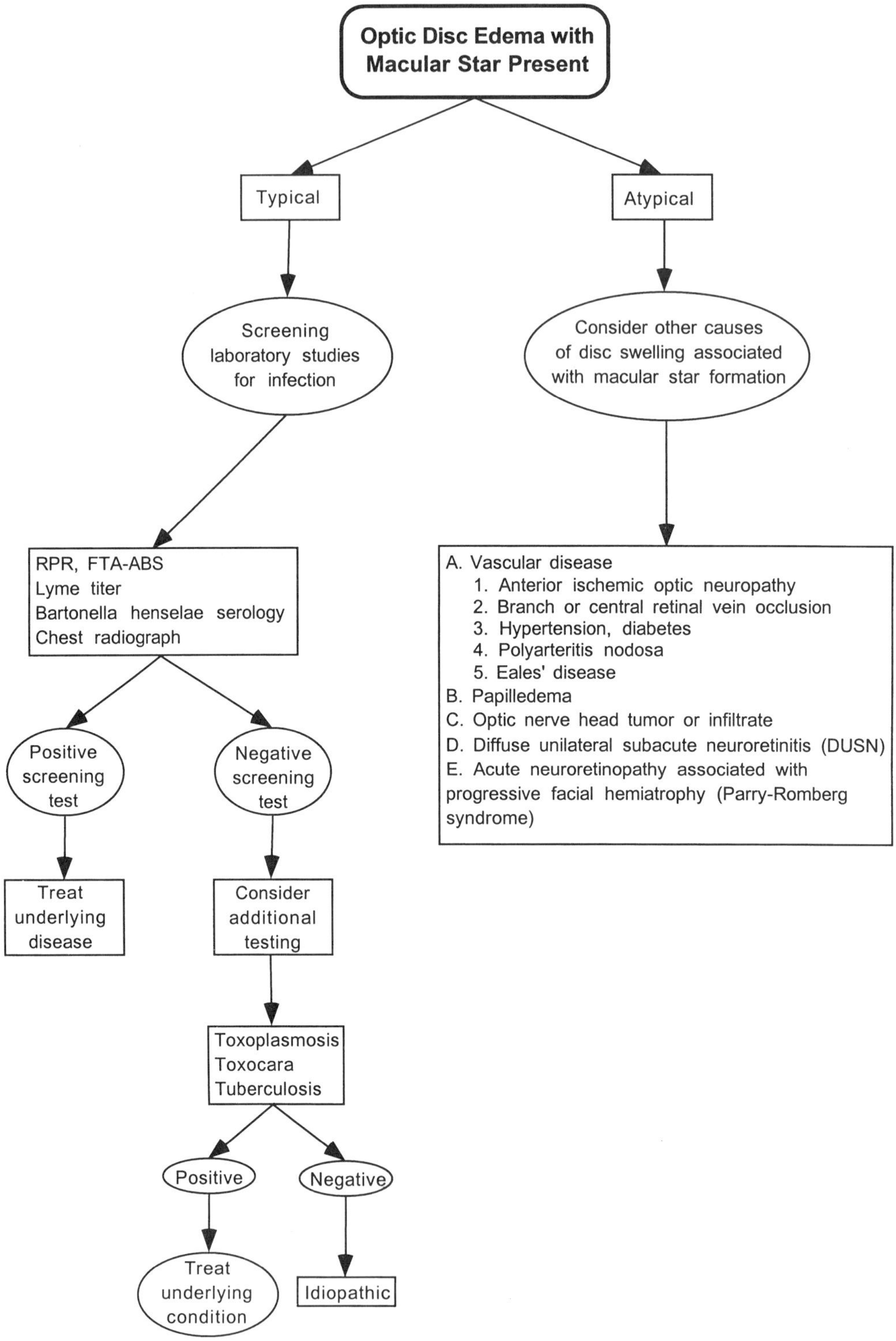

Figure 3–1. Evaluation of optic disc edema with a macular star (ODEMS) and neuroretinitis.

What Is the Prognosis in Cases of ODEMS?

ODEMS is usually a benign condition that resolves spontaneously without treatment. The disc edema and peripapillary retinal detachment tend to resolve over a period of 2 to 3 months while the macular star usually begins to disappear after one month (Dreyer, 1984). The macular star, however, may persist for up to one year. Optic atrophy and macular retinal pigment epithelial changes may be residuals of previous ODEMS. The prognosis for visual recovery in ODEMS is usually good, but significant residual visual disability may occasionally occur (Lee, 1997). Recurrences of ODEMS or neuroretinitis in the same or fellow eye have been described in idiopathic as well as infectious cases, especially in patients with toxoplasmosis (Dreyer, 1984; Fish, 1993; Purvin, 1994). Purvin and Chioran (Purvin, 1994) described an apparently distinct type of recurrent ODEMS in patients who experienced from two to seven attacks of ODEMS at intervals ranging from 1 to 10 years. The attacks often affected both eyes but never simultaneously. Visual field defects were of the nerve fiber bundle type instead of the central or cecocentral scotomas most often noted in benign ODEMS. Patients with the recurrent form of the disease may not experience significant improvement in optic nerve function.

Although optic neuritis is a risk factor for the development of multiple sclerosis (see Chapter 2), ODEMS or neuroretinitis is not (Parmley, 1987). Because a macular exudate may not develop in cases of ODEMS until 2 weeks after presentation, patients who demonstrate acute papillitis with a normal macula should be reevaluated within 2 weeks for the development of a macular star. Its presence makes the subsequent development of multiple sclerosis extremely unlikely.

Idiopathic ODEMS usually requires no treatment. Steroids have been used in some cases with unclear effect. If a specific infectious agent is discovered, appropriate antibiotics should be instituted. Aggressive immunosuppressive agents may be considered in the rare recurrent cases (Purvin, 1994).

References

Arruga J, Valentines J, Mauri F, et al. (1985). Neuroretinitis in acquired syphilis. *Ophthalmology 92:*262–270.

Audry-Chaboud D, Durnas R, Audry F, Guard O. (1981). Coxsackie B virus neuropapillitis. *Rev Otoneuro-ophthalmol 53:*473–482.

Bar S, Segal M, Shapira R, Savir H. (1990). Neuroretinitis associated with cat scratch disease. *Am J Ophthalmol 110:*703–705.

Beck RW, Sergott RC, Barr CC, Annesley WH. (1984). Optic disc edema in the presumed histoplasmosis syndrome. *Ophthalmology 91:*183–185.

Bialasiewicz AA. (1992). Augenbefunde bei Lyme-Borreliose. *Ophthalmologe 89:*W47–W59.

Bialasiewicz AA, Huk W, Druschky KF, Neumann GOH. (1989). Borrelia burgdorferi-Infektion mit beidseitiger Neuritis nervic optici und intrazerebralen Demyelinisierungsherden. *Klin Monatsbl Augenheilkd 195:*91–94.

Brazis PW, Lee AG. (1996). Optic disk edema with a macular star. *Mayo Clin Proc 71:*1162–1166.

Brazis PW, Stokes HR, Ervin FR. (1986). Optic neuritis in cat scratch disease. *J Clin Neuro-ophthalmol 6:*172–174.

Brown GC, Tasman WS. (1981). Retinal arterial obstruction in association with presumed toxocara canis neuroretinitis. *Ann Ophthalmol 13:*1385–1397.

Carroll DM, Franklin RM. (1982). Leber's idiopathic stellate retinopathy. *Am J Ophthalmol 93:*96–101.

Chrousos GA, Drack AV, Young M, et al. (1990). Neuroretinitis in cat scratch disease. *J Clin Neuro-ophthalmol 10:*92–94.

Cohen SM, Davis JL, Gass DM. (1995). Branch retinal arterial occlusions in multifocal retinitis with optic nerve edema. *Arch Ophthalmol 113:*1271–1276.

Cox TA, Haskins GE, Gangitano JL, Antonson DL. (1983). Bilateral toxocara optic neuropathy. *J Clin Neuro-ophthalmol 3:*267–274.

Dreyer RF, Hopen G, Gass JDM, Smith JL. (1984). Leber's idiopathic stellate neuroretinitis. *Arch Ophthalmol 102:*1140–1145.

Duke-Elder S, Dobree JH. (1967). Diseases of the retina. In Duke-Elder (ed). *System of Ophthalmology*. St Louis, Mosby, vol. 10, pp. 246–248.

Farthing CF, Howard RS, Thin RN. (1986). Papillitis and hepatitis B. *Br Med 292:*1712.

Fewell AG. (1932). Unilateral neuroretinitis of syphilitic origin with a striate figure in the macula. *Arch Ophthalmol 8:*615.

Fish RH, Hogan RN, Nightingale SD, Anand R. (1992). Peripapillary angiomatosis associated with cat-scratch neuroretinitis. *Arch Ophthalmol 110:*323.

Fish RH, Hoskins JC, Kline LB. (1993). Toxoplasmosis neuroretinitis. *Ophthalmology 100:*1177–1182.

Folk JC, Weingeist TA, Corbett JJ, et al. (1983). Syphilitic neuroretinitis. *Am J Ophthalmol 95:*480–486.

Foster RE, Lowder CY, Meisler DM, et al. (1990). Mumps neuroretinitis in an adolescent. *Am J Ophthalmol 110:*91–93.

Francois J, Verriest G, De Laey JJ. (1969). Leber's idiopathic stellate retinopathy. *Am J Ophthalmol 68:*340–345.

Frey T. (1973). Optic neuritis in children: Infectious mononucleosis as an etiology. *Doc Ophthalmol 34:*183–188.

Fusco R, Magli A, Guacci P. (1986). Stellate maculopathy due to salmonella typhi. A case report. *Ophthalmologica 192:*154–158.

Garcia-Arumi J, Salvador F, Corcostegui B, Mateo C. (1994). Neuroretinitis associated with melanocytoma of the optic disk. *Retina 14:*173–176.

Gass JDM. (1977). Diseases of the optic nerve that may simulate macular disease. *Trans Am Acad Ophthalmol Otolaryngol 83:*763–770.

Gass JDM, Harbin TS Jr, Del Piero EJ. (1991). Exudative stellate neuroretinopathy and Coat's syndrome in patients with progressive hemifacial atrophy. *Eur J Ophthalmol 1:*2–10.

Glaser JS. (1978). *Neuro-ophthalmology*. Hagerstown, MD, Harper & Row, p. 85.

Golnik KC, Marotto ME, Fanous MM, et al. (1994). Ophthalmic manifestations of Rochalimaea species. *Am J Ophthalmol 118:*145–151.

Graveson GS. (1950). Syphilitic optic neuritis. *J Neurol Neurosurg Psychiatry 13:*216–224.

Grehn F, Witschel H. (1984). Neuroretinitis. *Klin Monatsbl Augenheilkd 184:*94–98.

Halperin LS. (1992). Neuroretinitis due to seronegative syphilis associated with human immunodeficiency virus. *J Clin Neuro-ophthalmol 12:*171–172.

Hamard P, Hamard H, Ngohou S. (1994). La neuroretinite stellaire idiopathique de Leber. A propos de neuf cas. *J Francais d'Ophtalmologie 17:*116–123.

Jensen J. (1948). A case of herpes zoster ophthalmicus complicated with neuroretinitis. *Acta Ophthalmol 26:*551–555.

Johnson BL, Witsotzkey HM. (1977). Neuroretinitis associated with herpes simplex encephalitis in an adult. *Am J Ophthalmol 83:*481–489.

King MH, Cartwright MJ, Carney MD. (1991). Leber's idiopathic stellate neuroretinitis. *Ann Ophthalmol 23:*58–60.

Knapp A. (1916). Optic neuritis after influenza, with changes in the spinal fluid. *Arch Ophthalmol 45:*247–249.

Koch FLP. (1939). Herpes zoster ophthalmicus. A report of a case. *Arch Ophthalmol 21:*118–120.

Leber T. (1916). Die pseudonephritischen Netzhauterkrankungen, die Retinitis stellata: Die Purtschersche Netzhautaffektion nach schwere Schädelverletzung. In Graefe AC, Saemisch T (eds). *Graefe-Saemisch Handbuch der Gesamten Augenheilkunde.* 2nd ed. Leipzig, East Germany, Engelmann, vol 7, pt 2, chap 10.

Lee AG, Brazis PW: Poor visual outcome following optic disc edema with a macular star (neuroretinitis). *J Neuro-ophthalmol* in press.

Lesser RL, Kornmehl EW, Pachner AR, et al. (1990). Neuro-ophthalmologic manifestations of Lyme disease. *Ophthalmology 97:*699–706.

McCleish WM, Pulido JS, Holland S, et al. (1990). The ocular manifestations of syphilis in the human immunodeficiency virus type 1-infected host. *Ophthalmology 97:*196–203.

McCrary B, Cockerhan W, Pierce P. (1994). Neuroretinitis in cat-scratch disease associated with the macular star. *Ped Infect Dis J 13:*938–939.

Maitland CG, Miller NR. (1984). Neuroretinitis. *Arch Ophthalmol 102:*1146–1150.

Margo CE, Sedwick LA, Rubin ML. (1986). Neuroretinitis in presumed visceral larva migrans. *Retina 6:*95–98.

Margolis T, Irvine AR, Hoyt WF, Hyman R. (1988). Acute retinal necrosis syndrome presenting with papillitis and arcuate neuroretinitis. *Ophthalmology 95:*937–940.

Matsuda A, Chin S, Ohashi T. (1994). A case of neuroretinitis associated with long-standing polyarteritis nodosa. *Ophthalmologica 208:*168–171.

May EF, Levi L, Ng JD, Truxal AR. (1995). Rochalimaea neuroretinitis and retinal vasculitis. Presented at the Meeting of the North American Neuro-Ophthalmology Society, Tucson, AZ.

Miller NR. (1995). *Walsh and Hoyt's Clinical Neuro-ophthalmology*. Baltimore, Williams and Wilkins, pp. 4487–4489.

Miller NR. (1995). *Walsh and Hoyt's Clinical Neuro-ophthalmology*. Baltimore, Williams and Wilkins, pp. 3657–3658.

Molk R. (1982). Treatment of toxocaral optic neuritis. *J Clin Neuro-ophthalmol 2:*109–112.

Monroe LD. (1979). Optic neuritis in a child with herpes zoster. *Ann Ophthalmol 11:*405–406.

Moreno RJ, Weisman J, Waller S. (1992). Neuroretinitis: An unusual presentation of ocular toxoplasmosis. *Ann Ophthalmol 24:*68–70.

Ninomiya H, Hamada T, Akiya S, Kazama H. (1990). Three cases of acute syphilitic neuroretinitis. *Folia Ophthalmol Jpn 41:*2088–2094.

Papastratigakis B, Stavrakas E, Phanouriakis C, et al. (1981). Leber's idiopathic stellate maculopathy. *Ophthalmologic 183:*68–71.

Parmley VC, Schiffman JS, Maitland CG, et al. (1987). Does neuroretinitis rule out multiple sclerosis? *Arch Neurol 44:*1045–1048.

Perkin GD, Rose FC. (1979). *Optic Neuritis and its Differential Diagnosis.* Oxford, Oxford Medical Publications, pp. 109–110.

Purvin VA, Chioran G. (1994). Recurrent neuroretinitis. *Arch Ophthalmol 112:*365–371.

Ricci A. (1961). La retinite pseudo-albuminurigue de Leber (retinitis stellata). *Ann Ocul 194:*1038–1047.

Riffenburgh RS. (1961). Ocular manifestations of mumps. *Arch Ophthalmol 66:739–743.*

Roach ES, Zimmerman CF, Troost BT, Weaver RG. (1985). Optic neuritis due to acquired toxoplasmosis. *Pediatr Neurol 1:*114–116.

Schönherr U, Lang GE, Maythaler FH. (1991). Bilaterale Lebersche Neuroretinitis stellata bei Borrelia burgdorferi-Serokonversion. *Klin Monatsbl Augenheilkd 198:*44–47.

Schönherr U, Wilk CM, Lang GE, Naumann GOH. Intraocular manifestations of Lyme borreliosis. Presented at the Fourth International Conference on Borreliosis, Stockholm, Sweden, June 18–21, 1990.

Smith JL. (1968). Spirochetes in late seronegative syphilis despite penicillin therapy. In Smith JL (ed). *Neuro-ophthalmology Symposium of the University of Miami Bascom-Palmer Eye Institute.* St Louis, Mosby, vol. IV, pp. 1–14.

Spalton DJ, Murdoch I, Holder GE. (1989). Coxsackie B5 papillitis. *J Neurol Neurosurg Psychiatry 52:*1310–1359.

Sweeney VP, Drance SM. (1970). Optic neuritis and compressive optic neuropathy associated with cat scratch disease. *Can Med Assoc J 103:*1380–1381.

Ulrich GG, Waecker NJ Jr, Meister SJ, et al. (1992). Cat scratch disease associated with neuroretinitis in a 6-year-old girl. *Ophthalmology 99:*246–249.

Veldman E, Bos PJM. (1986). Neuroretinitis in secondary syphilis. *Doc Ophthalmol 64:*23–29.

Verm A, Lee AG. (1997). Bilateral optic disk edema with macular exudates as the manifesting sign of a cerebral arteriovenous malformation. *Am J Ophthalmol 123:*422–424.

Zhao X, Ge B. (1991). Treatment of papillo-retinitis and uveitis with cat scratch disease by combination of TCM and modern drugs. *J Trad Chin Med 11:*184–186.

◆ 4 ◆

Non-arteritic Ischemic Optic Neuropathy

What Are the Clinical Features for Typical NA-AION?

Anterior ischemic optic neuropathy (AION) is characterized clinically by the acute onset of usually painless (although pain may occur in up to 8 to 12% of patients) unilateral visual loss (Rizzo, 1991; Schwartz, 1995) in a middle aged to older patient (usually greater than age 50 years); an ipsilateral relative afferent pupillary defect; and edema of the optic nerve head with or without peripapillary hemorrhages (Arnold, 1994; Awai, 1986; Bastianensen, 1986; Beck, 1987; Beri, 1987; Boghen, 1975; Burde, 1973, 1976, 1985; Cullen, 1976; Eagling, 1974; Ellenberger, 1968, 1973; Friedland, 1996; Glaser, 1978a, 1978b; Goodwin, 1985; Grosvenor, 1993; Hayreh, 1974a, 1974b, 1975, 1978, 1981a, 1981b, 1984, 1990a; Hines, 1983; Ischemic Optic Neuropathy Decompression Trial, 1995, 1996; Johnson, 1987, 1993, 1994a,b, 1996a,b; Kay, 1991; Manor, 1985; Moro, 1989, 1990; Palimeris, 1979; Repka, 1983; Rizzo, 1991; Sanders, 1972; Sawle, 1990; Shults, 1977, 1980; Shoch, 1983; Smith, 1985; Traustason, 1988). The presence of optic disc edema in the acute phase allows the diagnosis of AION to be made. Usually the optic disc develops sector or diffuse pallor (Hayreh, 1969; Lepore, 1985) or glaucomatous-like cupping (Orgul, 1994; Quigley, 1977). The typical clinical features of non-arteritic (NA)-AION are outlined in Table 4–1.

Table 4–1. Typical Clinical Features of Non-arteritic Anterior Ischemic Optic Neuropathy

Age usually over 40 years
Unilateral variable loss of visual acuity and/or visual field
Visual field defects consistent with an optic neuropathy (e.g., central, cecocentral, arcuate, or altitudinal)
Optic disc edema (usually pallid edema) in the acute phase followed by optic atrophy that may be sector or diffuse
Relative afferent pupillary defect in unilateral or bilateral but asymmetric cases

(continued)

Table 4–1. *(continued)*

Small cup and cup to disc ratio (less than 0.2) (Beck, 1984, 1987; Burde, 1993; Doro, 1985; Feit, 1984; Green, 1980; Jonas, 1988; Lavin, 1994; Mansour, 1988; Naumann, 1989)
Often associated with underlying vasculopathic risk factors (e.g., hypertension, diabetes, smoking) (Chung, 1994; Hayreh, 1994)
Lack of premonitory symptoms (e.g., transient visual loss) (Boghen, 1975; Ellenberger, 1973; Repka, 1983)
Usually visual loss remains static but may progress (Burde, 1985; Boghen, 1975; Cullen, 1967; Ellenberger, 1973; Hayreh, 1975; Kline, 1988; Miller, 1966; Repka, 1983; Shults, 1977)

Ischemic optic neuropathy (ION) without acute disc edema is referred to as posterior ischemic optic neuropathy (PION). PION is an atypical presentation of ION but it may occur in several conditions as listed in Table 4–2.

Younger patients (less than 40 years of age) with diabetes (Appen, 1980a, 1980b; Barr, 1980; Hayreh, 1981; Lubow, 1971; Neuman, 1978; Pavan, 1980), migraine (Cowan, 1982; Katz, 1985a, 1985b; McDonald, 1971; O'Hara, 1984; Victor, 1977; Weinstein, 1982), severe hypertension including preeclampsia (Beck, 1980; Hulse, 1979; Kishi, 1985; Taylor, 1981), or oral contraceptive use (Varga, 1976) may also develop ION. We consider ION in patients less than 40 years old an atypical presentation (Rinaldi, 1990). A clinical presentation of AION may occur in young patients without any known vasculopathic risk factors and has been termed AION of the young (AIONY). AIONY differs from typical AION in that recurrent attacks are more common than with typical NA-AION (Dutton, 1983; Hamed, 1988; Josef, 1988).

Bilateral simultaneous involvement may occur in NA-AION (up to 15% of cases) (Eagling, 1974; Ellenberger, 1973; Hayreh, 1979, 1981; Kurz, 1969; Miller, 1982) but we consider this also an atypical finding. Giant cell arteritis (as well as other causes of a bilateral optic neuropathy) should be excluded in these cases (Boghen, 1975; Cullen, 1967, Hayreh, 1979; Meadows, 1968; Neuman, 1978).

Table 4–2. Conditions Associated with Posterior Ischemic Optic Neuropathy

Atherosclerosis and arteriosclerosis (Cullen, 1983)
Severe hypotension or blood loss
Collagen vascular disorders (e.g., systemic lupus erythematosus) (Hayreh, 1981)
Giant cell (temporal) arteritis (Boghen, 1975; Hayreh, 1981; Hollenhorst, 1967)
Hematologic disorders
Infection
  Aspergillus (Weinstein, 1989)
  Herpes zoster
Internal carotid artery occlusion (Sawle, 1987)
Malignant hypertension
Migraine
Surgical complication
Severe anemia
Radiation therapy (Fishman, 1976)
Thromboembolism (e.g., internal carotid artery disease) (Lieberman, 1978)

Source: Burde, 1992; Fishman, 1976; Hayreh, 1981; Lee, 1995; Isayama, 1983a, 1983b, 1983c; Johnson, 1987; Rizzo, 1987; Ross, 1973; Rootman, 1980.

What Other Conditions Are Associated with Ischemic Optic Neuropathy?

ION has been reported in association with a number of systemic conditions listed in Table 4–3.

Table 4–3. Conditions Associated with Anterior (and Posterior) Ischemic Optic Neuropathy

Systemic vasculopathy
- *Common*
  - Hypertension (Beri, 1987; Boghen, 1975; Ellenberger, 1979; Hayreh, 1986, 1990, 1994; Hulse, 1979; Kishi, 1985; Repka, 1983; Smith, 1975)
  - Hypotension
  - Diabetes mellitus (Appen, 1980a, 1980b; Barner, 1982; Barr, 1980; Beri, 1987; Brogelli, 1986; Cullen, 1967; Hayreh, 1971, 1981, 1994; Lubow, 1971; Moro, 1986; Neuman, 1978; Pavan, 1980; Slavin, 1987; Ward, 1984)
  - Arteriosclerosis, atherosclerosis, and ischemic heart disease (Beri, 1987; Boke 1980; Ellenberger, 1973, 1979; Francois, 1976; Hayreh, 1994; Miller, 1982; Repka, 1983)
- *Uncommon*
  - Female carrier of Fabry's disease (Abe, 1992)
  - Takayasu's arteritis (Leonard, 1983; Miller, 1982)
  - Carotid artery disease (Eagling, 1974; Knox, 1971)
    - Carotid occlusive disease (Brown, 1986; Knox, 1971; Walsh, 1969; Waybright, 1982)
    - Carotid dissection (Rivkin, 1990)
  - Thromboangiitis obliterans
  - Vasospasm (Hayreh, 1997; Kaiser, 1996)
    - Migraine
    - Raynaud's disease

Acute blood loss or hypotension (Ballen, 1985; Bogousslavsky, 1987; Brown, 1994; Chisholm, 1969; Connolly, 1994; Coyle, 1986; Drance, 1973; Foulds, 1969; Hayreh, 1987; Larkin, 1987; Lazaro, 1971; Lee, 1995; Klewin, 1978; Presencia, 1985; Rizzo, 1987; Rootman, 1980; Sundaram, 1986)
- Postsurgical (Wessells, 1987; Williams, 1995)
  - Cardiopulmonary bypass procedures (Alpert, 1987; Larkin, 1987; Lund, 1994; Rizzo, 1987; Shahian, 1989; Shapira, 1996; Spoor, 1991; Sweeney, 1982; Tomsak, 1985)
  - Lumbar spine surgery (Brown, 1994; Katz, 1994; Lee, 1995; Loftman, 1996; Smith, 1996)
  - Abdominal surgery (Hayreh, 1987; Johnson, 1987)
  - Radical neck dissection (Chutkow, 1973; Kirkali, 1990; Marks, 1990; Nawa, 1992; Schnobel, 1995; Wilson, 1991)
  - Mitral valve surgery
  - Nasal surgery (intranasal anesthetic) (Savino, 1990)
  - Cholecystectomy
  - Parathyroidectomy
  - Coronary angiography (Tomsak, 1985)
- After treatment for malignant hypertension (Connolly, 1994; Cove, 1979; Pryor, 1979; Taylor, 1981)
- Hemodialysis (Connolly, 1994; Hamed, 1989; Michaelson, 1989; Servilla, 1986)
- Nocturnal hypotension (Hayreh, 1981, 1993, 1994)
- Therapeutic phlebotomy

(continued)

Table 4–3. *(continued)*

Cardiac arrest (Slavin, 1987)
Surgical (nonhypotensive or anemic)
Cataract surgery (Garvin, 1982; Gass, 1969; Hayreh, 1980, 1982; Michaels, 1973; Perez-Santonja, 1993; Serrano, 1982; Slavin, 1985)
Secondary intraocular lens implantation (Spedick, 1984)
After general surgery without significant blood loss
Retinal surgery (Isayama, 1983c; Jaben, 1983; Jarrett, 1965)
Infectious
Aspergillus (Weinstein, 1989)
Herpes zoster (Ahmad, 1969; Borruat, 1992; Carroll, 1979; Kattah, 1978; Kothe, 1990; Ramsell, 1967)
Lyme disease
Recurrent herpes labialis (Johnson, 1996b)
Staphylococcal cavernous sinus thrombosis (Friberg, 1978)
Syphilis (Sanders, 1971)
Inflammatory disorders (Coppetto, 1992)
Allergic vasculitis (Miller, 1982)
Behçet's disease (Scouras, 1976)
Buerger's disease (Miller, 1982)
Churg-Strauss disease (Acheson, 1993; Kattah, 1994; Weinstein, 1983)
Crohn's disease (Heuer, 1982)
Mixed connective tissue disease (Gressell, 1983)
Polyarteritis nodosa (Herman, 1973; Killian, 1978; Kimbrell, 1967; McKay, 1974; Schults, 1984)
Postviral vasculitis
Relapsing polychondritis (Anderson, 1967; Herman, 1973; Killian, 1978; McKay, 1974)
Rheumatoid arthritis (Crompton, 1980)
Sjögren's syndrome (and antiphospholipid antibodies) (Rosler, 1995)
Systemic lupus erythematosus (Cinefro, 1978; Hackett, 1974; Miller, 1982)
Ocular
Hyperopia (Beck, 1987; Katz, 1993; Mansour, 1988)
Optic disc drusen (Beck, 1985; Cohen, 1971; Gittinger, 1984; Karel, 1972; Sarkies, 1987)
Papilledema
Elevated intraocular pressure (Begg, 1971; Kalenak, 1991; Katz, 1990, 1992; Tomsak, 1989)
Birdshot retinochoroidopathy (Caballero-Presencia, 1988)
Hematological abnormalities
Anemia (Golnik, 1990; Laibovitz, 1982)
Antiphospholipid antibodies (Briley, 1989; Galetta, 1991; Rosley, 1995)
G-6-P-D deficiency syndrome
Leukemia (Hayreh, 1975)
Lipid abnormalities (Giuffre, 1990; Talks, 1995)
Lupus anticoagulant (Levine, 1988)
Pernicious anemia
Polycythemia vera
Sickle cell trait and disease (Perlman, 1994; Slavin, 1988)
Thrombocytopenic purpura (Hayreh, 1975)
Waldenström's macroglobulinemia (Mansour, 1985)
Embolic (Burde, 1982; Horton, 1995; Lieberman, 1978; Portnoy, 1989; Tomsak, 1985)
Miscellaneous
Acute intermittent porphyria (DeFrancisco, 1979)

Allergic disorders (Hayreh, 1975)
  Serum sickness
  Bacille Calmette-Guérin (BCG) vaccination
  Urticaria
  Quincke's edema
Cardiac valvular disease (Hayreh, 1994)
Cavernous sinus thrombosis (Gupta, 1990)
Cervical discopathies and vasospasm (Hayreh, 1975)
Favism (Choremis, 1960; Miller, 1982)
Gastrointestinal ulcers (Hayreh, 1994)
Graves's disease (Dosso, 1994)
Human lymphocyte antigen-A29 (Johnson, 1993)
Medications
  Interferon alfa treatment (Farkkila, 1984; Purvin, 1995; Tang, 1995)
  Intracarotid carmustine (Pickrell, 1987)
  Sumatriptin for migraine (Chiari, 1994)
Lymphoma and sepsis (Guyer, 1990)
Migraine (Chiari, 1994; Cowan, 1982; Hupp, 1989; Katz, 1985a, 1985b; McDonald, 1971; O'Hara, 1984; Victor, 1977; Weinstein, 1982)
Postimmunization (Miller, 1982)
Radiation necrosis (Parsons, 1994)
Renal failure and uremia (Hamed, 1989; Knox, 1988)
Smoking (Chung, 1994; Johnson, 1994; Talks, 1995)
Trauma (Gadkari, 1990; Hedges, 1981; Wylie, 1972)

Source: Miller, 1980.

What Clinical Features Are Atypical for Anterior Ischemic Optic Neuropathy?

Patients with an atypical AION should undergo a complete evaluation to exclude other causes of an optic neuropathy (e.g., inflammatory, infiltrative, compressive optic neuropathies). The clinical features that are atypical for AION are listed in Table 4–4.

Table 4–4. Clinical Features Atypical for Non-arteritic Anterior Ischemic Optic Neuropathy

Age younger than 40 years
Bilateral simultaneous onset
Visual field defect not consistent with an optic neuropathy (e.g., bitemporal hemianopsia, homonymous hemianopsia)
Lack of optic disc edema in the acute phase
Lack of relative afferent pupillary defect
Large cup to disc ratio (Beck, 1987)
Lack of vasculopathic risk factors
Presence of premonitory symptoms of transient visual loss (amaurosis fugax)
Progression of visual loss beyond 2–4 weeks
Recurrent episodes in the same eye (Kao, 1989)
Anterior or posterior segment inflammation (e.g., vitreous cells)

Although it is uncommon for NA-AION to recur in the same eye (Beck, 1983, 1984; Boghen, 1975; Glaser, 1978b; Hayreh, 1975; Lavin, 1983; Miller, 1980; Repka, 1983; Smith, 1975), it may involve the fellow eye in 10 to 73% of cases (Boghen, 1975; Cullen, 1967; Ellenberger, 1973, 1979; Eagling, 1974; Hayreh, 1979; King, 1979; Kline, 1980; Kurz, 1969; Repka, 1983). Beri et al. evaluated 439 patients with AION (Beri, 1987); 388 had NA-AION and 50 had arteritic AION. The risk of bilateral involvement for the arteritic form was 1.9 times the risk for NA-AION. At 3 years, Beri et al. calculated an incidence of bilateral NA-AION of 26% (Beri, 1987).

The visual loss in NA-AION is usually acute and remains relatively static, but may spontaneously improve in up to 42.7% of patients (Aiello, 1992; Barrett, 1992; Cho, 1986; IONDT, 1995; Movsas, 1991; Rizzo, 1991). In up to 25% of patients, visual loss may be progressive over several weeks (Beck, 1983; Boghen, 1975; Borchert, 1988; Kline, 1988; Knox, 1971; Sergott, 1989). In our opinion, progression should prompt further evaluation, including neuroimaging, to exclude other causes of a continuing optic neuropathy (Borchert, 1988).

What Is the Evaluation and Treatment for AION?

Patients with typical features of AION (e.g., acute onset, unilateral visual loss, ipsilateral optic disc edema, older-aged patient) do not require neuroimaging. The major entity that must be excluded in AION is giant cell arteritis (GCA) (see chapter 5). An erythrocyte sedimentation rate and other appropriate evaluation for GCA should be performed in all cases of AION in patients over age 50. Patients with atypical features (see Table 4–4) should be evaluated for other etiologies of an optic neuropathy (see Chapter 1).

Unfortunately, although corticosteroids (systemic, retrobulbar, sub-Tenons), anticoagulation, dipyrimadole, acetazolamide, hemodilution, vasodilators, vasopressors, atropine, norepinephrine, diphenylhydantoin, and hyperbaric oxygen have been tried in the past, there is no proven therapy for NA-AION (Arnold, 1996; Becker, 1972; Boghen, 1975; Eagling, 1974; Ellenberger, 1973, 1974; Foulds, 1969; Hayreh, 1974b, 1975; Keltner, 1972; Kline, 1988; Kollarits, 1981; Miller, 1982; Sanders, 1971; Smith, 1981; Wolfe, 1993). The natural history of NA-AION in the past has been difficult to define. In the Ischemic Optic Neuropathy Decompression Trial (IONDT), there was an unexpectedly high rate of spontaneous (three or more lines from baseline at 6 months) improvement of 42.7%. This rate is higher than that noted in the literature on AION (Boghen, 1975, Repka, 1983) before 1989 (less than 10%). In the literature since then, visual improvement rates as high as 33% have been reported (Arnold, 1994; Rizzo, 1991; Yee, 1993).

We believe that any future treatments for NA-AION will have to prove better than the natural history data of the IONDT. Most previously published reports on treatment for NA-AION are limited by retrospective design, nonstandardized methods of data collection or measurement, small sample sizes, and variable (usually relatively short) lengths of follow-up.

Medical control of underlying hypertension, diabetes, and other presumed etiologic vasculopathic risk factors (such as smoking cessation) has been recommended (Chung, 1994; Hayreh, 1994), but no well-controlled data on the efficacy of such measures in reducing fellow-eye involvement exist. In addition, overaggressive control of arterial hypertension may be potentially dangerous in patients in whom acute and/or nocturnal hypotension is an underlying etiology for NA-AION (Burde, 1985; Hayreh, 1994). Patients with malignant hypertension in whom the blood pressure is lowered too rapidly may also be at risk for the precipitation of NA-AION in the fellow eye (Pitcher, 1979).

Are Any Additional Studies (e.g., Noninvasive Carotid Doppler Studies, Cardiac Studies, Neuroimaging) Warranted in Patients with NA-AION?

Although Guyer et al. (Guyer, 1985, 1988) reported a significantly higher incidence of cerebrovascular and cardiovascular disease in 200 patients with idiopathic AION, Hayreh et al. have found no increased risk for subsequent cerebrovascular or cardiovascular disease (Hayreh, 1994). Some authors have found no increased incidence of generalized cerebral vascular disease on magnetic resonance (MR) imaging of the head in 9 patients with NA-AION but Arnold et al. reported an increased number of central nervous system white matter lesions on MR brain imaging in patients with NA-AION (Arnold, 1995). Fry, et al. found no significant difference in carotid stenosis in 15 patients with AION versus controls (Fry, 1993). Several authors have reported no significant association between AION and extracranial carotid artery occlusive disease (Boghen, 1975; Ellenberger, 1973; Repka, 1983). AION has rarely been attributed to embolic disease (Burde, 1982; Horton, 1995; Lieberman, 1978; Portnoy, 1989; Tomsak, 1985). We do not perform additional noninvasive evaluation of the carotid or cardiac systems in patients with NA-AION unless there are other signs of carotid disease, such as ocular ischemic syndrome or retinal emboli, or a history of transient or persistent focal neurologic deficits (Brown, 1986; Burde, 1982; Horton, 1995; Lieberman, 1978; Portnoy, 1989; Tomsak, 1985). Neuroimaging studies of the head are not indicated in patients with typical unilateral NA-AION (Arnold, 1995; Schwartz, 1995).

Should the Patient with NA-AION Be Placed on Aspirin Therapy?

Aspirin is often given to patients following the development of NA-AION, but there does not seem to be any beneficial effect of treatment on eventual visual outcome (Botelho, 1996). Some authors, however, have suggested that aspirin therapy may reduce the risk of NA-AION in the fellow eye (Beck, 1997; Sanderson, 1995). Sanderson et al. performed a retrospective review of 101 patients with AION for over 3 years (Sanderson, 1995). Fellow eye involvement occurred in 33 cases, of which 23 did not take aspirin (compared with 47 patients on aspirin out of 68 patients without fellow eye involvement). These authors estimated a three-fold reduction of second eye involvement ($p = .0005$) in the aspirin-treated group and concluded that aspirin therapy significantly reduces the relative risk of NA-AION in the fellow eye. Beck reported in the results of a survey (270 of 350 neuro-ophthalmologist respondents) that among ophthalmologists ($N = 188$), 60% usually or always prescribed aspirin (usually 325 mg per day); 6% prescribed aspirin about half the time; and 34% occasionally or never prescribed aspirin. Among neurologists ($N = 82$), the percentages were 71%, 10%, and 19%, respectively (Beck, 1997). In light of the possible association between NA-AION and cerebrovascular and cardiac vasculopathic risk factors (e.g., hypertension, diabetes) and the recognized reduction in morbidity and mortality for patients with cerebrovascular disease and cardiac disease (e.g., myocardial infarction) (Roth, 1994) treated with aspirin, our current practice (until a prospective trial is performed) is to offer oral aspirin therapy to patients (who have no contraindications to aspirin) with NA-AION.

Are There Other Treatments for NA-AION?

Recently, a pilot clinical trial on the efficacy of levodopa in NA-AION was published with interesting results. Johnson, et al. reported a prospective, randomized, double-masked, placebo-controlled, clinical trial of 20 subjects with NA-AION of 30 months mean duration (Johnson, 1996). Subjects were randomized to low-dose levodopa and carbidopa or placebo for 3 weeks. At 12 weeks, the levodopa group was provided a higher, conventional dose of levodopa and carbidopa for 3 additional weeks. At 12 weeks, the levodopa group experienced a significant ($p = 0.16$) mean difference in improvement of visual acuity of 5.9 letters from the placebo group, and at 24 weeks the treatment effect remained ($p = 0.36$). There was a mean gain of 7.5 letters in the levodopa group compared to the placebo group, and 3 subjects experienced a doubling of the visual angle as denoted by a gain of at least 15 letters. No significant improvement was noted for color vision or visual field. Unfortunately, larger population studies and longer follow-up intervals are needed to confirm these initial promising results and it is premature to say with any certainty that levodopa is an effective treatment for NA-AION.

Does Optic Nerve Sheath Fenestration Improve Visual Outcomes in NA-AION?

Initial reports of visual improvement following optic nerve sheath fenestration (ONSF) for NA-AION were encouraging, but anecdotal (Kelman, 1991; Manor, 1990; Sergott, 1989, 1990; Spoor, 1991). Other reports followed with mixed results (Flaharty, 1993; Glaser, 1994; Hayreh, 1990a; Jablons, 1993; Kelman, 1991; Keltner, 1988; McHenry, 1993a, 1993b; Mutulhan, 1990; Sadun, 1993; Sergott, 1989, 1990; Spoor, 1991, 1993; Wall, 1991; Wilson, 1990; Yee, 1993). Subsequently, a well-designed, masked, prospective, randomized IONDT at 25 clinical centers was initiated with the support of the National Eye Institute (IONDT, 1995). The study inclusion criteria included a clinical syndrome consistent with NA-AION (e.g., acute, unilateral visual loss, relative afferent pupillary defect, swollen optic nerve, etc.); age greater than 50 years; visual symptoms for less than 14 days from onset; and visual acuity of 20/64 or worse. Patients were randomly assigned to either ONSF (119 patients) or a control group (125 patients). Surgery was performed by experienced, protocol-certified study surgeons. The primary outcome measure was a 3 or more line improvement of visual acuity after 6 months, and visual field mean deviation on the Humphrey Field Analyzer (Program 24-2) was a secondary outcome measure. Recruitment was halted in September, 1994 on the recommendation of the study's Data and Safety Monitoring Committee. After 6 months, 32.6% of the ONSF (surgery) group had improved 3 or more lines of visual acuity compared with 42.7% of the control group; but 23.9% of the ONSF group had lost 3 or more lines of visual acuity compared with only 12.4% of the control group. Likewise, visual field data confirmed a lack of benefit for surgery. The 3-month and 12-month data confirmed the findings of the 6-month data. In addition, there was no indication of benefit from ONSF in the subgroup of patients with progressive visual loss.

The authors concluded that "ONSF is not effective and may be harmful in NA-AION" (IONDT, 1995), but were careful to state that they could "offer no recommendation regarding the safety and efficacy of this surgery for other conditions" (IONDT, 1995). We agree that ONSF should not be performed for NA-AION (Beck, 1995; IONDT, 1995; Lessell, 1995; Smith, 1995).

Our approach to NA-AION is outlined in Figure 4–1.

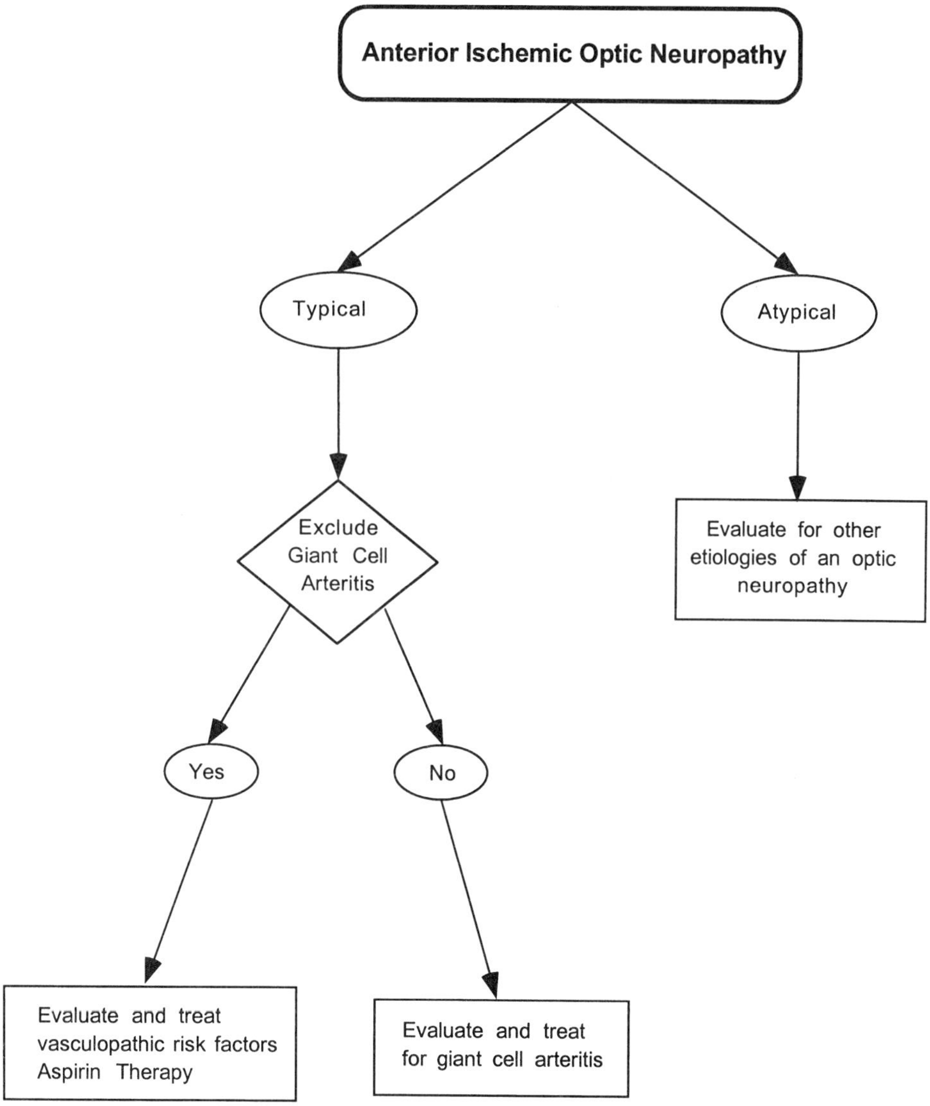

Figure 4–1. Anterior ischemic optic neuropathy.

References

Abe H, Sakai T, Sawaguchi S, et al. (1992). Ischemic optic neuropathy in a female carrier with Fabry's disease. *Ophthalmologica 205:*83–88.

Acheson JF, Cockrell OC, Bentley CR, Sanders MD. (1993). Churg-Strauss vasculitis presenting with severe visual loss due to bilateral sequential optic neuropathy. *Br J Ophthalmol 77:*118–119.

Ahmed M, Bowen SF, Burke R. (1969). Optic atrophy following herpes zoster ophthalmicus in a child. *Can J Ophthalmol 4:*387–389.

Aiello AL, Sadun AA, Feldon SE. (1992). Spontaneous improvement of progressive anterior ischemic optic neuropathy. Report of two cases. *Arch Ophthalmol 110:*1197–1199.

Alpert JN, Pena Y, Leachman DR. (1987). Anterior ischemic optic neuropathy after coronary bypass surgery. *Tex Med 83:*45–47.

Anderson B. (1967). Ocular lesions in relapsing polychondritis and other rheumatoid syndromes. *Trans Am Acad Ophthalmol Otolaryngol 71:*227–242.

Appen RE, DeVenencia G, Ferwerda J. (1980a). Optic disk vasculitis. *Am J Ophthalmol 90:*352–359.

Appen RE, Chandra SR, Klein R, Myers FL. (1980b). Diabetic papillopathy. *Am J Ophthalmol 90:*203–209.

Arnold AC. (1987). Anterior ischemic optic neuropathy following ocular pneumoplethysmography (letter). *J Clin Neuro-ophthalmol 7:*58–59.

Arnold AC, Badr MA, Hepler RS. (1996). Fluorescein angiography in nonischemic optic disc edema. *Arch Ophthalmol 114:*293–298.

Arnold AC, Hepler RS. (1994). Fluorescein angiography in acute nonarteritic anterior ischemic optic neuropathy. *Am J Ophthalmol 117:*222–230.

Arnold AC, Hepler RS. (1994). Natural history of nonarteritic anterior ischemic optic neuropathy. *J Neuro-ophthalmol 14:*66–69.

Arnold AC, Hepler RS, Hamilton DR, Lufkin RB. (1995). Magnetic resonance imaging of the brain in nonarteritic anterior ischemic optic neuropathy. *J Neuro-ophthalmol 15:*158–160.

Arnold AC, Hepler RS, Lieber M, Alexander JM. (1996). Hyperbaric oxygen therapy for nonarteritic anterior ischemic optic neuropathy. *Am J Ophthalmol 122:*535–541.

Awai T. (1986). Studies on the pathogenesis of anterior ischemic optic neuropathy. *Neuro-ophthalmology 6:*329.

Ballen PH, Fox MJ, Weissman GS. (1985). Ischemic optic neuropathy secondary to intestinal hemorrhage. *Ann Ophthalmol 17:*486–488.

Barner SS, Fledlius HC. (1982). Anterior ischemic optic neuropathy as an initial sign of diabetes mellitus: A case report. *Ann Ophthalmol 100:*1177–1178.

Barr CC, Glaser JS, Blankenship G. (1980). Acute disc swelling in juvenile diabetes. *Arch Ophthalmol 98:*2185–2192.

Barrett DA, Glaser JS, Schatz NJ, Winterkorn JMS. (1992). Spontaneous recovery of vision in progressive anterior ischemic optic neuropathy. *J Clin Neuro-ophthalmol 12:*219–225.

Bastiaensen LA, Keunen RW, Tijssen CC, Vandoninck JJ. (1986). Anterior ischemic optic neuropathy: Sense and nonsense in diagnosis and treatment. *Doc Ophthalmol 61:*205–210.

Beck RW. (1992). Optic neuritis or anterior ischemic optic neuropathy? *Arch Ophthalmol 110:*1357.

Beck RW. (1995). Optic nerve sheath fenestration for anterior ischemic optic neuropathy? The answer is in (editorial). *J Neuro-ophthalmol 15:*61–62.

Beck RW, Corbett JR, Thompson HS, et al. (1985). Decreased visual acuity from optic disc drusen. *Arch Ophthalmol 103:*1155–1159.

Beck RW, Gamel JW, Willcourt RJ, Berman G. (1980). Acute ischemic optic neuropathy in severe preeclampsia. *Am J Ophthalmol 90:*342–346.

Beck RW, Hayreh SS, Podhajsky PA, Tan E-S, Moke PS. (1997). Aspirin therapy in nonarteritic anterior ischemic optic neuropathy. *Am J Ophthalmol 123:*212–217.

Beck RW, Savino PJ, Repka MX, Schatz NJ, Sergott R. (1984). Optic disc structure in anterior ischemic optic neuropathy. *Ophthalmology 91:*1334–1337.

Beck RW, Savino PJ, Schatz NJ, Smith CH, Sergott R. (1983). Anterior ischemic optic neuropathy: Recurrent episodes in the same eye. *Br J Ophthalmol 67:*705–709.

Beck RW, Servais GE, Hayreh SS. (1987). Anterior ischemic optic neuropathy. IX. Cup-to-disc ratio and its role in pathogenesis. *Ophthalmology 94:*1503–1508.

Becker B. (1972). Effect of diphenylhydantoin on glaucomatous field loss: A preliminary report. *Trans Am Acad Ophthalmol Otolaryngol 76:*412–422.

Begg IS, Drance SM, Sweeney VP. (1971). Ischemic optic neuropathy in chronic simple glaucoma. *Br J Ophthalmol 55:*73–90.

Beri M, Klugman MR, Kohler JA, Hayreh SS. (1987). Anterior ischemic optic neuropathy VII. Incidence of bilaterality and various influencing factors. *Ophthalmology 94:*1020–1028.

Boghen DR, Glaser JS. (1975). Ischemic optic neuropathy: A clinical profile and natural history. *Brain 98:*689–708.

Bogousslavsky J, Regli F, Zografos L, Uske A. (1987). Optico-cerebral syndrome: Simultaneous hemodynamic infarction of optic nerve and brain. *Neurology 37:*263–268.

Boke W, Voigt GJ. (1980). Circulatory disorders of the optic nerve. *Ophthalmologica 180:*88–100.

Boone MI, Massry GG, Frankel RA, Holds JB, Chung SM. (1996). Visual outcome in bilateral nonarteritic anterior ischemic optic neuropathy. *Ophthalmology 103:*1223–1228.
Borchert M, Lessell S. (1988). Progressive and recurrent nonarteritic ischemic optic neuropathy. *Am J Ophthalmol 106:*443–449.
Borruat FX, Herbort CP. (1992). Herpes zoster ophthalmicus. Anterior ischemic optic neuropathy and acyclovir. *J Clin Neuro-ophthalmol 12:*37–40.
Botelho PJ, Johnson LN, Arnold AC. (1996) The effect of aspirin on the visual outcome of nonarteritic anterior ischemic optic neuropathy. *Am J Ophthalmol 121:*450–451.
Briley DP, Coull BM, Goodnight SH Jr. (1989). Neurological disease associated with antiphospholipid antibodies. *Ann Neurol 25:*221–227.
Brogelli S, Valentini G. (1986). Anterior ischemic optic neuropathy in type I diabetes. *Met Ped Syst Ophthalmol 9:*90–93.
Brown GC. (1986). Anterior ischemic optic neuropathy occurring in association with carotid artery obstruction. *J Clin Neuro-ophthalmol 6:*39–42.
Brown RH, Schauble JF, Miller NR. (1994). Anemia and hypotension as contributors to perioperative loss of vision. *Anesthesiology 80:*222–226.
Burde RM. (1973). Ischemic optic neuropathy. In Smith JL, Glaser JS. *Neuro-ophthalmology, Symposium of the University of Miami and the Bascom Palmer Eye Institute.* St. Louis, Mosby, vol. 7, p. 38.
Burde RM. (1976). Ischemic optic neuropathies. In Burde RM, Glaser JS, Hollenhorst RW, Jampolsky A, Schatz NJ, Udvarhelyi GB, van Dyk HJL, contributors. *Symposium on Neuro-ophthalmology, Trans New Orleans Acad Ophthalmol.* St. Louis, Mosby, pp. 25–37.
Burde RM. (1993). Optic disk risk factors for nonarteritic anterior ischemic optic neuropathy (Review). *Am J Ophthalmol 116:*759–764.
Burde RM, Savino PJ, Trobe JD. (1985). *Clinical Decisions in Neuro-ophthalmology.* St. Louis, Mosby, pp. 41–46.
Burde RM, Smith ME, Black JT. (1979). Retinal artery occlusion in the absence of a cherry red spot. *Surv Ophthalmol 27:*181.
Caballero-Presencia A, Diaz-Guia E, Lopez-Lopez JM. (1988). Acute anterior ischemic optic neuropathy in birdshot retinochoroidopathy. *Ophthalmologica, 196:*87–91.
Carroll WM, Mastaglia FL. (1979). Optic neuropathy and ophthalmoplegia in herpes zoster oticus. *Neurology 29:*726–729.
Chiari M, Manzoni GC, Van de Geijn EJ. (1994). Ischemic optic neuropathy after sumatriptan in a migraine with aura patient (letter). *Headache 34:*237–238.
Chisholm IA. (1969). Optic neuropathy of recurrent blood loss. *Br J Ophthalmol 53:*289–295.
Cho MH. (1986). Remission of visual field loss in nonarteritic anterior ischemic optic neuropathy. *Am J Optom Physiol Optics 63:*472–476.
Choremis C, Joannides T, Kyriakides B. (1960). Severe ophthalmologic complications following favism. *Br J Ophthalmol 44:*353.
Chung SM, Gay CA, McCrary JA, III. (1994). Nonarteritic ischemic optic neuropathy. The impact of tobacco use. *Ophthalmology 101:*779–782.
Chutkow JG, Sharbrough FW, Riley FC. (1973). Blindness following simultaneous bilateral neck dissection. *Mayo Clin Proc 48:*713–717.
Cinefro RJ, Frenkel M. (1978). Systemic lupus erythematosus presenting as optic neuritis. *Ann Ophthalmol 10:*559–563.
Cohen DN. (1971). Drusen of the optic disc and the development of field defects. *Arch Ophthalmol 85:*224–226.
Connolly SE, Gordon KB, Horton JC. (1994). Salvage of vision after hypotension-induced ischemic optic neuropathy. *Am J Ophthalmol 117:*235–242.
Coppetto JR, Greco TP. (1992). Autoimmune ischemic optic neuropathy associated with positive rheumatoid factor and transient nephrosis. *Ann Ophthalmol 24:*434–438.
Cove DH, Seddon M, Fletcher RF, Dukes DC. (1979). Blindness after treatment for malignant hypertension. *Br Med J 2:*245.
Cowan CL, Jr, Knox DL. (1982). Migraine optic neuropathy. *Ann Ophthalmol 14:*164–166.
Coyle JT. (1986). Ischemic optic neuropathy secondary to intestinal hemorrhage (letter). *Ann Ophthalmol 18:*149–150.
Crompton JL, Iyer P, Begg MW. (1980). Vasculitis and ischaemic optic neuropathy associated with rheumatoid arthritis. *Aust J Ophthalmol 8:*219–230.
Cullen JF. (1967). Ischaemic optic neuropathy. *Trans Ophthalmol Soc UK 87:*759–774.
Cullen JF, Duvall J. (1983). Posterior ischemic optic neuropathy. *Neuro-ophthalmology 3:*15–19.
DeFrancisco M, Savino PJ, Schatz NJ. (1979). Optic atrophy in acute intermittent porphyria. *Am J Ophthalmol 87:*221–224.
Diegel JT. (1994). The ischemic optic neuropathy decompression trial (letter). *Arch Ophthalmol 112:*1275–1276.
Doro S, Lessell S. (1985). Cup-disc ratio and ischemic optic neuropathy. *Arch Ophthalmol 103:*1143–1144.
Dosso A, Safran AB, Sunaric G, Burger A. (1994). Anterior ischemic optic neuropathy in Graves' disease. *J Neuro-ophthalmol 14:*170–174.
Drance SM, Morgan RW, Sweeney VP. (1973). Shock-induced optic neuropathy. *N Engl J Med 288:*392–395.
Dutton JJ, Burde RM. (1983). Anterior ischemic optic neuropathy of the young. *J Clin Neuro-ophthalmol 3:*135–144.

Eagling EM, Sanders MD, Miller SJH. (1974). Ischaemic papillopathy: Clinical and fluorescein angiographic review of forty cases. *Br J Ophthalmol 58:*990–1008.
Ellenberger CJ. (1979). Ischemic optic neuropathy as a possible early complication of vascular hypertension. *Am J Ophthalmol 88:*1045–1051.
Ellenberger CJ, Burde RM, Keltner JL. (1974). Acute optic neuropathy. Treatment with diphenylhydantoin. *Arch Ophthalmol 91:*435–438.
Ellenberger CJ, Keltner JL, Burde RM. (1973). Acute optic neuropathy in older patients. *Arch Neurol 28:*182–185.
Ellenberger CJ, Netsky MD. (1968). Infarction of the optic nerve. *J Neurol Neurosurg Psychiatr 31:*606–611.
Farkkila M, Livanainen M, Roine R, et al. (1984). Neurotoxic and other side effects of high-dose interferon in amyotrophic lateral sclerosis. *Acta Neurol Scand 69:*42–48.
Feit RH, Tomsak RL, Ellenberger CL, Jr. (1984). Structural factors in the pathogenesis of ischemic optic neuropathy. *Am J Ophthalmology 98:*105–108.
Fishman ML, Bean SC, Cogan DG. (1976). Optic atrophy following prophylactic chemotherapy and cranial radiation for acute lymphoblastic leukemia. *Am J Ophthalmol 82:*571.
Flaharty PM, Sergott RC, Lieb W, Bosley TM, Savino PJ. (1993). Optic nerve sheath decompression may improve blood flow in anterior ischemic optic neuropathy. *Ophthalmology 100:*297–302.
Foulds WS. (1969). Visual disturbances in systemic disorders. Optic neuropathy and systemic disease. *Trans Ophthalmol Soc UK 89:*125–147.
Francois J. (1976). Vascular pseudopapillitis: Ischemic optic neuropathy. *Ann Ophthalmol 8:*901–919.
Friberg TR, Sogg RL. (1978). Ischemic optic neuropathy in cavernous sinus thrombosis. *Arch Ophthalmol 96:*453–456.
Friedland S, Winterkorn JM, Burde RM. (1996). Luxury perfusion following anterior ischemic optic neuropathy. *J Neuro-ophthalmol 16:*163–171.
Fry CL, Carter JE, Kanter MC, Tegeler CH, Tuley MR. (1993). Anterior ischemic optic neuropathy is not associated with carotid artery atherosclerosis. *Stroke 24:*539–542.
Gadkari SS, Ladi DS, Gupta S, et al. (1990). Traumatic ischaemic optic neuropathy (a case report). *J Postgrad Med 37:*179–180.
Galetta SL, Plock GL, Kushner MJ, Wyszynski RE, Brucker AJ. (1991). Ocular thrombosis associated with antiphospholipid antibodies. *Ann Ophthalmol 23:*207–212.
Gartner S. (1964). Optic neuritis and macular edema following cataract extraction. *Eye Ear Nose Throat Monthly 43:*45–49.
Garvin CG, Weber PA. (1982). Intermediate postcataract extraction ischemic optic neuropathy associated with an intraocular lens implant. *Am Intraocular Soc Implant J 8:*144–146.
Gass JDM. (1969). Ischemic optic neuropathy in aphakia and phakia. In Welsh J, Welsh RC (eds). *The New Report on Cataract Surgery.* Miami, Miami Education Press, pp. 84–86.
Gittinger JW, Lessell S, Bondar RL. (1984). Ischemic optic neuropathy associated with optic disc drusen. *J Clin Neuro-ophthalmol 4:*79–84.
Giuffre G. (1990). Hematological risk factors for anterior ischemic optic neuropathy. *Neuro-ophthalmology 10:*197–203.
Glaser JS. (1978a). *Neuro-ophthalmology,* pp. 87–91. Hagerstown: Harper and Row.
Glaser JS. (1978b). How to recognize ischemic optic neuropathy—and what to do about it. *Geriatrics 33:*68–75.
Glaser JS. (1991). Optic neuritis and ischemic neuropathy: What we thought we already knew. *Arch Ophthalmol 109:*1666–1667.
Glaser JS, Teimory M, Schatz NJ. (1994). Optic nerve sheath fenestration for progressive ischemic optic neuropathy. *Arch Ophthalmol 112:*1047–1050.
Golnik KC, Newman SA. (1990). Anterior ischemic optic neuropathy associated with macrocytic anemia. *J Clin Neuro-ophthalmol 10:*244–247.
Goodwin J. (1985). Acute ischemic optic neuropathy. *JAMA 254:*951–952.
Green GJ, Lessell S, Lowenstein JI. (1980). Ischemic optic neuropathy in chronic papilledema. *Arch Ophthalmology 98:*502–504.
Gressell MF, Tomsak RL. (1983). Recurrent bilateral optic neuropathy in mixed connective tissue disease. *J Clin Neuro-ophthalmol 3:*101–104.
Grosvenor T, Malinovsky V, Gelvin J, Tonekaboni K. (1993). Diagnosis and management of temporal arteritis: A review and case report. *Optometry Vision Sci 70:771–777.*
Gupta A, Jalali S, Bansal RK, Grewal SP. (1990). Anterior ischemic optic neuropathy and branch retinal artery occlusion in cavernous sinus thrombosis. *J Clin Neuro-ophthalmol 10:*193–196.
Guyer DR, Green WR, Schachat AP, Bastacky S, Miller NR. (1990). Bilateral ischemic optic neuropathy and retinal vascular occlusions associated with lymphoma and sepsis. *Ophthalmology 97:*882–888.
Guyer DR, Miller NR, Enger CL, Fine SL. (1985). The risk of cerebrovascular and cardiovascular disease in patients with anterior ischemic optic neuropathy. *Arch Ophthalmol 103:*1136–1142.
Guyer DR, Miller NR, Enger CL, Fine SL. (1988). Incidence of subcortical lesions not increased in nonarteritic anterior ischemic optic neuropathy on magnetic resonance imaging (letter). *Am J Ophthalmol 105:*324.
Hackett ER, Martinez RD, Larson PF, Paddison RM. (1974). Optic neuritis in systemic lupus erythematosus. *Arch Neurol 31:*9–11.
Hamed LM, Purvin V, Rosenberg M. (1988). Recurrent anterior ischemic optic neuropathy in young adults. *J Clin Neuro-ophthalmol 8:*239–246.

Hamed LM, Winward KE, Glaser JS, Schatz NJ. (1989). Optic neuropathy in uremia. *Am J Ophthalmol 108:*30.
Hayreh SS. (1969). Blood supply of the optic nerve head and its role in optic atrophy, glaucoma, and edema of the optic disc. *Br J Ophthalmol 53:*721–747.
Hayreh SS. (1974a). Anterior ischemic optic neuropathy I. Terminology and pathogenesis. *Br J Ophthalmol 58:*981–989.
Hayreh SS. (1974b). Anterior ischemic optic neuropathy III. Treatment, prophylaxis, and differential diagnosis. *Br J Ophthalmol 58:*981–989.
Hayreh SS. (1975). *Anterior Ischemic Optic Neuropathy.* New York, Springer Verlag.
Hayreh SS. (1978). Ischemic optic neuropathy. *Int Ophthalmol 1:*9–18.
Hayreh SS. (1980). Anterior ischemic optic neuropathy IV. Occurrence after cataract extraction. *Arch Ophthalmol 98:*1410–1416.
Hayreh SS. (1981a). Anterior ischemic optic neuropathy. *Arch Neurol 38:*675–678.
Hayreh SS. (1981b). Anterior ischemic optic neuropathy. V. Optic disc edema as an early sign. *Arch Ophthalmol 99:*1030–1040.
Hayreh SS. (1982). Post cataract extraction ischemic optic neuropathy (Letter). *Arch Ophthalmol 100:*853–854.
Hayreh SS. (1987). Anterior ischemic optic neuropathy. VIII. Clinical features and pathogenesis of post-hemorrhagic amaurosis. *Ophthalmology 94:*1488–1502.
Hayreh SS. (1981). Posterior ischemic optic neuropathy. *Ophthalmologica 182:*29.
Hayreh SS. (1990a). The role of optic nerve sheath fenestration in management of anterior ischemic optic neuropathy (letter). *Arch Ophthalmol 108:*1063–1064.
Hayreh SS. (1990b). Anterior ischaemic optic neuropathy. Differentiation of arteritic from nonarteritic type and its management. *Eye 4:*25–41.
Hayreh SS. (1996). Acute ischemic disorders of the optic nerve: Pathogenesis, clinical manifestations, and management. *Ophthalmol Clin No Am 9:*407–442.
Hayreh SS, Baines JAB. (1984). Occlusion of the posterior ciliary artery. III. Effects on the optic nerve head. *Br J Ophthalmol 94:*1488–1502.
Hayreh SS, Joos KM, Podhajsky PA, Long CR. (1994). Systemic diseases associated with nonarteritic anterior ischemic optic neuropathy. *Am J Ophthalmol 118:*776–780.
Hayreh SS, Piegors DJ, Heistad DD. (1997). Serotonin-induced constriction of ocular arteries in atherosclerotic monkeys: Implications for ischemic disorders of the retina and optic nerve head. *Arch Ophthalmol 115:*220–228.
Hayreh SS, Podhajsky P. (1979). Visual field defects in anterior ischemic optic neuropathy. *Doc Ophthalmol Proc Ser, 19:*53–71.
Hayreh SS, Servais GE, Virdi PS. (1986). Fundus lesions in malignant hypertension: V. Hypertensive optic neuropathy. *Ophthalmology 93:*74–87.
Hayreh SS, Zahoruk RM. (1981). Anterior ischemic optic neuropathy. VI. In juvenile diabetics. *Ophthalmologica 182:*13–28.
Hayreh SS, Zimmerman BM, Podhajsky P, Alward WLM. (1994). Nocturnal arterial hypotension and its role in optic nerve head and ocular ischemic disorders. *Am J Ophthalmol 117:*603–624.
Hedges TR, III, Gragoudas ES. (1981). Traumatic anterior ischemic optic neuropathy. *Ann Ophthalmol 13:*625–628.
Henkind P, Charles NC, Pearson J. (1970). Histopathology of ischemic optic neuropathy. *Arch Ophthalmol 69:*78–90.
Herman JH, Dennis MV. (1973). Immunopathology studies in relapsing polychondritis. *J Clin Invest 52:*549–557.
Heuer DK, Gager WE, Reeser FH. (1982). Ischemic optic neuropathy associated with Crohn's disease. *J Clin Neuro-ophthalmol 2:*175–181.
Hines JL, Jones WL. (1983). Arteritic and idiopathic ischemic optic neuropathy. *J Am Optometr Assoc 54:*41–49.
Hollenhorst RW. (1967). Effect of posture on retinal ischemia from temporal arteritis. *Arch Ophthalmol 78:*569–577.
Horton JC. (1995). Embolic cilioretinal artery occlusion with atherosclerosis of the ipsilateral carotid artery. *Retina 15:*441–444.
Hoyt WF, Beeson D. (1966). *The Ocular Fundus in Neurologic Disease.* St. Louis, Mosby.
Hulse JA, Taylor DSI, Dillon MJ. (1979). Blindness and paraplegia in severe childhood hypertension. *Lancet 2:*553–556.
Hupp AL, Kline LB, Corbett JJ. (1989). Visual disturbances of migraine. *Surv Ophthalmol 33:*221–236.
Isayama Y, Hiramatsu K, Asakura S, et al. (1983a). Posterior ischemic optic neuropathy I. Blood supply of the optic nerve. *Ophthalmologica 186:*141–147.
Isayama Y, Takahashi T. (1983b). Posterior ischemic optic neuropathy II. Histopathology of the idiopathic form. *Ophthalmologica 187:*8–18.
Isayama Y, Takahashi T, Inoue M, Jimura T. (1983c). Posterior ischemic optic neuropathy III. Clinical diagnosis. *Ophthalmologica 187:*141.
Ischemic Optic Neuropathy Decompression Trial Research Group (IONDT). (1995). Optic nerve decompression for nonarteritic anterior ischemic optic neuropathy (AION) is not effective and may be harmful. *JAMA 273:*625–632.
Ischemic Optic Neuropathy Decompression Trial Research Group. (IONDT). (1996). Characteristics of patients with nonarteritic anterior ischemic optic neuropathy eligible for the Ischemic optic neuropathy decompression trial. *Arch Ophthalmol 114:*1366–1374.

Jaben SL, Glaser JS, Daily M. (1983). Ischemic optic neuropathy following general surgery procedures. *J Clin Neuro-ophthalmol 3:*239–244.
Jablons MM, Glaser JS, Schatz NJ, et al. (1993). Optic nerve sheath fenestration for treatment of progressive ischemic optic neuropathy: Results in 26 patients. *Arch Ophthalmol 111:*84–87.
Jarrett WH, Brockhurst RJ. (1965). Unexplained blindness and optic atrophy following retinal detachment surgery. *Arch Ophthalmol 73:*782.
Johnson LN, Arnold AC. (1994). Incidence of non-arteritic anterior ischemic optic neuropathy: Population based study in the state of Missouri and Los Angeles County, California. *J Neuro-ophthalmol 14:*38–44.
Johnson LN, Botelho PJ, Kuo HC. (1994). Is smoking a risk factor for NAAION? (letter). *Ophthalmol 101:*1322–1324.
Johnson LN, Gould TJ, Krohel GB. (1996a). Effect of levodopa and carbidopa on recovery of visual function in patients with nonarteritic anterior ischemic optic neuropathy of longer than six months duration. *Am J Ophthalmol 121:*77–83.
Johnson LN, Krohel GB, Allen SD, Mozayeni R. (1996b). Recurrent herpes labialis as a potential risk factor for nonarteritic anterior ischemic optic neuropathy. *J National Med Assoc 88:*369–373.
Johnson LN, Kuo HC, Arnold AC. (1993). HLA-A29 as a potential risk factor for nonarteritic anterior ischemic optic neuropathy (letter). *Am J Ophthalmol 115:*540–542.
Johnson MW, Kinkaid MC, Trobe JD. (1987). Bilateral retrobulbar optic nerve infarctions after blood loss and hypotension: A clinicopathologic case study. *Ophthalmology 94:*1577–1584.
Jonas JB, Gusek GC, Naumann GOH. (1988). Anterior ischemic optic neuropathy. Nonarteritic form in small and giant cell arteritis in normal sized optic discs. *Int Ophthalmol 12:*119–125.
Josef JM, Burde RM. (1988). Ischemic optic neuropathy of the young. *J Clin Neuro-ophthalmol 8:*247–248.
Kaiser HJ, Flammer J, Messerli J. (1996). Vasospasm—a risk factor for non-arteritic anterior ischemic optic neuropathy? *Neuro-ophthalmology 16:*5–10.
Kalenak JW, Kosmorsky GS, Rockwood EJ. (1991). Nonarteritic anterior ischemic optic neuropathy and intraocular pressure. *Arch Ophthalmol 109:*660–661.
Kao LY, Huang L, Chen TT. (1989). Anterior ischemic optic neuropathy—recurrent attacks in one eye in a bilateral case. *Ann Ophthalmol 21:*71–74.
Karel I, Otradovec J, Peleska M. (1972). Fluorescence angiography in circulatory disturbances in drusen of the optic disk. *Ophthalmologica 164:*449–462.
Kattah JC, Chrousos GA, Katz PA, McCasland B, Kolsky MP. (1994). Anterior ischemic optic neuropathy in Churg-Strauss syndrome. *Neurology 44:*2200–2202.
Kattah JC, Kennerdell JS. (1978). Orbital apex syndrome secondary to herpes zoster ophthalmicus. *Am J Ophthalmol 85:*378-382.
Katz B. (1985). Bilateral sequential migrainous ischemic optic neuropathy. *Am J Ophthalmol 99:*489.
Katz B. (1992). Anterior ischemic optic neuropathy and intraocular pressure (letter). *Arch Ophthalmol 110:*596–597.
Katz B, Bamford CR. (1985). Migrainous ischemic optic neuropathy. *Neurology 35:*112–114.
Katz B, Spencer WH. (1993). Hyperopia as a risk factor for nonarteritic anterior ischemic optic neuropathy. *Am J Ophthalmol 116:*754–758.
Katz B, Weinreb RN, Wheeler DT, Klauber MR. (1990). Anterior ischemic optic neuropathy and intraocular pressure. *Br J Ophthalmol 74:*99–102.
Katz B, Weinreb RN, Wheeler DT. (1987). Ischemic optic neuropathy and intraocular pressure. *Ophthalmology 94 (supp):*92.
Katz DM, Trobe JD, Cornblath WT, Kline LB. (1994). Ischemic optic neuropathy after lumbar spine surgery. *Arch Ophthalmol 112:*925–931.
Kay MC. (1991). Ischemic optic neuropathy. *Neurologic Clin 9:*115–129.
Kelman SE, Elman MJ. (1991). Optic nerve sheath decompression for nonarteritic ischemic optic neuropathy improves multiple visual function measurements. *Arch Ophthalmol 109:*667–671.
Keltner JL. (1988). Optic nerve sheath decompression: How well does it work? Has its time come? *Arch Ophthalmol 106:*1365–1369.
Keltner JL, Becker B, Gay AJ, Podos SM. (1972). Effect of diphenylhydantoin in ischemic optic neuritis. *Trans Am Ophthalmol Soc 70:*113–128.
Killian PJ, Susac J, Lawless OJ. (1978). Optic neuropathy in relapsing polychondritis. *JAMA 239:*49–50.
Kimbrell OC, Wheliss JA. (1967). Polyarteritis nodosa complicated by bilateral optic neuropathy. *JAMA 201:*61–62.
King J. (1979). Ischaemic optic neuropathy. *Clin Exp Neurol 16:*205–216.
Kirkali P, Kansu T. (1990). A case of unilateral posterior ischemic optic neuropathy after radical neck dissection. *Ann Ophthalmol 22:*297–298.
Kishi S, Tso MOM, Hayreh SS. (1985). Fundus lesions in malignant hypertension. II. A pathologic study of experimental hypertensive optic neuropathy. *Arch Ophthalmol 103:*1198–1206.
Klewin KM, Appen RE, Kaufman PL. (1978). Amaurosis and blood loss. *Am J Ophthalmol 86:*669–672.
Kline LB. (1980). Ischemic optic neuropathy. *Ala J Med Sci 17:*129–132.
Kline LB. (1988). Progression of visual defects in ischemic optic neuropathy. *Am J Ophthalmol 106:*199–203.
Knox DL, Duke JR. (1971). Slowly progressive ischemic optic neuropathy. A clinicopathologic case report. *Trans Am Acad Ophthalmol Otolaryngol 75:*1065–1068.

Knox DL, Hanneken AM, Holow FC, Miller NR, Schick HL, Jr, Gonzalez WL. (1988). Uremic optic neuropathy. *Arch Ophthalmol 106:*50–54.
Kollarits CR, McCarthy WR, Corrie WS, Swann ER. (1981). Norepinephrine therapy of ischemic optic neuropathy. *J Clin Neuro-ophthalmol 1:*283–288.
Kothe AC, Flanagan J, Trevino RC. (1990). True posterior ischemic optic neuropathy associated with herpes zoster ophthalmicus. *Optometry Vis Sci 67:*845–849.
Kurz O. (1969). Vascular opticopathy. *Doc Ophthalmol 26:*582–591.
Laibovitz RA. (1982). Reversible ischemic optic neuropathy in severe anemia. *Texas Med 78:*56–58.
Larkin DFP, Wood AE, Neligan M, Eustace P. (1987). Ischaemic optic neuropathy complicating cardiopulmonary bypass. *Br J Ophthalmol 71:*344–347.
Lavin PJ. (1994). Optic disk risk factors for nonarteritic anterior ischemic optic neuropathy (letter). *Am J Ophthalmol 117:*822.
Lavin PJM, Ellenberger C, Jr. (1983). Recurrent ischemic optic neuropathy. *Neuro-ophthalmology 3:*193–198.
Lazaro EJ, Cinotti AA, Eichler PN, Khawaja AA. (1971). Amaurosis due to massive gastrointestinal hemorrhage. *Am J Gastroenterol 55:*50–53.
Lee AG. (1995a). Reversible loss of vision due to posterior ischemic optic neuropathy. *Can J Ophthalmol 30:*327–329.
Lee AG. (1995b). Ischemic optic neuropathy following lumbar spine surgery. *J Neurosurg 83:*348–349.
Lee AG, Brazis PW, Miller NR. (1996). Posterior ischemic optic neuropathy associated with migraine. *Headache 36:*506–509.
Leonard TJK, Sanders MD. (1983). Ischaemic optic neuropathy in pulseless disease. *Br J Ophthalmol 67:*389–392.
Lepore FE, Yarian DL. (1985). A mimic of the "exact diagnostic sign" of Foster Kennedy. *Ann Ophthalmol 17:*411–412.
Lessell S. (1995). Surgery for ischemic optic neuropathy (editorial). *Arch Ophthalmol 113:*273–274.
Levine SR, Crofts JW, Lesser GR, Floberg J, Welch KM. (1988). Visual symptoms associated with the presence of a lupus anticoagulant. *Ophthalmology 95:*686–692.
Lichter PR, Henderson JW. (1978). Optic nerve infarction. *Am J Ophthalmol 85:*302–310.
Lieberman MF, Maumenee AE, Green WR. (1976). Histologic studies of the vasculature of the anterior optic nerve. *Am J Ophthalmol 82:*405–423.
Lieberman MF, Shahi A, Green WR. (1978). Embolic ischemic optic neuropathy. *Am J Ophthalmol 86:*206–210.
Loftman BA, Shapiro J. (1996). Ischemic optic neuropathy (letter). *J Neurosurg 84:*306.
Lubow M, Makely TA, Jr. (1971). Pseudopapilledema of juvenile diabetes mellitus. *Arch Ophthalmol 85:*417–422.
Lund PE, Madsen K. (1994). Bilateral blindness after cardiopulmonary bypass. *J Cardiothorac Vasc Anesth 8:*448–450.
McDonald WI, Sanders MD. (1971). Migraine complicated by ischaemic papillopathy. *Lancet 2:*521–523.
McHenry JG, Spoor TC. (1993a). Optic nerve sheath fenestration for treatment of progressive ischemic optic neuropathy. *Arch Ophthalmol 111:*1601–1602, 1602–1603.
McHenry JG, Spoor TC. (1993b). The efficacy of optic nerve sheath fenestration for anterior ischemic optic neuropathy and other optic neuropathies. (letter). *Am J Ophthalmol 116:*254–256.
McKay DAR, Watson PG, Lyne AJ. (1974). Relapsing polychondritis and eye disease. *Br J Ophthalmol 58:*600–606.
Manor RS. (1990). Nonarteritic ischemic optic neuropathy in identical female twins: Improvement of visual outcome in one by optic nerve decompression. (letter). *Arch Ophthalmol 108:*1067–1068.
Manor RS, Axer-Siegel R, Hart M. (1985). Anterior ischemic optic neuropathy. *Am J Ophthalmol 99:*608–609.
Mansour AM, Shoch D, Logani S. (1988). Optic disk size in ischemic optic neuropathy. *Am J Ophthalmol 106:*587–589.
Marks SC, Jaques DA, Hirata RM, Saunders JR. (1990). Blindness following bilateral radical neck dissection. *Head Neck 12:*342–345.
Michaels DD, Zugsmith GS. (1973). Optic neuropathy following cataract extraction. *Ann Ophthalmol 5:*303–306.
Michaelson C, Behrens M, Odel J. (1989). Bilateral anterior ischemic optic neuropathy associated with optic disc drusen and systemic hypotension. *Br J Ophthalmol 73:*762–764.
Miller GR, Smith JL. (1966). Ischemic optic neuropathy. *Am J Ophthalmol 62:*103–115.
Miller NR. (1980). Anterior ischemic optic neuropathy: Diagnosis and management. *Bull NY Acad Med 56:*643–654.
Miller NR. (1982). *Walsh and Hoyt's Clinical Neuro-ophthalmology,* 4th ed. Baltimore, Williams and Wilkins, pp. 212–226.
Moody TA, Irvine AR, Cahn PH, Susac JO, Horton JC. (1993). Sudden visual field constriction associated with optic disc drusen. *J Clin Neuro-ophthalmol 13:*8–13.
Moro F, Doro D. (1986). Diabetic optic neuropathies. *Metab Ped Syst Ophthalmol 9:*65–70.
Moro F, Doro D, Mantovani E, Sala M. (1989). Anterior ischemic optic neuropathy and aging. *Metab Ped Syst Ophthalmol 12:*46–57.
Moro F, Doro D, Mantovani E, Sala M. (1990). Ischemic optic neuropathies. *Metab Ped Syst Ophthalmol 13:*75–78.
Movsas T, Kelman SE, Elman MJ, Miller NR, Dickersin K, Min Y-I. (1991). The natural course of non-arteritic ischemic optic neuropathy (Abstract). *Invest Ophthalmol Vis Sci 42:*951.
Mutlukan E, Cullen JF. (1990). Can empty sella syndrome be mistaken for a progressive form of nonarteritic ischemic optic neuropathy? (letter) *Arch Ophthalmol 108:*1066–1067.

Naumann GO, Jonas J. (1989). Optic disk size in ischemic optic neuropathy (letter). *Am J Ophthalmol 107:*685–686.
Nawa Y, Jaques JD, Miller NR, et al. (1992). Bilateral posterior optic neuropathy after bilateral radical neck dissection and hypotension. *Graefes Arch Clin Exp Ophthalmol 230:*301–308.
Neuman RW, Maggiano JM, Frenkel M. (1978). Bilateral acute anterior ischemic neuropathy in diabetes: Case report. *Ann Ophthalmol 10:*1501–1504.
O'Hara M, O'Connor PS. (1984). Migrainous optic neuropathy. *J Clin Neuro-ophthalmol 4:*85–90.
Palimeris G, Chimonidou E, Droutsas D. (1979). Some observations on the treatment of ischemic optic neuropathy. *Ann Ophthalmol 11:*1539–1544.
Parsons JT, Bova FL, Fitzgerald CR, Mendenhall WM, Million RR. (1994). Radiation optic neuropathy after megavoltage external-beam irradiation: Analysis of time-dose factors. *Int J Rad Onc Biol Phy 30:*755–763.
Pavan PR, Aiello LM, Wafai Z, Briones JC, Sebestyen JG, Bradbury MJ. (1980). Optic disc edema in juvenile-onset diabetes. *Arch Ophthalmol 98:*2193–2195.
Perez-Santonja JJ, Bueno JL, Meza J, Garcia-Sandoval B, Serrano JM, Zato MA. (1993). Ischemic optic neuropathy after intraocular lens implantation to correct high myopia in a phakic patient. *J Cat Refract Surg, 19:*651–654.
Perlman JI, Forman S, Gonzalez ER. (1994). Retrobulbar ischemic optic neuropathy associated with sickle cell disease. *J Neuro-ophthalmol 14:*45–48.
Pickrell L, Purvin V. (1987). Ischemic optic neuropathy secondary to intracarotid infusion of BCNU. *J Clin Neuro-ophthalmol 7:*87–92.
Pitcher D, Curry P. (1979). Blindness after treatment for malignant hypertension. *Br Med J 2:*245–246.
Portnoy SL, Beer PM, Packer AJ, Van Dyk HJL. (1989). Embolic anterior ischemic optic neuropathy. *J Clin Neuro-ophthalmol 9:*21–25.
Presencia AC, Hernandez AM, Guia ED. (1985). Amaurosis following blood loss. *Ophthalmologica, 191:*119–121.
Pryor JS, Davies PD, Hamilton DV. (1979). Blindness and malignant hypertension. *Lancet 2:*803.
Purvin VA. (1995). Anterior ischemic optic neuropathy secondary to interferon alpha. *Arch Ophthalmol 113:*1041–1044.
Quigley HA, Anderson DR. (1977). Cupping of the optic disc in ischemic optic neuropathy. *Trans Am Acad Ophthalmol Otolaryngol 83:*755–762.
Quigley HA, Miller NR, Green WR. (1985). The pattern of optic nerve fiber loss in anterior ischemic optic neuropathy. *Am J Ophthalmol 109:*769–776.
Ramsell TG. (1967). Complications of herpes zoster ophthalmicus. *Am J Ophthalmol 63:*1796–1798.
Repka MX, Savino PJ, Schatz NJ, Sergott RC. (1983). Clinical profile and long-term implications of anterior ischemic optic neuropathy. *Am J Ophthalmol 96:*478–483.
Rinaldi G, Pastori G, Ammirati M, Bellavitis A. (1990). Considerations upon a non-typical anterior ischemic optic neuropathy. *Metab Ped Syst Ophthalmol 13:*92–95.
Rivkin MJ, Hedges TR III, Logigian EL. (1990). Carotid dissection presenting as posterior ischemic optic neuropathy. *Neurology 40:*1469.
Rizzo JF, III, Lessell S. (1991). Optic neuritis and ischemic optic neuropathy: Overlapping clinical profiles. *Arch Ophthalmol 109:*1668–1672.
Rizzo JF, III, Lessell S. (1987). Posterior ischemic optic neuropathy during general surgery. *Am J Ophthalmol 103:*808–811.
Rootman J, Butler D. (1980). Ischaemic optic neuropathy—a combined mechanism. *Br J Ophthalmol 64:*826–831.
Rosenberg MA, Savino PJ, Glaser JS. (1979). A clinical analysis of pseudopapilledema I. Population, laterality, acuity, refractive error, ophthalmoscopic characteristics, and coincident diseases. *Arch Ophthalmol 97:*65–70.
Rosler SH, Conway MD, Anaya JM, et al. (1995). Ischemic optic neuropathy and high-level anticardiolipin antibodies in primary Sjogren's syndrome. *Lupus 4:*155–157.
Ross HS, Rosenberg S, Friedman AH. (1973). Delayed radiation necrosis of the optic nerve. *Am J Ophthalmol 76:*683–686.
Roth GJ, Calverly DC. (1994). Aspirin, platelets, and thrombosis: Theory and practice. *Blood 83:*885–898.
Sadun AA. (1993). The efficacy of optic nerve sheath decompression for anterior ischemic optic neuropathy and other optic neuropathies. *Am J Ophthalmol 115:*384–389.
Sanders MD. (1971). Ischaemic papillopathy. *Trans Ophthalmol Soc UK 91:*369–386.
Sanderson M, Kupersmith M, Frohman L, et al. (1995). Aspirin reduces anterior ischemic optic neuropathy in the second eye. ARVO abstracts. *Invest Ophthalmol Vis Sci 36:*S196.
Sarkies NJC, Sanders MD. (1987). Optic disc drusen and episodic visual loss. *Br J Ophthalmol 71:*537–539.
Savino PJ, Burde RM, Mills RP. (1990). Visual loss following intranasal anesthetic injection. *J Clin Neuro-ophthalmol 10:*140–144.
Sawle GV, James CB, Ross-Russell RW. (1990). The natural history of nonarteritic anterior ischemic optic neuropathy. *J Neurol Neurosurg Psychiatr 53:*830–833.
Sawle GV, Sarkies NJC. (1987). Posterior ischaemic optic neuropathy due to internal carotid artery occlusion. *Neuro-ophthalmology 7:*349–353.
Schatz NJ, Smith JL. (1967). Non-tumor causes of the Foster Kennedy syndrome. *J Neurosurg 27:*37–44.
Schnobel GA, Schmidbauer M, Millesi W, Undt G. (1995). Posterior ischemic optic neuropathy following bilateral radical neck dissection. *Int J Oral Maxillofacial Surg 24:*283–287.
Scouras J, Koutroumanos J. (1976). Ischaemic optic neuropathy in Behcet's syndrome. *Ophthalmologica 173:*11–18.

Sebag J, Thomas JV, Epstein DL, Grant WM. (1986). Optic disc cupping in arteritic anterior ischemic optic neuropathy resembles glaucomatous cupping. *Ophthalmology 93:*357–361.

Segato T, Peirmarochhi S, Midena E. (1990). The role of fluorescein angiography in the interpretation of optic nerve head diseases. *Metab Pediatr Syst Ophthalmol 13:*111–114.

Sergott RC, Cohen MS, Bosley TM, Savino PJ. (1989). Optic nerve decompression may improve the progressive form of nonarteritic ischemic optic neuropathy. *Arch Ophthalmol 107:*1743–1754.

Serrano LA, Behrens MM, Carroll FD. (1982). Post-cataract extraction ischemic optic neuropathy (letter). *Arch Ophthalmol 100:*1177.

Servilla KS, Groggel GC. (1986). Anterior ischemic optic neuropathy as a complication of hemodialysis. *Am J Kidney Dis 8:*61–63.

Shahian DM, Speert PK. (1989). Symptomatic visual deficits after open heart operations. *Ann Thorac Surg 48:*275–279.

Shapira OM, Kimmel WA, Lindsey PS, Shahian DM. (1996). Anterior ischemic optic neuropathy after open heart operations. *Ann Thoracic Surg 61:*660–666.

Shoch D. (1983). Ischemic optic neuropathy. Common cause of visual loss in the elderly. *Postgrad Med 74:*74–75.

Shults WT. (1977). Ischemic optic neuropathy: Some interesting features. *Trans Pacific Coast Oto-ophthalmol Soc 58:*281–298.

Shults WT. (1984). Ischemic optic neuropathy: Still the ophthalmologist's dilemma. *Ophthalmology 91:*1338–1341.

Slavin ML. (1987). Chronic asymptomatic ischemic optic neuropathy. A report of two cases in adults with diabetes mellitus. *J Clin Neuro-ophthalmol 7:*198–201.

Slavin ML. (1987). Ischemic optic neuropathy after cardiac arrest. *Am J Ophthalmol 104:*435–436.

Slavin ML, Barondes MJ. (1988). Ischemic optic neuropathy in sickle cell disease. *Am J Ophthalmol 105:*212–213.

Slavin ML, Lopinto RJ, Prywes AS, Rosen DA. (1985). Optic disc edema with aphakic cystoid maculopathy masquerading as ischemic optic neuropathy. *J Clin Neuro-ophthalmol 5:*180–184.

Smith DB. (1995). Ischemic optic neuropathy decompression trial (letter). *JAMA 274:*612.

Smith FP. (1996). Ischemic optic neuropathy (letter). *J Neurosurg 84:*149–150.

Smith JL. (1981). Norepinephrine therapy of ischemic optic neuropathy (editorial). *J Clin Neuro-ophthalmol 1:*289–290.

Smith JL. (1985). Pseudohemangioma of the optic disc following ischemic optic neuropathy. *J Clin Neuro-ophthalmol 5:*81–89.

Smith JL, Goldhammer Y. (1975). Hypertensive optic neuropathy. *Trans Am Acad Ophthalmol Otolaryngol 79:*520–523.

Sonty S, Schwartz B. (1983). Development of cupping and pallor in posterior ischemic optic neuropathy. *Int Ophthalmol 6:*213–220.

Spedick MJ, Tomsak RL. (1984). Ischemic optic neuropathy following secondary intraocular lens implantation. *J Clin Neuro-ophthalmol 4:*255–257.

Spoor TC, McHenry JG, Lau-Sickon L. (1993). Progressive and static nonarteritic ischemic optic neuropathy treated by optic nerve sheath decompression. *Ophthalmology 100:*306–311.

Spoor TC, Wilkinson MJ, Ramocki JM. (1991). Optic nerve sheath decompression for the treatment of progressive nonarteritic ischemic optic neuropathy. *Am J Ophthalmol 111:*724–728.

Sundaram DM, Avram D, Cziffer A. (1986). Unilateral ischemic optic neuropathy following systemic hypotension. *J R Soc Med 79:*250.

Swartz NG, Beck RW, Savino RC, et al. (1995). Pain in anterior ischemic optic neuropathy. *J Neuro-ophthalmol 15:*9–10.

Sweeney PJ, Breuer AC, Selhorst JB, et al. (1982). Ischemic optic neuropathy: A complication of cardiopulmonary bypass surgery. *Neurology 32:*560–562.

Talks SJ, Chong NHV, Gibson JM, et al. (1995). Fibrinogen, cholesterol, and smoking as risk factors for non-arteritic anterior ischemic optic neuropathy. *Eye 9:*85.

Tang RA. (1995). Interferon: Friend or foe? *Arch Ophthalmol 113:*987.

Taylor D, Ramsay J, Day S, Dillon M. (1981). Infarction of the optic nerve head in children with accelerated hypertension. *Br J Ophthalmol 65:*153–160.

Tice DA. (1987). Ischemic optic neuropathy and cardiac surgery (letter). *Ann Thorac Surg 44:*677.

Tomsak RL. (1985). Ischemic optic neuropathy associated with retinal embolism. *Am J Ophthalmol 99:*590–592.

Tomsak RL, Remler BF. (1989). Anterior ischemic optic neuropathy and increased intraocular pressure. *J Clin Neuro-ophthalmol 9:*116–118.

Traustason OI, Feldon SE, Leemaster JE, Weiner JM. (1988). Anterior ischemic optic neuropathy: Classification of field defects by Octopus automated static perimetry. *Graefe's Arch Clin Exp Ophthalmol 226:*206–212.

Varga M. (1976). Recent experiences on the ophthalmologic complications of oral contraceptives. *Ann Ophthalmol 10:*925–934.

Victor DI, Welch RB. (1977). Bilateral retinal hemorrhages and disk edema in migraine. *Am J Ophthalmol 84:*555–558.

Wall M, Newman SA. (1991). Optic nerve sheath decompression for the treatment of progressive nonarteritic ischemic optic neuropathy (letter). *Am J Ophthalmol 112:*741–742.

Walsh FB, Hoyt WF. (1969). *Clinical Neuro-ophthalmology,* 3rd ed. Williams and Wilkins, Baltimore, vol. 2, pp. 673, 1828.

Ward SC, Woods DR, Gilstrap LC III, Hauth HC. (1984). Pregnancy and acute optic disc edema of juvenile-onset diabetes. *Obstet Gynecol 64:*816–818.
Waybright EA, Selhorst JB, Combs J. (1982). Anterior ischemic optic neuropathy with internal carotid artery occlusion. *Am J Ophthalmol 93:*42–47.
Weinstein JM, Chui H, Lane S, Corbett J, Towfighi J. (1983). Churg-Strauss syndrome (allergic granulomatous angiitis). Neuro-ophthalmologic manifestations. *Arch Ophthalmol 101:*1217–1220.
Weinstein JM, Feman SS. (1982). Ischemic optic neuropathy in migraine. *Arch Ophthalmol 100:*1097–1100.
Weinstein JM, Morris GL, ZuRhein GM, Gentry LR. (1989). Posterior ischemic optic neuropathy due to Aspergillus fumigatus. *J Clin Neuro-ophthalmol 9:*7–13.
Wessells IF. (1987). Posterior ischemic optic neuropathy during general surgery (letter). *Am J Ophthalmol 104:*555–556.
Williams EL, Hart WM, Jr, Tempelhoff R. (1995). Postoperative ischemic optic neuropathy. *Anesth Analges 80:*1018–1029.
Wilson JF, Freeman SB, Breene DP. (1991). Anterior ischemic optic neuropathy causing blindness in the head and neck surgery patient. *Arch Otolaryngol Head Neck Surg 117:*1304–1306.
Wilson WB. (1990). Does optic nerve sheath decompression help progressive ischemic optic neuropathy? (letter). *Arch Ophthalmol 108:*1065–1066.
Wolfe S, Schulte-Strake U, Bertram B, et al. (1993). Hemodilution therapy in patients with acute anterior ischemic optic neuropathy. *Ophthalmology 90:*21–26.
Wylie AM, McLeod D, Cullen JF. (1972). Traumatic ischaemic optic neuropathy. *Br J Ophthalmol 56:*851–853.
Yee RD, Selky AK, Purvin VA. (1993). Outcomes of surgical and nonsurgical management of nonarteritic ischemic optic neuropathy. *Trans Am Ophthalmol Soc 91:*227–243.

◆ 5 ◆

Arteritic Anterior Ischemic Optic Neuropathy and Giant Cell Arteritis

Giant cell (temporal or cranial) arteritis (GCA) is an inflammatory vasculopathy of the elderly that affects medium to large-sized arteries. GCA may present with numerous systemic and ocular manifestations (Aburahma, 1992, 1996; Aiello, 1993; Allison, 1984; Andrews, 1966; Astion, 1994; Barricks, 1977; Barton, 1991; Bengtsson, 1981a,b,c; Berlit, 1992; Buchbinder, 1992; Calamia, 1980; Clearkin, 1992b; Cohen, 1973; Cullen, 1967, 1972; Diamond, 1991, 1993; DiBartolomeo, 1992; Eshaghian, 1979; Evans, 1993; Fernandez-Herlighy, 1988; Gabriel, 1995; Gaynes, 1994; Goodman, 1979; Graham, 1980; Hart, 1967; Hayreh, 1991; Healey, 1977; Hellman, 1993; Hunder, 1985, 1986, 1990; Ishak, 1988; Jonasson, 1979; Kachroo, 1996; Keltner, 1982; Koorey, 1984; Kyle, 1993; Machado, 1988; Matzkin, 1992; McDonnell, 1986; Meadows, 1966; Mizen, 1991; Model, 1978; Myles, 1992; Nadeau, 1988; Nielsen, 1979; Nordborg, 1990; Ostberg, 1971; Postel, 1993; Pountain, 1995; Rosenfeld, 1986; Rousseau, 1994; Russell, 1966, 1969; Salvarani, 1995; Schmidt, 1994; Schneider, 1971; Siatkowski, 1993; Slavin, 1988; Sonnenblick, 1994; Stevens, 1995; Tang, 1988; Wagener, 1958; Wang, 1979; Weinberg, 1994; Wilkinson, 1972; Zion, 1974). Here we concentrate on the ocular manifestations, diagnosis, and treatment of GCA. Less emphasis is placed on nonocular involvement by GCA.

What Clinical Features Suggest Giant Cell Arteritis?

GCA usually causes visual loss due to anterior ischemic optic neuropathy (AION). All patients older than age 50 years with AION should be suspected of having GCA. The index of suspicion is greater with increasing numbers of typical features of GCA listed in Table 5–1. (Aburahma, 1992, 1996; Aiello, 1993; Allison, 1984; Andrews, 1966; Astion, 1994; Barricks, 1977; Barton, 1991; Bengtsson, 1981a; Berlit, 1992; Buchbinder, 1992; Calamia, 1980; Clearkin, 1992b; Cohen, 1973; Cullen, 1967, 1972; Diamond, 1991, 1993; DiBartolomeo, 1992; Eshaghian, 1979; Evans, 1993; Gabriel, 1995; Gaynes, 1994; Goodman,

Table 5–1. Typical Features of Giant Cell Arteritis

Age greater than 50 years (median 75 years)
Acute, often severe visual loss [usually anterior ischemic optic neuropathy (AION)]
Unilateral or bilateral visual loss (higher incidence of bilateral than non-arteritic-AION)
Pallid swelling of the optic nerve (may be "chalk white")
Optic atrophy eventually and some develop glaucomatous-like optic cupping (Sebag, 1986)
Constitutional signs and symptoms (Keltner, 1981)
Headache (4–100%)
Scalp or temporal artery tenderness (28–91%)
Weight loss (16–76%)
Jaw claudication (4–67%) (Lee, 1995; Selsky, 1985; Sofferman, 1980)
Anorexia (14–69%)
Fever (low grade) and diaphoresis (Esposito, 1978; Fife, 1994; Goodman, 1979)
Proximal muscle aches or weakness (28–86%)
Polymyalgia rheumatica (Chuang, 1982; Fessell, 1967; Hunder, 1967, 1989, 1973; Huston, 1978; Keltner, 1981)
Morning stiffness lasting 30 minutes or more
Proximal joint pain (e.g., shoulders, hips, neck or torso)
Fatigue and malaise (12–97%)
Leg claudication (2–43%) (Hamilton, 1971; Huston, 1978)
Elevated erythrocyte sedimentation rate (usually > 50 mm/hr by Westergren method)
Temporal artery biopsy positive

1979; Graham, 1980; Hart, 1967; Hayreh, 1991; Healey, 1977; Hellman, 1993; Hunder, 1985, 1986, 1990; Ishak, 1988; Jonasson, 1979; Kachroo, 1996; Kyle, 1993; Matzkin, 1992; McDonnell, 1986; Meadows, 1966; Mizen, 1991; Model, 1978; Myles, 1992; Nielsen, 1979; Nordborg, 1990; Ostberg, 1971; Postel, 1993; Pountain, 1995; Rosenfeld, 1986; Rousseau, 1994; Russell, 1966, 1969; Salvarani, 1995; Schneider, 1971; Siatkowski, 1993; Slavin, 1988; Sonnenblick, 1994; Stevens, 1995; Tang, 1988; Wagener, 1958; Wang, 1979; Weinberg, 1994; Wilkinson, 1972; Zion, 1974).

Is the Clinical Suspicion for GCA High?

In 1990 the American College of Rheumatology (Hunder, 1990a) analyzed 214 patients with GCA (196 proven by positive temporal artery biopsy) and compared them with 593 patients with other forms of vasculitis. In their analysis of 33 criteria, the highest sensitivity criteria for GCA were:

1. Age > 50 years (mean age 69 years, 90% > 60 years)
2. Westergren erythrocyte sedimentation rate (ESR) > 50 mm/hr
3. Abnormal temporal artery biopsy (TAB)

The highest specificity clinical criteria were:

1. Jaw and/or tongue claudication
2. Visual abnormalities (e.g., AION, amaurosis, optic atrophy)
3. Temporal artery abnormalities (e.g., decreased pulse, tenderness, or nodules)

If at least three or more criteria of the following five were met, the specificity of diagnosis was 91.2% and the sensitivity was 93.5%:

1. Age > 50 years
2. New headache (localized)
3. Temporal artery abnormality (see above)
4. Elevated ESR (> 50 mm/hr)
5. Abnormal temporal artery biopsy (e.g., necrotizing arteritis, multinucleated giant cells)

Fernandez-Herlihy increased the specificity for diagnosis of GCA by defining symptom clusters. (For example, jaw claudication with any of the following (Fernandez-Herlihy, 1988):

1. Recent headaches and scalp tenderness
2. Scalp tenderness and ESR > 50 mm/hr
3. Visual symptoms and ESR > 50 mm/hr

A specificity of 90 to 100% could be obtained if the cluster included elevated ESR, scalp tenderness, jaw claudication, recent visual changes, polymyalgia rheumatica, and a good response to steroid therapy. A 94.8% sensitivity and 100% specificity were obtained if the symptom cluster included new onset headache, jaw claudication, and abnormal temporal artery examination (Mizen, 1991). Vilaseca, et al. felt that simultaneous jaw claudication, abnormal temporal arteries on exam, and new headache had a specificity of 94.8% for positive TAB (Vilaseca, 1987). Chmelewski, et al. compared the initial clinical features of 30 patients with positive TAB and 68 with negative TAB (Chmelewski, 1992). TAB-positive patients had significantly increased incidence of headache (93% vs. 62%) and jaw claudication (50% vs. 18%). Jaw claudication had a specificity of 56% as a differentiating feature, but the specificity of headache was low (40%). Hayreh, et al. reported that jaw claudication ($p < 0.001$) and neck pain (mostly in the occipital and back parts of the neck; $p = .0003$) were significant indicators of a positive TAB independent of ESR and age, and that these clinical signs were more highly correlated to a positive TAB than anorexia, weight loss, fever, and scalp tenderness (Hayreh, 1997). Hayreh, et al. felt that the odds of a positive TAB were 9 times greater with jaw claudication, 3.3 times greater with neck pain, 3.2 times greater with a C-reactive protein (CRP) > 2.45 mg/dl, 2.1 times greater with an ESR of 47 to 107 mm/hr, 2.7 times greater with an ESR > 107 mm/hr, and 2.0 times greater when the patient was greater than 75 years old (compared with age below 75 years). The typical features of GCA are listed in Table 5–1.

Acute visual loss is reported in 7 to 60% (average 36%) of patients with GCA (Goodman, 1979). Although the usual cause of visual loss in GCA is AION or central retinal artery occlusion (CRAO) (Charness, 1991; Clearkin, 1992a; Graham, 1980; Jonasson, 1979; Liu, 1994; Wilkinson, 1972), posterior ischemic optic neuropathy (PION), choroidal or rarely occipital lobe ischemia may also occur (Miller, 1991; Wagener, 1958). Although visual loss and AION in GCA tends to be more severe than that seen in NA-AION, the severity of visual loss is not a differentiating feature. Up to 25% of GCA patients have visual acuities of 20/40 or better and 20% of NA-AION patients have initial visual acuities of counting fingers or worse (Hayreh, 1990). The clinical features favoring arteritic AION over NA-AION are listed in Table 5–2.

Other less common ocular features of GCA are indicated in Table 5–3.

The differential diagnosis for these ocular conditions (especially unexplained diplopia, retinal or choroidal ischemia, or transient visual loss) should include GCA. Goldberg reviewed the literature in 1983 on ocular motor paresis in GCA (Goldberg, 1983) and found ocular muscle involvement was reported in 59 patients. The duration of symptoms

Table 5–2. Features Suggestive of Arteritic AION Instead of NA-AION

Elderly patients with constitutional symptoms (Cullen, 1967, 1976; Hamilton, 1971) (especially scalp tenderness or jaw claudication)
Polymyalgia rheumatica
Elevated ESR and/or CRP
Amaurosis fugax (Ronchetto, 1992)
Ocular findings (Hayreh, 1990):
- Posterior ischemic optic neuropathy (PION)
- Cup to disc ratio greater than 0.2 in fellow eye
- Severe or bilateral simultaneous visual loss
- Markedly pallid optic disc edema (chalky white)
- Fluorescein angiography findings of choroidal nonperfusion (Eagling, 1974; Hayreh, 1974, 1990; Mack, 1991; Segato, 1990; Siatkowski, 1993)
- AION associated with choroidal nonfilling
- Simultaneous non-embolic CRAO or cilioretinal artery occlusion
- Simultaneous choroidal or retinal infarction

Table 5–3. Other Ocular Features of GCA

Visual loss
- Transient visual loss (Beevers, 1973; Healey, 1977; Hollenhorst, 1960; Hutson, 1978; Thystrup, 1994; Turner, 1974)
- Non-embolic branch or central retinal artery occlusion (Cohen, 1973; Cullen, 1967, 1976; Fineman, 1996; Miller, 1991; Wang, 1979)
- Combined central retinal artery and vein occlusion (Cullen, 1966)
- Ophthalmic artery occlusion (Macfaul, 1967)
- Choroidal or retinal ischemia (Fastenberg, 1982; Quillen, 1993; Slavin, 1994; Spolaore 1984; Tang, 1982)
- Cotton wool spots (Cohen, 1975; Hollenhorst, 1960; MacLeod, 1993, 1996; Melberg, 1995; Thystrup, 1994)
- Posture related retinal ischemia (Hollenhorst, 1967)
- General anesthesia induced ischemic optic neuropathy (Cullen, 1976; McGowan, 1967; Wessels, 1987)
- Pre- and perichiasmal ischemia and visual field defects (Boghen, 1975; Hayreh, 1981)
- Postchiasmal ischemic visual field defects (Chisholm, 1975; Goodman, 1979)

Anterior segment ischemia (Birt, 1994; Cullen, 1976; Verdich, 1975; Winter, 1977; Zion, 1974)
- Episcleritis and scleritis (Long, 1976)
- Iritis (Hamilton, 1971)
- Conjunctivitis (Hamilton, 1971)
- Glaucoma
- Transient bilateral corneal edema (Verdich, 1975)
- Acute hypotony (Radda, 1981)
- Marginal corneal ulceration (Gerstle, 1980; Tomsak, 1997)
- Uveitic glaucoma (Tomsak, 1997)

Autonomic pupil abnormalities (Rabinowich, 1988)
- Tonic pupil (Currie, 1984)
- Light-near dissociation (Bronster, 1983)

- Horner syndrome (Bromfield, 1988)
- Miosis (Desser, 1969)
- Mydriasis (Mehler, 1988)

Diplopia (Beevers, 1973; Graham, 1980; Healey, 1977; Hollenhorst, 1960; Huston, 1978; Jay, 1986; Lockshin, 1970, 1974; Mehler, 1988; Turner, 1974)

- Orbital ischemia (Andrews, 1966; Barricks, 1977; Goldberg, 1983)
- Ophthalmoplegia (Goadsby, 1991; Hollenhorst, 1960; Rush, 1979; Sibony, 1984) due to ischemia to cranial nerves III, IV, and/or VI (Diamond, 1991; Dimant, 1978; Goodman, 1979; Graham, 1980)
- Brainstem ischemia (rare) (Monteiro, 1984)
  - Internuclear ophthalmoplegia (Askari, 1993; Crompton, 1989; Johnston, 1992; Thomson, 1989; Trend, 1990)
  - Nystagmus (Meadows, 1966)
- Subjective diplopia by history (Hollenhorst, 1960)
  - Transient diplopia with or without ptosis (Cullen, 1967; Martin, 1970)
  - Transient oculomotor synkinesis (Sibony, 1984)
- Laboratory measures of ischemia
  - Color Doppler hemodynamics (Ho, 1994)
  - Decreased ocular pulse (Bienfang, 1989)
  - Decreased ocular pulse amplitudes (Bosley, 1989)
- Orbital involvement
  - Orbital pseudotumor (Chertok, 1990; Clark, 1987; Gibbs, 1974; Laidlaw, 1990)
  - Orbital infarction (Borruat, 1993; Chertok, 1990; Laidlaw, 1990)
  - Ocular ischemic syndrome (Hamed, 1992)
  - Reversible bruit (Gilbert, 1970)

---

was transitory to several months. Many cases had other signs to suggest GCA (e.g., headache, scalp tenderness, optic nerve or retinal involvement). The diplopia was often transient, variable, and sometimes not associated with motility examination abnormalities. The optic nerve or central retinal artery involvement followed within several days in many patients. Graham described ten patients with ophthalmoplegia (four pupil-sparing third nerve palsies, four sixth nerve palsies, and two multiple ocular motor nerve palsies) (Graham, 1980). We do not routinely obtain an ESR on patients with transient or persistent diplopia without systemic signs of GCA in whom there is a clear alternative etiology (e.g., other vasculopathic risk factors). Nevertheless, we consider the diagnosis of GCA in all patients over 55 years with unexplained diplopia.

Caselli and Hunder reviewed the neurologic aspects of GCA and emphasized the often underrecognized fact that GCA affects the aortic arch and its branches, not just the superficial temporal arteries. Although GCA does not cause a widespread intracranial vasculitis, it may involve the cervicocephalic arteries including the carotid artery and vertebral arteries (Caselli, 1993). Less commonly recognized findings of GCA are listed in Table 5–4.

Is the ESR Always Elevated in GCA?

Although the ESR is often elevated in GCA (Bedell, 1985; Brittain, 1967, 1991; Cullen, 1976; Eshaghian, 1979; Huston, 1978; Jonasson, 1979; Sox, 1986; Weinstein, 1994), patients with

Table 5–4. Less Common Features of GCA

- Large vessel involvement (Butt, 1991; Lambert, 1996)
  - Carotid siphon (Vincent, 1986)
  - Bruits (Caselli, 1988)
  - Facial artery (Achkar, 1995)
  - Occipital artery pain and occipital neuralgia (Blaiss, 1982; Jundt, 1991)
  - Subclavian or axillary artery (Ninet, 1990)
  - Aortitis or aortic rupture (Evans, 1995; Gersbach, 1993; Kent, 1967; Klein, 1975; Lagrand, 1996; Lie, 1995; Liu, 1995; Mitnich, 1990; Richardson, 1996)
  - Limb claudication or gangrene (Hunder, 1967; Lie, 1995; Walz-Leblanc, 1991)
  - Central nervous system arteritis (Caselli, 1988, 1990, 1993; Enzmann, 1977; Fulton, 1976; Hussein, 1990; Reich, 1990)
    - Acute encephalopathy (Caselli, 1990; Gibb, 1985; Tomer, 1992)
    - Aseptic meningitis (Fulton, 1976)
    - Cerebellar infarction (McLean, 1993)
    - Diabetes insipidus (Gentric, 1988)
    - Occipital infarction (McAlindon, 1989) and cortical blindness (Chisholm, 1975)
    - Myelopathy (Caselli, 1988)
      - Cervical radiculopathy (Rivest, 1995; Sanchez, 1983)
      - Quadriplegia (Brennan, 1982)
      - Transverse myelopathy
      - Spinal cord infarction (Gibb, 1985)
    - Neuropsychiatric syndromes (Cochran, 1978)
      - Hallucinations (Cullen, 1976; Hart, 1967)
      - Depression (Calamia, 1981; Caselli, 1988; Cherry, 1980; Hamilton, 1971)
      - Behavioral changes
      - Psychosis and confusion
    - Seizures (Fulton, 1976)
    - Transient ischemic attacks (Caselli, 1988)
    - Tremor
    - Neuro-otologic symptoms (Caselli, 1988)
      - Deafness (Caselli, 1988; Reich, 1990)
      - Tinnitus
      - Vertigo
    - Brainstem (Dick, 1991; Shenberger, 1981; Wilkinson, 1972)
      - Ataxia, nystagmus, upgaze palsy (Monteiro, 1984)
    - Vertebrobasilar involvement (Sheehan, 1993)
      - Acute confusional states (Caselli, 1988, 1990; Small, 1984)
- Pain syndromes (headache, neck pain, backache) (Calamia, 1980; Caselli, 1993)
- Peripheral neuropathies (Caselli, 1988; Golbus, 1987; Nesher, 1987; Warrell, 1968; Wilske, 1971)
  - Sciatic neuropathy (Massey, 1978)
  - Carpal tunnel syndrome (Ahmed, 1978; Dennis, 1996; Kovarsky, 1973)
- Respiratory tract (Gur, 1996; Hunder, 1989; Karam, 1982; Larson, 1984; Rischmueller, 1996; Zenone, 1994)
  - Cough
  - Hoarseness
  - Tongue ischemia (Arnung, 1979; Caselli, 1988)
- Seronegative polyarthritis (Ginsburg, 1985)

Coronary arteritis and myocardial infarction (Spencer, 1965)
Visceral involvement (Lie, 1978)
  Renal involvement (Klein, 1975; Lin, 1995; Truong, 1985)
  Visceral angiitis (O'Neill, 1976)
  Liver involvement (Ilan, 1993; von Knorring, 1972)
  Small bowel infarction (Phelan, 1993; Srigley, 1980)
  Tongue necrosis (Llorente, 1994)
  Submandibular swelling (Ruiz-Masera, 1995)
Ischemic skin lesions (Hansen, 1995) and scalp necrosis (Boghen, 1975)
Mortality (Bisgard, 1991; Graham, 1980, 1981; Matteson, 1996; Nordborg, 1989)
  Myocardial infarction and mesenteric infarction (Save-Soderbergh, 1986)
  GCA is rare in black individuals (Ballou, 1978; Bell, 1967; Dimant, 1978; Goodman, 1978; Lie, 1995; McDonnell, 1986; Sanford, 1977)

biopsy proven GCA may have a normal ESR (2–30%) (Bethlenfalvay, 1964; Biller, 1982; Brittain, 1991; Cohen, 1973; Cullen, 1967; Ellis, 1983; Espinoza, 1982; Gill, 1977; Ginsberg, 1985; Grodrum, 1990; Hamrin, 1968; Hayreh, 1997; Jundt, 1991; Kansu, 1977; Kattwinkel, 1970; Keltner, 1981; Litwin, 1992; Liu, 1994; Neish, 1991; Nelson, 1982; Permin, 1973; Sox, 1986; Turner, 1974; Watson, 1984; Weintreb, 1978; Wise, 1991; Wong, 1986; Zweegman, 1993). Cullen found an average ESR of 84 mm/hr in TAB proven GCA (Cullen, 1967).

What Is the Normal Value for an ESR?

The ESR rises with increasing age (Bottinger, 1967; Boyd, 1966; Miller, 1983; Sox, 1986). The Westergren method is preferred over the Wintrobe method because of the more limited scale of the Wintrobe ESR (Bull, 1974). Boyd and Hofbrand reported a Westergren ESR normal of 40 mm/hr for persons over age 65 years (Boyd, 1966). Bottiger and Svedberg felt that 30 mm/hr for women and 20 mm/hr for men was a reasonable limit (Bottiger, 1967). Hayreh felt that a patient with an ESR > 40 mm/hr should be considered to "suffer from temporal arteritis, unless proven otherwise" (Hayreh, 1975).

Miller et al. measured Westergren ESR in 27,912 adults aged 20 to 65 years (Miller, 1983). None of the subjects were anemic. A series of curves of ESR versus age were derived for men and women with maximum values for 98% of the population. An empiric formula (98% curve) for deriving the maximum ESR normal is listed below (Miller, 1983; Sox, 1986):

MEN: age divided by 2
WOMEN: age + 10 divided by 2

Hayreh et al. suggested a cut-off criteria for an elevated ESR of 33 mm/hr for men and 35 mm/hr for women with a sensitivity and specificity of 92% (Hayreh, 1997). In addition, the ESR value at the time of diagnosis may not correlate with the clinical features or prognosis for visual loss in GCA (Ellis, 1983; Jacobson, 1987). Other markers (e.g., CRP, von Willebrand factor) have also been proposed in the evaluation of GCA (Eshaghian, 1980; Federici, 1984). Jacobson and Slamovits found an inverse correlation between ESR and hematocrit and felt that the "ESR may not reliably indicate active disease in a patient with a normal hematocrit" (Jacobson, 1987). Finally, it should be emphasized that the diagnosis of GCA is a clinical diagnosis and reliance for such a diagnosis should not be placed on the ESR alone. If the clinical suspicion for GCA is high, a repeat ESR, TAB, and treatment with empiric prednisone should begin regardless of the initial ESR value (Hall, 1983; Ikard, 1988; Karanjia, 1989; Kent, 1989).

Are There Other Hematologic Tests for the Diagnosis of GCA?

Another acute phase reactant, CRP has also been advocated as a marker for GCA (Deodhar, 1989; Eshaghian, 1980; Espinoza, 1982; Hayreh, 1997). Hayreh et al. felt that an elevated CRP (above 2.45 mg/dl) was more sensitive (100%) than the ESR (92%) for the detection of GCA, and that a CRP combined with an ESR gave the best specificity for diagnosis (97%) (Hayreh, 1997).

Other hematologic tests listed in Table 5–5 have been reported in association with GCA, but are of uncertain significance [e.g., serum amyloid, von Willebrand's factor, plasma viscosity, antineutrophil cytoplasmic antibodies, and various human lymphocyte antigen (HLA) types].

Is a TAB Necessary in a Patient with a High Clinical Suspicion for GCA? Should a Unilateral or Bilateral TAB Be Performed?

TAB is a relatively easy and safe procedure to perform with a low morbidity (Hall, 1984; Ikard, 1988). There is one case of stroke after TAB, but this is a rare complication (Haist,

Table 5–5. Laboratory Abnormalities in GCA

Laboratory Abnormalities in GCA
Anticardiolipin antibodies (Kerleau, 1994; McHugh, 1990)
Antineutrophilic antibodies (Bosch, 1991; McHugh, 1990)
Mild to moderate normochromic, normocytic anemia (Healey, 1971; Weiss, 1995)
Elevated white blood cell count and platelet count
Elevated acute phase reactant proteins (Chess, 1983; Persellin, 1985; Pountain, 1994) (e.g., fibrinogen, von Willebrand factor)
Abnormal plasma viscosity (Gudmundsson, 1993; Orrell, 1993)
Serum protein electrophoresis abnormalities (Sorenson, 1977)
Hepatic dysfunction (Goodman, 1979; Knorring, 1976; Kosolcharoen, 1976)
Multiple immunologic abnormalities (Andersson, 1987, 1988; Armstrong, 1983; Banks, 1983; Bosch, 1991; Cid, 1989; Elling, 1985, 1989; Espinoza, 1982; Gallagher, 1982; Hazleman, 1975; Lowenstein, 1983; Papaioannou, 1979; Radda, 1991; Richardson, 1987; Salvarani, 1991; Shiiki, 1989; Smith, 1987; Wawryk, 1991; Weyand, 1992, 1994, 1995, 1997)
Immune complexes
T-cell abnormalities
Immunohistochemical abnormalities
HLA-DR4 and DR3 (Armstrong, 1983; Barrier, 1981; Calamia, 1981b)

1985). Several authors have reported various techniques (Brennan, 1975; Clearkin, 1991; Hedges, 1992; Tomsak, 1991). Temporal arteries that are difficult to locate may require the use of intraoperative Doppler for localization (Beckman, 1990; Bienfang, 1984). Hall, et al. performed 134 TAB and 46 (34%) showed GCA (Hall, 1983). Of the 88 TAB (66%) that were normal (over a 70 month follow-up period), only 8 patients required steroid therapy. Thus, a negative TAB predicted the absence of steroid therapy requirement in 91% and helped determine the appropriate treatment in 94% of cases. These and other authors felt that a TAB should be done before patients are committed to long-term corticosteroid therapy (Goodman, 1979; Hall, 1983) because of the associated significant side effects of chronic steroid use including Cushinghoid features, hypertension, diabetes, osteoporosis, compression fractures (up to 25% of patients), steroid myopathy, steroid psychosis, and fluid retention requiring diuretics (Allsop, 1981; Beevers, 1973; Huston, 1978; Kyle, 1989; Nescher, 1994; Rubinow, 1984; Spiera, 1978). Nadeau reviewed four different series (162 patients) of steroid therapy in GCA and found a 38% incidence of complications (range 12.7 to 60.6%) (Nadeau, 1988). Using a clinical decision analysis approach, Nadeau concluded that when steroid complications were likely, a TAB was useful even with "fairly high pre-biopsy probabilities of disease" (Nadeau, 1988). In addition, Hedges, et al. felt that no laboratory test (i.e., ESR) or frequently observed symptom or sign of GCA alone or in combination with other findings (e.g., jaw claudication) had the diagnostic specificity or sensitivity of the TAB (Hedges, 1983).

Patients with a negative unilateral TAB in whom there is a strong clinical suspicion (see clinical features and symptom clusters above) for GCA should undergo a TAB on the contralateral side (Coppetto, 1990; Fernandez-Herlihy, 1988; Hunder, 1990a). To minimize cost, some authors have advocated that a frozen section be performed on the symptomatic side TAB and, if it is normal, proceed at the same sitting with a contralateral TAB (Hall, 1984).

Ponge et al. analyzed 200 patients who underwent 200 bilateral TAB, all of which were preceded by Doppler flow studies. Forty-two TAB were positive, 20 bilaterally and 22 unilaterally (Ponge, 1988). In their analysis, they discovered that 4 patients with GCA would not have been diagnosed if only a unilateral TAB had been performed. Unilaterally positive TAB have been demonstrated in 8% to 14% of retrospective bilateral TAB series (Hall, 1984; Klein, 1976; Sorensen, 1977). Hall and Hunder retrospectively reviewed 652 TAB at Mayo Clinic (Hall, 1984). Of these, 234 (36%) revealed GCA, and 193 (82%) were positive on unilateral TAB. Bilateral TAB were performed in 41 cases (18%) because frozen section was normal on the first TAB. Of the 193 unilateral TAB, frozen section was abnormal in 188 TAB and normal in 5 TAB. Thus, 86% of the 234 cases would have been diagnosed by unilateral TAB alone and 14% were diagnosed only because a TAB was performed on the contralateral side. Hayreh et al. reported 76 of 363 patients who underwent a second TAB because of a strong clinical index of suspicion for GCA (Hayreh, 1997). Seven of these 76 patients had a positive contralateral TAB. Of the remaining 257 patients with a negative TAB, none developed signs of GCA on follow-up and these authors felt that this was indicative that a second TAB would not have been positive.

TAB has a variable sensitivity for GCA in the literature ranging from 56 to 93% (Allsop, 1981; Egge, 1966; Fauchald, 1972; Hauser, 1971; Hedges, 1983, Lie, 1970, Mizen, 1991; Roth, 1984; Wadman, 1972). The sensitivity improves to 85 to 90% when clear criteria for negative TAB are established (Nadeau, 1988). Skip lesions may occur pathologically (even in bilateral TAB) and may produce a false negative rate of at least 4 to 5% (Klein, 1976; McDonnell, 1986). A large segment TAB of a length of at least 2 to 5 cm is often recommended (Albert, 1976; Brennan, 1975; Brownstein, 1983; Cohen, 1974; Keltner, 1981; Klein, 1976; McDonnell, 1986; Mehler, 1988), but other authors have found that even TAB as short as 4 mm (if serially sectioned properly at 1 mm segments and with a minimum of nine sections from each segment) may result in a less than 1% false negative rate (99% probability of detecting any evidence of GCA) (Chambers, 1988). Short length TAB, insufficient sectioning (0.25–0.5 mm cross sections through the entire specimen are recommended) (McDonnell, 1986), and variability in the quality and availability of good ophthalmic pathologic interpretation of specimens contribute to a high false-negative rate of up to 9 to 61% (Allsop, 1981; Egge, 1966; Fauchald, 1972; Hauser, 1971; Hedges, 1983; Mizen, 1991; Roth, 1984; Wadman, 1972). In addition, although steroid therapy may produce a false negative result (Allison, 1984), TAB may be performed up to a few weeks (or more) of starting steroid treatment (Achkar, 1994; Allison, 1984; McDonnell, 1986; To, 1994). Thus, even in the setting of a negative unilateral (or bilateral) TAB, the patient with a high clinical suspicion for GCA should be treated with continued empiric corticosteroids (oral prednisone 80–120 mg/day). Consideration could be given toward a third biopsy of other arteries (e.g., occipital, facial, or frontal artery) if the clinical suspicion for GCA remains high and pathological confirmation is desired (Cohen, 1973; Kattah, 1991; Weems, 1992).

What Is the Evaluation for a Patient with a Moderate Clinical Suspicion for GCA?

Patients with moderate clinical suspicion for GCA should undergo an ESR and a TAB. Unfortunately, constitutional symptoms and signs may be absent in up to 18% of cases ("occult" GCA) (Desmet, 1990; Liu, 1994). If the ESR is elevated, and if a unilateral TAB is negative, then a contralateral TAB should be performed. Alternatively, a frozen section of the TAB on the symptomatic side could be performed and, if negative, a simultaneous contralateral TAB is done (Hall, 1984). If both TAB are negative, alternative etiologies of the elevated ESR should be considered, such as infections, connective tissue disease, renal disease (especially nephrotic syndrome and uremia) (Gruener, 1992), malignant neoplasm (21% of negative TAB were cancer in Hedges series), diabetes mellitus (Elias, 1989; Hedges, 1983; Roth, 1984), and diffuse disseminated atheroembolism (Coppetto, 1984). If the ESR (and/or CRP) are normal, and a unilateral TAB is negative, and the patient has few or nonspecific constitutional symptoms, then the steroid therapy can be tapered or a contralateral TAB can be performed. If both TAB are negative, the steroids can be tapered.

What Is the Evaluation of the Patient with a Low Clinical Suspicion for GCA?

In patients with low clinical suspicion for GCA (e.g., typical AION in a known vasculopathic patient with no constitutional signs or symptoms), alternative etiologies (e.g., infection, inflammation, collagen vascular disease, underlying malignancy, diabetes) for a

Table 5–6. Laboratory Evaluation for Markedly Elevated ESR

Complete blood count with differential
Blood urea nitrogen and creatinine
Alkaline phosphatase
Serum protein electrophoresis
Chest radiography
Consider mammogram and other evaluation for underlying malignancy
Urine analysis
Purified protein derivative (ppd) and control skin testing
Guaiac tests of stools (six determinations)

"high" or "borderline" ESR should be investigated (Hedges, 1983). Bedell and Bush suggested that patients with markedly elevated ESR (i.e., ESR > 100 mm/hr) should be evaluated for underlying disease (Bedell, 1985). Based in part on these recommendations, we suggest the evaluation outlined in Table 5–6 for patients with an elevated ESR and a low clinical suspicion for GCA. In patients with a low clinical suspicion for GCA and an elevated ESR, a unilateral TAB could be performed and, if negative, no further evaluation or treatment for GCA is needed.

What Is the Preferred Treatment Regimen for GCA?

Untreated GCA may result in significant visual loss in one or both eyes (Faarvang, 1989; Keltner, 1981; Rosenfeld, 1986). Therefore, it is imperative that corticosteroid therapy begin immediately upon clinical suspicion of GCA to prevent visual loss (i.e., before TAB and laboratory confirmation). Most authors have recommended an initial dose of oral prednisone of 1.0 mg/kg to 1.5 mg/kg/d (60 to 100 mg per day) (Bengtsson, 1982; Delecoeullerie, 1988; Herrick, 1980; Hugod, 1979; Hunder, 1989; Keltner, 1981; Kyle, 1989a,b; Laidlaw, 1992; Lundberg, 1990; Myles, 1992; Weisman, 1995). Although some authors (Aiello, 1993; Delecoeullerie, 1988; Kyle, 1989) have reported that an initial lower dose of 40 mg per day may be adequate to control clinical symptoms (Myles, 1992), patients with visual loss probably require higher doses. Some anecdotal cases of visual improvement have been reported following intravenous (IV) corticosteroids for patients with visual loss and GCA (Diamond, 1991; Liu, 1994; Matzkin, 1992; Model, 1978; Postel, 1993; Rosenfeld, 1986). Many patients note improvement in symptoms (Cohen, 1973; Cullen, 1967, 1976; Fenton, 1968) within 1 to 2 days of starting steroid therapy but other patients may continue to experience symptoms of GCA including visual loss despite adequate corticosteroid therapy (Aiello, 1993; Evans, 1994; Hugod, 1979; Liu, 1994; Rauser, 1995; Slavin, 1988). A rapid or premature reduction of steroid therapy in GCA may also precipitate visual loss (Cullen, 1967).

Should Oral or IV Corticosteroids Be Used for GCA?

Liu et al. reported a 34% chance of visual improvement after corticosteroid therapy. Additional visual loss occurred in 7 of 41 (17%) patients despite corticosteriods (Liu, 1994). Three patients experienced fellow eye involvement after oral therapy, but none of those treated with IV steroids developed fellow eye involvement. Based upon these results, these authors recommended IV therapy (methylprednisolone 250 mg 4 times daily for 3 to 5 days in patients with visual loss due to GCA [Liu, 1994]).

Matzkin et al. reported visual recovery in two patients with central retinal artery occlusions due to GCA after treatment with high dose IV methylprednisolone (Matzkin, 1992). Other authors have described anecdotal cases of visual improvement following IV corticosteroids for patients with visual loss and GCA (Aiello, 1993; Diamond, 1991; Liu, 1994; Matzkin, 1992; Model, 1978; Postel, 1993; Rosenfeld, 1986). Unfortunately, well-controlled prospective data is lacking (Clearkin, 1992a). Nevertheless, we favor IV steroids in patients with severe visual loss of less than 48 hours duration due to GCA, especially if there is bilateral involvement, if the patient is monocular, or if the patient has lost vision during oral steroid therapy (Hayreh, 1990; Slamovits, 1992).

Although the visual prognosis after AION or CRAO due to GCA is poor, significant visual improvement after steroid therapy has been reported in a small percentage of patients (Aiello, 1993; Clearkin, 1992a, 1992b; Diamond, 1991; Lipton, 1985; Model, 1978; Rosenfeld, 1986; Schneider, 1971). Aiello et al. reviewed 245 patients over a 5-year period at the Mayo Clinic (Aiello, 1993). Of these 245 patients, 34 (14%) permanently lost vision due to GCA. After 5 years, the probability of visual loss after starting steroid therapy (oral) was 1%. These authors reviewed an additional 857 patients from the literature. Of these 857 patients, 174 (20%) lost vision due to GCA, and 31 of these 174 patients had visual loss or progression on steroid therapy.

Consultation with an internist or rheumatologist is recommended for the detection of constitutional signs, monitoring of ESR, and management of steroid therapy and potential side effects in patients with GCA (Mizen, 1991). Hunder emphasized that the goal of therapy is to use the lowest dose of steroid over the shortest period of time to adequately control the symptoms of GCA. Unfortunately, the dosage and duration of therapy are variable among patients and must be determined on an individual and empirical basis (Hunder, 1986). Gradual tapering of the steroid dose by 10% per week as long as symptoms and ESR remain stable is a reasonable approach (Burde, 1992; Goodman, 1979). Most patients can be tapered off steroids within one year, but some patients (especially those with neurological or other systemic symptoms) may require prolonged (years) or indefinite therapy (Beevers, 1973; Bengtsson, 1981c; Kyle, 1989a,b; Graham, 1981). Recurrences may also occur years later (Beevers, 1973; Blumberg, 1980; Cohen, 1973; Cullen, 1976; Fulton, 1976). Turner reported a normalization of the ESR in 87% of 47 patients within 4 weeks of treatment (Turner, 1974). Huston reported a duration of steroid treatment of 1 to 77 months (median 7 months) (Huston, 1978). Cullen and Coleiro felt that an ESR of less than 20 mm/hr was a desirable goal (Cullen, 1976). Delecoeullerie, et al. reported a mean duration of therapy of 30.9 months in 210 patients (Delecoeullerie, 1988), but Andersson et al. reported an average duration of 5 years (Andersson, 1986). Tapering of steroids is equally important as starting therapy in GCA because the risk of fracture is increased sixfold and that of cataract formation fourfold after 5 years of steroid therapy (Robb-Nicholson, 1988). Recurrent symptoms and/or ESR elevation may prompt increase of the steroid dosage, but clinical symptoms may be a better indicator than the ESR alone (Beevers, 1973; Brittain, 1991; Kyle, 1989). As corticosteroid doses are lowered, the ESR may rise and, if it increases to above normal rates, the tapering schedule may be interrupted for 2 to 4 weeks to allow stabilization of the ESR. Although a rise in the ESR is often associated with clinical recurrence of GCA, ischemic complications may occur on steroid therapy despite a stable ESR (Rosenfeld, 1986; Rynes, 1977; Save-Soderbergh, 1986). Every other day steroid therapy does not seem to sufficiently control disease activity (Hunder, 1975, 1986) but may eventually be used once active GCA is under control (Bengtsson, 1981c; Hunder, 1986).

If Major Steroid Complications Occur, Therapy Is Prolonged, or the Disease Is Still Active, What Should Be Done?

A repeat TAB could be considered, but subjects the patient to a second surgical procedure. In addition, as already stated, a negative TAB (first or second), especially after prolonged steroid therapy, does not exclude GCA. Nevertheless, Cohen reported 13 patients with known GCA and a rising ESR with any attempt at tapering steroid therapy (Cohen, 1973). Nine of these patients underwent a second TAB and one of those had a third TAB to determine if active GCA was present histologically or whether the ESR was elevated due to alternative etiologies. Steroid related complications (e.g., Cushingoid appearance, melena, hematuria, osteoporosis) had developed in nine patients. Five of the ten second TAB (50%) continued to show active inflammation and patients were continued on steroid therapy whereas the five (50%) patients with inactive TAB were tapered off steroids.

If a second TAB is not performed or the clinical suspicion for active disease remains high, then patients with significant contraindications to steroid therapy, those who fail steroid therapy (Wilke, 1995), or patients who develop steroid complications may benefit from other immunosuppressive agents. Steroid derivatives such as deflazacort (Cimmino, 1994), and other immunosuppressive regimens such as cyclophosphamide (Cytoxan), azathioprine (Imuran), dapsone (Doury, 1983), and cyclosporine (Sandimmune) have been employed in GCA, but there is little controlled clinical data regarding their efficacy in GCA (DeSilva, 1986; de Vita, 1992; Reinitz, 1988; Wendling, 1985). Several authors (Hernandez-Garcia, 1994; Krall, 1989; van der Veen, 1996) have reported variable responses to methotrexate in addition to steroid therapy in GCA, and this agent may prove to be a useful steroid-sparing medication for GCA in the future. In addition, DeSilva and Hansleman reported the use of azathioprine in a double-blind placebo-controlled study. There was a statistically significant reduction in mean prednisolone dose after 52 weeks in the azathioprine treated group (DeSilva, 1986).

Our approach to the patient with GCA is outlined in Figure 5–1.

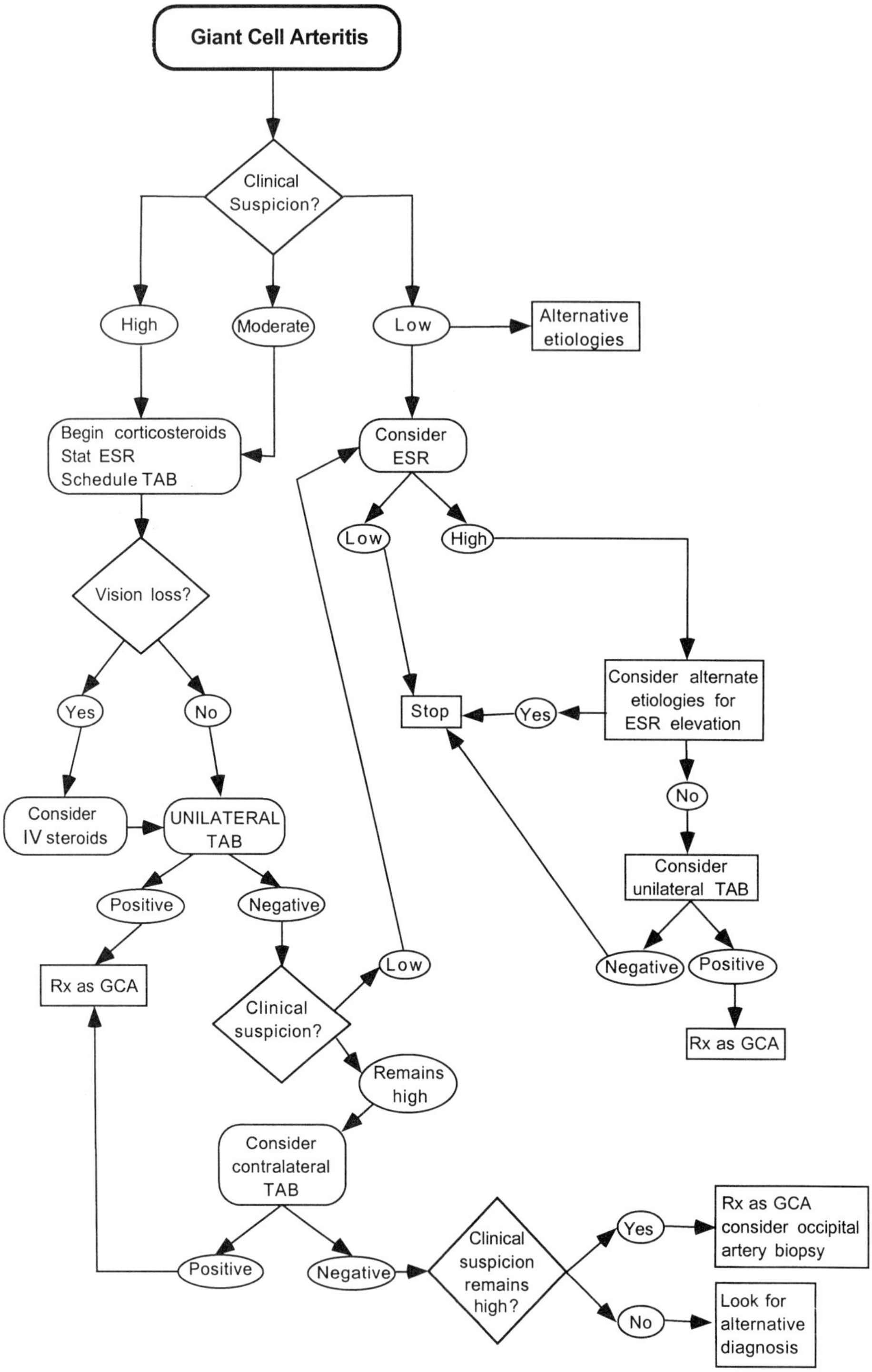

Figure 5–1. Giant cell arteritis.

References

Aburahma AF, Thaxton L. (1996). Temporal arteritis: Diagnostic and therapeutic considerations. *Am Surg 62:*449–451.

Aburahma AF, Wistberger TA. (1992). Diagnosing giant cell temporal arteritis. *West Virginia Med J 88:*188–193.

Achkar AA, Lie JT, Gabriel SE, Hunder GG. (1995). Giant cell arteritis involving the facial artery. *J Rheum 22:*360–362.

Achkar AA, Lie JT, Hunder GG, et al. (1994). How does previous corticosteroid treatment affect the biopsy findings in giant cell (temporal arteritis). *Ann Intern Med 120:*987.

Ahmed T, Braun A. (1978). Carpal tunnel syndrome with polymyalgia rheumatica. *Arthr Rheum 21:*22.

Aiello PD, Trautmann JC, McPhee TJ, et al. (1993). Visual prognosis in giant cell arteritis. *Ophthalmology 100:*550–555.

Albert DM, Ruchman MC, Keltner JL. (1976). Skip areas in temporal arteritis. *Arch Ophthalmol 94:*2072–2076.

Albert DM, Searl SS, Craft JL. (1982). Histologic and ultrastructural characteristics of temporal arteritis. *Ophthalmology 89:*1111–1126.

Allison MC, Gallagher PJ. (1984). Temporal artery biopsy and corticosteroid treatment. *Ann Rheum Dis 43:*416–417.

Allsop CJ, Gallagher PJ. (1981). Temporal artery biopsy in giant-cell arteritis: A reappraisal. *Am J Surg Pathol 5:*317–323.

Anderson R, Malwall B, Bengtsson B-A. (1986). Long-term survival in giant cell arteritis including temporal arteritis and polymyalgia rheumatica. *Acta Med Scand 220:*361–364,

Anderson R, Malwall B, Bengtsson B-A. (1988). Long-term corticosteroid treatment in giant cell arteritis. *Clin Exp Immunol 73:*82.

Andersson R, Hansson GK, Soderstrom T, et al. (1988). HLA-DR expression in the vascular lesion and circulating T lymphocytes of patients with giant cell arteritis. *Clin Exp Immunol 73:*82–87.

Andersson R, Jonsson R, Tarkowski A, Bengtsson BA, Malvall BE. (1987). T cell subsets and expression of immunological activation markers in the arterial walls of patients with giant cell arteritis. *Ann Rheum Dis 46:*915–923.

Andrews JM. (1966). Giant cell arteritis. *Neurology 16:*963–971.

Appenzeller O. (1974). Temporal arteritis. *Postgrad Med 56:*133.

Armstrong RD, Behn A, Myles A, Panayi GS, Welsh KI. (1983). Histocompatibility antigens in polymyalgia rheumatica and giant cell arteritis. *J Rheumatol 10:*659–661.

Arnung K, Nielsen IL. (1979). Temporal arteritis and gangrene of the tongue. *Acta Med Scand 206:*239–240.

Askari A, Jolobe OM, Shepherd DI. (1993). Internuclear ophthalmoplegia and Horner's syndrome due to presumed giant cell arteritis. *J Roy Soc Med 86:*362.

Astion ML, Wener MH, Thomas RG, Hunder GG, Bloch DA. (1994). Application of neural networks to the classification of giant cell arteritis. *Arthr Rheum 37:*760–770.

Atkins SD. (1978). Giant cell arteritis—a systemic spectrum including temporal arteritis and polymyalgia rheumatica. *J Fam Pract 7:*1109.

Ballou SP, Muhammad AK, Kushner I. (1978). Giant-cell arteritis in a black patient. *Ann Intern Med 88:*659–660.

Banks PM, Cohen MD, Ginsburg WW, Hunder GG. (1983). Immunohistologic and cytochemical studies of temporal arteritis. *Arthritis Rheum 26:*1201–1207.

Barricks ME, Traviesa DB, Glaser JS, Levy IS. (1977). Ophthalmoplegia in cranial arteritis. *Brain 100:*209–221.

Barrier J, Bignon J-D, Soulillou JP, et al. (1981). Increased prevalence of HLA-DR4 in giant cell arteritis. *N Engl J Med 305:*104–105.

Barton JJ, Corbett JJ. (1991). Neuro-ophthalmologic vascular emergencies in the elderly. *Clin Geriatr Med 7:*525–548.

Beckman RL, Hartmann BM. (1990). The use of a Doppler flow meter to identify the course of the temporal artery (letter). *J Clin Neuro-ophthalmol 10:*304.

Bedell SE, Bush BT. (1985). Erythrocyte sedimentation rate: From folklore to facts. *Am J Med 78:*1001–1009.

Beevers DG, Harpur JE, Turk KAD. (1973). Giant cell arteritis: The need for prolonged treatment. *J Chronic Dis 26:*571–584.

Bell WR, Klinefelter HF. (1967). Polymyalgia rheumatica. *Johns Hopkins Med J 121:*175–187.

Bengtsson B-A. (1982). Eye complications in giant cell arteritis. *Acta Med Scand Supp 658:*38–43.

Bengtsson B-A, Malmvall B-E. (1981a). The epidemiology of giant cell arteritis including temporal arteritis and polymyalgia rheumatica: Incidences of different clinical presentations and eye complications. *Arthritis Rheum 24:*899–904.

Bengtsson B-A, Malmvall B-E. (1981b). Prognosis of giant cell arteritis including temporal arteritis and polymyalgia rheumatica: A follow-up study on ninety patients treated with corticosteroids. *Acta Med Scand 209:*337–345.

Bengtsson B-A, Malmvall B-E. (1981c). An alternate day corticosteroid regimen in maintenance therapy of giant cell arteritis. *Acta Med Scand 209:*347–350.

Berlit P. (1992). Clinical and laboratory findings with giant cell arteritis. *J Neurol Sci 111:*1–12.

Bethlenfalvay NC, Nusynowitz ML. 1964. Temporal arteritis: A rarity in the young adult. *Arch Intern Med 114:*487–489.

Bevan AT, Dunhill MS, Harrison MJG. 1968. Clinical and biopsy findings in temporal arteritis. *Ann Rheum Dis 27*:271.
Bienfang D. (1989). Loss of the ocular pulse in the acute phase of temporal arteritis. *Acta Ophthalmol 67*:35–37.
Bienfang DC. (1984). Use of the Doppler probe to detect the course of the superficial temporal artery. *Am J Ophthalmol 97*:526–527.
Biller J, Asconape J, Weinblatt E, Toole JF. (1982). Temporal arteritis associated with normal sedimentation rate. *JAMA 247*:486–487.
Birt CM, Slomovic A, Motolko M, Buncic R. (1994). Anterior segment ischemia in giant cell arteritis. *Can J Ophthalmol 29*:93–94.
Bisgard C, Sloth H, Keiding N, Juel K. (1991). Excess mortality in giant cell arteritis. *J Intern Med 230*:119–123.
Blaiss MS, Waxman J, Lange RK. (1982). Occipital headache as a manifestation of giant cell arteritis. *South Med J 75*:887–888.
Blodi FC. (1970). The temporal artery biopsy as a diagnostic procedure in ophthalmology. *Trans Ophthalmol Soc NZ 22*:26–33.
Blumberg S, Giansiracusa DF, Docken WP, Kantrowitz FG. (1980). Recurrence of temporal arteritis: Clinical recurrence 9 years after initial illness. *JAMA 244*:1713–1718.
Boghen DR, Glaser JS. (1975). Ischemic optic neuropathy: A clinical profile and natural history. *Brain 98*:689–708.
Borruat FX, Bogousslavsky J, Uffer S, Klainguti G, Schatz NJ. (1993) Orbital infarction syndrome. *Ophthalmology 100*:562–568.
Bosch X, Font J, Mirapeix E, et al. (1991). Antineutrophil cytoplasmic antibodies in giant cell arteritis (letter). *J Rheumatol 18*:787.
Bosley TM, Savino PJ, Sergott RC, Eagle RC, Sandy R, Gee W. (1989). Ocular pneumoplethysmography can help in the diagnosis of giant-cell arteritis. *Arch Ophthalmol 107*:379–381.
Bottiger LE, Svedberg CA. (1967). Normal erythrocyte sedimentation rate and age. *Br Med J 2*:85–87.
Boyd RV, Hoffbrand BI. (1966). Erythrocyte sedimentation rate in elderly hospital in-patients. *Br Med J 1*:901–902.
Brennan MJW, Sandyk R. (1982). Reversible quadriplegia in a patient with giant cell arteritis (letter). *S Afr Med J 62*:81–82.
Brennan J, McCrary JA. (1975). Diagnosis of superficial temporal arteritis. *Ann Ophthalmol 7*:1125–1129.
Brittain GP, McIlwaine GG, Bell JA, Gibson JM. (1991). Plasma viscosity or erythrocyte sedimentation rate in the diagnosis of giant cell arteritis? *Br J Ophthalmol 75*:656–659.
Bromfield EB, Slakter JS. (1988). Horner syndrome in temporal arteritis (letter). *Arch Neurol 45*:604.
Bronster DJ, Rudolph SH, Shanzer S. (1983). Pupillary light-near dissociation in cranial arteritis: A case report. *Neuro-ophthalmol 3*:65–70.
Brownstein S, Nicolle DA, Codere F. (1983). Bilateral blindness in temporal arteritis with skip areas. *Arch Ophthalmol 101*:388–391.
Buchbinder R, Detsky AS. (1992). Management of suspected giant cell arteritis: A decision analysis. *J Rheum 19*:1220–1228.
Bull BS, Brecher G. (1974). An evaluation of the relative merits of the Wintrobe and Westergren sedimentation methods, including hematocrit correction. *Am J Clin Pathol 62*:502–510.
Butt Z, Cullen JF, Mutlukan E. (1991). Pattern of arterial involvement of the head, neck and eyes in giant cell arteritis: Three case reports. *Br J Ophthalmol 75*:368–371.
Calamia KT, Hunder GG. (1980). Clinical manifestations of giant cell arteritis. *Clin Rheum Dis 6*:389–403.
Calamia KT, Hunder GG. (1981a). Giant cell arteritis presenting as fever of unknown origin. *Arthritis Rheum 24*:1414–1418.
Calamia KT, Moore SB, Elveback LR, et al. (1981b). HLA–DR locus antigens in polymyalgia rheumatica and giant cell arteritis. *J Rheumatol 8*:993–996.
Caselli RJ. (1990). Giant cell (temporal) arteritis: A treatable cause of multi-infarct dementia. *Neurology 40*:753–755.
Caselli RJ, Hunder GG. (1993). Neurologic aspects of giant cell (temporal) arteritis. *Rheum Dis Clin No Amer 19*:941–953.
Caselli RJ, Hunder GG, Whisnant JP. (1988). Neurologic disease in biopsy-proven giant cell arteritis. *Neurology 38*:352–359.
Chambers W, Bernardino V. (1988). Specimen length in temporal artery biopsies. *J Clin Neuro-ophthalmol 8*:121–125.
Charness ME, Liu GT. (1991). Central retinal artery occlusion in giant cell arteritis. Treatment with nitroglycerin. *Neurol 41*:1698–1699.
Cherry JE, Pearce JMS. (1980). Unusual variants in the presentation of temporal arteritis. *Postgrad Med J 56*:88–91.
Chertok P, Leroux JL, LeMarchand M, et al. (1990). Orbital pseudotumor in temporal arteritis revealed by computed tomography. *Clin Exp Rheumatol 8*:587–589.
Chess J, Albert DM, Bhan AK, Paluck EI, Robinson N, Collins B, Kaynor B. (1983). Serologic and immunopathologic findings in temporal arteritis. *Am J Ophthalmol 96*:283–289.
Chisholm IH. (1975). Cortical blindness in cranial arteritis. *Br J Ophthalmol 95*:332–333.
Chmelewski WL, McKnight KM, Agudelo CA, Wise CM. (1992). Presenting features and outcome in patients undergoing temporal artery biopsy: A review of 98 patients. *Arch Intern Med 152*:1690–1695.

Chuang T-Y, Hunder GG, Hstrup DM, Kurland LT. (1982). Polymyalgia rheumatica: A 10 year epidemiologic and clinical study. *Ann Intern Med 97*:672–680.

Cid MC, Campo E, Ercilla G, et al. (1989). Immunohistochemical analysis of lymphoid and macrophage cell subsets and their immunologic activation markers in temporal arteritis. *Arthritis Rheum 32*:884–893.

Cimmino MA, Moggiana G, Montecucco C, et al. (1994). Long term treatment of polymyalgia rheumatica with deflazacort. *Ann Rheum Dis 43*:331.

Clark AE, Victor WH. (1987). An unusual presentation of temporal arteritis. *Ann Ophthalmol 19*:343–346.

Clearkin LG. (1992a). IV steroids for central retinal artery occlusion in giant-cell arteritis (letter). *Ophthalmology 99*:1482–1483.

Clearkin LG, Caballero J. (1992b). Recovery of visual function in anterior ischemic optic neuropathy due to giant cell arteritis. *Am J Med 92*:703–704.

Clearkin LG, Watts MT. (1991). How to perform a temporal artery biopsy. *Br J Hosp Med 46*:172–174.

Cochran JW, Fox JH, Kelly MP. (1978). Reversible mental symptoms in temporal arteritis. *J Nerv Ment Dis 166*:446.

Cohen DN. (1973). Temporal arteritis: Improvement in visual prognosis and management with repeat biopsies. *Trans Am Acad Ophthalmol Otolaryngol 77*:74–85.

Cohen DN, Damaske MM. (1975). Temporal arteritis: A spectrum of ophthalmic complications. *Ann Ophthalmol 7*:1045–1054.

Cohen DN, Smith TR. (1974). Skip areas in temporal arteritis. *Trans Am Acad Ophthalmol Otolaryngol 78*:772–783.

Coppetto JR, Lessell S, Lessell IM, Greco TP, Eisenberg MS. (1984). Diffuse disseminated atheroembolism. Three cases with neuro-ophthalmic manifestations. *Arch Ophthalmol 102*:224–228.

Coppetto JR, Monteiro M. (1990). Diagnosis of highly occult temporal arteritis by repeat temporal artery biopsies. *Neuro-ophthalmol 10*:217–218.

Costa MM, Romeu JC, da Silva P, de Queiroz V. (1995). Successful treatment of ischaemic optic neuropathy secondary to giant cell arteritis with intravenous pulse of methylprednisolone. (letter). *Clin Rheum 14*:713–714.

Crompton JL, Burrow DJ, Lyer PV. (1989). Bilateral internuclear ophthalmoplegia—an unusual initial presenting sign of giant cell arteritis. *Aust N Z J Ophthalmol 17*:71.

Cullen JF. (1967). Occult temporal arteritis. A common cause of blindness in old age. *Br J Ophthalmol 51*:513–525.

Cullen JF. (1972). Temporal arteritis. Occurrence of ocular complications 7 years after diagnosis. *Br J Ophthalmol 56*:584–588.

Cullen JF, Coleiro JA. (1976). Ophthalmic complications of giant cell arteritis. *Surv Ophthalmol 20*:247–260.

Currie J, Lessell S. (1984). Tonic pupil in giant cell arteritis. *Br J Ophthalmol 68*:135–138.

Delecoeullerie G, Joly P, DeLara AC, et al. (1988). Polymyalgia rheumatica and temporal arteritis: A retrospective analysis of prognostic features and different corticosteroid regimens (11 year survey of 210 patients). *Ann Rheum Dis 47*:733–739.

Dennis RH II, Ransome JR. (1996). Giant cell arteritis presenting as a carpal tunnel syndrome. *J Nat Med Assoc 88*:524–525.

Deodhar SD. (1989). C-reactive protein: The best laboratory indicator for monitoring disease activity. *Cleve Clin J Med 56*:126–130.

DeSilva M, Hazleman BL. (1986). Azathioprine in giant cell arteritis/polymyalgia rheumatica: A double-blind study. *Ann Rheum Dis 45*:136–138.

Desmet GD, Knockaert DC, Bobbaers HJ. (1990). Temporal arteritis: The silent presentation and delay in diagnosis. *J Intern Med 227*:237–240.

Desser EJ. (1969). Miosis, trismus and dysphagia: An unusual presentation of temporal arteritis. *Ann Intern Med 71*:961–962.

de Vita S, Tavoni A, Jeracitano G, Gemignani G, Dolcher MP, Bombardieri S. (1992). Treatment of giant cell arteritis with cyclophosphamide pulses (letter). *J Intern Med 232*:373–375.

Diamond JP. (1991). Treatable blindness in temporal arteritis. *Br J Ophthalmol 75*:432.

Diamond JP. (1993). IV steroid treatment in giant cell arteritis (letter). *Ophthalmology 100*:291–292.

DiBartolomeo AG, Brick JE. (1992). Giant cell arteritis and polymyalgia rheumatica. *Postgrad Med 91*:107–109.

Dick AD, Millar A, Johnson N. (1991). Brainstem vascular accidents and cranial arteritis. *Scott Med J 36*:85.

Dimant J, Farmer PM, Sobol N. (1978). Giant cell arteritis in a black person. *Arthritis Rheum 21*:391–393.

Doury P, Pattin S, Eulry F, Thabaut A. (1983). The use of dapsone in the treatment of giant cell arteritis and polymyalgia rheumatica (letter). *Arthritis Rheum 26*:689–690.

Egge K, Midtbo A, Westby R. (1996). Arteritis temporalis. *Acta Ophthalmol 44*:49–56.

Elias AN, Domurat E. (1989). Erythrocyte sedimentation rate in diabetic patients: Relationship to glycosylated hemoglobin and serum proteins. *J Med 20*:297–302.

Elling H, Elling P. (1985). Decreased level of suppressor/cytotoxic T cells (OKT8) in polymyalgia rheumatica and temporal arteritis: Relation to disease activity. *J Rheumatol 9*:306–309.

Elling H, Elling P, Olsson A. (1989). CD8+ lymphocyte subset in polymyalgia rheumatica and giant cell arteritis: Circulating immune complexes. *Clin Exp Rheumatol 7*:627–630.

Elliot DL, Watts WJ, Reuler JB. (1983). Management of suspected temporal arteritis. A decision analysis. *Med Decis Making 3*:63–68.

Ellis JD, Munro P, McGettrick P. (1994). Blindness with a normal erythrocyte sedimentation rate in giant cell arteritis. *Br J Hosp Med 52*:358–359.

Ellis ME, Ralston S. (1983). The ESR in the diagnosis and management of the polymyalgia rheumatica/giant cell arteritis syndrome. *Ann Rheum Dis 42*:168–170.

Enzmann D, Scott WR. (1977) Intracranial involvement of giant-cell arteritis. *Neurology 27:*794–797.
Eshaghian J. (1979). Controversies regarding giant cell (temporal, cranial) arteritis. *Doc Ophthalmol 47:*43–67.
Eshaghian J, Goeken JA. (1980). C-reactive protein in giant cell (cranial, temporal) arteritis. *Ophthalmology 87:*1160–1166.
Espinoza LR, Bridgeford P, Lowenstein M, et al. (1982). Polymyalgia rheumatica and giant cell arteritis: Circulating immune complexes. *J Rheumatol 9:*556–560.
Esposito AL, Gleckman RA. (1978). Fever of unknown origin in the elderly. *J Am Geriatr Soc 26:*498.
Evans JM, Batts KP, Hunder GG. (1994). Persistent giant cell arteritis despite corticosteroid treatment. *Mayo Clin Proc 69:*1060–1061.
Evans JM, O'Fallon WM, Hunder GG. (1995). Increased incidence of aortic aneurysm and dissection in giant cell (temporal) arteritis. A population-based study. *Ann Intern Med 122:*502–507.
Evans JM, Vukov LF, Hunder GG. (1993). Polymyalgia rheumatica and giant cell arteritis in emergency department patients. *Ann Emerg Med 22:*1633–1635.
Faarvang KL, Thyssen EP. (1989). Case report. Giant cell arteritis: Loss of vision during corticosteroid therapy. *J Intern Med 225:*215.
Fastenberg DM, Feldon SE. (1982). Reversible choroidal vascular insufficiency without infarction in temporal arteritis. *Graefes Arch Clin Exp Ophthalmol 218:*327.
Fauchald P, Rygvold O, Oystese B. (1972). Temporal arteritis and polymyalgia rheumatica. *Ann Intern Med 77:*845–852.
Federici AB, Fox RI, Espinoza LR, Zimmerman TS. (1984). Elevation of von Willebrand factor is independent of erythrocyte sedimentation rate and persists after glucocorticoid treatment in giant cell arteritis. *Arthritis Rheum 27:*1046–1049.
Fenton M. (1968). Giant cell arteritis—a spectrum of disease. *Trans Ophthalmol Soc UK 88:*751–756.
Fernandez-Herlihy L. (1988). Temporal arteritis: Clinical aids to diagnosis. *J Rheumatol 15:*1797.
Fessel WJ, Pearson CM. (1967). Polymyalgia rheumatica and blindness. *N Engl J Med 276:*1403–1405.
Fife A, Dorrell L, Snow MH, Ong EL. (1994). Giant cell arteritis—A cause of pyrexia of unknown origin. *Scott Med J 39:*114–115.
Fineman MS, Savino PJ, Federman JL, Eagle RC, Jr. (1996). Branch retinal artery occlusion as the initial sign of giant cell arteritis. *Am J Ophthalmol 122:*428–430.
Fischer CM. In discussion. Schlezinger N, Schatz NJ. (1971). Giant-cell arteritis (temporal arteritis). *Trans Am Neurolog Assoc 96:*12–15.
Fulton AB, Lee RV, Keltner JL, Albert DM. (1976). Active giant cell arteritis with cerebral involvement. *Arch Ophthalmol 94:*2068–2071.
Gabriel SE, O'Fallon WM, Achkar AA, Lie JT, Hunder GG. (1995). The use of clinical characteristics to predict the results of temporal artery biopsy among patients with suspected giant cell arteritis. *J Rheum 22:*93–96.
Galetta SL, Raps EC, Wulc AE, et al. (1990). Conjugal temporal arteritis. *Neurology 40:*1839–1842.
Gallagher P, Jones K. (1982). Immunohistochemical findings in cranial arteritis. *Arthritis Rheum 25:*75–79.
Gaynes BI. (1994). Occult giant cell arteritis: A diagnosis of suspicion. *J Amer Optom Assoc 65:*564–571.
Gentric A, Baccino E, Mottier D, Islam S, Cledes J. (1988). Temporal arteritis revealed by a syndrome of inappropriate secretion of antidiuretic hormone. *Am J Med 85:*559–560.
Gersbach P, Lang H, Kipfer B, Meyer R, Schupbach P. (1993). Impending rupture of the ascending aorta due to giant cell arteritis. *Eur J Cardio-Thoracic Surg 7:*667–670.
Gerstle CC, Frideman AH. (1980). Marginal corneal ulceration (limbal guttering) as a presenting sign of temporal arteritis. *Ophthalmology 87:*1173–1176.
Gibb WRG, Urry PA, Lees AJ. (1985) Giant cell arteritis with spinal cord infarction and basilar artery thrombosis. *J Neurol Neurosurg Psychiatr 48:*945.
Gibbs P. (1974). Temporal arteritis: Onset with pseudotumor orbit or red eye. *Practitioner 213:*205–211.
Gilbert GJ. (1970). Eyeball bruits in temporal arteritis. *Dis Nerv Syst 31:*130–132.
Gill CR. (1977). Temporal arteritis with normal sedimentation rate. *J Ky Med Assoc 75:*483–485.
Ginsberg WW, Cohen MD, Hall S, Vollertsen R, Hunder GG. (1985). Seronegative polyarthritis in giant cell arteritis. *Arth Rheum 28:*1362–1365.
Goadsby PJ, Mossman S. (1991). Giant cell arteritis and ophthalmoplegia. (letter). *Aust N Z J Med 21:*930.
Golbus J, McCune WJ. (1987). Giant cell arteritis and peripheral neuropathy: A report of 2 cases and review of the literature. *J Rheumatol 14:*129–134.
Goldberg RT. (1983). Ocular muscle paresis and cranial arteritis—an unusual case. *Ann Ophthalmol 15:*240–243.
Goodman BW, Jr. (1979). Temporal arteritis. *Am J Med 67:*839–852.
Goodman LJ, Layfer LF, Banner BF. (1978). Polymyalgia rheumatica and giant-cell arteritis in a black woman. *N Engl J Med 298:*113.
Gouet D, Marechaud R, Alcalay M, et al. (1985). Survival in giant cell arteritis: A 14-year survey of 87 patients (letter). *J Rheumatol 12:*1209–1210.
Graham E. (1980). Survival in temporal arteritis. *Trans Ophthalmol Soc UK 100:*108–110.
Graham E, Holland A, Avery A, Russell RWR. (1981). Prognosis in giant cell arteritis. *Br Med J 282:*269–271.
Grodum E, Petersen HA. (1990). Temporal arteritis with normal erythrocyte sedimentation rates presenting as occipital neuralgia. *J Intern Med 227:*279–280.
Grosvenor T, Malinovsky V, Gelvin J, Tonekaboni K. (1993). Diagnosis and management of temporal arteritis: A review and case report. *Optom Vis Sci 70:*771–777.

Gruener G, Merchut MP. (1992). Renal causes of elevated sedimentation rate in suspected temporal arteritis. *J Clin Neuro-ophthalmol 12:*272–274.
Gudmundsson M, Nordborg E, Bengtsson B-A, et al. (1993). Plasma viscosity in giant cell arteritis as a predictor of disease activity. *Ann Rheum Dis 52:*104.
Gur H, Whrenfeld M, Izsak E. (1996). Pleural effusion as a presenting manifestation of giant cell arteritis. *Clin Rheum 15:*200–203.
Haist SA. (1985). Stroke after temporal artery biopsy. *Mayo Clin Proc 60:*538.
Hall S, Hunder GG. (1984) Is temporal artery biopsy prudent? *Mayo Clin Proc 59:*793–796.
Hall S, Lie JT, Kurland LT, Persellin S, O'Brien PC, Hunder GG. (1983). The therapeutic impact of temporal artery biopsy. *Lancet 2:*1217–1220.
Hamed LM, Guy JR, Moster ML, Bosley T. (1992). Giant cell arteritis in the ocular ischemic syndrome. *Am J Ophthalmol 113:*702–705.
Hamilton CR, Shelley WM, Tumulty PA. (1971). Giant cell arteritis: Including temporal arteritis and polymyalgia rheumatica. *Medicine 50:*1–27.
Hamrin B, Jonsson N, Kellsten S. (1968). Polymyalgia arteritica. *Ann Rheum Dis 27.*397.
Hansen BL, Junker P. (1995). Giant cell arteritis presenting with ischaemic skin lesions of the neck. *Br J Rheumatol 34:*1182–1184.
Harrison MJG, Bevan AT. (1967). Early symptoms of temporal arteritis. *Lancet 1:*628.
Hart CT. (1967). Formed visual hallucinations: A symptom of cranial arteritis. *Br Med J 3:*643–644.
Hauser WA, Ferguson RH, Holly KE. (1971). Temporal arteritis in Rochester 1951–1967. *Mayo Clin Proc 46:*597–602.
Hayreh SS. (1990). Anterior ischaemic optic neruopathy. Differentiation of arteritic from nonarteritic type and its management. *Eye 4:*25–41.
Hayreh SS. (1981). Posterior ischemic optic neuropathy. *Ophthalmologica 182:*29–41.
Hayreh SS. (1991). Ophthalmic features of giant cell arteritis. *Baillieres Clin Rheum 5:*431–459.
Hayreh SS, Podhajsky PA, Raman R, Zimmerman B. (1997). Giant cell arteritis: Validity and reliability of various diagnostic criteria. *Am J Ophthalmol 123:*285–296.
Hazleman BL, Maclennan ICM, Esiri MM. (1975). Lymphocyte proliferation to artery antigen as a positive diagnosis test in polymyalgia rheumatica. *Ann Rheum Dis 34:*122–127.
Healey LA, Wilske KR. (1977). Manifestations of giant cell arteritis. *Med Clin No Am 61:*261–270.
Healey LA, Wilske KR. (1980). Presentation of occult giant cell arteritis. *Arthr Rheum 23:*641–643.
Healey LA, Wilske KR. (1971). Anemia as a presenting manifestation of giant cell arteritis. *Arthr Rheum 14:*27.
Hedges TR III. (1992). The importance of temporal artery biopsy in the diagnosis of giant cell arteritis. *Arch Ophthalmol 110:*1377.
Hedges TR III, Gieger GL, Albert DM. (1983). The clinical value of negative temporal artery biopsy specimens. *Arch Ophthalmol 101:*1251–1254.
Hellman DB. (1993). Immunopathogenesis, diagnosis, and treatment of giant cell arteritis, temporal arteritis, polymyalgia rheumatica and Takayasu's arteritis. *Curr Opin Rheum 5:*25–32.
Hernandez-Garcia C, Soriano C, Morado C, et al. (1994). Methotrexate treatment in the management of giant cell arteritis. *Scand J Rheum 23:*295–298.
Herrick PC. (1980). Cranial arteritis. A preventable cause of blindness. *Trans Ophthalmol Soc N Z 32:*106–109.
Hintzpeter EN, Naumann G. (1976). Ischemic papilledema in giant-cell arteritis. *Arch Ophthalmol 94:*624–628.
Ho AC, Sergott RC, Regillo CD, et al. (1994). Color Doppler hemodynamics of giant cell arteritis. *Arch Ophthalmol 112:*938–945.
Hollenhorst RW. (1967). Effect of posture on retinal ischemia from temporal arteritis. *Arch Ophthalmol 78:*569–577.
Hollenhorst RW, Brown JR, Wagener HP, Shick RM. (1960). Neurologic aspects of temporal arteritis. *Neurology 10:*490–498.
Howard GF III, Ho SU, Kim KS, Wallach J. (1984). Bilateral carotid artery occlusion resulting from giant cell arteritis. *Ann Neurol 15:*204–207.
Hugod C, Scheibel M. (1979). Temporal arteritis—progressive affection of vision during high-level corticosteroid therapy. A case report. *Acta Med Scand 205:*445–446.
Hunder GG. (1986). Polymyalgia rheumatica and giant cell arteritis. *Drug Therapy* 73–83.
Hunder GG. (1989a). Giant cell arteritis and polymyalgia rheumatica. In Kelly WN, Harris ED, Ruddy S, et al. (eds). *Textbook of Rheumatology*. Philadelphia, WB Saunders, p. 1200.
Hunder GG. (1989b). Giant cell arteritis: Improving your patients' prognosis. *J Musculoskel Med 6:*94–105.
Hunder GG. (1990a). Giant cell (temporal) arteritis. *Rheum Disc Clin North Am 16:*399.
Hunder GG, Allen GL. (1973). The relationship between polymyalgia rheumatica and temporal arteritis. *Geriatrics 28:*124–142.
Hunder GG, Bloch DA, Michel BA, et al. (1990b). The American College of Rheumatology, 1990 criteria for the classification of giant cell arteritis. *Arthritis Rheum 33:*1122–1128.
Hunder GG, Michet CJ. (1985). Giant cell arteritis and polymyalgia rheumatica. *Clin Rheum Dis 11:*471–483.
Hunder GG, Sheps SG. (1967). Intermittent claudication and polymyalgia rheumatica. *Arch Intern Med 119:*638.
Hussein AMA, Hay N. (1990). Case report: Cerebral arteritis with unusual distribution. *Clin Radiol 41:*353.
Huston KA, Hunder GG, Lie JT, Kennedy RH, Elveback LR. (1978). Temporal arteritis: A 25-year epidemiologic, clinical, and pathologic study. *Ann Int Med 88:*162–167.

Ikard RW. (1988). Clinical efficacy of temporal artery biopsy in Nashville, Tennessee. *South Med J 81:*1222.
Ilan Y, Ben-Chetrit E. (1993). Liver involvement in giant cell arteritis. *Clin Rheum 12:*219–222.
Imakita M, Yutani C, Ishibashi-Ueda H. (1993). Giant cell arteritis involving the cerebral artery. *Arch Pathol Lab Med 117:*729–733.
Ishak AW, Persak GC, Mitchell PC, Warwick S. (1988). Giant cell arteritis. *J Am Optom Assoc 59:*864–868.
Jacobson DM, Slamovits TL. (1987). Erythrocyte sedimentation rate and its relationship to hematocrit in giant cell arteritis. *Arch Ophthalmol 105:*965–967.
Jay WM, Nazarian SM. (1986). Bilateral sixth nerve pareses with temporal arteritis and diabetes. *J Clin Neuro–ophthalmol 6:*91–95.
Johnston JL, Thomson GT, Sharpe JA, Inman RD. (1992). Internuclear ophthalmoplegia in giant cell arteritis (letter). *J Neurol Neurosurg Psychiatr 55:*84–85.
Jonasson F, Cullen JF, Elton RA. (1979). Temporal arteritis: A 14-year epidemiologic, clinical, and prognostic study. *Scott Med J 24:*111–117.
Jundt JW, Mock D. (1991). Temporal arteritis with normal erythrocyte sedimentation rates presenting as occipital neuralgia. *Arthritis Rheum 34:*217–219.
Kachroo A, Tello C, Bais R, Panush RS. (1996). Giant cell arteritis: Diagnosis and management. *Bull Rheumatc Dis 45:*2–5.
Kansu T, Corbett JJ, Savino PJ, Schatz NJ. (1977). Giant cell arteritis with normal sedimentation rate. *Arch Neurol 34:*624–625.
Karam GH, Fulmer JD. (1982). Giant cell arteritis presenting as interstitial lung disease. *Chest 82:*781–784.
Karanjia ND, Giddings AEB. (1989). Too few, too late. Temporal artery biopsy in cranial arteritis. *J Cardiovasc Surg 30:*882–884.
Kattah JC, Cupps T, Manz HJ, el Khodary A, Caputy A. (1991). Occipital artery biopsy: A diagnostic alternative in giant cell arteritis. *Neurol 41:*949–950.
Kattwinkel N, Fernandez-Herlihy L. (1970). Polymyalgia rheumatica and temporal arteritis. *Lahey Clin Foundation Bull 19:*41.
Keltner JL. (1981). Giant-cell arteritis: Signs and symptoms. *Ophthalmology 89:*1101–1110.
Kent DC, Arnold H. (1967). Aneurysm of the aorta due to giant cell arteritis. *J Thorac Cardiovasc Surg 53:*572.
Kent RB, Thomas L. (1989). Temporal artery biopsy. *Am Surg 56:*16–21.
Kerleau JM, Levesque H, Delpech A, et al. (1994). Prevalence and evolution of anticardiolipin antibodies in giant cell arteritis during corticosteroid therapy. A prospective study of 20 cases. *Br J Rheumatol 33:*648.
Klein RG, Campbell RJ, Hunder GG, Carney JA. (1976). Skip lesions in temporal arteritis. *Mayo Clin Proc 51:*504–510.
Klein RG, Hunder GG, Stanson AW, Sheps SG. (1975). Large artery involvement in giant cell (temporal) arteritis. *Ann Intern Med 83:*806–812.
Knorring JV, Waastjerna C. (1976). Liver involvement in polymyalgia rheumatica. *Scand J Rheumatol 5:*50.
Koorey DJ. (1984). Cranial arteritis: A twenty-year review of cases. *Aust N Z J Med 14:*143–147.
Kosolcharoen P, Magrin GE. (1976). Liver dysfunction and polymyalgia rheumatica. *J Rheumatol 2:*50.
Kovarsky J, Baum J, Goldstein MN. (1973). Carpal tunnel syndrome in temporal arteritis. *J Rheum 2:*108.
Krall PL, Mazanec DJ, Wilke WS. (1989). Methotrexate for corticosteroid-resistant polymyalgia rheumatica and giant cell arteritis. *Clev Clin J Med 56:*253.
Kyle V, Hanzleman BL. (1993). The clinical and laboratory course of polymyalgia rheumatica/giant cell arteritis after the first two months of treatment. *Ann Rheum Dis 52:*847–850.
Kyle V, Hanzleman BL. (1989a). Treatment of polymyalgia rheumatica and giant cell arteritis. I. Steroid regimens in the first two months. *Ann Rheum Dis 48:*658.
Kyle V, Hanzleman BL. (1989b). Treatment of polymyalgia rheumatica and giant cell arteritis. II. Relation between steroid dose and steroid associated side effects. *Ann Rheum Dis 48:*662–666.
Lagrand WK, Hoogendoorn M, Bakker K, teVelde J, Labrie A. (1996). Aortoduodenal fistula as an unusual manifestation of giant-cell arteritis. *Eur J Vascul Endovasc Surg 11:*502–503.
Laidlaw PAH, Smith PEM, Hudgson P. (1990). Orbital pseudotumor secondary to giant cell arteritis: An unreported condition. *Br Med J 300:*784.
Lambert M, Weber A, Boland B, DePlaen JF, Donckier J. (1996). Large vessel vasculitis without temporal artery involvement: Isolated form of giant cell arteritis? *Clin Rheum 15:*174–180.
Larson TS, Hall S, Hepper NGG, Hunder GG. (1984). Respiratory tract symptoms as a clue to giant cell arteritis. *Ann Intern Med 101:*594–597.
Lee AG. (1995). Jaw claudication: A sign of giant cell arteritis. *JADA 126:*1028–1029.
Lessell S. (1995). Surgery for ischemic optic neuropathy (editorial). *Arch Ophthalmol 113:*273–274.
Levin LA. (1995). Clarifying the treatment of nonarteritic anterior ischemic optic neuropathy (editorial). *JAMA 273:*666–667.
Lie JT. (1995). Aortic and extracranial large vessel giant cell arteritis: A review of 72 cases with histopathologic documentation. *Sem Arthr Rheum 24:*422–431.
Lie JT, Brown AL Jr, Carter ET. (1970). Spectrum of aging changes in temporal arteries: Its significance in interpretation of biopsy of temporal artery. *Arch Pathol 90:*278–285.
Lie JT, Tokugawa DA. (1995). Bilateral lower limb gangrene and stroke as initial manifestations of systemic giant cell arteritis in an African-American. *J Rheum 22:*363–366.
Lin JL, Hsueh S. (1995). Giant cell arteritis induced renal artery aneurysm (letter). *Clin Nephr 43:*66–68.

Lipton RB, Solomon S, Wertenbaker C. (1985). Gradual loss and recovery of vision in temporal arteritis. *Arch Intern Med 145:*2252–2253.

Litwin MS, Henderson DR, Kirkham B. (1992). Normal sedimentation rates and giant cell arteritis. *Arch Intern Med 152:*209.

Liu GT, Glaser JS, Schatz NJ, Smith JL. (1994). Visual morbidity in giant cell arteritis. *Ophthalmology 101:*1779–1785.

Liu G, Shupak R, Chiu BK. (1995). Aortic dissection in giant-cell arteritis. *Sem Arthr Rheum 25:*160–171.

Llorente Pendas S, DeVicente Rodriguez JC, et al. (1994). Tongue necrosis as a complication of giant cell arteritis. *Oral Surg Oral Med Oral Pathol 78:*448–451.

Lockshin MD. (1970). Diplopia as an early sign of temporal arteritis. *Arthr Rheum 13:*419.

Long RG, Friedmann AI, James DG. (1976). Scleritis and temporal arteritis. *Postgrad Med J 52:*689–692.

Lowenstein MB, Brideford PH, Vasey FB, Germain BG, Espinoza LR. (1983). Increased frequency of HLA-DR3 and DR4 in polymyalgia rheumatica and giant cell arteritis. *Arthritis Rheum 26:*925–927.

Lundberg I, Hedfors E. (1990). Restricted dose and duration of corticosteroid treatment in patients with polymyalgia rheumatica and temporal arteritis. *J Rheumatol 17:*1340–1345.

Macfaul PA. (1967). Ciliary artery involvement in giant cell arteritis. *Br J Ophthalmol 51:*505–512.

Machado EBV, Michet CJ, Ballard DJ, et al. (1988). Trends in incidence and clinical presentation of temporal arteritis in Olmstead County, Minnesota, 1950–1985. *Arthritis Rheum 31:*745.

Mack HG, O'Day J, Currie JN. (1991) Delayed choroidal perfusion in giant cell arteritis. *J Clin Neuro-ophthalmol 11:*221–227.

MacLeod JD, Rizk SN. (1993). Cotton-wool spots in giant cell arteritis (letter). *Eye 7:*715–716.

Martin EA. (1970). Double vision and temporal arteritis. *J Ir Med Assoc 63:*191–193.

Massey EW, Weed T. (1978). Sciatic neuropathy with giant-cell arteritis. *N Engl J Med 298:*917.

Matteson EL, Gold KN, Block DA, Hunder GG. (1996). Long-term survival of patients with giant cell arteritis in the American College of Rheumatology giant cell arteritis classification criteria cohort. *Am J Med 100:*193–196.

Matzkin DC, Slamovits TL, Sachs R, Burde RM. (1992). Visual recovery in two patients after intravenous methylprednisolone treatment of central retinal artery occlusion secondary to giant-cell arteritis. *Ophthalmology 99:*68–71.

McAlindon TE, Ferguson IT. (1989). Mononeuritis multiplex and occipital infarction complicating giant cell arteritis. *Br J Rheumatol 28:*257–258.

McDonnell PJ, Moore GW, Miller NR, Hutchins GM, Green WR. (1986). Temporal arteritis: A clinicopathologic study. *Ophthalmology 93:*518–530.

McGowan BL. (1967). Active temporal arteritis as a contraindication to elective surgery with general anesthesia. *Am J Ophthalmol 64:*455.

McHugh NJ, James IE, Plant GT. (1990). Anticardiolipin and antineutrophil antibodies in giant cell arteritis. *J Rheumatol 17:*916–922.

McLean CA, Gonzales MF, Dowling JP. (1993). Systemic giant cell arteritis and cerebellar infarction. *Stroke 24:*899–902.

McLeod D, Kohner EM. (1996). Cotton-wool spots and giant cell arteritis (letter). *Ophthalmology 103:*701–702.

McLeod D, Oji EO, Kohner EM, Marshall J. (1978). Fundus signs in temporal arteritis. *Br J Ophthalmol 62:*591–594.

Meadows SP. (1968). Temporal or giant-cell arteritis, ophthalmic aspects. In Smith JL (ed). *Neuro-ophthalmology Symposium of the University of Miami.* St. Louis, Mosby, Vol. 4, pp. 148–157.

Meadows SP. (1966). Temporal or giant cell arteritis. *Proc R Soc Med 59:*329–333.

Mehler MF, Rabinowich L. (1988). The clinical neuro-ophthalmologic spectrum of temporal arteritis. *Am J Med 85:*839–844.

Melberg NS, Grand MG, Diekert JP, et al. (1995). Cotton-wool spots and the early diagnosis of giant cell arteritis. *Ophthalmology 102:*1611–1614.

Miller A, Green M. (1983). Simple rule for calculating normal erythrocyte sedimentation rate. *Br Med J 286:*266.

Miller NR. (1991). *Walsh and Hoyt's Clinical Neuro-ophthalmology.* 4th ed. Baltimore, William and Wilkins, pp. 2601–2627.

Mitnich HJ, Tunick PA, Rotterdam H, et al. (1990). Antemortem diagnosis of giant cell aortitis. *J Rheumatol 17:*708.

Mizen TR. (1991). Giant cell arteritis: Diagnostic and therapeutic considerations. *Ophthalmol Clin No Amer 4:*547–556.

Model DG. (1978). Reversal of blindness in temporal arteritis with methylprednisolone. *Lancet 1:*340.

Monteiro MLR, Coppetto JR, Greco P. (1984). Giant cell arteritis of the posterior cerebral circulation presenting with ataxia and ophthalmoplegia. *Arch Ophthalmol 102:*407–409.

Myles AB, Perera T, Ridley MG. (1992). Prevention of blindness in giant cell arteritis by corticosteroid treatment. *Br J Rheumatol 31:*103–105.

Nadaeu SE. (1988). Temporal arteritis: A decision-analytical approach to temporal artery biopsy. *Acta Neurol Scand 78:*90–100.

Neisch PR, Sergent JS. (1991). Giant cell arteritis: a case with unusual neurologic manifestations and a normal sedimentation rate. *Arch Intern Med 151:*378–380.

Nelson MW, Kunath AM, Welton RC, et al. (1982). Temporal arteritis presenting with jaw claudication and normal erythrocyte sedimentation rate. *South Med J 75:*1014–1016.

Nesher G, Rosenberg P, Shorer Z, Gilai A, Solomowovich A, Sunnerblick M. (1987). Involvement of the peripheral nervous system in temporal arteritis-polymyalgia rheumatica. Report of 3 cases and review of the literature. *J Rheumatol 14:*355–360.

Nesher G, Sonnenblick M, Friedlander Y. (1994). Analysis of steroid related complications and mortality in temporal arteritis: a 15 year survey of 43 patients. *J Rheumatol 21:*1283.

Nielsen NV, Eriksen JS. (1979). Unusual ocular manifestation in temporal arteritis. A case report. *Acta Ophthalmol 57:*362–368.

Ninet JP, Bachet P, Dumontet CM, et al. (1990). Subclavian and axillary involvement in temporal arteritis and polymyalgia rheumatica. *Am J Med 88:*13.

Nordborg E, Bengtsson BA. (1989). Death rates and causes of death in 284 consecutive patients with giant cell arteritis confirmed by biopsy. *Br Med J 299:*549–550.

Nordborg E, Bengtsson BA. (1990). Epidemiology of biopsy-proven giant cell arteritis (GCA). *J Intern Med 227:*233.

O'Neill WM, Jr., Hammar SP, Bloomer HA. (1976). Giant cell arteritis with visceral angiitis. *Arch Intern Med 136:*1157–1160.

Orgull S, Gass A, Flammer J. (1994). Optic disc cupping in arteritic anterior ischemic optic neuropathy. *Ophthalmologica 208:*336–338.

Orrell RW, Johnson MH. (1993). Plasma viscosity and the diagnosis of giant cell arteritis. *Br J Clin Practice 47:*71–72.

Ostberg G. (1971) Temporal arteritis in a large necropsy series. *Am J Rheum Dis 30:*224,.

Papaioannou CC, Hunder GG, McDuffie FC. (1979). Cellular immunity in polymyalgia rheumatica and giant cell arteritis: Lack of response to muscle or artery homogenates. *Arthritis Rheum 22:*740–745.

Pedro-Botet J, Coll J, Lopez MJ, Grau JM. (1996). Pericardial effusion and giant cell arteritis (letter). *Br J Rheumatol 35:*194–195.

Permin H, Juhl F, Wiik A, Balslov JT. (1973). Immunoglobulin deposits in the dermo-epidermal junction zone in patients with systemic lupus erythematosus, rheumatoid arthritis and temporal arteritis compared by serological testing including a2 macroglobulin. *Scand J Rheumatol 6:*105–110.

Persillin ST, Daniels TM, Riggs LJ, et al. (1985). Factor VIII-von Willebrand factor in giant cell arteritis and polymyalgia rheumatica. *Mayo Clin Proc 60:*457–462.

Phelan MJ, Kok K, Burrow C, Thompson RN. (1993). Small bowel infarction in association with giant cell arteritis. *Br J Rheum 32:*63–65.

Ponge T, Barrier JH, Grolleau JY, et al. (1988). The efficacy of selective unilateral temporal artery biopsy versus bilateral biopsies for diagnosis of giant cell arteritis. *J Rheumatol 15:*997.

Postel EA, Pllock SC. (1993). Recovery of vision in a 47-year-old man with fulminant giant cell arteritis. *J Clin Neuro-ophthalmol 13:*262–270.

Pountain G, Calvin J, Hazleman BL. (1994). Alpha 1-antichymotrypsin, C-reactive protein and erythrocyte sedimentation rate in polymyalgia rheumatica and giant cell arteritis. *Br J Rheum 33:*550–554.

Pountain G, Hazleman B. (1995). ABC of rheumatology. Polymyalgia rheumatica and giant cell arteritis. *BMJ 310:*1057–1059.

Quillen DA, Cantore WA, Schwartz SR, Brod RD, Saddani JW. (1993). Choroidal nonperfusion in giant cell arteritis. *Am J Ophthalmol 116:*171–175.

Rabinowich L, Mehler MF. (1988). Parasympathetic involvement in biopsy-proven temporal arteritis. *Ann Ophthalmol 20:*400–402.

Radda TM, Bardach H, Riss B. (1981a). Acute ocular hypotony. A rare complication of temporal arteritis. *Ophthalmologica 182:*148.

Radda TM, Pehamberger H, Smolen J, Menzel J. (1981b). Ocular manifestations of temporal arteritis: Immunological studies. *Arch Ophthalmol 99:*487–488.

Rauser M, Rismondo V. (1995). Ischemic optic neuropathy during corticosteroid therapy for giant cell arteritis (letter). *Arch Ophthalmol 113:*707–708.

Reich KA, Giansiracusa DF, Strongwater SL. (1990). Neurologic manifestations of giant cell arteritis. *Am J Med 89:*67–72.

Reinitz E, Aversa A. (1988). Long-term treatment of temporal arteritis with dapsone. *Am J Med 85:*457.

Richardson JE, Gladmann DD, Fam A, Keystone EC. (1987). HLA-DR4 in giant cell arteritis: Association with polymyalgia rheumatica syndrome. *Arthritis Rheum 30:*1293–1297.

Richardson MP, Lever AM, Fink AM, Dixon AK, Hazleman BL. (1996). Survival after aortic dissection in giant cell arteritis (letter). *Ann Rheum Dis 55:*332–333.

Rischmueller M, Davies RP, Smith MD. (1996). Three year follow-up of a case of giant cell arteritis presenting with a chronic cough and upper limb ischaemic symptoms. *Br J Rheumatol 35:*800–802.

Rivest D, Brunet D, Desbiens R, Bouchard JP. (1995). C-5 radiculopathy as a manifestation of giant cell arteritis. *Neurology 45:*1222–1224.

Robb-Nicholson C, Chang RW, Anderson S, et al. (1988). Diagnostic value of history and examination in giant cell arteritis: A clinical pathological study of 81 temporal artery biopsies. *J Rheumatol 15:*1793.

Ronchetto F. (1992). Transient monocular blindness in a patient with giant-cell arteritis. Pathogenetic and therapeutic considerations (letter). *Recenti Progressi in Medicina 83:*241–242.

Rosenfeld SI, Kosmorsky GS, Klingele TG, Burde RM, Cohen EM. (1986). Treatment of temporal arteritis with ocular involvement. *Am J Med 80:*143–145.

Roth AM, Milsow L, Keltner JL. (1984). The ultimate diagnosis of patients undergoing temporal artery biopsies. *Arch Ophthalmol 102*:901.

Rousseau P. (1994). Giant cell arteritis. *Arch Fam Med 3*:628–632.

Rubinow A, Brandt KD, Cohen AS, et al. (1984). Iatrogenic morbidity accompanying suppression of temporal arteritis by adrenal corticosteroids. *Ann Ophthalmol 16*:258.

Ruiz-Masera JJ, Alamillos-Granados FJ, Dean-Ferrer A, et al. (1995). Submandibular swelling as the first manifestation of giant cell arteritis. Report of a case. *J Cranio-Maxillo-Facial Surgery 23*:119–121.

Rush JA, Kramer LD. (1979). Biopsy-negative cranial arteritis with complete oculomotor palsy. *Ann Ophthalmol 11*:209.

Russell RUR. (1969). Giant cell arteritis: Review of 35 cases. *Qtr J Med 28*:471–489.

Russell RW. (1996). Giant cell arteritis—a clinical review. *Curr Med Drugs 7*:3–8.

Rynes RI, Mika P, Bartholomew LE. (1977). Development of giant cell (temporal) arteritis in a patient "adequately" treated for polymyalgia rheumatica. *Ann Rheum Dis 36*:88–90.

Salvarani C, Gabriel SE, O'Fallon WM, Hunder GG. (1995). The incidence of giant cell arteritis in Olmsted County, Minnesota: Apparent fluctuations in cyclic pattern. *Ann Intern Med 123*:192 194.

Salvarani C, Macchioni P, Zizzi F, et al. (1991). Epidemiologic and immunogenic aspects of polymyalgia rheumatica and giant cell arteritis in northern Italy. *Arthritis Rheum 34*:351–356.

Sanchez MC, Arenillas JIC, Guitierrez DA, Alonso JLG, Alvarez JP. (1983). Cervical radiculopathy: A rare symptom of giant cell arteritis. *Arthritis Rheum 26*:207–210.

Sanford RG, Berney SN. (1977). Polymyalgia rheumatica and temporal arteritis in blacks—clinical features and HLA typing. *J Rheumatol 4*:493–496.

Save-Soderbergh J, Malmvall BE, Anderson R, et al. (1986). Giant cell arteritis as a cause of death: Report of nine cases. *JAMA 255*:493–496.

Schmidt D, Loffler KU. (1994). Temporal arteritis. Comparison of histological and clinical findings. *Acta Ophthalmologica 72*:319–325.

Schneider HA, Weber AA, Ballen PH. (1971). The visual prognosis in temporal arteritis. *Ann Ophthalmol 3*:1215–1230.

Schwartz NG, Beck RW, Savino PJ, et al. (1995). Pain in anterior ischemic optic neuropathy. *J Neuro-ophthalmol 15*:9–10.

Sebag J, Thomas JV, Epstein DL, Grant WM. (1986). Optic disc cupping in arteritic anterior ischemic optic neuropathy resembles glaucomatous cupping. *Ophthalmol 93*:357–361.

Sehgal M, Swanson JW, DeRemee RA, Cobly TV. (1995). Neurologic manifestations of Churg-Strauss syndrome. *Mayo Clin Proc 70*:337–341.

Selsky IJ, Nirankari VS. (1985). Temporomandibular joint pain as a manifestation of temporal arteritis. *South Med J 78*:249–251.

Sheehan MM, Keohane C, Twomey C. (1993). Fatal vertebral giant cell arteritis. *J Clin Pathol 46*:1129–1131.

Shenberger KN, Meharg JG, Lane CD. (1981). Temporal arteritis presenting as ataxia and dementia. *Postgrad Med 69*:246–249.

Shiiki H, Shimokama T, Watanabe T. (1989). Temporal arteritis: cell composition and the possible pathogenetic role of cell mediated immunity. *Hum Pathol 20*:1057–1064.

Siatkowski RM, Gass JDM, Glaser JS, Smith JL, Schatz NJ, Schiffman J. (1993). Fluorescein angiography in the diagnosis of giant cell arteritis. *Am J Ophthalmol 115*:57–63.

Sibony PA, Lessell S. (1984). Transient oculomotor synkinesis in temporal arteritis. *Arch Neurol 41*:87–88.

Slamovits TL, Matzkin SC, Burde RM, Sachs R. (1992). IV steroids for central retinal artery occlusion in giant cell arteritis. (letter). *Ophthalmology 99*:1482–1484.

Slavin ML, Barnondes MJ. (1994). Visual loss caused by choroidal ischemia preceding anterior ischemic optic neuropathy in giant cell arteritis. *Am J Ophthalmol 117*:81–86.

Slavin ML, Margolis AJ. (1988). Progressive anterior ischemic optic neuropathy due to giant cell arteritis despite high-dose intravenous corticosteroids (letter). *Arch Ophthalmol 106*:1167.

Small P. (1984). Giant cell arteritis presenting as a bilateral stroke. *Arthritis Rheum 27*:819.

Smith AJ, Kyle V, Cawston ET, Hazleman BL. (1987). Isolation and analysis of immune complexes from sera of patients with polymyalgia rheumatica and giant cell arteritis. *Ann Rheum Dis 46*:468–474.

Sofferman RA. (1980). Cranial arteritis in otolaryngology. *Ann Otol 89*:215–219.

Sonnenblick M, Nesher G, Friedlander Y, Rubinow A. (1994). Giant cell arteritis in Jerusalem: A 12-year epidemiologic study. *Br J Rheum 33*:938–941.

Sorensen PS, Lorenzen I. (1977). Giant-cell arteritis, temporal arteritis and polymyalgia rheumatica. *Acta Med Scand 201*:207–213.

Sox HC, Liang MH. (1986). The erythrocyte sedimentation rate: Guidelines for rational use. *Ann Intern Med 104*:515–523.

Spencer WF, Hoyt WF. (1965). A fatal case of giant-cell arteritis (temporal or cranial) with ocular involvement. *Arch Ophthalmol 64*:862–867.

Spiera H, Davidson S. (1978). Long-term follow-up of polymyalgia rheumatica. *Mt Sinai J Med 45*:225–229.

Spiotta EF, Blumenfeld HB, Hayes WT. (1975). Temporal arteritis. Clinicopathologic conference. *J Tenn Med Assoc 68*:19–21.

Spolaore R, Gaudric A, Coscas G, De Margerie J. (1984). Acute sectorial choroidal ischemia. *Am J Ophthalmol 98*:707.

Srigley JR, Gardner GW. (1980). Giant cell arteritis with small bowel infarction. A case report and review of the literature. *Am J Gastroenterol 73:*157–161.
Stevens RJ, Hughes RA. (1995). The aetiopathogenesis of giant cell arteritis. *Br J Rheumatol 34:*960.
Tang RA. (1988). Giant cell arteritis diagnosis and management. *Semin Ophthalmol 3:*244.
Tang RA, Kaldis RC. (1982). Retinopathy in temporal arteritis. *Ann Ophthalmol 14:*652–654.
Thompson GTD, Johnston JL, Sharpe JA, et al. (1989). Internuclear ophthalmoplegia in giant cell arteritis. *J Rheumatol 16:*693.
Thystrup J, Knudsen GM, Mogensen AM, Fledelius HC. (1994) Atypical visual loss in giant cell arteritis. *Acta Ophthalmol 72:*759–764,.
To KW, Enzer YR, Tsiaras WG. (1994). Temporal artery biopsy after one month of corticosteroid therapy. *Am J Ophthalmol 117:*265.
Tomer Y, Neufeld MY, Shoenfeld Y. (1992). Coma with triphasic wave pattern in EEG as a complication of temporal arteritis. *Neurology 42:*439.
Tomsak RL. (1997). *Handbook of treatment in Neuro-ophthalmology.* Newton, MA, Butterworth-Heineman.
Tomsak RL. (1991). Superficial temporal artery biopsy: A simplified technique. *J Clin Neuro-ophthalmol 11:*202–204.
Townes DE, Blodi FC. 1968. The diagnostic value of temporal artery biopsy. *Trans Am Ophthalmol Soc 66:*33–44.
Trend P, Graham E. (1990). Internuclear ophthalmoplegia in giant cell arteritis (letter). *J Neurol Neurosurg Psychiatr 53:*532.
Truong L, Kopelman RG, Williams GS, Pirani CL. (1985). Temporal arteritis and renal disease. *Am J Med 78:*171–175.
Turner RG, Henry J, Friedmann AI, et al. (1974). Giant cell arteritis. *Postgrad Med J 50:*265.
van der Veen MJ, Dinant HJ, van Booma-Frankfort C, van Albada-Kuipers GA, Biljsma JW. (1996). Can methotrexate be used as a steroid sparing agent in the treatment of polymyalgia rheumatica and giant cell arteritis? *Ann Rheum Dis 55:*219–223.
Verdich M, Nielsen NV. (1975). Acute transient ophthalmomalacia in giant-cell arteritis. Report of a case. *Acta Ophthalmol 53:*875–878.
Vilaseca J, Gonzalez A, Cid MC, Lopez-Vivancos J, Ortega A. (1987). Clinical usefulness of temporal artery biopsy. *Ann Rheum Dis 46:*282–285.
Vincent FM, Vincent T. (1986). Bilateral carotid siphon involvement in giant cell arteritis. *Neurosurgery 18:*773–776.
Von Knorring J, Wassatjerna C. (1976). Liver involvement in polymyalgia rheumatica. *Scand J Rheumatol 5:*197–204.
Wadman B, Werner I. (1972). Observations on temporal arteritis. *Acta Med Scand 192:*377–383.
Wagener HP, Hollenhorst RW. (1958). The ocular lesions of temporal arteritis. *Am J Ophthalmol 45:*617–630.
Walz-Leblanc BA, Ameli FM, Keystone EC. (1991). Giant cell arteritis presenting as limb claudication. Report and review of the literature. *J Rheum 18:*470–472.
Wang FM, Henkind P. (1979). Visual system involvement in giant cell (temporal) arteritis. *Surv Ophthalmol 69:*78–90.
Warrell DA, Godfrey S, Olsen EGJ. (1968). Giant-cell arteritis with peripheral neuropathy. *Lancet 1(550):* 1010–1013.
Wawryk SO, Ayberk H, Boyd AW, Rode J. (1991). Analysis of adhesion molecules in the immunopathogenesis of giant cell arteritis. *J Clin Pathol 44:*497–501.
Watson P. (1984). Temporal arteritis: Dysphagia and a normal ESR. *JAMA 252:*1280–1281.
Weems JJ Jr. (1992). Diagnosis of giant cell arteritis by occipital artery biopsy (letter). *Am J Med 93:*231–232.
Weinberg DA, Savino PJ, Sergott RC, Bosley TM. (1994). Giant cell arteritis. Corticosteroids, temporal artery biopsy and blindness. *Arch Fam Med 3:*623–627.
Weinstein A, Del Guidice J. (1994). The erythrocyte sedimentation rate—time honored and tradition bound. *J Rheumatol 21:*1177.
Weintreb MI. (1978). Temporal arteritis. *Arch Neurol 35:*183.
Weiss LM, Gonzalez E, Miller SB, Agudelo CA. (1995). Severe anemia as the presenting manifestation of giant cell arteritis. *Arthr Rheum 38:*434–436.
Weisman MH. (1995). Corticosteroids in the treatment of rheumatologic diseases. *Curr Opin Rheum 7:*183–190.
Wendling D, Hory B, Blanc D. (1985). Cyclosporine: A new adjuvant therapy for giant cell arteritis (letter). *Arthritis Rheum 28:*1078–1079.
Wessels IF. (1987). Posterior ischemic optic neuropathy during general surgery. *Am J Ophthalmol 104:*555–556.
Weyand CM, Bartley GB. (1997). Editorial: Giant cell arteritis: New concepts in pathogenesis and implications for management. *Am J Ophthalmol 123:*392–395.
Weyand CM, Gorozny JJ. (1995). Giant cell arteritis as an antigen driven disease. *Rheum Dis Clin No Amer 21:*1027–1039.
Weyand CM, Hicok KC, Hunder GG, Goronzy JJ. (1992). The HLA-DRB1 locus as a genetic component in giant cell arteritis: Mapping of a disease-linked sequence motif to the antigen-binding site of the HLA-DR molecule. *J Clin Invest 90:*2355–2361.
Weyand CM, Schonberger J, Ippitz U, Hunder NNH, Hicok KC, Goronzy JJ. (1994). Distinct vascular lesions in giant cell arteritis share identical T cell clonotypes. *J Exp Med 179:*695–703.

Wilke WS, Hoffman GS. (1995). Treatment of corticosteroid-resistant giant cell arteritis. *Rheum Dis Clin No Amer 21*:59–71.
Wilkinson IMS, Russell RWR. (1972). Arteries of the head and neck in giant cell arteritis. A pathological study to show the pattern of arterial involvement. *Arch Neurol 27*:378–391.
Wilske KR, Healey LA. (1971). Clinical manifestations of biopsy-proven giant cell arteritis. *Arthritis Rheum 14*:424.
Winter BJ, Cryer TH, Hameroff SB. (1977). Anterior segment ischemia in temporal arteritis. *South Med J 70*:1479.
Wise CM, Agudelo CA, Chmeleski WL, McKnight KM. (1991). Temporal arteritis with low erythrocyte sedimentation rate: A review of five cases. *Arthritis Rheum 34*:217–219.
Wong RL, Korn JH. (1986). Temporal arteritis without an elevated erythrocyte sedimentation rate. Case report and review of the literature. *Am J Med 80*:959.
Zenone T, Souquet PJ, Bohas C, Vital Durand D, Bernard JP. (1994). Unusual manifestations of giant cell arteritis: Pulmonary nodules, cough, conjunctivitis and otitis with deafness. *Eur Resp J 7*:2252–2254.
Zion VM, Goodside V. (1974) Anterior segment ischemia with ischemic optic neuropathy. *Surv Ophthalmol 19*:19–30.
Zweegman S, Makkink B, Stehouwer CD. (1993). Giant-cell arteritis with normal erythrocyte sedimentation rate: Case report and review of the literature. *Netherlands J Med 42*:128–131.

6

Traumatic Optic Neuropathy

What Is the Traumatic Optic Neuropathy?

Traumatic optic neuropathy (TON) is a clinical diagnosis. Table 6–1 summarizes the clinical features and Table 6–2 lists the proposed mechanisms for TON.

Table 6–1. Clinical Features of Traumatic Optic Neuropathy

History of direct or indirect impact injury to the head, face, or orbit
Unilateral or bilateral visual loss
Variable loss of visual acuity (range 20/20 to no light perception)
Variable loss of visual field
Relative afferent pupillary defect (unilateral or bilateral but asymmetric cases)
Commonly normal or less commonly swollen optic nerve (Brodsky, 1995)
Eventual ipsilateral optic atrophy
Exclusion of other etiologies of visual loss in the setting of trauma:
Open globe
Traumatic cataract
Vitreous hemorrhage
Retinal detachment

Table 6–2. Proposed Mechanisms of Traumatic Optic Neuropathy

Compressive or direct mechanical injury
Laceration
Optic nerve contusion, edema, and swelling
Avulsion or transection
Bone fragment or fracture
Hemorrhage
Retrobulbar with increased intraorbital pressure
Subperiosteal hematoma
Optic nerve sheath hematoma
Vascular injury
Vasospasm
Ischemia
Infarction

Source: Aitken, 1991; Anderson, 1982; Feist, 1987; Frenkel, 1987; Guy, 1989; Hedges, 1981; Holt, 1983; Keane, 1989; Lessell, 1989; Manor, 1986; Matsuzaki, 1982; Mauriello, 1992; Miller, 1990; Millesi, 1988; Nau, 1987; Obenchain, 1973; Steinsapir, 1994; Sullivan, 1969; Ticho, 1973; Venable, 1978; Volpe, 1991; Wolin, 1990; Wyllie, 1972.

What Is the Evaluation of Traumatic Optic Neuropathy?

Once the clinical diagnosis of TON is made, neuroimaging should be performed if possible. The incidence of visible canal fracture in TON is variable and does not correlate well with the severity of visual loss (Goldberg, 1992; Lessell, 1989; Manfredi, 1981; Ramsay, 1979; Seiff, 1984, 1990; Steinsapir, 1994). Computed tomography (CT) may be the best imaging study for the evaluation of TON, detailed examination for bone fractures, evaluation of bone anatomy (Goldberg, 1992), and detection of acute hemorrhage (Knox, 1990; Lipkin, 1987; Manfredi, 1981, Seiff, 1984, 1990). Crowe et al. described a case of an intrasheath and intrachiasmal hemorrhage and delayed visual loss (Crowe, 1989). Chou et al. in 1996 summarized the literature on TON from 1922 to 1990 and reported optic canal fracture in 92 of 431 cases (21%) (Chou, 1996).

The role of magnetic resonance (MR) imaging in TON has yet to be clearly defined (Takehara, 1994). In addition, MR imaging is generally not available in the acute setting and is less useful than CT imaging for the detection of acute hemorrhage, canal fractures, and bone anatomy.

What Is the Treatment of Traumatic Optic Neuropathy?

The natural history of TON is unknown. Hughes described 56 cases of untreated TON of which 44% were permanently blind and 16% gained useful vision (Hughes, 1962). There

Table 6–3. Grades of Traumatic Optic Neuropathy

Grade 1:	Acuity better than 20/200 without posterior orbital fracture
Grade 2:	Acuity 20/200 to light perception (LP) without a posterior orbital fracture
Grade 3:	Acuity of no light perception (NLP) or presence of nondisplaced posterior orbital fracture and some remaining vision
Grade 4:	NLP and a displaced posterior orbital fracture

Source: Cook, 1996.

is, however, no large, well-controlled randomized prospective data regarding the treatment of TON. The literature on medical and surgical treatment of TON is thus difficult to summarize accurately because of the variations in clinical presentation, treatment modalities (e.g., steroids alone, steroids with surgery, surgery alone), variable surgical techniques and approaches, variable study inclusion criteria, recruitment bias, small sample sizes, and different outcome measures. Cook, et al. in 1996 reviewed all cases of TON published in the English language literature and performed a meta-analysis of treatment results (Cook, 1996). Patients were classified into one of four grades (see Table 6–3) depending on visual acuity and the location and type of fracture.

Recovery of vision was significantly better in patients who underwent treatment compared with observation alone. No significant difference in improvement was noted in patients treated with corticosteroids alone, surgical decompression alone, or a combination of those modalities. The prognosis for visual recovery worsened with increasing severity of grade. Recovery of vision was better in patients without orbital fractures and in those with anterior rather than posterior fractures.

Chou et al. in 1996 summarized the treatment results from the literature (28 reports) and found improvement in 94 (53%) of 176 medical treatment patients; 219 (46%) of 477 surgical treatment patients; and 25 of 81 (31%) patients without treatment (Chou, 1996). These authors divided the patients undergoing medical and surgical treatment into two groups: patients with no light perception (NLP) vision and those with better than light perception (LP) vision. They reported that the NLP group had an improvement rate of 36% (14 of 39 patients) following medical treatment and 34% (19 of 56 patients) following surgical treatment, versus the better than LP group that had an improvement rate of 70% (55 of 79) after medical treatment and 70% (69 of 98) after surgical treatment (Chou, 1996).

How Much and What Dose of Corticosteroids Should Be Used?

Although the mainstay of medical treatment for TON has been corticosteroids, there is no prospective well-controlled study to support the efficacy of treatment or the validity of the various steroid preparations, dosages, or duration of therapy (Anderson, 1982; Lam, 1990; Mauriello, 1992; Volpe, 1991). Anderson, et al. proposed dexamethasone 3 to

5 mg/kg/day for all patients with TON and advocated surgery for patients with delayed visual loss who failed medical treatment or those with initial visual improvement followed by worsening despite medical treatment (Anderson, 1982). Three (50%) of six patients had visual recovery after steroids, and four patients underwent transethmoidal-sphenoidal decompression with return of vision in one case (25%). Seiff reported a nonconsecutive, nonrandomized retrospective series of 36 patients with TON (Seiff, 1990). Eighteen patients experienced visual improvement, including 5 of 15 (33%) patients who did not receive corticosteroids, and 13 of 21 (62%) patients treated with dexamethasone 1 mg/kg/day. This difference was not found to be statistically significant. Spoor et al. reported an uncontrolled, nonconsecutive, retrospective series of 22 eyes in 21 patients with TON (Spoor, 1990). Of these 21 patients, 8 received intravenous (IV) dexamethasone 20 mg every 6 hours and 13 received IV methylprednisolone (MP) 30 mg/kg load followed by 15 mg/kg every 6 hours. Visual improvement occurred in 7 of 9 patients in the dexamethasone group and 12 of the 13 patients in the MP group. Lessell described 33 cases of TON. Vision improved in 5 of 25 untreated cases, 1 of 4 treated with corticosteroids, and 3 of 4 treated with transethmoidal decompression (Lessell, 1989).

Since there are no double-masked, placebo-controlled, prospective, randomized data for the treatment of TON, many authors have advocated high doses of IV corticosteroids for TON, extrapolating the data on the use of higher dose MP for central nervous system (CNS) injury (Bracken, 1984, 1985, 1990, 1993). The first National Acute Spinal Cord Injury Study (NASCIS 1) (Bracken, 1993) was a non-placebo-controlled study that concluded there was no beneficial effect of MP 1000 mg bolus followed by 1000 mg per day for 10 days ("high dose") compared with MP 100 mg bolus, then 100 mg per day for 10 days ("standard dose"). NASCIS 2 was a multicenter, placebo-controlled, randomized, double-masked study of acute spinal cord injury that showed that treatment within 8 hours with MP 30 mg/kg bolus followed by 5.4 mg/kg/hr for 24 hours resulted in significant improvement in motor and sensory function compared to placebo. MP delivered after 8 hours did not improve neurologic outcome. It was felt that MP in the 15 to 30 mg/kg dose range had a different pharmacologic effect on CNS injury parameters including blood flow, calcium homeostasis, energy metabolism, and clinical outcome (Bracken, 1984, 1985, 1990, 1993). The traditional dose calculation for

Table 6–4. Traumatic Optic Neuropathy Protocol

Diagnose TON appropriately
Perform canthotomy or cantholysis if the orbit is tense. Drain subperiosteal hematoma if present (Gillum, 1981; Katz, 1983; Wolter, 1978)
Institute MP (30 mg/kg IV bolus, then 5.4 mg/kg/hr IV for 48 hours or 15 mg/kg every 6h) even in patients with NLP (Feist, 1987; Joseph, 1990; Lessell, 1989; Marouf, 1985; Spoor, 1990)
If vision improves on IV MP after 48 hours, then start rapid oral taper of prednisone
If there is no clinical response after 48 hours or if vision deteriorates during the steroid taper, then surgical decompression of the optic canal is offered.

Source: Modified from Steinsapir, 1994.

an equivalent dose of dexamethasone compared with MP has been based on the glucocorticoid potency of 5:1. Steinsapir and Goldberg have emphasized that the potency ratio for dexamethasone to MP in CNS injury may be closer to 2:1 and therefore that dexamethasone 15 mg/kg may be required (compared to the dose of 3 to 6 mg/kg recommended by Anderson and other authors) for the adequate treatment of TON (Steinsapir, 1994).

Table 6–4 outlines a protocol for the treatment of TON.

What Is the Surgical Treatment of Traumatic Optic Neuropathy?

Multiple surgical approaches (e.g., lateral facial, transantral, transconjunctival/intranasal endoscopic, sublabial transnasal, transfrontal, transethmoidal, or a combination of these approaches, extracranial versus intracranial, etc.) and surgical indications have been offered for the treatment of TON. Unfortunately, there is no well-controlled prospective data to support the use of any one surgical approach to the optic nerve over another (Anand, 1991; Call, 1986; Fernandez, 1994; Friedman, 1991; Fujitani, 1986; Fukado, 1975, Girard, 1992; Guyer, 1985; Joseph, 1990; Karnik, 1981; Kennerdell, 1976; Knox, 1990; Kuppersmith, 1997; Levin, 1994; Lipkin, 1987; Niho, 1970; Sofferman, 1981; Spoor, 1986; Steinsapir, 1994; Takahashi, 1989; Walsh, 1966). Of particular interest is the literature from Japan concerning TON. Several papers have suggested that TON is much more common in Japan and more responsive to surgical treatment. Fukado reported 460 canal fractures on stereoscopic radiography of the optic canal in 500 patients with loss of vision following head trauma. Of 400 patients who underwent transethmoidal canal decompression, almost 100% had improvement. Several authors have raised serious questions about these studies, including the validity of the diagnostic criteria for canal fracture; the lack of complete ocular examination data including visual field information; the paucity of bilateral cases; the high percentage of improvement after surgery; and the suspiciously high frequency of canal fracture (Kennerdell, 1976). Niho et al. reported an 80% success rate in 25 patients with TON and transsphenoidal decompression of the canal (Niho, 1970). Matsuzaki et al. reported optic canal fractures in 51% of 33 patients with TON (Matsuzaki, 1982). Vision improved in 36% of the 11 cases undergoing surgical decompression of the canal (8 transcranial and 3 transethmoidal). Vision improved in 50% of the 22 patients treated medically with prednisone (40–100 mg/day for 5–7 days), mannitol, and urokinase (if perineural hematoma was suspected). Fujitani, et al. reported 110 cases of TON, of which 43 cases underwent medical therapy with prednisone 60 mg/day and 70 eyes underwent transethmoidal decompression. The medically treated group had a 44% improvement rate versus a 47% improvement rate after surgery (Fujitani, 1986).

Joseph, et al. reported 14 patients in a retrospective, nonconsecutive study with TON treated with transethmoidal-sphenoidal canal decompression and dexamethasone pre- and post-operatively. Eleven of the 14 patients improved including 3 of 5 patients who presented with NLP vision (Joseph, 1990).

Unfortunately, until a randomized, prospective, double-masked, placebo-controlled clinical trial is performed, the treatment of TON will remain controversial. The approach to TON is outlined in Figure 6–1.

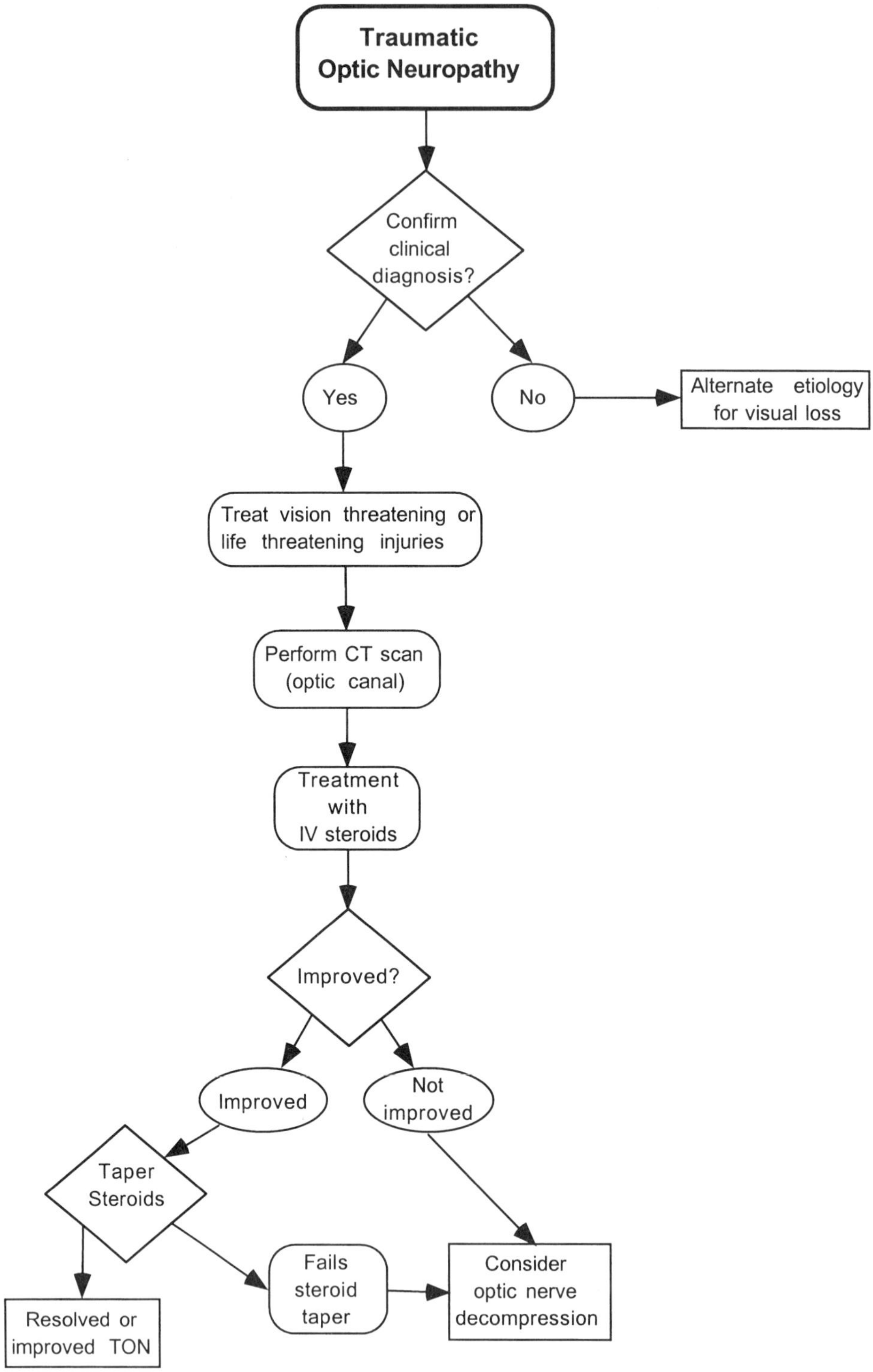

Figure 6–1. Traumatic optic neuropathy.

References

Aitken P, Sofferman R. (1991). Traumatic optic neuropathy. *Ophthalmol Clin North Amer 4:*479–490.

Anand VK, Sherwood C, Al-Mefty O. (1991). Optic nerve decompression via transethmoidal and supraorbital approaches. *Op Tech Otolaryngol Head Neck Surg 2:*157–166.

Anderson RL, Panje WR, Gross CE. (1982). Optic nerve blindness following blunt forehead trauma. *Ophthalmology 89:*445–455.

Berestka JS, Rizzo JF, III. (1994). Controversy in the management of traumatic optic neuropathy. *Int Ophthalmol Clin 34(3):*87–96.

Bracken MB, Collins WF, Freeman DF, et al. (1984). Efficacy of methylprednisolone in acute spinal cord injury. *JAMA 251:*45–52.

Bracken MB, Holford TR. (1993). Effects of timing of methylprednisolone or naloxone administration on recovery of segmental and long-tract neurologic function in NASCIS 2. *J Neurosurg 79:*500–507.

Bracken MB, Shepard MJ, Collins WF, et al. (1990). A randomized controlled trial of methylprednisolone or naloxone in the treatment of acute spinal cord injury. Results of the Second National Acute Spinal Cord Injury Study. *N Engl J Med 322:*1405–1411.

Bracken MB, Shepard MJ, Hellenbrand KG, et al. (1985). Methylprednisolone and neurological function 1 year after spinal cord injury. Results of the National Acute Spinal Cord Injury Study. *J Neurosurg 63:*713.

Brodsky MC, Wald KJ, Chen S, Weiter JJ. (1995). Protracted posttraumatic optic disc swelling. *Ophthalmology 192:*1628–1631.

Call N. (1986). Decompression of the optic nerve in the optic canal. *Ophthalmic Plast Reconstr Surg 2:*133–137.

Chou PI, Sadun AA, Chen YC, Su WY, Lin SZ, Lee CC. (1996). Clinical experiences in the management of traumatic optic neuropathy. *Neuro-ophthalmology 18:*325–336.

Cook MW, Levin LA, Joseph MP, Pinczower EF. (1996). Traumatic optic neuropathy. A meta-analysis. *Arch Otolaryngol Head Neck Surg 122:*389–392.

Crowe NW, Nickles TP, Troost T, Elster AD. (1989). Intrachiasmal hemorrhage: A cause of delayed post-traumatic blindness. *Neurology 39:*863–865.

Davis WH, Nevins RC, Williot JH. (1972). Optic atrophy after ocular contusion. *Am J Ophthalmol 73:*278–280.

Elisevich KV, Ford RM, Anderson DP, et al. (1984). Visual abnormalities with multiple trauma. *Surg Neurol 22:*565–575.

Feist RM, Kline LB, Morris RE, et al. (1987). Recovery of vision after presumed direct optic nerve injury. *Ophthalmology 94:*1567–1569.

Fernandez CIS, Rollon A, Padilla JDG. (1994). Posttraumatic amaurosis with partial return of visual acuity. *J Oral Maxillofacial Surg 52:*1077–1079.

Frenkel R, Spoor T. (1987). Diagnosis and management of traumatic optic neuropathies. *Adv Ophthalmic Plast Reconstr Surg 6:*71–90.

Friedman M. (1991). Optic nerve decompression. *Op Tech Otolaryngol Head Neck Surg 2:*149.

Fujitani T, Inoue K, Takahashi T, et al. (1986). Indirect traumatic optic nerve neuropathy—visual outcome of operative and non-operative cases. *Jpn J Ophthalmology 30:*125–134.

Fukado Y. (1972). Results in 350 cases of surgical decompression of the optic nerve. *Trans Asia Pacif Acad Ophthalmol 4:*96–99.

Fukado Y. (1975). Results in 400 cases of surgical decompression of the optic nerve. *Mod Prob Ophthalmol 14:*474–481.

Gillum WN, Anderson RL. (1981). Reversible visual loss in subperiosteal hematoma of the orbit. *Ophthalmic Surg 12:*203–209.

Girard BC, Bouzas EA, Lama SG, et al. (1992). Visual improvement after transethmoidal-sphenoid decompression in optic nerve injuries. *J Clin Neuro-ophthalmol 12:*142.

Goldberg RA, Hannani K, Toga AW. (1992). Microanatomy of the orbital apex: Computed tomography and microplanning of soft and hard tissue. *Ophthalmology 99:*1447–1452.

Gross C, DeKock J, Panje W, Hershowitz N, Newman J. (1981). Evidence for orbital deformation that may contribute to monocular blindness following minor frontal head trauma. *J Neurosurg 55:*963–966.

Guy J, Sherwood M, Day AL. (1989). Surgical treatment of progressive visual loss in traumatic optic neuropathy. Report of two cases. *J Neurosurg 70:*799–801.

Guyer DR, Miller NR, Long DM, et al. (1985). Visual function following optic nerve decompression. *J Neurosurg 62:*631–638.

Guyon JJ, Brandt-Zawadzki M, Seiff SR. (1984). CT demonstration of optic canal fractures. *AJNR 143:*1031–1034.

Hedges TR, Gragoudas ES. (1981). Traumatic anterior ischemic optic neuropathy. *Ann Ophthalmol 13:*625–628.

Holt GR, Holt JE. (1983). Incidence of eye injuries in facial fractures: An analysis of 727 cases. *Otolaryngol Head Neck Surg 91:*276–279.

Hughes B. (1962). Indirect injury of the optic nerve and chiasm. *Bull Johns Hopkins Hosp 111:*98–126.

Joseph MP, Lessell S, Rizzo J, Momose KJ. (1990). Extracranial optic nerve decompression for traumatic optic neuropathy. *Arch Ophthalmol 108:*1091–1093.

Karnik PP, Maskati BT, Kirtane MV, Tonsekar KS. (1981). Optic nerve decompression in head injuries. *J Laryngol Otol 95:*1135–1140.

Katz B, Herschler J, Brick D. (1983). Orbital haemorrhage and prolonged blindness: A treatable posterior optic neuropathy. *Br J Ophthalmol 67*:549–553.

Keane JR. (1989). Neurologic eye signs following motorcycle accidents. *Arch Neurol 46*:761–762.

Kennerdell JS, Amsbaugh GA, Myers EN. (1976). Transantral-ethmoidal decompression of optic canal fracture. *Arch Ophthalmol 94*:1040–1043.

Kersten R, Rice C. (1987). Subperiosteal orbital hematoma: Visual recovery following delayed drainage. *Ophthalmic Surg 18*:423–427.

Kline LB, Morawetz RB, Swaid NS. (1984). Indirect injury of the optic nerve. *Neurosurgery 14*:756–764.

Knox BE, Gates GA, Berry SM. (1990). Optic nerve decompression via the lateral facial approach. *Laryngoscope 100*:458–462.

Krausen AS, Ogura JH, Burde RM, Ostrow DE. (1981). Emergency orbital decompression: A reprieve from blindness. *Otolaryngol Head Neck Surg 89*:252–256.

Kuppersmith RB, Alford EL, Patrinely JR, Lee AG, Parke RB, Holds JB. (1997). Combined transconjunctival/intranasal endoscopic approach to the optic canal in traumatic optic neuropathy. *Laryngoscope 107*:311–315.

Lam BL, Weingeist TA. (1990). Corticosteroid-responsive traumatic optic neuropathy. *Am J Ophthalmol 109*:99–101.

Lessell S. (1989). Indirect optic nerve trauma. *Arch Ophthalmol 107*:382–386.

Levin LA, Joseph MP, Rizzo JF III. (1994). Optic canal decompression in indirect optic nerve trauma. *Ophthalmology 101*:566.

Lipkin AF, Woodson GE, Miller RH. (1987). Visual loss due to orbital fracture. The role of early reduction. *Arch Otolaryngol Head Neck Surg 113*:82–83.

Mahapatra AK, Tandon DA. (1993). Traumatic optic neuropathy in children—a prospective study. *Pediatr Neurosurg 19*:34.

Manfredi SJ, Mohammad RR, Sprinkle PS, et al. (1981). Computerized tomographic scan findings in facial fractures associated with blindness. *Plast Reconstr Surg 68*:479–490.

Manor RS, Cohen S, Svetliza E, BenSira I. (1986). Papilledema in traumatic lesion of optic nerve with amaurosis. *J Clin Neuro-ophthalmol 6*:100–105.

Marouf LK, Azar DT. (1985). Reversible visual loss following optic nerve injury. *Ann Ophthalmol 17*:582–584.

Matsuzaki H, Kunita M, Kawai K. (1982). Optic nerve damage in head trauma: Clinical and experimental studies. *Jpn J Ophthalmol 26*:447–461.

Mauriello JA, DeLuca J, Krieger A, Schulder M, Frohman L. (1992). Management of traumatic optic neuropathy—a study of 23 patients. *Br J Ophthalmol 76*:349–352.

Miller NR. (1990). Editorial: The management of traumatic optic neuropathy. *Arch Ophthalmol 108*:1086–1087.

Millesi W, Hollmann K, Funder J. (1988). Traumatic lesion of the optic nerve. *Acta Neurochir 93*:50–54.

Nau HE, Gerhard L, Foerster M, et al. (1987). Optic nerve trauma: Clinical, electrophysiological and histological remarks. *Acta Neurochir 89*:16–27.

Niho S, Murakami I, Sugita S, Sugita Y, Kawabe Y. (1966). Decompression of the optic canal by the transethmoidal route. *Acta Soc Ophthalmol Jpn 70*:343–352.

Niho S, Niho M, Niho K. (1970). Decompression of the optic canal by the transethmoidal route and decompression of the superior orbital fissure. *Can J Ophthalmol 5*:22–40.

Noble MJ, McFadzean R. (1987). Indirect injury to the optic nerves and optic chiasm. *Neuro-ophthalmology 7*:341–348.

Obenchain TG, Killefer FA, Stern WE. (1973). Indirect injuries of the optic nerve and chiasm with closed head injury. *Bull Los Angeles Neurol Soc 38*:12–20.

Purvin V. (1988). Evidence of orbital deformation in indirect optic nerve injury. *J Clin Neuro-ophthalmol 8*:9–11.

Ramsay J. (1979). Optic nerve injury in fracture of the canal. *Br J Ophthalmol 63*:607–610.

Seiff RR. (1990). High dose corticosteroids for treatment of vision loss due to indirect injury to the optic nerve. *Ophthalmic Surg 21*:389–395.

Seiff RR, Berger MS, Guyon J, Pitts LH. (1984). Computerized tomographic evaluation of the optic canal in sudden traumatic blindness. *Am J Ophthalmol 98*:751–755.

Sofferman R. (1981). Sphenoethmoid approach to the optic nerve. *Laryngoscope 91*:184–196.

Spoor TC, Hartel WC, Lensink DB, Wilkinson MJ. (1990). Treatment of traumatic optic neuropathy with corticosteroids. *Am J Ophthalmol 110*:665–669.

Spoor TC, Mathog RH. (1986). Restoration of vision after optic canal decompression (letter). *Arch Ophthalmol 104*:804–806.

Steinsapir KD, Goldberg RA. (1994). Traumatic optic neuropathy. *Surv Ophthalmol 38*:487–518.

Sullivan G, Helveston EM. (1969). Optic atrophy after seemingly trivial trauma. *Arch Ophthalmol 81*:159–161.

Takahashi M, Itoh M, Kaneko M, Shiii J, Yoshida A. (1989). Microscopic intracranial decompression of the optic nerve. *Arch Otorhinolaryngol 246*:113–116.

Takehara S, Tanaka T, Uemura K, et al. (1994). Optic nerve injury demonstrated by MRI with STIR sequences. *Neuroradiology 36*:512.

Tang RA, Li HK, Regner LV, Bridges MB, Prager TC. (1986). Traumatic optic neuropathy: Analysis of 37 cases (abstract). *Invest Ophthalmol Vis Sci 27*:102.

Ticho U, Feinsod M. (1973). Traumatic optic neuritis. *Ann Ophthalmol 5*:430–432.

Venable H, Wilson S, Allan S, Prensky A. (1978). Total blindness after trivial frontal head trauma: Bilateral indirect optic nerve injury. *Neurology 28*:1066–1068.

Volpe N, Lessell S, Kline L. (1991). Traumatic optic neuropathy: Diagnosis and management. *Int Ophthalmol Clin 31:*142–156.

Walsh FB. (1966). Pathological-clinical correlations. I. Indirect trauma to the optic nerves and chiasm. II. Certain cerebral involvements associated with defective blood supply. *Invest Ophthalmol 5:*443–449.

Weymuller EA. (1984). Blindness and LeFort III fractures. *Ann Otol Rhinol Laryngol 93:*2.

Wolin M, Lavin P. (1990). Spontaneous visual recovery from traumatic optic neuropathy after blunt head injury. *Am J Ophthalmol 109:*430–435.

Wolter JR, Vanderveen GJ, Wacksman RL. (1978). Posttraumatic subgaleal hematoma extending into the orbit as a cause of permanent blindness. *J Pediatr Ophthalmol 15:*151–153.

Wyllie AM, McLeod D, Cullen JF. (1972). Traumatic ischemic optic neuropathy. *Br J Ophthalmol 56:*851–853.

7

Optic Disc Swelling and Papilledema

The term "papilledema" is frequently applied to optic disc swelling from any cause, but should be used only for disc swelling that results from increased intracranial pressure. Other forms of disc swelling due to local or systemic etiologies should be named according to their presumed etiology (e.g., optic neuritis, anterior ischemic optic neuropathy, etc). It is usually not possible to determine the etiology of disc swelling from the ophthalmoscopic appearance of the disc alone; the history and neuro-ophthalmologic examination, especially the visual fields, are necessary to reach an etiologic diagnosis. It is also important to note that optic disc swelling may not develop if optic atrophy is present.

The symptoms associated with optic disc swelling depend on the underlying etiology. In general, swollen optic discs from any cause may be associated with transient visual obscurations (see Chapter 8)(Sadun, 1984). These are typically unilateral or bilateral dimming or blacking out of vision that usually last seconds and may be precipitated by changes in posture (e.g., bending or straightening).

True disc swelling must be distinguished from pseudopapilledema and anomalously elevated discs caused by optic nerve head drusen (Lorentzen, 1966; Rosenberg, 1979). Pseudopapilledema, with or without optic disc drusen, is not an uncommon condition. Drusen of the disc may be obvious, tiny, or buried. Ophthalmoscopic criteria that distinguish pseudopapilledema form true papilledema include (Glaser, 1990):

1. An absent central cup with disc diameter toward small.
2. Vessels arise from the central apex of the disc.
3. Anomalous branching of vessels, increased number of disc vessels, venous pulsations present.
4. Disc may be transilluminated, with glow of drusen when present.
5. Disc margins irregular with derangement of peripapillary retinal pigment epithelium.
6. Absence of superficial capillary telangiectasia.
7. No hemorrhages (rare exceptions).
8. No exudates or cotton-wool spots.

Drusen may also be detected by autofluorescence, noted prior to the injection of dye with fluorescein angiography, and by computed tomography (CT) imaging in which small calcified masses may be noted in the optic nerve. Drusen may also be observed with orbital ultrasound, but are not seen on MR imaging. Although central visual acuity is usually preserved in patients with disc drusen, 70 to 75% of them have visual field defects, including blind spot enlargement, arcuate defects, and infero-nasal defects.

Other disc anomalies that may be mistaken for papilledema include "crowded" discs and tilted discs. In these cases, the peripapillary nerve fiber layer and the retinal vessels that traverse it remain normal, venous pulsations are usually present, there is no vascular engorgement or hemorrhages, there are no cotton-wool spots, and the discs do not leak dye on fluorescein angiography. Myelinated nerve fibers may occasionally resemble disc swelling but are characterized by a white feathery appearance.

Is the Disc Swelling Caused by Optic Neuropathy or Papilledema?

Disc swelling due to raised intracranial pressure (papilledema) is usually bilateral and approximately equal in both eyes. Unilateral disc swelling is most commonly caused by local pathology within the optic nerve or orbit. Unilateral papilledema can, however, occur, although most of these cases are actually bilateral but asymmetric disc swelling (Bruntse, 1970; Chari, 1991; Kirkham, 1973; Lepore, 1992; Maxner, 1987; Sher, 1983; Strominger, 1992; To, 1990). As noted, if one optic nerve is atrophic it will not swell, so that unilateral disc swelling may occur from increased intracranial pressure in these cases [e.g., in the Foster Kennedy syndrome, although many of these latter cases may be due to direct bilateral optic nerve compression rather than increased intracranial pressure per se (Watnick, 1989)]. An important feature that helps distinguish papilledema from other causes of disc swelling, such as optic neuritis or anterior ischemic optic neuropathy, is that during the initial presentation of papilledema, optic nerve function is usually preserved even in the presence of marked disc swelling. Patients with optic neuropathies usually have impaired visual acuity, impaired color vision, visual field defects, and, if unilateral or bilateral but asymmetric, a relative afferent pupillary defect. These optic neuropathies are discussed in Chapters 1 through 6. Processes causing optic neuropathies associated with disc swelling are usually unilateral, but may be bilateral, and are listed in Table 7–1.

Other processes that may mimic papilledema and that may present with bilateral optic disc swelling with little or no visual acuity impairment, color vision loss, or visual field defects and normal intracranial pressure are listed in Table 7–2.

Table 7–1. Bilateral Optic Neuropathies with Disc Edema

Infectious and inflammatory conditions, including optic neuritis, optic disc edema with macular star (ODEMS or neuroretinitis), uveitis, and sarcoidosis.
Vascular conditions, including arteritic and nonarteritic anterior ischemic optic neuropathy, disc swelling in diabetics, central retinal vein occlusion, and carotid-cavernous sinus fistula.
Infiltrative, compressive, and neoplastic processes, including sarcoidosis, lymphoma, optic nerve sheath meningioma, glioma, orbital pseudotumor, thyroid ophthalmopathy, and other intraorbital tumors.
Leber's hereditary optic neuropathy.
Trauma and mechanical causes, including hypotony.

Table 7–2. Etiologies for Bilateral Optic Disc Edema with Normal Visual Function

Hypertensive retinopathy—these patients usually have other funduscopic changes suggestive of hypertension (e.g., arteriolar narrowing, etc). However, the blood pressure should be measured in all patients presenting with bilateral disc swelling.
Cyanotic congenital heart disease—disc swelling may be due to decreased arterial oxygen saturation and polycythemia (Peterson, 1972).
Sleep apnea—probably by a mechanism similar to that in congenital cyanotic heart disease (Bucci, 1988).
Spinal cord tumors (Raynor, 1969)—these patients will have symptoms and signs of myelopathy (e.g., back pain, leg weakness, sensory changes, bladder involvement, etc).
Guillain-Barré syndrome (Ropper, 1984)—some of these patients may have increased intracranial pressure. Patients with Guillain-Barré syndrome have clinical evidence for a polyradiculoneuropathy (e.g., extremity paresis, areflexia, etc).
POEMS (peripheral neuropathy, organomegaly, endocrinopathy, monoclonal gammopathy, and skin changes) or the Crow-Fukase syndrome—these patients have evidence for a peripheral polyneuropathy, organomegaly (especially hepatomegaly), lymphadenopathy with the pathologic changes of Castleman's disease, endocrinopathy (including diabetes, thyroid dysfunction, gonadal failure), gammopathy or myeloma (often osteosclerotic myeloma), and skin changes (including diffuse hyperpigmentation, thickening of the skin, hypertrichosis, finger clubbing, white fingernails, verrucous angiomas of the skin, and peripheral edema) (Bolling, 1990).
Uremia—these patients may have normal or increased intracranial pressure.
Hypoxemia and anemia
Certain inflammatory or infectious processes, such as syphilis, sarcoidosis, and viral meningoencephalitis, affecting the meninges-disc swelling here is not due to papilledema but to perineuritis (Dutton, 1985; Hykin, 1991; Margo, 1989; Rush, 1981; Silverstein, 1974).

What Studies Should Be Performed to Investigate the Patient with Papilledema?

All patients with papilledema require a thorough neurologic and neuro-ophthalmologic history and physical examination. In general, the syndromes causing increased intracranial pressure are listed in Table 7–3.

In all patients with bilateral optic disc swelling, blood pressure should be checked to evaluate for possible malignant hypertension. Neuroimaging is required in all patients. CT imaging is the study of choice in the acute setting in evaluating the patient with a possible acute vascular processes (e.g., subarachnoid, epidural, subdural, or intracerebral hemorrhage, acute infarction) or after head trauma. CT studies are also indicated in patients with contraindications to MR imaging (e.g., pacemakers, metallic clips in head, metallic foreign bodies, etc.) or in those who are too large to fit into the machine or too claustrophobic to obtain an adequate study. Otherwise, magnetic resonance (MR) imaging, with and without contrast, is the modality of choice. In selected cases, we also obtain MR angiography or MR venography at the same time to evaluate the patient for arterial disease or venous obstruction. If neuroimaging shows no structural lesion or hydrocephalus, then lumbar puncture is warranted. Studies should include an accurate opening pressure, to evaluate for intracranial hypertension, as well as cell count and differential, glucose, protein, cytology, VDRL, and appropriate studies for microbial agents. As noted, optic disc swelling with normal intracranial pressure may result from optic perineuritis that is often infectious or inflammatory in nature; spinal fluid studies in these patients usually show elevated white cells in the spinal fluid.

Table 7–3. **Syndromes Causing Increased Intracranial Pressure**

Primary causes
Idiopathic intracranial hypertension (IIH, idiopathic pseudotumor cerebri syndrome) with papilledema
IIH without papilledema
Secondary causes
Hydrocephalus
Mass lesions—tumor, hemorrhage, large infarction, abscess
Meningitis/encephalitis
Subarachnoid hemorrhage
Trauma
Arteriovenous malformations with high blood flow overloading venous return
Intracranial or extracranial venous obstruction
Secondary pseudotumor cerebri syndrome due to certain systemic diseases, drugs, or pregnancy

Source: Adapted from JJ Corbett, personal communication.

What Is the Pseudotumor Cerebri Syndrome?

If neuroimaging studies are normal or reveal no structural lesion, cerebrospinal fluid contents are normal, and lumbar puncture opening pressures are elevated, the patient, by definition, has a pseudotumor cerebri syndrome. Pseudotumor cerebri is often idiopathic intracranial hypertension (IIH), but may result from certain systemic diseases, drugs, pregnancy, and intracranial or extracranial venous obstruction.

Obstruction or impairment of intracranial venous drainage may result in cerebral edema with increased intracranial pressure and papilledema. Tumors that occlude the posterior portion of the superior sagittal sinus or other cerebral venous sinuses may cause increased intracranial pressure as may septic or aseptic thrombosis or ligation of the cavernous sinus, lateral sinus, sigmoid sinus, or superior sagittal sinus (Couban, 1991; Cremer, 1996; Daif, 1995; Gills, 1967; Greer, 1967; Horton, 1992; Lam, 1992; Mones, 1965; Morantz, 1980; Powers, 1986; Schonsted-Madsen, 1984; Van den Brink, 1996). Ligation of one or both jugular veins (e.g., during radical neck dissection for regional tumors), thrombosis of a central intravenous catheter in the chest or neck, subclavian vein catheterization and arteriovenous fistula, the superior vena cava syndrome, or a glomus jugulare tumor impairing venous drainage may also cause increased intracranial pressure (Ageli, 1994; Beck, 1979; Blervacque, 1965; Brookes, 1984; Fitz-Hugh, 1966; Kiers, 1991; Lam, 1992; Rotellar, 1987; Tobin, 1971). Venous sinus thrombosis may be the mechanism of pseudotumor cerebri syndrome reported with systemic lupus erythematosus, essential thrombocythemia, protein S deficiency, antithrombin III deficiency, the antiphospholipid antibody syndrome, paroxysmal nocturnal hemoglobinuria, Behçet's disease, meningeal sarcoidosis, hypervitaminosis A, mastoiditis, and other disease processes associated with the secondary pseudotumor cerebri syndromes (Akova, 1993; Byrne, 1983; Daif, 1995; Hauser, 1996; Kaplan, 1985; Krausz, 1978; Mitchell, 1986; Mokri, 1993; Parnass, 1987). In fact, elevated intracranial venous pressure is thought by some authors to be the "universal mechanism" of pseudotumor cerebri of varying etiologies, including IIH (Karahalios, 1996; King, 1995). Increased blood flow and venous hypertension have also been implicated as the mechanism of papilledema noted in some patients with cerebral arteriovenous malformations (AVMs), especially dural AVMs (Chimowitz, 1990; Cockerell, 1993; David, 1995; Forman, 1975; Kuhner, 1976; Lamas, 1977; Nazarian, 1987; Rosenfeld, 1991; Takahashi, 1983; Van den

Bergh, 1980; Vassilouthis, 1979; Weisberg, 1977; Zabramski, 1988). Thus, we consider MR venography (and, in selected cases, MR angiography) is warranted to investigate the possibility of venous sinus occlusion in patients with pseudotumor cererbi, especially in patients with features not typical for IIH (e.g., in thin patients, men, elderly).

Many systemic diseases, drugs, vitamin deficiencies and excesses, pregnancy, and hereditary conditions have been associated with the pseudotumor cerebri syndrome (secondary pseudotumor cerebri). These reported etiologies are listed in Table 7–4.

In general, many of these reported associations may be coincidental and anecdotal. Of those listed in Table 7–4, the etiologies most firmly associated with pseudotumor cerebri include (Ireland 1990):

Table 7–4. Reported Etiologies of Secondary Pseudotumor Cerebri

Etiology or Association	References
Nutritional Causes	
Hypervitaminosis A	Alemayehu, 1995; Bhettay, 1988; Fedotin, 1970; Feldman, 1970; Gerber, 1954; Hawkins, 1974; James, 1982; Krausz, 1978; Lascari, 1970; Lombaert, 1976; Morrice, 1960; Moskowitz, 1993; Narayanan, 1972; Oliver, 1958; Pasquariello, 1977; Restak, 1972; Selhorst, 1984; Sharieff, 1996; Sirdofsky, 1994; Spector, 1984; Vollbracht, 1976
Hypovitaminosis A	Edmunds, 1973; Kasarskis, 1982; Roos 1985
Vitamin D deficient rickets	Alpan, 1991; DeJong, 1985; Hanafy, 1967
Multiple vitamin deficiencies	Van Gelder, 1991
Parenteral hyperalimentation	Saxena, 1976
Drugs and other exogenous agents	
Nalidixic acid	Boreus, 1967; Cohen, 1973; Deonna, 1974; Fisher, 1967; Gedroyc, 1982; Kilpatrick, 1982; Mukherjee, 1990; Rao, 1974
Tetracycline	Cuddihy, 1994; Folsom, 1966; Gardner, 1995; Giles, 1971; Jay, 1978; Köch-Weser, 1967; Maroon, 1971; Minutello, 1988; Ohlrich, 1977; O'Doherty, 1965; Olson, 1966; Pearson, 1981; Pierog, 1986; Sharma, 1975; Stuart, 1978; Walters, 1981
Minocycline	Beran, 1980; Donnet, 1992; Landers, 1989; Monaco, 1978; Moskowitz, 1993; Torres, 1997
Nitrofurantoin	Korzets, 1988; Mushet, 1977; Sharma, 1974
Penicillin	Grant, 1974
Ofloxacin	Getenet, 1993
Ciprofloxacin	Winrow, 1990
Amiodarone	Ahmad, 1996; Borruat, 1993; Cordon, 1985; Fikkers, 1986; Grogan, 1987
Lithium	Ames, 1994; Dommisse, 1991; Levine, 1990; Lobo, 1978; Saul, 1985
Phenytoin	Kalanie, 1986
Cytosine arabinoside	Evers, 1992
Cyclosporine	Avery, 1991; Cruz, 1996; Katz, 1997
Danazol or danazol withdrawal	Fanoous, 1991; Hamed, 1989; Pears, 1990; Shah, 1987
All-trans-retinoic acid (ATRA), tretinoin, isotretinoin	Mahmoud, 1993; Roytman, 1988; Selleri, 1996; Varadi, 1995; Visani, 1996; Yokokura, 1994
Etretinate	Bonnetblanc, 1983

(continued)

Table 7–4. *(continued)*

Leuprorelin acetate	Arber, 1990
Ketamine	Fontana, 1980
Indomethicin in Bartter's syndrome	Konomi, 1978
Ketoprofen in Bartter's syndrome	Larizza, 1979
Insecticide exposure—lindane, chlordecone (Kepone)	Jenkyn, 1979; Heuser, 1976; Sanborn, 1979; Verderber, 1991
Steroids, including topical steroids and anabolic steroids	Cohn, 1963; Dees, 1959; Fardal, 1982; Greer, 1963; Hosking, 1978; Laurence, 1960; Sakamaki, 1990; Vyas, 1981; Walker, 1964; Wigglesworth, 1967
Steroid withdrawal	Fourie, 1977; Liu, 1994; Neville, 1970; Roussounis, 1976
Oxytocin	Mayer-Hubner, 1996
Growth hormone	Price, 1995, Blethen, 1995; Malozowski, 1995
Beta-human chorionic gonadotropin	Haller, 1993
Depo-provera (depo-medroxyprogrogesterone	Bahemuka, 1981
L-thyroxine therapy for juvenile hypothyroidism	Campos, 1995; Huseman, 1984; McVie, 1984; Misra, 1992; Prendes, 1978; VanDop, 1983
Endocrine and metabolic dysfunction and pregnancy	
Pregnancy and postpartum	Alderson, 1983; Caroscio, 1978; Daif, 1995; Digre, 1984; Elian, 1968; Greer, 1963; Gupta, 1980; Henry, 1979; Kassam, 1983; Katz, 1989; Koontz, 1983; Koppel, 1990; Nickerson, 1965; Palop, 1979; Peterson, 1985; Powell, 1972; Shapiro, 1995; Shekleton, 1980; Thomas, 1986; Wheatley, 1986
Menarche	Greer, 1964; Tessler, 1985a, 1985b
Turner syndrome	Disckman, 1980; Donaldson, 1981; Sybert, 1985
Hyperthyroidism	Disckman, 1980; Roos, 1985
Hypothyroidism	Adams, 1994; Press, 1983
Addison's disease and crisis	Alexandrakis, 1993; Jefferson, 1956; Leggio, 1995; Walsh, 1952
Hypoparathyroidism and pseudohypoparathyroidism	Asplund, 1980; Grant, 1953; Kralik, 1976; Mada, 1993; Mor, 1988; Palmer, 1959; Sambrook, 1977; Sheldon, 1987
Cushing's disease and post-pituitary surgery for Cushing's disease	Newman, 1980; Parfitt, 1994; Weissman, 1983
Systemic illnesses (including some causing venous occlusion)	
Systemic lupus erythematosus	Abramsky, 1972; Bettman, 1968; Carlow, 1974; Chevalier, 1992; Daif, 1995; Gibson, 1976; Green, 1995; Horoshovski, 1995; Kaplan, 1985; Lessell, 1979; Li, 1989; Maiuri, 1983; Parnass, 1987; Shiozawa, 1986; Silberberg, 1973; Vachvanichsanong, 1992
Behçet's syndrome	Bank, 1984; Bosch, 1995; Bousser, 1985; Cobby, 1988; Daif, 1995; Graham, 1980; Kalbian, 1970; Kansu, 1991; Kozin, 1977; Masheter, 1959; Pamir, 1981; Reza, 1978; Schell, 1988; Stern, 1989; Wilkins, 1986
Cystic fibrosis	Bikangaga, 1996; Bray, 1973; Katznelson, 1978; Lucidi, 1993; Nasr, 1995
Reye syndrome	Massey, 1974
Antiphospholipid antibody syndrome	Daif, 1995; Mokri, 1993; Orefice 1995

Hematologic abnormalities and malignancies	
Iron deficiency anemia	Capriles, 1963; Ikkala, 1963; Lubeck, 1959; Parag, 1983; Schwaber, 1961; Tugal, 1994
Pernicious anemia and other megaloblastic anemias	Murphy, 1969; Van Gelder, 1991
Thrombocythemia and thrombocytosis	Mitchell, 1986; Sussman, 1997; Tehindrazanarivelo, 1990
Cryofibrinogenemia	Dunsker, 1970
Abnormal fibrinogen or increased serum fibrinogen	D'Souza, 1979; Sussman, 1997
Cryoglobulinemia	Mdrucker, 1985
Hodgkin's disease	Thomas, 1986
Castleman's disease	Black, 1988
Leukemia	Guymer, 1993; Watkins, 1941
Myeloma	Wasan, 1992
Protein S deficiency	Daif, 1995
Antithrombin III deficiency	Daif, 1995; Sussman, 1997
Multicentric angiofollicular lymph node hyperplasia	Feigert, 1990
Paroysmal nocturnal hemoglobinuria	Hauser, 1996
Thrombocytopenic purpura	Nover, 1963; Simpson, 1948
Polycythemia	Sussman, 1997
Chronic respiratory insufficiency and the Pickwickian syndrome	Chrispen, 1961; Freedman, 1963; Imari, 1962; Manfredi, 1961; Meyer, 1961; Miller, 1962; Spalter, 1964; Stevens, 1963; Westlake, 1954; Wolin, 1995
Chronic renal failure and uremia	Chang, 1992; Guy, 1990
Renal or bone marrow transplantation	Avery, 1991; Katz, 1997; Sheth, 1994
HIV infection and AIDS	Gross, 1991; Javeed, 1995; Schwarz, 1995; Travero, 1993
Lyme disease	Jacobson, 1989; Raucher, 1985
Neurosarcoidosis	Akova, 1993; Byrne, 1978; Phanthumchinda, 1984; Redwood, 1990; Vyrne, 1983
Typhoid fever	Moodley, 1990; Vargas, 1990
Familial Mediterranean fever	Gokalp, 1992
Tolosa-Hunt syndrome	Nezu, 1995
Mucopolysaccaridoses	Sheridan, 1994
After occipitocervical arthrodesis and immobilization in a halo vest	Daftari, 1995
Guillain-Barré syndrome	Macaya, 1988; Ropper, 1984; Weiss, 1991
Familial pseudotumor cerebri (possible autosomal recessive or dominant transmission)	Bucheit, 1969; Coffey, 1982; Howe, 1973; Kharode, 1992; Rothner, 1974; Shapiro, 1980; Torlai, 1989; Traviesa, 1976

Drugs: Hypervitaminosis A, steroid withdrawal, anabolic steroids, lithium, nalidixic acid, the insecticide chlordecone (Kepone), isoretinoin, ketaprofen (Orudis) or indomethacin in Bartter's syndrome, thyroid replacement in hypothyroid children, danazol, all-transretinoic acid (ATRA) or tretinoin cyclosporine, exogenous growth hormone, and, probably, tetracycline.

Table 7–5. Criteria for the Diagnosis of IIH

Increased intracranial pressure must be documented in an alert and oriented patient without localizing neurologic findings (except for cranial nerve VI palsy). Spinal fluid pressures between 200 and 250 mm H_2O may occur normally in obese patients and when elevated spinal fluid pressure is suspected, confirmation requires values greater than 250 mm H_2O (Corbett, 1983).
The cerebrospinal fluid should have normal contents (including protein and glucose) with no cytologic abnormalities. Occasionally the cerebrospinal fluid protein level may be low (Chandra, 1986).
Neuroimaging (CT imaging with and without contrast or, preferably, MR imaging with and without contrast and, possibly MR venography) should be normal with no evidence of hydrocephalus, mass lesion, meningeal enhancement, or venous occlusive disease. Neuroimaging my show enlarged optic nerve sheaths, empty sellae, and reversal of the optic nerve head in some patients with pseudotumor cerebri (Berke, 1975; Britton, 1980; Foley, 1975; Gibby, 1993; Jacobson, 1990; Manfre, 1995; Shapiro, 1980; Silbergleit, 1989; Vassilouthis, 1979; Weisberg, 1975; Wessel, 1987).
No secondary cause (secondary pseudotumor cerebri syndrome) is evident.

Systemic diseases: Behçet's syndrome, renal failure, Addison's disease, hypoparathyroidism, systemic lupus erythematosus, sarcoidosis (most of these likely cause pseudotumor cerebri syndrome by venous sinus obstruction or impairment of venous sinus drainage).

Idiopathic intracranial hypertension (IIH, idiopathic pseudotumor cerebri syndrome) is a disease typically of obese women in the childbearing years (Ahlskog, 1982; Arseni, 1992; Bodie, 1974; Bulens, 1979; Corbett, 1982; Ireland, 1990; Jain, 1992; Johnston, 1974a, 1974b; Orefice, 1984; Radhakrishnan, 1994; Rush, 1980; Wall, 1991). Approximately 10 to 15% of cases are male (Digre, 1988), and, when it occurs in children, there is no gender preference (Amacher, 1985; Baker, 1985; Lessell, 1986, 1992). Even though men with pseudotumor cerebri are less likely to be obese than woman, they tend to be more obese than control subjects (Digre, 1988). The occurrence of pseudotumor cerebri in a man, especially a thin man, should raise the possibility of venous occlusive disease or a secondary pseudotumor cerebri syndrome. Afro-American men appear to be at greater risk of visual loss. The incidence of IIH is approximately 1 to 2 per 100,000, with a higher incidence in obese women between the ages of 15 and 44 years (8 to 21 per 100,000) (Durcan, 1988; Radhakrishnan, 1991, 1993).

Table 7–5 lists the diagnostic criteria for IIH.

What Are the Risk Factors and Symptoms of IIH?

The most important risk factors for the development of IIH include female sex, obesity, and recent weight gain (Giuseffi, 1991; Ireland, 1990). Several conditions previously associated with IIH are no more common in IIH than in controls. For example, in a retrospective case-control study of 40 patients with IIH and 39 age- and sex-matched controls, all forms of menstrual abnormalities, incidence of pregnancy, antibiotic use, and oral contraceptive use were equal in both groups (Ireland, 1990). In another study comparing 50 IIH patients with 100 age-matched controls, iron deficiency anemia, thyroid dysfunction, pregnancy, antibiotic intake, and the use of oral contraceptives were no more common in IIH patients than in controls (Manfre, 1995).

The most common symptoms of IIH include headache, transient obscurations of vision, pulsatile tinnitus, and diplopia (Giuseffi, 1991; Ireland, 1990). In a prospective study of 50 IIH patients (92% women; mean age, 32 years; 92% obese), symptoms included headache (94%), transient visual obscurations (68%), intracranial noises (58%), sustained visual loss (26%), photopsia (54%), diplopia (38%), and retrobulbar pain (44%) (Wall, 1991). The headaches in patients with IIH may be constant or intermittent and in 93% of patients they are reported to be the most severe headache ever (Wall, 1990). The headache may often be pulsatile, be of gradually increasing intensity during the day, awaken the patient at night, may be precipitated by changes in posture, and is often transiently relieved by lumbar puncture (Wall, 1990). Pain in a cervical nerve root distribution (possibly from a dilated nerve root sleeve) or retro-ocular pain with eye movement, uncommon with other headache disorders, may help to differentiate this headache syndrome (Bortoluzzi, 1982; Bulens, 1988; Wall, 1990). There is no clear correlation between the height of cerebrospinal fluid pressure and the severity of the headache. Transient visual obscurations last seconds, may be unilateral or bilateral, related to changes in posture, do not correlate with the degree of intracranial hypertension or the extent of disc swelling, and are not considered harbingers of permanent visual loss (Corbett, 1982; Giuseffi, 1991; Rush, 1990). Intracranial noises are common with IIH and are perhaps due to transmission of intensified vascular pulsations via cerebrospinal fluid under high pressure to the walls of the venous sinuses (Sismanis, 1990). In fact, IIH without papilledema has been reported in patients with pulsatile tinnitus (Felton, 1995). Diplopia is often mild and usually results from a sixth cranial nerve palsy, presumably a nonlocalizing sign of raised intracranial pressure. In a study of 101 patients with IIH, other "minor symptoms" included neck stiffness in 31 patients, distal extremity paresthesias in 31, tinnitus in 27, joint pains in 13, low back pain in 13, and gait instability in 4 (Round, 1988). These "minor symptoms" resolved promptly with lowering of the intracranial pressure. Other rare and exceptional clinical abnormalities that have been described in patients with IIH are listed in Table 7–6.

Papilledema is found in most cases of IIH. It may be asymmetric, rarely unilateral, and even occasionally absent (Chari, 1991; Greenfield, 1997; Lipton, 1972; Marcelis, 1991; Mathew, 1996; Scanarini, 1979; Tourn, 1996). If optic atrophy is present unilaterally, the disc swelling will be unilateral in the opposite eye, thus mimicking the Foster-Kennedy syndrome (Tourn, 1996). If no papilledema is evident, there is no risk of visual loss no matter how high the intracranial pressure; in the individual patient, the severity of papilledema cannot predict the severity of visual loss.

Visual field and, eventually, visual acuity loss are the major causes of morbidity in IIH (Corbett, 1982; Krogsaa, 1985; Rush, 1980; Sorensen, 1988; Wall, 1983, 1987, 1991). Complete blindness and optic atrophy may occur. Hypertension and recent weight gain have been reported to be significant risk factors for visual loss (Corbett, 1982). Often the patient is unaware of peripheral visual field dysfunction and Snellen acuity testing is a poor indicator of early visual deficit in IIH. The papilledema causes optic nerve fiber attrition that results in field constriction and nerve fiber bundle defects (Corbett, 1982; Wall, 1983, 1991). Optic nerve diameter changes on ultrasound in IIH are associated with perimetric threshold loss; IIH functional deficits may thus be related to the degree of distension of optic nerve sheaths as a result of an increased cerebrospinal fluid pressure (Salgarello, 1996). Blind spot enlargement is commonly encountered, yet it is more a reflection of the disc swelling itself instead of optic nerve damage and is improved with refraction (Corbett, 1988; Wall, 1983). Visual field defects in IIH patients are typically "disc-related" defects—most commonly loss of the inferonasal field or general constriction of isopters, followed by arcuate defects, central loss, or altitudinal defects (Wall,

Table 7–6. Rare and Exceptional Findings described with IIH

Finding	References
Fourth cranial nerve palsy	Baker, 1985; Lee, 1995
Third cranial nerve palsy	McCammon, 1981; Sperry, 1979
Skew deviation	Baker, 1985; Frohman, 1985; Merikangas, 1978
Complete external ophthalmoplegia	Landan, 1987
Bilateral total internal and external ophthalmoplegia	Snyder, 1979
Internuclear ophthalmoplegia with vertical gaze paresis with or without ptosis	Friedman, 1997
Trigeminal neuropathy	Davenport, 1994
Unilateral or bilateral facial nerve palsy	Bakshi, 1992; Capobianco, 1997; Chutorian, 1977; Kiwak, 1984; Selky, 1994; Snyder, 1979
Hemifacial spasm	Mayer, 1996; Selky, 1994
Cerebrospinal fluid rhinorrhea	Clark, 1994
Transient partial pituitary deficiency	De Paepe, 1993
Fatal tonsillar herniation after lumbar puncture	Sullivan, 1991
Atypical ophthalmoscopic findings and visual abnormalties	
Gaze-evoked amaurosis	Pascual, 1988
Acute visual loss secondary to anterior ischemic optic neuropathy	Green, 1984
Acute visual loss due to central retinal artery occlusion	Baker, 1984
Acute visual loss due to branch retinal artery occlusion	Lam, 1992; Liu, 1994
Acute visual loss due to central retinal vein occlusion	Chern, 1991
Visual loss (occasionally acute) due to macular disease, including chorioretinal striae, pigmentary disturbances, exudates, subretinal hemorrhages from neovascular membranes, or subretinal scars	Akova, 1994; Carter, 1995; Coppeto, 1985; Gittinger, 1989; Jamison, 1978; Liu, 1994; Mitchell, 1989; Morse, 1981; Troost, 1979
Acquired hyperopia with choroidal folds	Jacobson, 1995

1983). Changes in the retinal nerve fiber layer observed in patients with IIH provide objective information regarding the status of the optic nerve (Hedges, 1995). In general, the visual loss is insidious and progressive, but acute visual loss may occur, especially by the mechanisms listed in Table 7–6 (e.g., anterior ischemic optic neuropathy, retinal artery or vein occlusion, or subretinal hemorrhage from neovascular membranes) . The frequency of visual field loss and acuity loss with IIH is variable, but in one study field loss was noted in 75% of eyes using manual strategies and 77.5% using automated threshold perimetry (Wall, 1987). Motion perimetry abnormalities correlate well with static perimetry abnormalities in patients with IIH, and, indeed, may identify nerve fiber bundle defects not detected with conventional perimetry (Wall, 1995). Contrast sensitivity testing is also a relatively accurate means of assessing optic nerve damage in patients with IIH (Bulens, 1988; Wall, 1986).

We recommend that all patients with atypical pseudotumor cerebri syndrome undergo MR venography to evaluate for venous occlusive disease. If venous occlusive disease is discovered, then evaluation for a hypercoagulable state and vasculitis should be performed. Otherwise, patients require a thorough history, especially attending to medication use, pregnancy, intercurrent illnesses, and recent weight gain. Secondary pseudotumor cerebri should be considered in men, thin patients, and those younger than 15 or older than 45 years. We suggest that the initial evaluation also include blood work (sedimentation rate, complete blood count, syphilis serology, calcium, phosphate, creatinine, and electrolytes), perimetry (Goldmann and/or automated), and optic disc stereo photography.

What Is the Treatment for IIH?

The treatment of pseudotumor cerebri has two major goals: the alleviation of symptoms and preservation of visual function. We suggest a management plan, adapted from that recommended by Corbett and Thompson, that is outlined in Table 7–7.

Some patients require no treatment so long as symptoms are minimal and visual function is normal, but all require serial monitoring of visual function, especially visual fields, to observe closely for signs of visual impairment. Visual evoked responses and repeated measurements of intracranial pressure by lumbar puncture do not provide data that help guide therapeutic decisions (Corbett, 1989). Weight reduction, including surgically induced weight reduction in morbidly obese patients, may improve the papilledema and

Table 7–7. Management of IIH

- Return monthly for 6–12 months—visual fields, stereo optic disc photos, visual acuity, relative afferent pupillary defect (RAPD) testing
- Above until papilledema has regressed
- Medical treatment:
  - Acetazolamide (e.g., Diamox sequels 500 mg qHS for three days then 500 mg BID—up to 2 to 4 grams per day; paresthesias, anorexia, malaise, tin-like taste, fatigue may limit); ? methazolamide (Neptazane) as alternate; ? consider concomitant use of furosemide (Lasix) in children
  - Weight reduction
  - Treat headaches symptomatically if they do not respond to acetazolamide
  - Consider high-dose methylprednisolone and acetazolamide if acute, severe visual loss; if fails, consider surgery (below)
  - During pregnancy, acetazolamide use contraindicated, especially during first 20 weeks, due to potential teratogenicity; also avoid diuretics and caloric restriction
- Surgical treatment—optic nerve sheath fenestration or lumboperitoneal shunt procedure if:
  - New visual field defect **
  - Enlargement of previously existing visual field defect **
  - Reduced visual acuity not due to macular edema
  - Presence of severe visual loss (20/40 or worse) in one or both eyes at time of initial examination
  - Anticipated hypotension induced by treatment of high blood pressure or renal dialysis
  - Psychosocial reasons, such as patient's inability to perform visual field studies, noncompliance with medications, an itinerant lifestyle, or a functional (nonorganic) component to the presentation
  - Headache unresponsive to standard headache medications

**Blind spot enlargement should not be considered significant visual loss (refractive).
Source: Corbett, 1989.

reduce intracranial pressure (Amaral, 1987; Kupersmith, 1997; Newborg, 1974; Noggle, 1986; Sugerman, 1995). For example, in one study, all nine patients placed on a salt-restricted, rapid weight reduction rice diet showed improvement in papilledema (mean wt. 261 lb. before treatment and 187 lb. after treatment) (Newborg, 1974). In another study, all eight morbidly obese patients with IIH who underwent gastric surgery had complete resolution of their papilledema, resolution or marked reduction in headache, resolution of tinnitus, and a decrease in cerebrospinal fluid pressure from a mean of 353 to a mean of 168 mm of H_2O following a mean wt. loss of 57 kg when measured at 34 months after surgery (Sugerman, 1995). In another retrospective study, weight reduction sped recovery from pseudotumor cerebri in women, but may not have definitely improved the eventual visual outcome (Kupersmith, 1997).

Medical treatments for IIH include carbonic anhydrase inhibitors, loop diuretics, corticosteroids, and repeat lumbar punctures. Acetazolamide in doses of 2 to 4 gs per day has proven effective in some patients with IIH (Schoeman, 1994; Tomsak, 1988). Acetazolamide should not be used during pregnancy, especially during the first 20 weeks, because of potential teratogenic effects; caloric restriction and the use of other diuretics are also relatively contraindicated during pregnancy (Digre, 1983). Other carbonic anhydrase inhibitors, such as methazolamide (Neptazane), are often used in acetazolamide-intolerant patients but their efficacy has not been proven. Furosemide (Lasix) inhibits cerebrospinal fluid production and may have an additive effect with acetazolamide; the use of this agent alone has not been systematically studied but in one report of eight children treated with combined therapy of acetazolamide and furosemide, all patients had a rapid clinical response with resolution of papilledema, reduction in the mean cerebrospinal fluid pressure after the first week of treatment, and normalization of pressure within six weeks of starting therapy (Schoeman, 1994). Digoxin has also been reported to be a successful treatment in one small group of patients (Goodwin, 1990). Corticosteroids may be efficacious in the short run, but the complications of this medication, especially in the chronic treatment of an already obese individual, have resulted in most clinicians suggesting that their use be avoided (Corbett, 1989). Liu et al. treated four patients with acute, severe visual loss associated with IIH with a combination of high-dose methylprednisolone (250 mg four times a day for 5 days followed by an oral taper), acetazolamide and ranitidine (Liu, 1994). In addition to severe disc edema, one patient had a serous detachment of both maculas and lipid deposition, one had unilateral macular star, and one had a monocular branch retinal artery occlusion. These three patients experienced rapid and lasting improvement in visual acuity, visual fields, papilledema, and symptoms, while the fourth patient did not improve and required optic nerve sheath fenestration. The authors suggested this combination treatment for patients with acute, severe visual loss associated with florid papilledema and surgical treatment if no immediate improvement occurs (Liu, 1994).

Repeated lumbar punctures have never been systematically studied for the treatment of IIH. Because these procedures are uncomfortable, of questionable benefit, and potentially associated with complications (e.g., infection, intraspinal epidermoid tumors [Corbett, 1983]), we feel they should not be performed therapeutically. Finally, if acetazolamide does not control the headache associated with IIH, symptomatic headache treatments are warranted.

When medical therapy fails or when visual dysfunction deteriorates, surgical therapies for IIH should be considered (Corbett, 1989). The indications for surgical therapy, as suggested by Corbett and Thompson (Corbett, 1989), are outlined in Table 7–7. The two main procedures performed include lumboperitoneal shunt (LPS) and optic nerve sheath fenestration (ONSF). Various authorities have vehemently advocated one or the other procedure; both have their advantages and disadvantages, but there has been no prospective study comparing their efficacy.

Lumboperitoneal shunt (LPS) can relieve headache, diplopia, and papilledema and can reverse visual loss (Angiari, 1992; Cornblath, 1989; Eggenberger, 1996; Johnston, 1988a, 1988b; Lundar, 1990; Repka, 1984; Rosenberg, 1993; Vander Ark, 1971). This procedure may be performed if warranted in pregnancy (Shapiro, 1995). Eggenberger et al. retrospectively studied 27 patients with pseudotumor cerebri treated with at least one LPS to ascertain the efficacy of this treatment (Eggenberger, 1996). The indications for LPS were intractable headache in 18 patients (67%) and progressive optic neuropathy in 14 patients (52%). Visual function returned to normal in both eyes of six patients, showed no change in either eye in four patients, and improved in at least one eye in the remaining four. Four patients had unilateral and one had bilateral sixth nerve palsies; all completely resolved post surgery. The average duration of follow-up for this population was 77 months (mean 47 months). A functioning LPS was successful in alleviating symptoms in all the patients studied and no patient with a functioning shunt complained of shunt-related symptoms, such as low-pressure headache or abdominal pain, within 2 months after the shunt was performed. Twelve patients (44%) required no revisions while the number of revisions among the 15 patients (56%) who needed them ranged from one (5 patients) to 14 (one patient). Six patients (40%) required one revision and two (13%) required two revisions; the average revisions per patient was 2.4. Three of these patients required 35 of the 66 total shunt revisions (53%). The main reason for LPS revision was shunt obstruction with recurrence of signs and symptoms of increased intracranial pressure (43/66 procedures or 65% of the total number of revisions). Other reasons for revisions were valve malfunction with development of low-pressure symptoms (10 revisions or 15.1% of total), lumbar radiculopathy (3 revisions, 4.5% of total), shunt-related infection (1 revision, 1.5% of total), and abdominal pain (1 revision, 1.5% of total). There were no major complications from LPS, other than failure of the shunt, even in patients who required multiple shunts. The authors concluded that placement of a LPS is a satisfactory treatment for the majority of patients with pseudotumor cerebri who require surgical therapy for the disorder even though some patients ultimately require multiple shunt revisions.

Rosenberg et al. reviewed the efficacy of cerebrospinal diversion procedures for pseudotumor cerebri in patients from six different institutions (Rosenberg, 1993). Thirty-seven patients underwent a total of 73 LPS and 10 ventricular shunts. Only 14 patients remained "cured" after a single surgical procedure. The average time between shunt insertion and shunt replacement was 9 months, although 64% of the shunts lasted less than 6 months. Shunt failure (recurrent papilledema or increased cerebrospinal fluid pressure on lumbar puncture) (55%) and low-pressure headaches (21%) were the most common indications for reoperation. Other reasons for shunt replacement included infection, abdominal pain, radicular pain, operative complications, and cerebrospinal fluid leak. The vision of most patients improved (13) or stabilized (13) postoperatively. However, three patients who had initially improved subsequently lost vision, six had a postoperative decrease in vision, two patients improved in one eye but worsened postoperatively in the other, and four lost vision despite apparently adequate shunt function. Shunt failure with relapse of pseudotumor cerebri occurred as late as 7 years after insertion. The authors concluded that cerebrospinal fluid diversion procedures have a significant failure rate as well as a high frequency of side effects. Johnston et al. reported 36 patients who during follow-up required a total of 85 shunting procedures with an overall complication rate of 52% and a failure rate of 48% (Johnston, 1988a).

Thus, cerebrospinal fluid diversion procedures, especially LPS, are often effective in controlling IIH and, although placement of the shunt is in general safe, any operation performed under general anesthesia carries some risk and there is at least one perioperative death reported following LPS (Eisenbergm, 1971). Shunt obstruction is the most common complication (Chumas, 1993; Cornblath, 1989; Eggenberger, 1996; Rosenberg, 1993) followed by secondary intracranial hypotension caused by excessive drainage of the cerebrospinal fluid via the LPS (Bret, 1986; Chumas, 1993; Eggenberger, 1996; Johnston, 1988a, 1988b, 1988c; Rosenberg, 1993; Sell, 1995; Selman, 1980; Spetzler, 1975). Symptoms of intracranial hypotension include nausea and vomiting, nuchal rigidity, disturbances of vision, vertigo, tinnitus, and reduced hearing (the latter three are thought to result from a decreased intralabyrinthine pressure gradient across the cochlear aqueduct). Other complications include lumbar radiculopathy (Eggenberger, 1996; Johnston, 1988; Rosenberg, 1993; Selman, 1980), shunt infection and disc space infection (Bret, 1986; Cabezudo, 1990; Eggenberger, 1993; Eisenberg, 1971; James, 1981; Johnston, 1988a, 1988b; Rosenberg, 1993; Selman, 1980), abdominal pain, bowel perforation, or migration or dislocation of the peritoneal end of the catheter (Bret, 1986; Chumas, 1993; Eggenberger, 1996; Eisenberg, 1971; Fischer, 1969; Jackson, 1954; James, 1981; Murtagh, 1967; Spetzler, 1975, 1977; Wilson, 1966), tonsillar herniation and syringomyelia (symptomatic or asymptomatic) (Chumas, 1993a, 1993b; Fisher, 1977; Sullivan, 1988; Welch, 1981), subdural hemorrhage (Jones, 1967; Murtagh, 1967), visual loss from retinal ischemia (Brew, 1987), and bilateral visual loss and simultagnosia from bilateral parieto-occipital infarction related to rupture of a previously asymptomatic intracranial aneurysm after LPS (Miller, 1997).

ONSF has been proven to prevent deterioration in vision and, in some cases, improve visual function in patients with IIH (Acheson, 1994; Anderson, 1992; Bourman, 1988; Brazier, 1996; Burde, 1974; Carter, 1995; Corbett, 1988; Davies, 1976; Galbraith, 1973; Hamed, 1992; Horton, 1992; Kaye, 1981; Kelman, 1991, 1992; Keltner, 1988; Kilpatrick, 1981; Knight, 1986; Liu, 1996; Mauriello, 1995; Mittra, 1993; Pearson, 1991; Sergott, 1988; Spoor, 1991a, 1993b, 1995c; Tomkins, 1984; Tse, 1988). For example, in one study 26 patients underwent 40 ONSFs for relief of visual loss or to preserve vision (16 unilateral and 12 bilateral operations) (Knight, 1986). Papilledema disappeared or was strikingly reduced in 24 of 28 patients. The other four patients had gliotic discs (two patients) or were followed up for only a short time. Visual acuity improved in 12 of 40 eyes and remained the same in 22 of 40 eyes. In 6 eyes, the visual acuity decreased. The visual fields improved in 21 of 40 eyes and remained the same in ten eyes; five of the ten eyes that did not change had poor vision before surgery. Eight eyes in five patients continued to lose acuity postoperatively. An additional two eyes developed visual field loss with preserved visual acuity. In another study, 23 patients with chronic papilledema had ONSF and 21 of the 23 patients demonstrated improvement in visual function (Sergott, 1988). Twelve of 21 patients with bilateral visual loss had improved visual function bilaterally after unilateral surgery and six of 21 patients needed bilateral surgery. ONSF improved vision in six patients who failed to recover vision after LPS.

Kelman et al. performed ONSF on 17 patients with severe visual acuity or field loss (Kelman, 1992). Postoperatively, visual acuity improved or stabilized in 33 of 34 eyes (97%) and the visual fields improved in 20 of 21 eyes that underwent surgery. Kelman et al. also performed ONSF in 12 patients (16 eyes) with functioning LPS and progressive visual loss (Kelman, 1991) and all patients demonstrated improvement in visual function. Liu et al. reported a woman with pseudotumor cerebri treated with a LPS who developed acute pallid disc swelling with peripapillary hemorrhages and visual acuity of NLP OD and 20/70 OS in association with LPS failure (Liu, 1991). The patient underwent ONSF and LPS revision and her visual acuity improved to 20/20 OU and the papilledema resolved. Pearson et al. operated on nine patients (14 eyes) and visual function showed significant improvement or stabilized in all but one (Pearson, 1991). Spoor et al. performed ONSF in 53 patients (101 eyes) with pseudotumor cerebri and visual loss (Spoor, 1991). Sixty-nine eyes (85 patients) with acute papilledema uniformily had improved visual function after ONSF. Of the 32 eyes with chronic papilledema (18 patients), only ten improved. Thirteen eyes required secondary or tertiary ONSF after an initial successful result. Eleven of 13 eyes had improved visual function after repeat ONSF.

Mittra et al. examined changes in color Doppler imaging before and after ONSF for pseudotumor cererbi (Mittra, 1993). Their results suggest that some of the visual loss from chronic papilledema may be due to ischemia, and worsening visual acuity correlates with greater impairment of the retrobulbar circulation. One of the mechanisms by which ONSF improves visual function may thus be reversal of this ischemic process.

Headaches may be relieved in over half of the patients with IIH undergoing ONSF (Corbett, 1989). For example, with unilateral decompression, headaches were improved or relieved in 13 of 17 patients in one series (Sergott, 1988) and in 10 of 16 patients in another study (Corbett, 1988), while 91% of patients (10/11) had relief of headache after (ONSD) in a third study (Kosmorsky, 1993). ONSF may also relieve papilledema and improve vision when performed on patients with pseudotumor cerebri secondary to occlusion of the dural sinuses (Horton, 1992; Mittra, 1993).

Thus, some reports have suggested that ONSF is more effective and associated with fewer complications than LPS (Corbett, 1988; Davies, 1976; Keltner, 1988; Sergott, 1988). Because of these reports, many physicians have abandoned LPS in favor of ONSF for the majority of their patients with IIH who require surgery (Eggenberger, 1996). However, long-term follow-up data suggest that ONSF may not be as effective as originally claimed and up to 33% of patients undergoing ONSD for pseudotumor cererbri who show initial improvement in visual function later show deterioration in visual field and acuity (Spoor, 1993, 1995). In a study of the long-term effectiveness of ONSF for IIH, Spoor and McHenry reviewed 32 series of postoperative visual fields in patients who were undergoing ONSF for pseudotumor cerebri who had stable visual acuity and four or more fields during 6 to 60 months of follow-up (Spoor, 1993). The authors then extended the review to include all patients (54 patients, 75 eyes) who underwent ONSF for pseudotumor cerebri, who were followed up with serial automated perimetry. Fifty-two eyes (68%) showed improvement (36%) or stabilization (32%) of visual function while 24 eyes (32%) experienced deterioration of visual function after an initially successful ONSF. The probability of failure from 3 to 5 years was .35 by life-table analysis. The authors concluded that ONSF effectively stabilizes or improves visual function in the majority of patients with pseudotumor cerebri and visual loss. However, it may fail at any time after surgery and patients need to be followed up routinely with automated perimetry to detect deterioration of visual function. Some of these late failures may be prevented by better and different operative techniques (Sergott, 1988; Spoor, 1995). Also, Acheson et al. reported 14 patients (11 with IIH and 3 with dural venous sinus occlusion) who underwent 8 unilateral and 6 bilateral ONSF (Acheson, 1994). Visual acuity and fields either improved or stabilized in 17 out of 20 eyes and 3 deteriorated. Of the eight patients undergoing unilateral surgery, the other eye remained stable in seven and deteriorated in one. Four patients required ONSF despite previous shunting or subtemporal decompression. Five patients required shunting or subtemporal decompression after ONSF because of persistent headache in three cases and for uncontrolled visual failure in two cases. No patient lost vision as a direct complication of surgery.

Thus, vision can be saved after shunt failure and, in other cases, may be maintained without the need for a shunt. Shunting may still be required, however, after ONSF, especially for persistent headache. Mauriello et al. reviewed the records of 108 patients with pseudotumor who underwent ONSF and showed visual loss within 1 month of surgery (Mauriello, 1995). Five patients, including two with renal failure and hypertension, had visual loss within 1 month of ONSF. The first had an abrupt decrease in vision 6 days after ONSF and a vessel on the nerve sheath bled into the surgical site. After high dose IV steroids failed to improve vision, emergency LPS resulted in full visual recovery. An apparent infectious optic neuropathy developed in the second patient 3 days after surgery. After 72 hours of IV antibiotics, visual acuity improved from 20/600 to 20/15. The other three patients had gradual visual loss after ONSF, which stabilized after LPSs. These authors reviewed ONSF failures in the literature and showed that four of seven patients with abrupt visual loss within the first 2 weeks of ONSF had no improvement in vision despite various treatments, including shunts. Corbett, et al's series of 40 ONSF in 28 patients included six patients who lost vision within the first 2 weeks of surgery (Corbett, 1988b). Only one of these six patients had return of vision and this patient had a dramatic decrease of vision from 20/30 in the involved eye to NLP 3 hours postoperatively after retrobulbar hemorrhage with acuity improving to 20/20 after surgical drainage of the retrobulbar hematoma. The other five patients had no visual recovery despite LPS, continuous lumbar drainage, and repeat ONSF in one patient described who had intrasheath hemorrhage due to coughing (this patient went from 20/30 to 20/200 10 days postoperatively). Intravenous steroids appeared to enhance visual recovery in one patient of Flynn, et al. who went from 20/400 to NLP 5 hours postoperatively but who improved to 20/800 after intravenous dexamethasone (Anderson, 1992). Mauriello, et al. concluded that avoidance of bleeding during ONSF may prevent fibrous occlusion of the surgical site and that patients with no identifiable cause for visual loss after ONSF, who do not respond to IV steroids, should be evaluated for emergency LPS (Mauriello, 1995). Also, postoperative infectious optic neuropathy should be considered in the differential of abrupt visual loss after ONSF. If ONSF fails, the authors favor LPS rather than repeat ONSF.

Numerous complications have also been reported after ONSF (Bourman, 1988; Corbett, 1988b; Flynn, 1994; Hupp, 1987; Kellen, 1987; Plotnik, 1993; Rizzo, 1994; Smith, 1992). Plotnik and Kosmorsky reported postoperative complications in 15 of the 38 eyes (40%) undergoing ONSF (Plotnik, 1993). Temporary motility disorders (resulting from extraocular muscle damage or damage to their nerve or blood supply) occurred in 29 percent and all resolved, the longest by 9 weeks. Pupillary dysfunction occurred in 4 eyes (11%) and consisted of sectoral tonic pupils (due to damage to short ciliary nerves or their blood supply causing iris sphincter palsy) which lasted 2 to 8 weeks in 3 eyes but persisted in one eye for 12 weeks. Four eyes (11%) had postoperative vascular complications including two with central retinal artery occlusions, one supertemporal branch retinal artery occlusion, and one episode of transient outer retinal ischemia. Both eyes with the central retinal artery occlusions had poor visual outcomes and eyes that had undergone prior ONSF were significantly more likely to have vascular complications than those without a previous operation. The incidence of vascular complications was 67% in eyes that had undergone prior ONSF and 6% in those that had never undergone a previous ONSF. The complications reported with ONSF are listed in Table 7–8.

From the above summary, it is evident that both ONSF and LPS may improve vision and prevent deterioration of vision in patients with IIH. Both procedures have their advantages and disadvantages and either may fail with time no matter what procedure is used. Approximately one-third of patients undergoing ONSF will not experience

Table 7–8. Complications of ONSF

Ocular motility disorders (e.g., temporary horizontal motility disorder caused by disinsertion of the medial rectus muscle or combined third and sixth nerve palsies)
Transient or permanent diffuse or sector tonic pupils
Conjunctival blebs with dellen formation
Chemosis
Chorioretinal scar from excessive traction on the globe
Peripapillary hemorrhages thought secondary to short ciliary vessel injury
Orbital hemorrhage
Trauma to the optic nerve
Myelinated nerve fibers (noted 5 months and 6 years postoperatively thought stimulated by trauma associated with surgery dellen)
Microhyphemas
Subconjunctival Tenon's cysts
Streptococcal corneal ulcers
Dacryocystitis
Intraoperative angle closure glaucoma
Deterioration of visual function, transient blindness, choroidal infarction (fundus changes with choroidal infarction may not be evident for several weeks after operation)
Central or branch retinal artery occlusion
Death

Source: Bourman 1988; Corbett 1988; Flynn 1994; Hupp 1987; Kellen 1987; Plotnik 1993; Rizzo 1994; Smith 1992

headache relief and only about 75% of ONSFs appear to be functioning 6 months after surgery. The probability of functioning of ONSF steadily decreases thereafter such that 66% are functioning at 12 months, 55% at 3 years, 38% at 5 years, and 16% at 6 years after surgery (Spoor, 1993). Thus, these patients must have their visual function followed for years as deterioration may require repeat procedures for ONSF failures. Although patients may be treated with a second ONSF after initial failure, eyes that have more than one ONSF are less likely to improve after surgery and more likely to experience significant vascular complication than are eyes that undergo a single surgery (Plotnik, 1993). On the other hand, LPS is fraught with many complications, although headache due to IIH is probably better controlled by LPS. LPS failure is also common, although most shunt failures occur within 2 to 3 months of the initial LPS (cumulative risk, 37%) and only rarely is the first shunt revision required more than one year after initial LPS (Eggenberger, 1996). Thus, a patient with IIH who undergoes a LPS and maintains a functioning shunt for more than one year has a lower risk of requiring a shunt revision over subsequent years (Eggenberger, 1996). However, patients undergoing LPS also need careful follow-up after their procedure because of the possibility of late failures. LPS failure has been reportedly successfully treated by repeat LPS or by ONSF, just as ONSF failure has been reported to be successfully treated with repeat ONSF or LPS. Until a prospective, randomized study comparing ONSF with LPS for IIH is performed, the question of which surgical procedure is best for the treatment of IIH remains unanswered.

The evaluation of the patient with optic disc swelling is summarized in Figure 7–1.

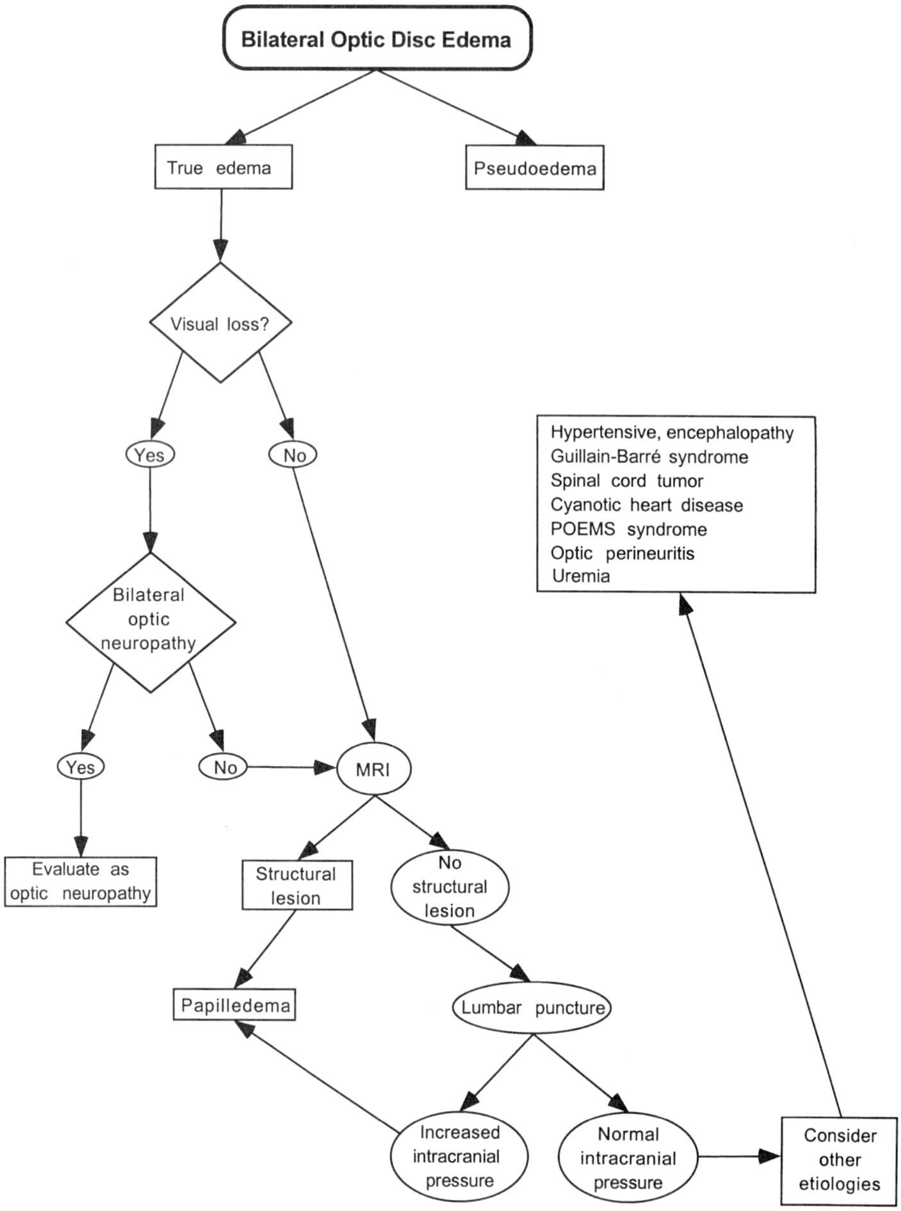

Figure 7–1. Bilateral optic disc edema.

References

Abramsky O, Melemd E, Sofer S. (1972). Involvement of the nervous system in lupus erythematosus. *Harefuah 83:*313–316.

Acheson JF, Green WT, Sanders MD. (1994) Optic nerve sheath decompression for the treatment of visual failure in chronic raised intracranial pressure. *J Neurol Neurosurg Psych 57:*1426–1429.

Adams C, Dean HJ, Israels SJ, et al. (1994). Primary hypothyroidism with intracranial hypertension and pituitary hyperplasia. *Ped Neurology 10:*166–168.

Ageli SI, Sato Y, Gantz BJ. (1994). Glomus jugulare tumors masquerading as benign intracranial hypertension. *Arch Otolaryngol 120:*1277–1280.

Ahlskog JE, O'Neill BP. (1982). Pseudotumor cerebri. *Ann Int Med 97:*249–256.

Ahmad S. (1996). Amiodarone and reversible benign intracranial hypertension. *Cardiology 87:*90.

Akova YA, Kansu T, Duman S. (1993). Pseudotumor cerebri secondary to dural sinus thrombosis in neurosarcoidosis. *J Clin Neuro-ophthalmol 13:*188–189.

Akova YA, Kansu T, Yazar Z, et al. (1994). Macular subretinal neovascular membrane associated with pseudotumor cerebri. *J Neuro-ophthalmol 14:*193–195.

Alderson TL. (1983). Nonrecurrent pseudotumor cererbi in pregnancy: report of case. *J American Osteopath Assoc 82 (9 Suppl):*728–731.

Alemayehu W. (1995). Pseudotumor cerebri (toxic effect of the "magic bullet"). *Ethiopian Med J 33:*265–270.

Alexandrakis G, Filatov V, Walsh T. (1993). Pseudotumor cerebri in a 12-year-old boy with Addison's disease. *Am J Ophthalmol 116:*650–651.

Alpan G, Glick B, Peleg O, Eyal F. (1991). Pseudotumor cerebri and coma in vitamin D-dependent rickets. *Clin Pediatr 30:*254–256.

Amacher AL, Spence JD. (1985). Spectrum of benign intracranial hypertension in children and adolescents. *Childs Nervous System 1:*81–86.

Amaral JF, Tsiaris W, Morgan T, Thompson WR. (1987). Reversal of benign intracranial hypertension by surgically induced weight loss. *Arch Surg 122:*946–949.

Ames D, Wirshing WC, Cokely HT, Lo LL. (1994). The natural course of pseudotumor cerebri in lithiuk-treated patients. *J Clin Psychphar 14:*286–287.

Anderson RL, Flaharty PM. (1992). Treatment of pseudotumor cerebri by primary and secondary optic nerve sheath decompression. *Am J Ophthalmol 113:*599–601.

Angiari P, Corradini L, Corsi M, Merli GA. (1992). Pseudotumor cerebri. Lumboperitoneal shunt in long lasting cases. *J Neurosurg Sci 36:*145–149.

Arber N, Shirin H, Fadial R, et al. (1990). Pseudotumor cerebri associated with leuprorelin acetate. *Lancet 335:*668.

Arseni C, Simoca I, Jipescu I, et al. (1992). Pseudotumor cerebri: Risk factors, clinical course, prognostic criteria. *Romanian J Neurol Psych 30:*115–132.

Asplund J. (1980). Pseudotumor cerebri in pseudohypoparathyroidism. *Acta Medica Scand 208:*331–332.

Avery R, Jabs D, Wingard J, et al. (1991). Optic disk edema after bone marrow transplantation. Possible role of cyclosporine toxicity. *Ophthalmology 98:*1294–1301.

Bahemuka M. (1981). Bengn intracranial hypertension associated with the use of depo-provera (depot medroxyprogesterone): A case report. *East African Med J 58:*140–141.

Baker RS, Buncic JR. (1984). Sudden visual loss in pseudotumor cerebri due to central retinal artery occlusion. *Arch Neurol 41:*1274–1276.

Baker RS, Buncic JR. (1985). Vertical ocular motility disturbance in pseudotumor cerebri. *J Clin Neuro-ophthalmol 5:*41–44.

Baker RS, Carter D, Hendrick EB, Buncic JR. (1985). Visual loss in pseudotumor cerebri of childhood. A follow-up study. *Arch Ophthalmol 103:*1681–1686.

Bakshi SK, Oak JL, Chawla KP, et al. (1992). Facial nerve involvement in pseudotumor cerebri. *J Postgrad Med 38:*144–145.

Bank I, Weart C. (1984). Dural sinus thrombosis in Behçet's disease. *Arthritis Rheum 27:*816–818.

Beck DW, Kassell NF, Drake CG. (1979). Glomus jugulare tumor presenting with increased intracranial pressure. *J Neurosurg 50:*823–825.

Beran RG. (1980). Pseudotumor cerebri associated with minocycline therapy for acne. *Med J Australia 1:*323–324.

Berke JP, Buxton LF, Kokmen E. (1975). The empty sella. *Neurology 25:*1137–1143.

Bettman JW Jr, Daroff RB, Sanders MD, Hoyt WF. (1968). Papilledema and asymptomatic intracranial hypertension in systemic lupus erythematosus. A Fluorescein angiographic study of resolving papilledema. *Arch Ophthalmol 80:*189–193.

Bhettay EM, Bakst CM. (1988). Hypervitaminosis A causing benign intracranial hypertension. A case report. *South African Med J 74:*584–585.

Bikangaga P, Canny GJ. (1996). Benign intracranial hypertension in infants with cystic fibrosis. *Arch Pediatr Adolesc Med 150:*551–552.

Black DA, Forgacs I, Davies DR, Thompson RP. (1988). Pseudotumor cerebri in a patient with Castleman's disease. *Postgrad Med J 64:*217–219.

Blervacque A, Béal F, Malbrel P. (1965). Papilledema after an operation at the level of the neck. *Bull Soc Ophthalmol Fr 65:*135–136.

Blethen SL. (1995). Complications of growth hormone therapy in children. *Curr Opin Ped 7:*466–471.

Bodie HG, Banna M, Bradley WG. (1974). "Benign" intracranial hypertension. A survey of the clinical and radiological features, and long-term prognosis. *Brain 97:*313–326.

Bolling JP, Brazis PW. (1990). Optic disk swelling with peripheral neuropathy, organomegaly, endocrinopathy, monoclonal gammopathy, and skin changes (POEMS syndrome). *Am J Ophthalmol 109:*503–510.

Bonnetblanc JM, Hugon J, Dumas M, Rupin D. (1983). Intracranial hypertension with etretinate. *Lancet 2:*974.

Boreus LO, Sundstrom B. (1967). Intracranial hypertension in a child during treatment with nalidixic acid. *Br Med J 2:*744–745.

Borruat FX, Regli F. (1993). Pseudotumor cerebri as a complication of amiodarone therapy. *Am J Ophthalmol 116:*776–777.

Bortoluzzi M, Di Lauro L, Marini G. (1982). Benign intracranial hypertension with spinal and radicular pain. Case report. *J Neurosurg 57:*833–836.

Bosch JA, Valdes M, Solans R, et al. (1995). Skin hyper-reactivity in a patient with benign intracranial hypertension as an early manifestation of Behçet's disease. *Br J Rheumatol 34:*184.

Bourman ND, Spoor TC, Ramocki JM. (1988). Optic nerve sheath decompression for pseudotumor cerebri. *Arch Ophthalmol 106:* 1378–1383.

Bousser M-G, Chiras J, Bories J, Castaigne P. (1985). Cerebral venous thrombosis—a review of 38 cases. *Stroke 16:*199–213.

Bray PF, Herbst JJ. (1973). Pseudotumor cerebri as a sign of "catch-up" growth in cystic fibrosis. *Am J Dis Children 126:*78–79.

Brazier DJ, Sanders MD. (1996). Disappearance of optociliary shunt vessels after optic nerve sheath decompression. *Br J Ophthalmol 80:*186–187.

Bret P, Huppert J, Massini B, et al. (1986). Lumbar peritoneal shunt in non-hydrocephalic patients: A review of 41 cases. *Acta Neurochir 80:*90–92.

Brew BJ, Garrick R, Connelley TJ. (1987). Lumboperitoneal shunting as a cause of visual loss in benign intracranial hypertension. *Clin Exper Neurology 23:*233–235.

Britton C, Boxhill C, Brust JCM, et al. (1980). Pseudotumor cerebri, empty sella syndrome, and adrenal adenoma. *Neurology 30:*292–296.

Brookes GB, Graham MD. (1984). Benign intracranial hypertension complicating glomus jugulare tumor surgery. *Am J Otol 5:*350–354.

Bruntse E. (1970). Unilateral papilloedema in neurosurgical patients. *Acta Ophthalmol 48:*759–764.

Bucci FA Jr, Krohel GB. (1988). Optic nerve swelling secondary to the obstructive sleep apnea syndrome. *Am J Ophthalmol 105:*428–430.

Bucheit WA, Burton C, Haag B, Shaw D. (1969). Papilledema and idiopathic intracranial hypertension. *New Eng J Med 280:*938–942.

Bulens C, De Vries WA, Van Crevel H. (1979). Benign intracranial hypertension. A retrospective and follow-up study. *J Neurol Sci 40:*147–57.

Bulens C, Meerwaldt JD, Koudstaal PJ, Van der Wildt GJ. (1988). Spatial contrast sensitivity in benign intraccranial hypertension. *J Neurol Neurosurg Psych 51:*1323–1329.

Burde RM, Karp JS, Miller NR. (1974). Reversal of visual deficit with optic nerve decompression in long-standing pseudotumor cerebri. *Am J Ophthalmol 77:*770–772.

Byrne JV, Lawton CA. (1983). Meningeal sarcoidosis causing intracranial hypertension secondary to dural sinus thrombosis. *Br J Radiol 56:*755–757.

Cabezudo JM, Olabe J, Bacci F. (1990). Infection of the intervertebral disc space after placement of a percutaneous lumboperitoneal shunt for benign intracranial hypertension. *Neurosurg 26:*1008–1009.

Campos SP, Olitsky S. (1995). Idiopathic intracranial hypertension after L-thyroxine therapy for acquired primary hypothyroidism. *Clin Pediatrics 34:*334–337.

Capobianco DJ, Brazis PW, Chesire WP. (1997). Idiopathic intracranial hypertension and seventh nerve palsy. *Headache,* in press.

Capriles LF. (1963). Intracranial hypertension in iron-deficiency anemia: Report of four cases. *Arch Neurol 9:* 147–153.

Carlow TJ, Glaser JS. (1974). Pseudotumor cererbi syndrome in systemic lupus erythematosus. *JAMA 228:*197–200.

Caroscio JT, Pellmar M. (1978). Pseudotumor cerebri: occurrence during the third trimester of pregnancy. *Mount Sinai J Med 45:*539–541.

Carter SR, Seiff SR. (1995). Macular changes in pseudotumor cerebri before and after optic nerve sheath fenestration. *Ophthalmology 102:*937–941.

Chandra V, Bellur SN, Anderson RJ. (1986). Low CSF protein in idiopathic pseudotumor cerebri. *Ann Neurol 19:*80–82.

Chang D, Nagamoto G, Smith WE. (1992). Benign intracranial hypertension and chronic renal failure. *Cleveland Clinic J Med 59:*419–422.

Chari C, Rao NS. (1991). Benign intracranial hypertension—its unusual manifestations. *Headache 31:*599–600.

Chern S, Margargal LE, Brav SS. (1991). Bilateral central retinal vein occlusion as an initial manifestation of pseudotumor cerebri. *Ann Ophthalmol 23:*54–57.

Chevalier X, de Bandt M, Bourgeois P, Kahn MF. (1992). Primary Sjogern's syndrome preceding the presentation of systemic lupus erythematosus as a benign intracranial hypertension syndrome. *Ann Rheumatic Dis 51:*808–809.

Chimowitz MI, Little JR, Awad IA, et al. (1990). Intracranial hypertension associated with unruptured cerebral arteriovenous malformations. *Ann Neurol 27:*474–479.

Chrispen AR, Darke CS. (1962). Papilloedema and polycythaemia. *Br Med J 1:*989–990.

Chumas PD, Armstrong DC, Drake JM, et al. (1993a). Tonsillar herniation: The rule rather than the exception after lumboperitoneal shunting in the pediatric population. *J Neurosurg 78:*568–573.

Chumas PD, Kulkarni AV, Drake JM, et al. (1993b). Lumboperitoneal shunting: A retrospective study in the pediatric population. *Neurosurgery 32:*376–383.

Chutorian AM, Gold AP, Braun CW. (1977). Benign intracranial hypertension and Bell's palsy. *New Eng J Med 296:*1214–115.

Clark D, Bullock T, Hui T, Firth J. (1994). Benign intracranial hypertension: A cause of CSF rhinorrnea. *J Neurol Neurosurg Psychiatr 57*:847–849.

Cobby M, Higgs CM, Hall CL. (1988). Behçet's syndrome presenting as intracranial hypertension in a Caucasian. *J Royal Soc Med 81*:478–479.

Cockerell OC, Lai HM, Ross-Russell RW. (1993). Pseudotumor cerebri associated with arteriovenous malformations. *Postgrad Med J 69*:637–640.

Coffey CE, Ross DR, Massey EW, Olanow CW. (1982). Familial benign intracranial hypertension and depression. *Canadian J Neurol Sci 9*:45–47.

Cohen DN. (1973). Intracranial hypertension and papilledema associated with nalidixic acid therapy. *Am J Ophthalmol 76*:680–682.

Cohn GA. (1963). Pseudotumor cerebri in children secondary to administration of adrenal steroids. *J Neurosurg 20*:784–786.

Coppeto JR, and Monteiro ML. (1985). Juxtapapillary subretinal hemorrhages in pseudotumor cerebri. *J Clin Neuro-ophthalmol 5*:45–53.

Corbett JJ. (1983). Problems in the diagnosis and treatment of pseudotumor cerebri. *Can J Neurol Sci 10*:221–229.

Corbett JJ, Mehta MP. (1983). Cerebrospinal fluid pressure in normal obese subjects and patients with pseudotumor cerebri. *Neurology 33*:1386–1388.

Corbett JJ, Thompson HS. (1989). The rational management of idiopathic intracranial hypertension. *Arch Neurol 46*:1049–1051.

Corbett JJ, Jacobson DM, Maurer RC, et al. (1988a). Enlargement of the blind spot caused by papilledema. *Am J Ophthalmol 105*:261–265.

Corbett JJ, Nerad JA, Tse D, et al: (1988b). Result of optic nerve sheath fenestration for pseudotumor cerebri. The lateral orbitotomy approach. *Arch Ophthalmol 106*: 1391–1397.

Corbett JJ, Savino PJ, Thompson HS, et al. (1982). Visual loss in pseudotumor cerebri: Follow-up of 57 patients from 5 to 41 years and a profile of 14 patients with permanent severe visual loss. *Arch Neurol 39*:461–474.

Cordon Lopez A, Munoz lopez A, Fernandez Jimenez S, Ruiz de Elvira MJ. (1985). Acute intracranial hypertension during amiodarone infusion. *Critical Care Med 13*:688–689.

Cornblath W, Miller NR. (1989). Pseudotumor cerebri treated with lumbo-peritoneal shunt (abstract). *Ann Neurol 26*:183.

Couban S, Maxner CE. (1991). Cerebral venous sinus thrombosis presenting as idiopathic intracranial hypertension. *Canadian Med Assoc J 145*:657–659.

Cremer PD, Thompson EO, Johnston IH, Halmagyi GM. (1996). Pseudotumor cerebri and cerebral venous hypertension. *Neurology 47*:1602–1603.

Cruz OA, Fogg SG, Roper-Hall G. (1996). Pseudotumor cerebri associated with cyclosporine use. *Am J Ophthalmol 122*:436–437.

Cuddihy J. (1994). Case report of benign intracranial hypertension secondary to tetracycline. *Irish Med J 87*:90.

D'Souza L, Coots MC, Glueck HI. (1979). An acquired abnormal fibrinogen associated with thromboembolic disease and pseudotumor cerebri. *Thrombosis Haemostasis 42*:994–1008.

Daftari TK, Heller JG, Newman NJ. (1995). Pseudotumor cerebri after occipiocervical arthrodesis and immobilization in a halo vest. A case report. *J Bone Joint Surg—Amer Vol 77*:455–458.

Daif A, Awada A, al-Rajeh S, et al. (1995). Cerebral venous thrombosis in adults. A study of 40 cases from Saudi Arabia. *Stroke 26*:1193–1195.

Davenport RJ, Will RG, Galloway PJ. (1994). Isolated intracranial hypertension presenting with trigeminal neuropathy. *J Neurol Neurosurg Psych 57*:381.

David CA, Peerless SJ. (1995). Pseudotumor syndrome resulting from cerebral arteriovenous malformation: Case report. *Neurosurgery 36*:588–590.

Davies G, Zilkha KJ. (1976). Decompression of the optic nerve in benign intracranial hypertension. *Trans Ophthalmol Soc United Kingdom 96*:427–429.

De Paepe L, Abs R, Verlooy J, et al. (1993). Benign intracranial hypertension as a cause of transient partial pituitary deficiency. *J Neurol Sci 114*:152–155.

Dees SC, McKay HW Jr. (1959). Occurrence of pseudotumor cerebri during treatment of children with asthma by adrenal steroids. *Pediatrics 23*:1143–1151.

DeJong AR, Callahan CA, Weiss J. (1985). Pseudotumor cerebri and nutritional rickets. *European J Pediatr 143*:219–220.

Deonna T, Guigard JP. (1974). Acute intracranial hypertension after nalidixic acid administration. *Arch Dis Childhood 49*:743.

Digre KB, Corbett JJ. (1988). Pseudotumor cerebri in men. *Arch Neurol 45*:866–872.

Digre KB, Varner MW, Corbett JJ. (1984). Pseudotumor cerebri and pregnancy. *Neurology 34*:721–729.

Disckman MS, Somasundaram M, Brzozowski L. (1980). Pseudotumor cerebri and hyperthyroidism. *New York J Med 80*:1118–1120.

Dommisse J. (1991). Pseudotumor cerebri associated with lithium therapy in two patients. *J Clin Psych 52*:239.

Donaldson JO, Binstock ML. (1981). Pseudotumor cerebri in an obese woman with Turner syndrome. *Neurology 31*:758–760.

Donnet A, Dufour H, Graziani N, Grisoli F. (1992). Minocycline and benign intracranial hypertension. *Biomed Pharmacother 46*:171–172.

Dunsker SB, Torres-Reyes E, Peden JC Jr. (1970). Pseudotumor cerebri associated with idiopathic cryofibrinogenemia. Report of a case. *Arch Neurol 23:*120–127.

Durcan FJ, Corbett JJ, Wall M. (1988). The incidence of pseudotumor cerebri. Population studies in Iowa and Louisiana. *Arch Neurol 45:*875–877.

Dutton JJ, Anderson RL. (1985). Idiopathic inflammatory perioptic neuritis simulating optic nerve sheath meningioma. *Am J Ophthalmol 100:*424–430.

Edmunds C, Behrens M, Lewis L, Lennon R. (1973). Pseudotumor cerebri and low vitamin-A intake. *JAMA 226:*674.

Eggenberger ER, Miller NR, Vitale S. (1996). Lumboperitoneal shunt for the treatment of pseudotumor cerebri. *Neurology 46:*1524–1530.

Eisenberg HM, Davidson RI, Shillito J. (1971). Lumboperitoneal shunts: Review of 34 cases. *J Neurosurg 35:*427–431.

Elian M, Ben-Tovim N, Bechar M, Bornstein B. (1968). Recurrent benign intracranial hypertension (pseudotumor cerebri) during pregnancy. *Obstet Gynecol 31:*685–688.

Evers JP, Jacobson RJ, Pincus J, Zwiebel JA. (1992). Pseudotumor cerebri following high-dose cytosine arabinside. *Br J Haematol 80:*559–560.

Fanoous M, Hamed LM, Margo CE. (1991). Pseudotumor cerebri associated with danazol withdrawal. *JAMA 266:*1218–1219.

Fardal RW. (1982). Pseudotumor cerebri following steroid injections. *Hawaii Med J 41:*414.

Fedotin MS. (1970). Hypervitaminosis causing pseudotumor cerebri. *JAMA 212:*628.

Feigert JM, Sweet DL, Coleman M, et al. (1990). Multicentric angiofollicular lymph node hyperplasia with peripheral neuropathy, pseudotumor cerebri, IgA dysproteinemia, and thrombocytosis in women. A distinct syndrome. *Ann Int Med 113:*362–367.

Feldman MH, Schlezinger NS. (1970). Benign intracranial hypertension associated with hypervitaminosis A. *Arch Neurol 22:*1–7.

Felton WL, Sismanis A. (1995). Idiopathic intracranial hypertension without papilledema in patients with pulsatile tinnitus. Presented at the North American Neuro-Ophthalmology Meeting, Tucson, AZ.

Fikkers BG, Bogousslavsky J, Reglii F, Glasson S. (1986). Pseudotumor cerebri with amiodarone. *J Neurol Neurosurg Psych 49:*606.

Fischer ED, and Spillito J. (1969). Large abdominal cysts. A complication of peritoneal shunts. *J Neurosurg 31:*441–444.

Fischer EG, Welch K, Shillito J. (1977). Syringomyelia following lumboperitoneal shunting for communicating hydrocephalus: Report of three cases. *J Neurosurg 47:*96–100.

Fisher OD. (1967). Nalidix acid and intracranial hypertension. *Br Med J 3:*370–371.

Fitz-Hugh GS, Robins RB, Craddock WD. (1966). Increased intracranial pressure complicating unilateral neck dissection. *Laryngoscope 76:*893–906.

Flynn WJ, Westfall CT, Weisman JS. (1994). Transient blindness after optic nerve sheath fenestration. *Am J Ophthalmol 117:*678–679.

Foley KM, Posner JB. (1975). Does pseudotumor cerebri cause the empty sella syndrome? *Neurology 25:*565–569.

Folsom C. (1966). Increased intracranial pressure in infants. *J Oklahoma Med Assoc 68:*228–230.

Fontana M, Mastrostefano R, Pietrangeli A, Madonna V. (1980). Acute intracranial hypertenson syndrome due to ketamine in a patient with delayed radionecrosis simulating an expansive process. *J Neurol Sci 24:*93–98.

Forman AR, Luessenhop AJ, Limaye SR. (1975). Ocular findings in patients with arteriovenous malformations of the head and neck. *Am J Ophthalmol 79:*626–633.

Fourie DT. (1977). Benign intracranial hypertension after topical steroid withdrawal. *South African Med J 52:*301.

Freedman BJ. (1963). Papilloedema, optic atrophy, and blindness due to emphysema and chronic bronchitis. *Br J Ophthalmol 47:*290–294.

Friedman DI, Forman S, Levi L, et al. (1997). Unusual ocular motility disturbances in pseudotumor cererbi. Presented at the 23rd Annual Meeting of the North American Neuro-Ophthalmology Society, Keystone, CO, February 9–13.

Frohman LP, Kupersmith MJ. (1985). Reversible vertical ocular deviations associated with raised intracranial pressure. *J Clin Neuro-ophthalmol 5:*158–163.

Galbraith JE. (1973). Optic nerve decompression in benign intracranial hypertension. *Trans Ophthalmol Soc New Zealand 25:*165–170.

Gardner K, Cox T, Digre KB. (1995). Idiopathic intracranial hypertension associated with tetracycline use in fraternal twins: Case report and review. *Neurology 45:*6–10.

Gedroyc W, Shorvon SD. (1982). Acute intracranial hypertension and nalidixic acid therapy. *Neurology 32:*212–215.

Gerber A, Raab AP, Sobel AE. (1954). Vitamin A poisoning in adults. *Am J Med 16:*729–745.

Getenet JC, Croisile B, Vighetto A, et al. (1993). Idiopathic intracranial hypertension after ofloxacin treatment. *Acta Neurol Scandina 87:*503–504.

Gibby WA, Cohen MS, Goldberg HI, Sergott RC. (1993). Pseudotumor cerebri: CT findings and correlation with vision loss. *Am J Radiol 160:*143–146.

Gibson T, Meyers AR. (1976). Nervous system involvement in systemic lupus erythematosus. *Ann Rheum Dis 35:*298–406.

Giles CL, Soble AR. (1971). Intracranial hypertension and tetracycline therapy. *Am J Ophthalmol 72:*981–982.

Gills JP Jr, Kapp JP, Odom GL. (1967). Benign intracranial hypertension. Pseudotumor cerebri from obstruction of dural sinuses. *Arch Ophthalmol 78:*592–595.
Gittinger JW Jr, Asdourian GK. (1989). Macular abnormalities in papilledema from pseudotumor cerebri. *Ophthalmology 96:*192–194.
Giuseffi V, Wall M, Siegel PZ, Roojas PB. (1991). Symptoms and disease associations in idiopathic intracranial hypertension (pseudotumor cerebri): A case-control study. *Neurology 41:*239–244.
Glaser JS. (1990). *Neuro-ophthalmology,* p. 106. 2 ed. Philidelphia, JP Lippincott.
Gokalp HZ, Baskaya MK, Aydin V. (1992). Pseudotumor cerebri with familial Mediterranean fever. *Clin Neurology Neurosurg 94:*261–263.
Goodwin JA. (1990). Treatment of idiopathic intracranial hypertension with digoxin. *Ann Neurol 28:*248.
Graham EM, Al-Ashkar AF, Sanders MD, Hilton P. (1980). Benign intracranial hypertension in Behçet's syndrome. *Neuro-ophthalmology 1:*73–76.
Grant DK. (1953). Papilloedema and fits in hypoparathyroidism. *Quat J Med 22:*243–259.
Grant WM. (1974). *Toxology of the eye.* 2nd ed. Springfield, Il, Charles C Thomas.
Green GJ, Lessell S, Lowenstein JI. (1980). Ischemic optic neuropathy in chronic papilledema. *Arch Ophthalmol 98:*502–504.
Green L, Vinker S, Amital H, et al. (1995). Pseudotumor cerebri in systemic lupus erythematosus. *Seminars Arthritis Rheum 25:*103–108.
Greenfield DS, Wanichwecharungruang B, Liebman JM, Ritch R. (1997). Pseudotumor cerebri appearing with unilateral papilledema after trabeculectomy. *Arch Ophthalmol 115:*423–426.
Greer M. (1963). Benign intracranial hypertension III: Pregnancy. *Neurology 13:*670–672.
Greer M. (1967). Benign intracranial hypertension in children. *Pediatr Clin North Am 14:*819–830.
Greer M. (1963). Benign intracranial hypertension. II. Following corticosteroid therapy. *Neurology 13:*439–441.
Greer M. (1964). Benign intracranial hypertension: IV Menarche. *Neurology 14:*569–573.
Grogan WA, Narkun DM. (1987). Pseudotumor cerebri with amiodarone. *J Neurol Neurosurg Psychiatry 50:*651.
Gross FJ and Mindel JS. (1991). Pseudotumor cerebri and Guillain-Barré syndrome associated with human immunodeficiency virus infection. *Neurology 41:*1845–1846.
Gupta HL, Venkateswar N, Prakash SK. (1980). Benign intracranial hypertension in pregnancy. *J Indian Med Assoc 75:*93–94.
Guy J, Johnston PK, Corbett JJ, et al. (1990). Treatment of visual loss in pseudotumor cerebri associated with uremia. *Neurology 40:*28–32.
Guymer RH, Cairns JD, O'Day J. (1993). Benign intracranial hypertension in chronic myeloid leukemia. *Australian New Zealand J Ophthalmol 21:*181–185.
Haller JS, Meyer DR, Cromie W, et al. (1993). Pseudotumor cerebri following beta-human chorionic gonadotropin hormone treatment for undescended testicles. *Neurology 43:*448–449.
Hamed LM, Glaser JS, Schatz NJ, Perez TH. (1989). Pseudotumor cerebri induced by danazol. *Am J Ophthalmol 107:*105–110.
Hamed LM, Tse DT, Glaser JS, et al. (1992). Neuroimaging of the optic nerve fenestration for management of pseudotumor cerebri. *Arch Ophthalmol 110:*636–639.
Hanafy MM, Hassanein ES, Khateeb S. (1967). Benign intracranial hypertension in vitamin D deficiency rickets associated with malnutrition. *J Tropical Pediatr African Chil Health 13:*19–22.
Hauser D, Barzilai N, Zalish M, et al. (1996). Bilateral papilledema with retinal hemorrhages in association with cerebral venous sinus thrombosis and paroxysmal nocturnal hemoglobinuria. *Am J Ophthalmol 122:*592–593.
Hawkins TE, Burlon DT. (1974). Vitamin A intoxication. *J Amer Osteopath Assoc 73:*371–375.
Hedges TR III, Legge RH, Peli E, Yardley CJ. (1995). Retinal nerve fiber layer changes and visual field loss in idiopathic intracranial hypertension. *Ophthalmology 102:*1242–1247.
Henry SD, Jacques S. (1979). Benign intracranial hypertension in pregnancy. *JACEP 8:*323–325.
Heuser M, Heuser H. (1976). Pseudotumor cerebri following insecticide (lindane) intoxication. *Acta Universitatis Carolinae Medica Monographia 75:*133–135.
Horoshovski D, Amital H, Katz M, Shoenfeld Y. (1995). Pseudotumor cerebri in SLE. *Clin Rheum 14:*708–710.
Horton JC, Seiff SR, Pitts LH, et al. (1992). Decompression of the optic nerve sheath for vision-threatening papilledema caused by dural sinus occlusion. *Neurosurgery 31:*203–212.
Hosking GP, Elliston H. (1978). Benign intracranial hypertension in a child with eczema treated with topical steroids. *Br Med J 1:*550–551.
Howe J, Saunders M, Clarke P. (1973). Familial benign intracranial hypertension. *Acta Neurochir 29:*173–175.
Hupp SL, Glaser JS, and Frazier-Byrne S. (1987). Optic nerve sheath decompression: Review of seventeen cases. *Arch Ophthalmol 105:*386–389.
Huseman CA, Torkelson RD. (1984). Pseudotumor cerebri following treatment of hypothalamic and primary hypothyroidism. *Am J Dis Children 138:*927–931.
Hykin PG, Spalton DJ. (1991). Bilateral perineuritis of the optic nerves. *J Neurol Neurosurg Psych 54:*375–376.
Ikkala E, Laitinen L. (1963). Papilloedema due to iron deficiency anemia. *Acta Haematol 29:*368–370.
Imari AJ. (1962). Papilledema in chronic cor pulmonale. *Dis Chest 41:*671–675.
Ireland B, Corbett JJ, Wallace RB. (1990). The search for the cause of idiopathic intracranial hypertension: A preliminary case-control study. *Arch Neurol 47:*315–320.

Jackson IJ, Snodgrass SR. (1954). Peritoneal shunts in the treatment of hydrocephalus and increased intracranial pressure. *J Neurosurg 12:*216–222.
Jacobson DM. (1995). Intracranial hypertension and the syndrome of acquired hyperopia with choroidal folds. *J Neuro-ophthalmol 15:*178–185.
Jacobson DM, Frens DB:(1989). Pseudotumor cerebri syndrome associated with Lyme disease. *Am J Ophthalmol 107:*81–82.
Jacobson DM, Karanjia PN, Olson KA, Warner JJ. (1990). Computed tomography ventricular size has no predictive valua in diagnosing pseudotumor cerebri. *Neurology 40:*1454–1455.
Jain N, Rosner F. (1992). Idiopathic intracranial hypertension: report of seven cases. *Am J Med 93:*391–395.
James HE, Tibbs PA. (1981). Diverse clinical applications of percutaneous lumboperitoneal shunts. *Neurosurgery 8:*39–42.
James MB, Leonard JC, Fraser JJ Jr, Stuemky JH. (1982). Hypervitaminosis A: A case report. *Pediatrics 69:*112–115.
Jamison RR. (1978). Subretinal neovascularization and papilledema associated with pseudotumor cerebri. *Am J Ophthalmol 85:*78–81.
Javeed N, Shaikh J, Jayaram S. (1995). Recurrent pseudotumor cerebri in an HIV-positive patient. *AIDS 9:*817–819.
Jay WM, Jay S. (1978). Benign intracranial hypertension with tetracycline therapy. *J Pediatr 93:*901–902.
Jefferson A. (1956). A clinical correlation between encephalopathy and papilloedema in Addison's disease. *J Neurol Neurosurg Psychiatry 19:*2–27.
Jenkyn LR, Budd RC, Fein SH, Cornell CJ. (1979). Insecticide/herbicide exposure, aplastic anaemia, and pseudotumor cerebri. *Lancet 2:*368.
Johnston I, Besser M, Morgan M. (1988a). Cerebrospinal fluid diversion in the treatment of benign intracranial hypertension. *J Neurosurg 69:*195–202.
Johnston I, Paterson A. (1974a). Benign intracranial hypertension. I. Diagnosis and prognosis. *Brain 97:*289–300.
Johnston I, Paterson A. (1974b). Benign intracranial hypertension. II. CSF pressure and circulation. *Brain 97:*301–312.
Johnston I, Paterson A, Besser M. (1988b). The treatment of benign intracranial hypertension: A review of 134 cases. *Surg Neurol 69:*195–202.
Jones RFC. (1967). Long-term results in various treatments of hydrocephalus. *J Neurosurg 26:*313–315.
Kalanie H, Niakan E, Harati Y, Rolak LA. (1986). Phentoin-induced benign intracranial hypertension. *Neurology 36:*443.
Kalbian VV, Challis MT. (1970). Behçet's disease: Report of twelve cases with three manifesting as papilledema. *Am J Med 49:*823–829.
Kansu T, Kansu E, Zileli T, Kirkali P. (1991). Neuro-ophthalmologic mnifestations of Behçet's disease. *Neuro-Ophthalmology 11:*7–11.
Kaplan RE, Springate JE, Feld LG, Cohen ME. (1985). Pseudotumor cerebri associated with cerebral venous sinus thrombosis, internal jugular vein thrombosis, and systemic lupus erythematosus. *J Pediatr 107:*266–268.
Karahalios D, Rekate HL, Khayata MH, Apostolides, PJ. (1996). Elevated intracranial venous pressure as a universal mechanism in pseudotumor cerebri of varying etiologies. *Neurology 46:*198–202.
Kasarskis EJ, Bass NH. (1982). Benign intracranial hypertension induced by deficiency of vitamin A during infancy. *Neurology 32:*1292–1295.
Kassam SH, Hadi HA, Fadel HE, et al. (1983). Benign intracranial hypertension in pregnancy: Current diagnostic and therapeutic approach. *Obstet Gynecol 38:*314–321.
Katz B, Moster ML, Slavin ML. (1997). Disk edema subsequent to renal transplantation. *Survey Ophthalmol 41:*315–320.
Katz VL, Peterson R, Cefalo RC. (1989). Pseudotumor cerebri and pregnancy. *Am J Perinatology 6:*442–445.
Katznelson D. (1978). Increased intracranial pressure in cystic fibrosis. *Acta Paediatr Scand 67:*607–609.
Kaye AH, Galbraith JE, King J. (1981). Intracranial pressure following optic nerve sheath decompression for benign intracranial hypertension. Case report. *J Neurosurg 55:*453–456.
Kellen RI, Burde RM. (1987). Optic nerve decompression. *Arch Ophthalmol 105:*889.
Kelman SE, Heaps R, Wolf A, Elman MJ. (1992). Optic nerve decompression surgery improves visual function in patients with pseudotumor cerebri. *Neurosurgery 30:*391–395.
Kelman SE, Sergott RC, Cioffi GA, et al. (1991). Modified optic nerve sheath decompression in patients with functioning lumboperitoneal shunts and progressive visual loss. *Ophthalmology 98:*1449–1453.
Keltner JL. (1988). Optic nerve sheath decompression. How does it work? Has its time come? *Arch Ophthalmol 106:* 1365–1369.
Kharode C, McAbee G, Sherman J, Kaufman M. (1992). Familial intracranial hypertension: Report of a case and review of the literature. *J Child Neurol 7:*196–198.
Kiers L, King JO. (1991). Increased intracranial pressure following bilateral neck dissection and radiotherapy. *Australian New Zealand J Surg 61:*459–461.
Kilpatrick C, Ebeling P. (1982). Intracranial hypertensioin in nalidixic acid therapy. *Med J Australia 1:*252.
Kilpatrick CJ, Kaufman DV, Galbraith JE, King JO. (1981). Optic nerve decompression in benign intracranial hypertension. *Clin Exp Neurol 18:*161–168.
King JO, Mitchell PJ, Thompson KR, Tress BM. (1995). Cerebral venography and manometry in idiopathic intracranial hypertension. *Neurology 45:*2224–2228.

Kirkham TH, Sanders MD, Sapp GA. (1973). Unilateral papilloedema in benign intracranial hypertension. *Can J Ophthalmol 8:*533–538.

Kiwak KJ, Levine SE. (1984). Benign intracranial hypertension and facial diplegia. *Arch Neurol 41:*787–788.

Knight RS, Fielder AR, Firth JL. (1986). Benign intracranial hypertension: Visual loss and optic nerve sheath fenestration. *J Neurol Neurosurg Psych 49:*243–250.

Köch-Weser J, Gilmore EB. (1967). Benign intracranial hypertension in an adult after tetracycline therapy. *JAMA 200:*345–347.

Konomi H, Imai M, Nihei K, et al. (1978). Indomethicin causing pseudotumor cerebri in Bartter's syndrome. *New Eng J Med 298:*855.

Koontz WL, Herbert WN, Cefalo RC. (1983). Pseudotumor cerebri in pregnancy. *Obstet Gynecol 62:*324–327.

Koppel BS, Kaunitz AM, Tuchman AJ. (1990). Pseudotumor cerebri following eclampsia. *European Neurology 30:*6–8.

Korzets A, Rathaus M, Chen B, Bernheim J. (1988). Pseudotumor cerebri and nitrofurantoin Drug Intelligence *Clin Pharm 22:*345.

Kosmorsky GS, Boyle KA. (1993). Relief of headache after ONSD. 19th Annual Meeting of the North American Neuro-Ophthalmologic Society, Big Sky, MT.

Kozin F, Haughton V, Bernhard GC. (1977). Neuro-Behçet's disease: Two cases and neuroradiologic findings. *Neurology 27:*1148–1152.

Kralik M, Beno P, Tischler V. (1976). The idiopathic hypoparathryroidism as the cause of the intracranial hypertension in an infant. *Acta Universitatis Crolinae Medica Mono 75:*139–140.

Krausz MM, Feinsod M, Beller AJ. (1978). Bilateral tranverse sinus obstruction in benign intracranial hypertension due to hypervitaminosis A. *Israel J Med Sci 14:*858–861.

Krogsaa B, Soelberg Sorensen P, Seedorf HH, et al. (1985). Ophthalmologic prognosis in benign intracranial hypertension. *Acta Ophthalmologica 173 (Suppl):*62–64.

Kuhner A, Krastal A, Stoll W. (1976). Arteriovenous malformations of the transverse dural sinuses. *J Neurosurg 45:*12–19.

Kupersmith MJ, Gemell L, Turbin R, et al. (1997). Effect of weight loss on pseudotumor cerebri in women. *Neurology 48 (Supplement):*A386.

Lam BL, Schatz NJ, Glaser JS, Bowen BC. (1992). Pseudotumor cerebri from cranial venous obstruction. *Ophthalmology 99:*706–712.

Lam BL, Siatkowski RM, Fox GM, Glaser JS. (1992). Visual loss in pseudotumor cerebri from branch retinal artery occlusion. *Am J Ophthalmol 113:*334–336.

Lamas E, Lobato RD, Esparza J, Escudero L. (1977) Dural posterior fossa AVM producing raised sagittal sinus pressure. *J Neurosurg 46:*804–810.

Landan I, Policherla H, McLaurin J. (1987). Complete external ophthalmoplegia in a case of pseudotumor cerebri. *Headache 27:*573–574.

Landers CM. (1989). Minocycline-induced benign intracranial hypertension. *Clin Exp Neurology 26:*161–167.

Larizza D, Colombo A, Lorini R, Severi F. (1979). Ketoprofen causing pseudotumor cerebri in Bartter's syndrome. *New Eng J Med 300:*796.

Lascari AD, Bell WE. (1970). Pseudotumor cerebri due to hypervitaminosis A. Toxic consequence of self-medication for acne in an adolescent girl. *Clin Pediatr 9:*627–628.

Laurence BM, Matthews WB, Shepard RH. (1960). Raised intracranial pressure associated with triamcinolone. *Lancet 1:*701–702.

Lee AG. (1995). Fourth nerve palsy in pseudotumor cerebri. *Strabismus 3:*57–59.

Leggio MG, Cappa A, Molinari M, et al. (1995). Pseudotumor cerebri as presenting syndrome of Addisonian crisis. *Italian J Neurol Sci 16:*387–389.

Lepore FE. (1992). Unilateral and highly asymmetric papilledema in pseudotumor cerebri. *Neurology 42:*676–678.

Lessell S. (1979). The neuro-ophthalmology of systemic lupus erythematosus. *Doc Ophthalmol 47:*13–42.

Lessell S. (1992). Pediatric pseudotumor cerebri (Idiopathic intracranial hypertension). *Survey Ophthalmol 37:*155–166.

Lessell S, Rosman NP. (1986). Permanent visual impairment in childhood pseudotumor. *Arch Neurol 43:*801–804.

Levine SH, Puchalski C. (1990). Pseudotumor cerebri associated with lithium therapy in two patients. *J Clin Psychiatry 51:*251–253.

Li EK, Ho PC. (1989). Pseudotumor cerebri in systemic lupus erythematosus. *J Rheumatol 16:*113–116.

Lipton HL, Michelson PE. (1972). Pseudotumor cerebri without papilledema. *JAMA 220:*1591–1592.

Liu GT, Kay MD, Bienfang DC, Schatz NJ. (1994). Pseodotumor cerebri associated with corticosteroid withdrawel in inflammatory bowel disease. *Am J Ophthalmol 117:*352–357.

Liu GT, Volpe NJ, Schatz NJ, et al. (1996). Severe sudden visual loss caused by pseudotumor cerebri and lumboperitoneal shunt failure. *Am J Ophthalmol 122:*129–131.

Liu, GT, Glaser, JS, Schatz NJ. (1994). High-dose methylprednisolone and acetazolamide for visual loss in pseudotumor cerebri. *Am J Ophthalmol 118:*88–96.

Lobo A, Pilek E, Stokes PE. (1978). Papilledema following therapeutic dosages of lithium carbonate. *J Nerv Ment Dis 166:*526–529.

Lombaert A, Carton H. (1976). Benign intracranial hypertension due to A-hypervitaminosis in adults and adolescents. *European Neurology 14:*340–350.

Lorentzen SE: (1966). Drusen of the optic disc. A clinical and genetic study. *Acta Ophthalmol 90:*1–181.
Lubeck MJ. (1959). Papilledema caused by iron deficiency anemia. *Trans Amer Acad Ophthalmol 63:*306–310.
Lucidi V, Di Capua M, Rosati P, et al. (1993). Benign intracranial hypertension in an older child with cystic fibrosis. *Pediatr Neurology 9:*494–495.
Lundar T, Nornes H. (1990). Pseudotumor cerebri—neurosurgical considerations. *Acta Neurochir 51:*366–368.
Macaya A, Roig M, Fernandez JM, Boronat M. (1988). Pseudotumor cererbri, spinal and radicular pain, and hyporeflexia: a clinical variant of the Guillain-Barré syndrome? *Pediatr Neurol 4:*120–121.
McCammon A, Kaufman HH, Sears ES. (1981). Transient oculomotor paralysis in pseudotumor cerebri. *Neurology 31:*182–184.
McVie R. (1984). Abnormal TSH regulation, pseudotumor cerebri, and empty sella after replacement therapy in juvenile hypothyroidism. *J Pediatrics 105:*768–770.
Mada Mohan P, Noushad TP, Sarita P, et al. (1993). Hypoparathyroidism with benign intracranial hypertension. *J Assoc Physicians India 41:*752–753.
Mahmoud HH, Hurwitz CA, Roberts WM, et al. (1993). Tretinoin toxicity in children with acute promyelocytic leukaemia. *Lancet 342:*1394–1395.
Maiuri F, De Chiara A, Benvenui D, Stella L. (1983). Benign intracranial hypertension and Guillain-Barré syndrome in systemic lupus erythematosus. A case report. *Acta Neurologica 5:*475–478.
Malozowski S, Tanner LA, Wysowski DK, et al. (1995). Benign intracranial hypertension in children with growth hormone deficiency treated with growth hormone. *J Pediatrics 126:*996–999.
Manfre L, Lagalla R, Mangiameli A, et al. (1995). Idiopathic intracranial hypertension: Orbital MRI. *Neuroradiology 37:*459–461.
Manfredi F, Merwarth CR, Buckley CE III, Sieker HO. (1961). Papilledema in chronic respiratory acidosis. *Am J Med 30:*175–180.
Marcelis J, Silberstein SD. (1991). Idiopathic intracranial hypertension without papilledema. *Arch Neurol 48:*392–399.
Margo CE, Levy MH, Beck RW. (1989). Bilateral idiopathic inflammation of the optic nerve sheaths. *Ophthalmology 96:*200–206.
Maroon JC, Mealy J Jr. (1971). Benign intracranial hypertension. Sequel to tetracycline therapy in a child. *JAMA 216:*1479–1480.
Masheter HC. (1959). Behçet's syndrome complicated by intracranial thrombophlebitis. *Proc Royal Soc Med 52:*1039–1040.
Massey JY, Roy H, Bornhofen JH. (1974). Ocular manifestations of Reye syndrome. *Arch Ophthalmol 91:*441–444.
Mathew NT, Ravishankar K, Sanin LC. (1996). Coexistence of migraine and idiopathic intracranial hypertension without papilledema. *Neurology 46:*1226–1230.
Mauriello JA, Shaderowfsky P, Gizzi M, Frohman L. (1995). Management of visual loss after optic nerve sheath decompression in patients with pseudotumor cerebri. *Ophthalmology 102:*441–445.
Maxner CE, Freedman MI, Corbett JJ. (1987). Asymmetric papilledema and visual loss in pseudotumour cerebri. *Canadian J Neurol Sci 14:*593–596.
Mayer Benegas N, Volpe NJ, Liu GT, Galetta SL. (1996). Hemifacial spasm and idiopathic intracranial hypertension. *J Neuro-ophthalmol 16:*70.
Mayer-Hubner B. (1996). Pseudotumor cerebri from intranasal oxytocin and excessive fluid intake. *Lancet 347:*623
Mdrucker DJ, Bookman AA. (1985). Pseudotumor cerebri in association with polyarthritis, urticaria, and cryoglobulinemia. *Canadian Med Assoc J 132:*147–149.
Merikangas JR. (1978). Skew deviation in pseudotumor cerebri. *Ann Neurol 4:*583.
Meyer JS, Gotham J, Tazaki Y, Gotah F. (1961). Cardiorespiratory syndrome of extreme obesity with papilledema. *Neurology 11:*950–958.
Miller NR. (1997). Bilateral visual loss and simultagnosia after lumboperitoneal shunt for pseudotumor cerebri. *J Neuro-Ophthalmol 17:*36–38.
Miller SJH, Bastron JA, Kearns TP. (1962). Papilledema in patients with severe pulmonary emphysema. *Dis Chest 37:*350–355.
Minutello JS, Dimayuga RG, Carter J. (1988). Pseudotumor cerebri, a rare adverse reaction to tetracycline therapy. A case report. *J Periodontol 59:*848–851.
Misra M, Khan GM, Rath S. (1992). Eltroxin induced pseudotumor cerebri—a case report. *Indian J Ophthalmol 40:*117.
Mitchell D, Fisher J, Irving D, et al. (1986). Lateral sinus thrombosis and intracranial hypertension in thrombocythaemia. *J Neurol Neurosurg Psychiatr 49:*218–219.
Mitchell DJ, Steahly LP. (1989). Pseudotumor cerebri and macular disease. *Retina 9:*115–117.
Mittra RA, Sergott RC, Flaharty PM, et al. (1993). Optic nerve decompression improves hemodynamic parameters in papilledema. *Ophthalmology 100:*987–997.
Mokri B, Jack CR Jr, Petty GW. (1993). Pseudotumor syndrome associated with cerebral venous sinus occlusion and antiphospholipid antibodies. *Stroke 24:*469–472.
Monaco F, Agnetti V, Mutani R. (1978). Benign intracranial hypertension after minocycline therapy. *European Neurology 17:*48–49.
Mones RJ. (1965). Increased intracranial pressure due to metastatic disease of venous sinuses. *Neurology 15:*1000–1007.

Moodley M, Coovadia HM. (1990). Benign intracranial hypertension in typhoid fever. A case report. *South African Med J 78:*608–609.

Mor F, Wysenbeek AJ. (1988). Evidence on computed tomography of pseudotumor cerebri in hypoparathyroidism. *Br J Radiol 61:*158–160.

Morantz RA, Lansky L, Batnitzky S. (1980). Non-operative management of pseudotumor cerebri caused by lateral sinus thrombosis. *J Kansas Med Soc 81:*465–466.

Morrice G Jr, Havener WH, Kapetansky F. (1960). Vitamin A intoxication as a cause of pseudotumor cerebri. *JAMA 173:*1802–1805.

Morse PH, Leveille AS, Antel JP, Burch JV. (1981). Bilateral juxtapapillary subretinal neovascularization associated with pseudotumor cerebri. *Am J Ophthalmol 91:*312–317.

Moskowitz Y, Leibowitz E, Ronen M, Aviel E. (1993). Pseudotumor cerebri induced by vitamin A combined with minocycline. *Ann Ophthalmol 25:*306–308.

Mukherjee A, Dutta P, Lahiri M, et al. (1990). Benign intracranial hypertension after naldixic acid overdose in infant. *Lancet 335:*1602.

Murphy TE, Costanzi JJ. (1969). Pseudotumor cerebri associated with pernicious anemia. *Ann Int Med 70:*777–782.

Murtagh F, Lehman R. (1967). Peritoneal shunts in the management of hydrocephalus. *JAMA 202:*1010–1014.

Mushet GR. (1977). Pseudotumor and nitrofurantoin therapy. *Arch Neurol 34:*257.

Narayanan I, Puri RK, Balakrishnan S. (1972). Pseudotumor cerebri due to hypervitaminosis A (a case report). *Neurology India 20:*231–232.

Nasr SZ, Schaffert D. (1995). Symptomatic increase in intracranial pressure following pancreatic enzyme replacement therapy for cystic fibrosis. *Pediatr Pulmonology 19:*396–397.

Nazarian SM, Janati A, Angtuaco EJ, Jay WM. (1987). Oculomotor palsy and papilledema with pial-dural arteriovenous malformations. *J Clin Neuro-ophthalmol 7:*98–103.

Neville BG, Wilson J. (1970). Benign intracranial hypertension following corticosteroid withdrawal in childhood. *Br Med J 3:*554–556.

Newborg B. (1974). Pseudotumor cerebri treated with rice reduction diet. *Arch Int Med 133:*802–807.

Newman PK, Snow M, Hudgson P. (1980). Benign intracranial hypertension and Cushing's disease. *Br Med J 281:*113.

Nezu A, Kimura S, Osaka H. (1995). Tolosa-Hunt syndrome with pseudotumor cerebri. Report of an unusual case. *Brain Development 17:*216–218.

Nickerson CW, Kirk RF. (1965). Recurrent pseudotumor cerebri in pregnancy: Report of 2 cases. *Obstet Gynecol 26:*811–813.

Noggle JD, Rodning CB. (1986). Rapidly advancing pseudotumor cerebri associated with morbid obesity: An indication for gastric exclusion. *Southern Med J 79:*761–763.

Nover A. (1963). Papilledema in blood and vascular disease. *Fortschr Neurol Psychiatr 31:*267–274.

O'Doherty NJ. (1965). Acute benign intracranial hypertension in an infant receiving tetracycline. *Dev Med Child Neurol 7:*677–680.

Ohlrich GD, Ohlrich JG. (1977). Papilledema in an adolescent due to tetracycline. *Med J Australia 1:*334–335.

Oliver TK Jr, Havener WH. (1958). Eye manifestations of chronic vitamin A intoxication. *Arch Ophthalmol 60:*19–22.

Olson CA, Riley HD Jr. (1966). Complications of tetracycline therapy. *J Pediatr. 68:*783–791.

Orefice G, De Joanna G, Coppola M, et al. (1995). Benign intracranial hypertension: A non-thrombotic complication of the primary antiphospholipid syndrome? *Lupus 4:*324–326.

Orefice G, Strianoo S, Carrieri PB, et al. (1984). Benign intracranial hypertension of obese women. A twenty case report. *Acta Neurol 6:*186–192.

Palmer RF, Searles HH, Boldrey EB. (1959). Papilledema and hypoparathyroidism simulating brain tumor. *J Neurosurg 16:*378–384.

Palop R, Choed-Amphai E, Miller R. (1979). Epidural anesthesia for delivery complicated by benign intracranial hypertension. *Anesthesiology 50:*159–160.

Pamir MN, Kansu T, Erbengi A, Zileli T. (1981). Papilledema in Behçet's syndrome. *Arch Neurol 38:*643–645.

Parag KB, Omar MA. (1983). Benign intracranial hypertension associated with iron deficiency anaemia. A case report. *South African Med J 63:*981–982.

Parfitt VJ, Dearlove JC, Savage D, et al. (1994). Benign intracranial hypertension after pituitary surgery for Cushing's disease. *Postgrad Med J 70:*115–117.

Parnass SM, Goodwin JA, Patel DV, et al. (1987). Dural sinus thrombosis: A mechanism for pseudotumor cerebri in systemic lupus erythematosus. *J Rheumatology 14:*152–155.

Pascual J, Combarros O, Berciano J. (1988). Gaze-evoked amaurosis in pseudotumor cerebri. *Neurology 38:*1654–1655.

Pasquariello PS Jr, Schut L, Borns P. (1977). Benign increased intracranial hypertension due to chronic vitamin A overdosage in a 26-month-old child. The increased intracranial pressure subsided promptly with steroid therapy and cessation of vitamin A. *Clin Pediatr 16:*379–382.

Pears J, Sandercock PA. (1990). Benign intracranial hypertension associated with danazol. *Scottish Med J 35:*49.

Pearson MG, Littlewood SM, Bowden AN. (1981). Tetracycline and benign intracranial hypertension. *Br Med J Clin Res Ed 282:*568–569.

Pearson PA, Baker RS, Khorram D, Smith TJ. (1991). Evaluation of optic nerve sheath fenestration in pseudotumor cerebri using automated perimetry. *Ophthalmology 98:*99–105.

Peterson CM, Kelly JV. (1985). Pseudotumor cerebri in pregnancy. Case reports and review of literature. *Obstet Gynecol Survey 40:*323–329.
Peterson RS, Rosenthal A. (1972). Retinopathy and papilledema in cyanotic congenital heart disease. *Pediatrics 49:*243–249.
Phanthumchinda K, Hemachudha T, Swasdikul D, et al. (1984). Sarcoidosis presenting with pseudotumor cerebri and the nephrotic syndrome. *J Med Assoc Thailand 67:*694–700.
Pierog SH, Al-Salihi FL, Cinotti D. (1986). Pseudotumor cerebri—a complication of tetracycline treatment of acne. *J Adolescent Health Care 7:*139–140.
Plotnik, JL, Kosmorsky, GS. (1993). Operative complications of optic nerve sheath decompression. *Ophthalmology 100:*683–690.
Powell JL. (1972). Pseudotumor cerebri and pregnancy. *Obstet Gynecol 40:*713–718.
Powers JM, Schnur JA, Baldree ME. (1986). Pseudotumor cerebri due to partial obstruction of the sigmoid sinus by a cholesteatoma. *Arch Neurol 43:*519–521.
Prendes JL, McLean WT Jr. (1978). Pseudotumor cerebri during treatment for hypothyroidism. *Southern Med J 71:*977.
Press OW, Ladenson PW. (1983). Pseudotumor cerebri and hypothyroidism. *Arch Int Med 143:*167–168.
Price DA, Clayton PE, Lloyd IC. (1995). Benign intracranial hypertension induced by growth hormone treatment. *Lancet 345:*458–459.
Radhakrishnan K, Ahlskog JE, Cross SA, et al. (1993). Idiopathic intracranial hypertension (pseudotumor cerebri). Descriptive epidemiology in Rochester, Minn, 1976 to 1990. *Arch Neurol 50:*78–80.
Radhakrishnan K, Ahlskog JE, Garrity JA, Kurland LT. (1994). Idiopathic intracranial hypertension. *Mayo Clin Proc 69:*169–180.
Radhakrishnan K, Thacker AK, Bohlaga NH, et al. (1993). Epidemiology of idiopathic intracranial hypertension: A prospective and case-control study. *J Neurol Sci 116:*18–28.
Rao KG. (1974). Pseudotumor cerebri associated with nalidixic acid. *Urology 4:*204–207.
Raucher HS, Kaufman DM, Goldfarb J, et al. (1985). Pseudotumor cerebri and Lyme disease: A new association. *J Pediatr 107:*931–933.
Raynor RB. (1969). Papilledema associated with tumors of the spinal cord. *Neurology 19:*700–704.
Redwood MD, Winer JB, Rossor M. (1990). Neurosarcoidosis presenting as benign intracranial hypertensioin. *European Neurology 30:*282–283.
Repka MX, Miller NR, Savino PJ. (1984). Pseudotumor cerebri. *Am J Ophthalmol 98:*741–746.
Restak RM. (1972). Pseudotumor cerebri, psychosis, and hypervitaminosis A. *J Nervous Mental Dis 155:*72–75.
Reza MJ, Demanes DJ. (1978). Behçet's disease: A case with hemoptysis, pseudotumor cerebri, and arteritis. *J Rheumatol 5:*320–326.
Rizzo JF, Lessell, S. (1994). Choroidal infarction after optic nerve sheath decompression. *Ophthalmology 101:*1622–1626.
Roos RA, van der Blij JF. (1985). Pseudotumor cerebri associated with hypovitaminosis A and hyperthyroidism. *Develo Med Child Neurol 27:*246–248.
Ropper AH, Marmarou A. (1984). Mechanism of pseudotumor in Guillain-Barré syndrome. *Arch Neurol 41:*259–261.
Rosenberg MA, Savino PJ, Glaser JS. (1979). A clinical analysis of pseudopapilledema. I. Population, laterality, acuity, refractile error, ophthalmoscopic characteristics, and coincident disease. *Arch Ophthalmol 97:*65–70.
Rosenberg, ML, Corbett, JJ, Smith, C, et al. (1993). Cerebrospinal fluid diversion procedures in pseudotumor cerebri. *Neurology 43:*1071–1072.
Rosenfeld JV, Widaa HA, Adams CB. (1991). Cerebral arteriovenous malformation causing benign intracranial hypertension—case report. *Neurologia Medico-Chirurgica 31:*523–525.
Rotellar C. (1987). Benign intracranial hypertension: A complication of subclavian vein catheterization and arteriovenous fistula. *Am J Kidney Dis 9:*242.
Rothner A, Burst J. (1974). Pseudotumor cerebri: Report of a familial occurrence. *Arch Neurol 30:*110–111.
Round R, Keane JR. (1988). The minor symptoms of increased intracranial pressure: 101 patients with benign intracranial hypertension. *Neurology 38:*1461–1464.
Roussounis SH. (1976). Benign intracranial hypertension after withdrawal of topical steroids in an infant. *Br Med J 2:*564.
Roytman M, Frumkin A, Bohn TG. (1988). Pseudotumor cerebri caused by isoretinoin. *Cutis 42:*399–400.
Rush JA, Ryan EJ. (1981). Syphilitic optic perineuritis. *Am J Ophthalmol 91:*404–406.
Rush JA. (1980). Pseudotumor cerebri. Clinical profile and visual outcome in 63 patients. *Mayo Clin Proc 55:*541–546.
Sadun AA, Currie JN, Lessell S. (1984). Transient visual obscurations with elevated discs. *Ann Neurol 16:*489–494.
Sakamaki Y, Nakamura R, Uchida M, et al. (1990). A case of pseudotumor cerebri following glucocorticoid therapy in which warfarin prevented recurrence. *Japanese J Med 29:*566–570.
Salgarello T, Tamburrelli C, Falsini B, et al. (1996). Optic nerve diameters and perimetric thresholds in idiopathic intracranial hypertension. *Br J Ophthalmol 80:*509–514.
Sambrook MA, Hill LF. (1977). Cerebrospinal fluid absorption in primary hypoparathyroidism. *J Neurol Neurosurg Psych 40:*1015–1017.
Sanborn GE, Selhorst JB, Calabrese VP, Taylor JR. (1979). Pseudotumor cerebri and insecticide intoxication. *Neurology 29:*1222–1227.

Saul RF, Hamburger HA, Selhorst JB. (1985). Pseudotumor cerebri secondary to lithium carbonate. *JAMA 253*:2869–2870.

Saxena VK, Heilpern J, Murphy SF. (1976). Pseudotumor cerebri. A complication of parenteral hyperalimentation. *JAMA 235*:2124.

Scanarini M, Mingrino S, d'Avella D, Della Corte V. (1979). Benign intracranial hypertension without papilledema: case report. *Neurosurgery 5*:376–377.

Schell CL, Rathe RJ. (1988). Superior sagittal sinus thrombosis. Still a killer. *West J Med 149*:304–307.

Schoeman JF. (1994). Childhood pseudotumor cerebri: Clinical and intracranial pressure response to acetazolamide and furosemide treatment in a case series. *J Child Neurol 9*:130–134.

Schonsted-Madsen U, Sehested P, Brask T. (1984). Benign intracranial hypertension caused by mastoiditis and lateral sinus obstruction: The value of computerized tomography in diagnosis. *J Laryngol Otol 98*:395–398.

Schwaber JR, Blumberg AG. (1961). Papilledema associated with blood loss anemia. *Ann Int Med 55*:1004–1010.

Schwarz S, Husstedt IW, Georgiadis D, et al. (1995). Benign intracranial hypertension in an HIV-infected patient: Headache as the only presenting sign. *AIDS 9*:657–658.

Selhorst JB, Waybright EA, Jennings S, Corbett JJ. (1984). Liver lover's headache: Pseudotumor cerebri and vitamin A intoxication. *JAMA 252*:3365.

Selky AK, Purvin VA. (1994). Hemifacial spasm. An unusual manifestation of idiopathic intracranial hypertension. *J Neuro-ophthalmol 14*:196–198.

Selky AK, Dobyns WB, Yee, RD. (1994). Idiopathic intracranial hypertension and facial diplegia. *Neurology 44*:457.

Sell JJ, Ruppe FW, Orrison WW Jr. (1995). Iatrogenically induced intracranial hypotension syndrome. *Am J Radiol 165*:1513–1515.

Selleri C, Pane F, Notaro R, et al. (1996). All-trans-retinoic acid (ATRA) responsive skin relapses of acute promyelocytic leukaemia followed by ATRA-induced pseudotumor cerebri. *Br J Haematol 92*:937–940.

Selman WR, Spetzler RF, Wilson CB, Grollmus J. (1980). Percutaneous lumboperitoneal shunts: Review of 130 cases. *Neurosurgery 6*:255–257.

Sergott RC, Savino PJ, Bosley TM. (1988). Optic nerve sheath decompression provides long-term visual improvement for pseudotumor cerebri. *Arch Ophthalmol 106*:1384–1390.

Shah A, Roberts T, McQueen IN, et al. (1987). Danazol and benign intracranial hypertension. *Br Med J Clin Res Ed 294*:1323.

Shapiro I, Shapiro SK. (1980). Familial pseudotumor cerebri and the empty sella syndrome. *Ann Ophthalmol 12*:1045–1048.

Shapiro S, Yee R, Brown H. (1995). Surgical management of pseudotumor cerebri in pregnancy: Case report. *Neurosurgery 37*:829 – 831.

Sharieff GQ, Hanten K. (1996). Pseudotumor cerebri and hypercalcemia resulting from vitamin A toxicity. *Ann Emergency Med 27*:518–521.

Sharma DB, James A. (1974). Benign intracranial hypertension associated with nitrofurantoin therapy. *Br Med J 4*:771.

Sharma DB, Lahori UC. (1975). Benign intracranial hypertension following tetracycline therapy. *Indian Pediatr 12*:609–610.

Shekleton P, Fidler J, Grimwade J. (1980). A case of benign intracranial hypertension in pregnancy. *Br J Obstet Gynecol 87*:345–347.

Sheldon RS, Becker WJ, Hanley DA, Culver RL: (1987). Hypoparathyroidism and pseudotumor cerebri: An infrequant clinical association. *Canadian J Neurol Sci 14*:622–625.

Sher NA, Wirtschafter J, Shapiro SK, et al. (1983). Unilateral papilledema in 'benign' intracranial hypertension (pseudotumor cerebri). *JAMA 250*:2346–2347.

Sheridan M, Johnston I. (1994). Hydrocephalus and pseudotumor cerebri in the mucopolysaccharidoses. *Childs Nervous System 10*:148–150.

Sheth KJ, Kivlin JD, Leichter HE, et al. (1994). Pseudotumor cerebri with vision impairment in two children with renal transplantation. *Pediatr Nephrology 8*:91–93.

Shiozawa Z, Yoshida M, Kobayashi K, et al. (1986). Superior sagittal sinus thrombosis and systemic lupus erythematosus. *Ann Neurol 20*:272.

Silberberg DH, Laties AM. (1973). Increased intracranial pressure in disseminated lupus erythematosus. *Arch Neurol 29*:88–90.

Silbergleit R, Junck L, Gebarski SS, Hatfield MK. (1989). Idiopathic intracranial hypertension (pseudotumor cerebri): MR imaging. *Radiology 170*:207–220.

Silverstein A. (1974). Papilledema with acute viral infections of the brain. *Mt Sinai Med J 41*:435–443.

Simpson T. (1948). Papilloedema in emphysema. *Br Med J 2*:639–641.

Sirdofsky M, Kattah J, Macedo P. (1994). Intracranial hypertension in a dieting patient. *J Neuro-ophthalmology 14*:9–11.

Sismanis A, Butts FM, Hughes GB. (1990). Objective tinnitus in benign intracranial hypertension. An update. *Laryngoscope 100*:33–36.

Smith KH, Wilkinson JT, Brindley GO. (1992). Combined third and sixth nerve paresis following optic nerve sheath fenestration. *J Clin Neuro-ophthalmol 12*:85–87.

Snyder DA, Frenkel M. (1979). An unusual presentation of pseudotumor cerebri. *Ann Ophthalmol 11*: 1823–1827.

Sorensen PS, Krogsaa B, Gjerris F. (1988). Clinical course and prognosis of pseudotumor cerebri. A prospective study of 24 patients. *Acta Neurologica Scand 77:*164–172.
Spalter HF, Bruce GM. (1964). Ocular changes in pulmonary insufficiency. *Trans Amer Acad Ophthalmol 68:*661–676.
Spector RH, Carlisle J. (1984). Pseudotumor cerebri caused by a synthetic vitamin A preparation. *Neurology 34:*1509–1511.
Sperry B. (1979). Benign intracranial hypertension associated with palsy of the third cranial nerve. *J Amer Osteopath Assoc 78:*816–821.
Spetzler RF, Weinstein PR, Chater N, Wilson CB. (1977). Cisternoatrial, ventriculocisternal, and other cisternal shunts simplified: A percutaneous technique. *J Neurosurg 47:*299–302.
Spetzler R, Wilson C, Grollmus J. (1975). Percutaneous lumboperitoneal shunts. *J Neurosurg 43:*770–773.
Spoor TC, McHenry JG: (1993). Long-term effectiveness of optic nerve sheath decompression for pseudotumor cerebri. *Arch Ophthalmol 111:*632–635.
Spoor TC, McHenry JG, Shin DH. (1995). Long-term results using adjunctive mitomycin C in optic nerve sheath decompression for pseudotumor cerebri. *Ophthalmology 102:*2024–2028.
Spoor TC, Ramocki JM, Madison, MP, et al: (1991). Treatment of pseudotumor cerebri by primary and secondary optic nerve sheath decompression. *Am J Ophthalmol 112:* 177–185.
Stern JM, Kesler SM. (1989). Raised intracranial pressure in a 16-year-old boy. Report of a case of Behçet's disease. *South African Med J 75:*243–244.
Stevens PM, Austen F, Knowles JH. (1963). Prognostic significance of papilledema in course of respiratory insufficiency. *JAMA 183:*61–164.
Strominger MB, Weiss GB, Mehler MF. (1992). Asymptomatic unilateral papilledema in pseudotumor cerebri. *J Clin Neuro-ophthalmol 12:*238–241.
Stuart BH, Litt IF. (1978). Tetracycline-associated intracranial hypertension in an adolescent: Complication of systemic acne therapy. *J Pediatr 92:*679–680.
Sugerman HJ, Felton WL 3rd, Salvant JB Jr, et al. (1995). Effects of surgically induced weight loss on idiopathic intracranial hypertension in morbid obesity. *Neurology 45:*1655–1659.
Sullivan HC. (1991). Fatal tonsiilar herniation in pseudotumor cerebri. *Neurology 41:*1142–1144.
Sullivan LP, Stears JC, Ringel SP. (1988). Resolution of syringomyelia and Chiari I malformation by ventriculatrial shunting in a patient with pseudotumor cerebri and a lumboperitoneal shunt. *Neurosurgery 22:*744–747.
Sussman J, Leach M, Greaves M, et al. (1997). Potentially prothrombotic abnormalities of coagulation in benign intracranial hypertension. *J Neurol Neurosurg Psych 62:*229–233.
Sybert VP, Bird TD, Salk DJ. (1985). Pseudotumor cerebri and the Turner syndrome. *J Neurol Neurosurg Psych 48:*164–166.
Takahashi T, Okukubo K, Tagami Y, et al. (1983). A case of dural arteriovenous malformation with papilledema. *Neuro-ophthalmology 3:*199–204.
Tehindrazanarivelo A, Bousser MG. (1990). Possible benign intracranial hypertension and essential thrombocythaemia. *J Neurol Neurosurg Psych 53:*819.
Tessler Z, Biedner B, Yassur Y. (1985a). Benign intracranial hypertension in menarche. *Compr Ther 11:*16–18.
Tessler Z, Biedner B, Yassur Y. (1985b). Papilloedema: Benign intracranial hypertension in menarche. *Annals Ophthalmol 17:*76–77.
Thomas CV, Kennedy BJ. (1986). Primary Hodgkin's disease of the skull following a 3-year history of pseudotumor cerebri. *Cancer 58:*318–320.
Thomas E. (1986). Recurrent benign intracranial hypertension associated with hemoglobin SC disease in pregnancy. *Obstet Gynecol 67 (3 Suppl):*7S–9S.
To KW, Warren FA. (1990). Unilateral papilledema in pseudotumor cerebri. *Arch Ophthalmol 108:*644–645.
Tobin H. (1971). Increased cerebrospinal fluid pressure following unilateral neck dissection. *Laryngoscope 82:*817–820.
Tomkins CM, Spalton DJ. (1984). Benign intracranial hypertension treated by optic nerve sheath decompression. *J Royal Soc Med 77:*141–144.
Tomsak RL, Niffenegger AS, Remler BF. (1988). Treatment of pseudotumor cerebri with Diamox (acetazolamide). *J Clin Neuro-ophthalmol 8:*93–98.
Torlai F, Galassi G, Debbia A, et al. (1989). Familial pseudotumor cerebri in male heterozygous twins. *European Neurol 29:*106–108.
Torres M, May E, Watanabe F, et al. (1997). Intracranial hypertension associated with minocycline. Presented at the 23rd Annual Meeting of the North American Neuro Ophthalmology Society, Keystone, CO, February 9–13.
Tourn N, Sharpe JA. (1996). Pseudotumor cerebri mimicking Foster Kennedy syndrome. *Neuro-ophthalmology 16:*55–57.
Travero F, Stagnaro R, Fazio B. (1993). Benign intracranial hypertension with HIV infection. *European Neurology 33:*191–192.
Traviesa DC, Schwartzman RJ, Glaser JS, Savino P. (1976). Familial benign intracranial hypertension. *J Neurol Neurosurg Psych 39:*420–423.
Troost BT, Sufit RL, Grand MG. (1979). Sudden monocular visual loss in pseudotumor cerebri. *Arch Neurol 36:*440–442.
Tse DT, Nerad JA, Anderson RL, Corbett JJ. (1988). Optic nerve sheath fenestration in pseudotumor cerebri. A lateral orbitotomy approach. *Arch Ophthalmol 106:*1458–1462.

Tugal O, Jacobson R, Berezin S, et al. (1994). Recurrent benign intracranial hypertension due to iron deficiency anemia. Case report and review of the literature. *Amer J Pediatr Hematol-Oncol 16:*266–270.

Vachvanichsanong P, Dissaneewate P, Vasikananont P. (1992). Pseudotumor cerebri in a boy with systemic lupus erythematosus. *Am J Dis Children 146:*1417–1419.

Van den Bergh R, Dralands G, Crolla D, van den Bergh P. (1980). Pseudotumor cerebri due to intracranial arteriovenous malformation. *Clin Neurol Neurosurg 82:*119–125.

Van den Brink WA, Pieterman H, Avezaat CJ. (1996). Sagittal sinus occlusion, caused by an overlying depressed cranial fracture, presenting with late signs and symptoms of intracranial hypertension: Case report. *Neurosurgery 38:*1044–1046.

Van Dop C, Conte FA, Koch TK, et al. (1983). Pseudotumor cerebri associated with initiation of levothyroxine therapy for juvenile hypothyroidism. *New Eng J Med 308:*1076–1080.

Van Gelder T, van Gemert HM, Tjiong HL. (1991). A patient with megaloblastic anaemia and idiopathic intracranial hypertension. Case history. *Clin Neurol Neurosurg 93:*321–322.

Vander Ark GD, Kempe LG, Smith DR. (1971). Pseudotumor cerebri treated with lumbar-peritoneal shunt. *JAMA 217:*1832–1834.

Varadi G, Lossos A, Or R, et al. (1995). Successful allogenic bone marrow transplantation in a patient with ATRA-induced pseudotumor cerebri. *Am J Hematol 50:*147–148.

Vargas JA, Garcia-Merino A, Rodriguez E, Villagra A. (1990). Pseudotumor cerebri complicating typhoid fever. *European Neurology 30:*345–346.

Vassilouthis J, Uttley D. (1979). Benign intracranial hypertension: clinical features and diagnosis using computed tomography and treatment. *Surg Neurol 12:*389–392.

Vassilouthis J. (1979). Cerebral arteriovenous malformation with intracranial hypertension. *Surg Neurol 11:*402–404.

Verderber L, Lavin P, Wesley R. (1991). Pseudotumor cerebri and chronic benzene hexacloride (lindane) exposure. *J Neurol Neurosurg Psych 54:*113.

Verm A, Lee AG. (1997). Bilateral optic disk edema with macular exudates as the manifesting sign of a cerebral arteriovenous malformation. *Am J Ophthalmol 123:*422–424.

Visani G, Bontempo G, Manfroi S, et al. (1996). All-trans-retinoic acid and pseudotumor cerebri in a young adult with acute promyelocytic leukemia: A possible disease association. *Haematologica 81:*152–154.

Vollbracht R, Gilroy J. (1976). Vitamin A induced benign intracranial hypertension. *Canadian J Neurol Sci 3:*59–61.

Vyas CK, Talwar KK, Bhatnager V, Sharma BK. (1981). Steroid-induced benign intracranial hypertension. *Postgrad Med J 57:*181–182.

Walker AE, Adamkiewicz JJ. (1964). Pseudotumor cerebri associated with prolonged corticosteroid therapy. *JAMA 188:*779–784.

Wall M. (1986). Contrast sensitivity testing in pseudotumor cerebri. *Ophthalmology 93:*47.

Wall M. (1990). The headache profile of idiopathic intracranial hypertension. *Cephalgia 10:*331–335.

Wall M, George D. (1991). Idiopathic intracranial hypertension. A prospective study of 50 patients. *Brain 114:*155–180.

Wall M, George D. (1987). Visual loss in pseudotumor cerebri. Incidence and defects related to visual field strategy. *Arch Neurol* 170–175.

Wall M, Montgomery EB. (1995). Using motion perimetry to detect visual field defects in patient s with idiopathic intracranial hypertension: A comparison with conventional automated perimetry. *Neurology 45:*1169–1175.

Wall M, Hart WM Jr, Burde RM. (1983). Visual field defects in idiopathic intracranial hypertension (pseudotumor cerebri). *Am J Ophthalmol 96:*654–669.

Walsh FB. (1952). Papilledema associated with increased intracranial pressure in Addison's disease. *Arch Ophthalmol 47:*86.

Walters BN, Gubbay SS. (1981). Tetracycline and benign intracranial hypertension: Report of five cases. *Br Med J Clin Res Ed 282:*19–20.

Wasan H, Mansi JL, Benjamin S, et al. (1992). Myeloma and benign intracranial hypertension. *Br Med J 304:*685.

Watkins CH, Wagener HP, Brown RW. (1941). Cererbal symptoms accompanied by choked discs in types of blood dyscrasia. *Am J Ophthalmol 24:*1374–1383.

Watnick RL, Trobe JD. (1989). Bilateral optic nerve compression as a mechanism for the Foster-Kennedy syndrome. *Ophthalmology 96:*1793–1798.

Weisberg LA, Housepian EM, Saur DP. (1975). Empty sella synsrome as complication of benign intracranial hypertension. *J Neurosurg 43:*177–180.

Weisberg LA, Pierce JF, Jabbari B. (1977). Intracranial hypertension resulting from a cerebrovascular malformation. *South Med J 70:*624–626.

Weiss GB, Bajwa ZH, Mehler MF. (1991). Co-occurrence of pseudotumor cerebri and Guillain-Barré syndrome in an adult. *Neurology 41:*603–604.

Weissman MN, Page LK, Bejar RL. (1983). Cushing's disease in childhood: Benign intracranial hypertension after trans-sphenoidal adenomectomy. Case report. *Neurosurgery 13:*195–198.

Welch K, Shillito J, Strand R, et al. (1981). Chiari I "malformation"—an acquired disorder? *J Neurosurg 55:*604–609.

Wessel K, Thron A, Linden D, et al. (1987). Pseudotumor cerebri: Clinical and neuroradiological findings. *European Arch Psych Neurol Sci 237:*54–60.

Westlake EK, Kaye M. (1954). Raised intracranial pressure in emphysema. *Br Med J 1:*302–304.

Wheatley T, Clark JD, Edwards OM, Jordan K. (1986). Retinal haemorrhage and papilloedema due to benign intracranial hypertension in a pregnant diabetic. *Diabetic Med 3:*482–484.
Wigglesworth R. (1967). Pituitary-adrenal function after topical steroids. *Lancet 2:*1209.
Wilkins MR, Gove RI, Roberts SD, Kendall MJ. (1986). Behçet's disease presenting as benign intracranial hypertension. *Postgrad Med J 62:*39–41.
Wilson CB, Bertan V. (1966). Perforation of the bowel complicating peritoneal shunt for hydrocephalus: Report of two cases. *Am Surg 32:*601–603.
Winrow AP, Supramaniam G. (1990). Benign intracranial hypertension after ciprofloxacin administration. *Arch Dis Child 65:*1165–1166.
Wolin MJ, Brannon WL. (1995). Disk edema in an overweight woman. *Survey Ophthalmol 39:*307–314.
Yokokura M, Hatake K, Komatsu N, et al. (1994). Toxicity of tretinoin in acute promyelocytic leukaemia. *Lancet 343:*361–362.
Zabramski JM, Spetzler RF. (1988). AVMs and intracranial hypertension. *Neurosurgery 23:*48.

◆ 8 ◆

Transient Visual Loss

What Questions Should be Asked of a Patient with Transient Visual Loss?

The most important questions that need to be addressed in the assessment of the patient with transient visual loss (TVL) include:

1. Is the visual loss monocular or binocular? Monocular TVL implies disease of the eye, retina, optic nerve, orbit, circulation to the eye (heart, aorta, carotid artery, ophthalmic artery, central retinal artery, etc.), or migraine. Binocular TVL implies bilateral eye disease, disease affecting the circulation to both eyes (e.g., bilateral carotid stenosis), increased intracranial pressure with papilledema, brain tumor, or, most often, disease of the vertebrobasilar circulation (especially vertebrobasilar transient ischemic attacks [TIAs]) or migraine.
2. What is the temporal profile of the transient loss of vision? For example, TVL in one eye lasting seconds is characteristic of transient obscurations of vision resulting from optic nerve ischemia or papilledema, while monocular TVL lasting 2 to 30 minutes is characteristic of TVL associated with carotid artery disease.
3. What are the precipitants of the visual loss? For example, patients with an intraorbital mass may develop TVL only in certain eye positions due to the mass compressing the ipsilateral optic nerve or optic nerve circulation (gaze-evoked amaurosis). Monocular or binocular TVL due to carotid disease may occur following exposure to bright light.
4. Are any optic nerve or retinal vessel abnormalities evident on funduscopic examination? For example, fundus exam may well reveal papilledema in a patient with transient obscurations of vision, retinal vessel emboli in a patient with carotid or cardiac disease, and disc anomalies in a patient with monocular TVL.

In this chapter we will discuss various entities that may cause monocular or binocular TVL. An approach to the patient with monocular or binocular transient visual loss is given in Figures 8–1 and 8–2, respectively.

Does Monocular TVL Only Occur in Certain Positions of Gaze (Gaze-Evoked TVL) or Only After Prolonged Reading (Reading-Evoked TVL)?

Patients who experience TVL evoked by eccentric position of gaze (gaze-evoked TVL) usually have an intraorbital mass that intermittently compresses the circulation to the optic nerve or retina (Bradbury, 1987; Brown, 1981; Hampton, 1983; Knapp, 1992; Kohmoto, 1993; Levy, 1986; Miller, 1988; Orcutt, 1986, 1987; Unsold, 1979; Wilkes, 1979; Wright, 1977). The visual loss immediately clears when the direction of gaze is changed. The most common lesions are cavernous hemangiomas or optic nerve sheath meningiomas, but other lesions have included osteomas, neurofibromas, gliomas, medial rectus granular myoblastoma, varices, orbital trauma, and metastases. The examination may be normal or show evidence of an optic neuropathy with an afferent pupil defect, color vision impairment, disc edema, and optociliary shunt vessels. Other signs of orbital tumor, such as proptosis, limitation of extraocular muscle movement, swelling of the eyelids, chemosis, and conjunctival congestion, may be evident. Evaluation requires magnetic resonance (MR) or computed tomography (CT) imaging of the orbital structures. Gaze-evoked monocular TVL has also been noted in a patient with pseudotumor cerebri (Pascual,1988). The pathogenesis of the TVL in this case is unclear, but may have been related to kinking of the swollen nerve sheath with secondary compression of the vascular supply to the optic nerve during eccentric gaze (Miller, 1991a). Thus, if neuroimaging fails to reveal an orbital lesion as cause of gaze-evoked TVL, lumbar puncture is probably warranted, especially if other signs or symptoms are suggestive of pseudotumor cerebri.

Reading may also induce monocular TVL. Manor et al. described a 49-year-old man with a five year history of dimming of central vision in the left eye provoked only during reading (Manor, 1996). An orbital apex tumor situated lateral to and above the optic nerve was found. This reading-evoked visual dimming may well be a variant of gaze-evoked TVL. The optic nerve, displaced laterally and superiorly and stretched by the act of reading, may be compressed between the tumor above and the contracted inferior rectus muscle inferiorly. Thus, orbital neuroimaging is appropriate in patients with reading-induced TVL. However, intermittent angle closure glaucoma may cause a similar phenomena (O'Sullivan, 1995). O'Sullivan et al. described a 66-year-old patient with episodes of monocular TVL lasting 3 minutes to several hours that were precipitated by reading, writing, or watching television. Ophthalmologic exam was normal but reading over 4 hours induced corneal edema, a poorly reactive semidilated pupil, and a shallow anterior chamber with intraocular pressure 50 mm Hg. The intermittent angle closure glaucoma and the patient's symptoms were treated successfully by iridotomies. Thus, angle closure glaucoma attacks must also be considered in the differential of reading-induced monocular TVL.

Do the Episodes of Monocular TVL Last Seconds?

Episodes of TVL lasting less than 60 seconds may occur in patients with papilledema (Cogan, 1961; Wall, 1991). These transient obscurations of vision may occur in one or both eyes (individually or simultaneously) and typically last only a few seconds. In rare cases they may last for hours. The episodes may be precipitated by changes in position and are thought to be related to the effects of increased intracranial pressure on the flow of blood to the eye, perhaps where the central retinal artery penetrates the optic nerve sheath to enter the substance of the nerve (Miller, 1991a). Similar monocular episodes of TVL lasting seconds may occur in patients with optic nerve sheath meningiomas and are probably unrelated to increased intracranial pressure (Sibony, 1984). The pathogenesis of these episodes in meningioma patients is unknown and may be caused by the effect of the meningioma on the central retinal artery where it enters the optic nerve (Miller, 1991a). Transient obscurations of vision may also occur in an eye with congenital abnormalities of the optic disc, such as peripapillary staphyloma (see below), or optic disc drusen (Beck, 1985; Lorentzen, 1966). Finally, carotid atherosclerotic disease may rarely cause very brief episodes of transient visual loss, but more often attacks of TVL with carotid disease last 2 to 15 minutes (see below).

Patients with transient visual obscurations first require ophthalmologic examination. If papilledema is evident, these patients must have a magnetic resonance imaging (MRI) scan of the brain. If this study is normal, a spinal tap is indicated to investigate the possibility of infection or pseudotumor cerebri (idiopathic intracranial hypertension). Patients with drusen or other optic disc anomalies causing monocular TVL may require no further evaluation. If there are signs of an optic neuropathy on the side of the TVL (e.g., relative afferent pupillary defect, ipsilateral swollen or atrophic optic nerve, etc.), then MR imaging with attention to the orbit is warranted to evaluate a compressive lesion. Patients without apparent disc abnormalities should be screened for carotid atherosclerotic disease or other sources of emboli (see below) and MR imaging should be performed to investigate the possibility of a structural brain lesion such as optic nerve sheath meningioma.

Do the Episodes of Monocular TVL Last Minutes?

Monocular TVL lasting 5 to 60 minutes (usually 2 to 30 minutes) is strongly suggestive of thromboembolic disease. These episodes are most often due to emboli, involving the retinal arterial system, which may arise from aortic or carotid artery atherosclerotic disease or a cardiogenic source. Patients often describe a veil or shade descending or ascending over a portion or the whole of their visual field. Other patients complain of patchy visual loss ("Swiss cheese" pattern) or peripheral constriction with central visual sparing (Bruno, 1990; Ehrenfield, 1966; Venables, 1984). Some episodes of monocular TVL are accompanied by a sensation of color or other photopsias, similar to migraine, consisting of showers of stationary flecks of light that disperse quickly (Ashby, 1963; Bruno, 1990; Ehrenfield, 1966; Goodwin, 1984, 1987; Pessin, 1977; Venables, 1984). Most episodes of monocular TVL last 2 to 30 minutes. Marshall and Meadows found that in 51 of 67 patients (75%) episodes lasted 30 minutes or less, with 29 patients (43%) experiencing episodes lasting 5 minutes or less (Marshall, 1968). Pessin et al. noted that attacks lasted less than 15 minutes in 30 of 33 patients, and in 14 patients (42%) the episodes lasted 5 minutes or less (Pessin, 1977). Among 35 patients evaluated by Goodwin et al., 22 patients (63%) had attacks lasting 5 minutes or less, 8 (23%) had episodes lasting 6 to 15 minutes, and 6 patients (14%) had episodes lasting more than 15 minutes (Goodwin, 1987). Episodes of monocular TVL due to thromboembolic disease rarely last several hours (Fujino, 1983; Longfellow, 1962b).

Patients with TVL from thromboembolic disease may demonstrate emboli lodged within the retinal vessels. In general, emboli may be composed of clotted blood, fibrin, platelets, atheromatous tissue, white cells, calcium, infectious organisms (septic emboli), air, fat, tumor cells, amniotic fluid, or foreign materials (e.g., talc, artificial valve material, catheters, silicone, cornstarch, mercury, corticosteroids). The most common types of emboli seen in patients with atherosclerotic disease of the aorta/carotid arteries or cardiac disease include the following:

1. Cholesterol emboli (Hollenhorst plaques) are bright, glistening, yellow or copper-colored fragments, most often seen in peripheral arterioles in the temporal fundus. These emboli most often arise from atheromatous plaques in the aorta or carotid bifurcation.
2. Platelet-fibrin emboli are dull, white, gray, often elongated, and subject to fragmentation and distal movement. These emboli most often lodge at bifurcations of retinal vessels and arise from the walls of atherosclerotic arteries or from the heart, especially from heart valves. They may also be seen in patients with coagulopathies.
3. Calcific emboli, which tend to be large, ovoid or rectangular, and chalky-white. These emboli often occur over or adjacent the optic disc and usually arise from cardiac (aortic or mitral) valves, less often from the aorta or carotid artery. Unlike cholesterol emboli, which often disappear in a few days, calcific emboli may remain permanently visible.

TVL may also occur from ocular hypoperfusion rather than embolization. In some patients, monocular TVL may occur when the patient is exposed to bright light (Donnan, 1982; Furlan, 1979; Ross Russell, 1983). These patients usually have severe, ipsilateral carotid occlusive disease. Bilateral, simultaneous TVL induced by exposure to bright light may rarely occur with bilateral severe carotid stenosis or occlusion (Wiebers, 1989). The light-induced TVL probably reflects the inability of a borderline ocular circulation to sustain the increased retinal metabolic activity associated with light exposure. Postprandial transient visual loss has also been decribed (Levin, 1997). In one patient, episodes of splotchy visual loss occured unilaterally on the left one hour after eating her largest meal of the day with episodes lasting approximately three hours. These episodes were occasionally accompanied by numbness and weakness of the contralateral arm and were found to be due to severe left carotid stenosis. In a second patient, blotchy bilateral transient visual loss episodes lasting two minutes to one-and-a-half hours were precipitated by eating or standing from a sitting or lying position. This second patient was found to have complete occlusion of the right carotid artery and moderate stenosis of the left carotid artery. The authors proposed that postprandial visual loss may be a symptom of critical carotid stenosis, with retinal and choroidal hypoperfusion probably caused by a combination of mesenteric steal, decreased cardiac output, and abnormal vasomotor control (Levin, 1997).

Venous stasis retinopathy (hypotensive retinopathy), associated with severe carotid or ophthalmic artery occlusive disease, may also be associated with TVL (Brown, 1988; Carter, 1985; Fisher, 1952; Gass, 1997a; Hedges, 1962; Kahn, 1986; Kearns, 1963, 1983; McCrary, 1989; Ross Russell, 1983). This syndrome is characterized by visual loss and ischemic retinal infarction often accompanied by signs of ciliary artery obstruction, pallor of the disc, and hypotony. Venous stasis retinopathy may simulate Purtscher's retinopathy (multifocal areas of ischemia) and be associated with a variety of fundus pictures (Gass, 1997a):

1. Minimal or no ophthalmoscopic changes in some patients with monocular TVL.
2. Few widely scattered blot and dot hemorrhages and mild dilation of retinal veins (venous stasis retinopathy), usually in patients with minimal visual complaints.
3. Dilation of the retinal arterial tree, dilation of the retinal veins, and cotton-wool patches.
4. Retinal capillary changes, including microaneurysms, cystoid macular edema, and angiographic evidence of areas of capillary nonperfusion that may be confined to the areas along the horizontal raphe.
5. Larger areas of peripheral capillary nonperfusion, retinal neovascularization, and hemorrhage.
6. Any degree of branch retinal vein occlusion, branch retinal vein occlusion, branch retinal artery occlusion, and central retinal artery occlusion.

7. Ischemic optic neuropathy.
8. Any of the above associated with panuveitis, neovascular glaucoma, and a rapidly progressing cataract (ocular ischemic syndrome).

The ocular ischemic syndrome (Brown, 1988; Carter, 1985; Dhooge, 1989; Gass, 1997; Higgins, 1984; Jacobs, 1985; Kearns, 1979, 1983; Kerty, 1989; Knox, 1965; Mills, 1989; Ros, 1987; Sturrock, 1984) is a progressive disorder due to hypoperfusion of eye that may be associated with TVL and ocular discomfort or frank pain localized to the orbit and upper face that is often decreased when the patient lies down. Rubeosis iridis in the eye of an older nondiabetic, with no evidence of venous obstructive disease or other predisposing cause, is suggestive of the ocular ischemic syndrome. In persons over the age of 50 with a new-onset iritis, the possibility of ocular ischemic syndrome should be considered. Although usually due to atherosclerotic carotid or ophthalmic artery disease, venous stasis retinopathy and the ocular ischemic syndrome may also occur with giant cell arteritis, carotid artery dissection, cavernous sinus thrombosis, Takayasu's disease, fibromuscular dysplasia, mucormycosis, herpes zoster ophthalmicus, myelofibrosis, and post-aneurysm repair (Borruat, 1993; Ducker, 1988; Gupta, 1990; Hamed, 1992; Lewis, 1993; McLeod, 1978; Meire, 1991; Qingli, 1989; Zimmerman, 1995).

Giant cell arteritis may produce attacks of TVL lasting minutes to hours indistinguishable from those produced by atheromatous disease (Boghen, 1975; Hollenhorst, 1960). TVL probably results from intermittent inflammatory occlusion of the ophthalmic, posterior ciliary, or central retinal arteries. A postural form of TVL has been described in patients with giant cell arteritis and a tenuous optic disc perfusion (Wykes, 1984). TVL may also occur in association with increased antiphospholipid antibodies, hyperviscosity and hypercoaguable states, polycythemia vera, systemic lupus erythematosus, and arteriovenous malformations that divert blood flow from or reduce blood flow in the ophthalmic artery (ophthalmic steal syndrome) (Bougousslavsky, 1985; Briley, 1989; Digre, 1989; Fritz, 1989; Frohman, 1989; Kosary, 1973; Levine, 1989, 1990; Mundall, 1972; Shuaib, 1989).

Vasospasm, especially associated with migraine, may also produce TVL without any of the visual phenomena typically seen during a migraine attack (Booy, 1990; Burger, 1991; Cogan, 1961; Cohen, 1984; Fisher, 1951, 1952; Kline, 1980; Marshall, 1968; O'Sullivan, 1992; Poole, 1987; Tippin, 1989; Tomsak, 1987; Winterkorn, 1993). Vasospasm of the retinal vessels has been documented by ophthalmoscopy during some attacks of monocular TVL. TVL, likely due to vasospasm and migraine, may be induced by exercise or sexual intercourse (Imes, 1989; Teman, 1995). TVL in young individuals is often benign and related to migraine. For example, Tippin, et al. reviewed the records of 83 patients who had symptoms of TVL or ocular infarction before age 45 and found that cerebral transient ischemic attacks occurred in 9 of these but no case of stroke was found (Tippin, 1989). Forty-one percent of the patients had headaches or orbital pain accompanying their TVL spells and an additional 25.3% had severe headaches independent of the visual loss. Of the original 83 patients, 42 were reexamined after a mean period of 5.8 years. None of the patients in this group had a stroke and the clinical status at follow-up did not correlate with duration of visual loss (TVL vs. ocular infarction), frequency (single vs. recurrent episodes), gender, presence of headache or heart disease, cigarette smoking, use of oral contraceptives, or abnormal findings on echocardiogram or blood studies. The authors concluded that TVL and ocular infarction occurring in the younger patient are probably associated with a more benign clinical course than that seen in older persons and that migraine is a likely cause for visual loss in a majority in this group. O'Sullivan et al. described nine young adults (median age 19.5 years) who suffered from TVL (O'Sullivan, 1992). The attacks of

TVL were short in duration and preceded by premonitory symptoms in five cases and by a migrainous headache in two. In five patients the visual loss progressed in a lacunar pattern (vision was lost in a series of blobs) unlike the "curtain" pattern characteristic of TVL in older patients. Investigation revealed no evidence of an embolic or atheromatous etiology. In two cases a minor abnormality was found on echocardiography. The authors conclude that TVL in young adults has a different clinical pattern and may have a different etiology, possibly migrainous, compared with that seen in older patients. The pattern of visual loss in some of the cases suggests that the choroidal circulation rather than the retinal circulation is primarily affected.

TVL lasting 15 to 20 minutes (occasionally up to seven hours) may occur during episodes of spontaneous anterior chamber hemorrhage (hyphema) (Kosmorsky, 1985; Miller, 1991). In these patients TVL may be associated with erythropsia (seeing red) and color desaturation. Such hemorrhages are most likely to occur in patients who have undergone cataract extraction and are particularly apt to occur after placement of an iris fixation lens implant. Other potential causes of spontaneous anterior chamber hemorrhages include vascular anomalies of the iris (e.g., in myotonic dystrophy or Sturge-Weber syndrome), microhemangiomas, diffuse hemangiomatosis of childhood, neoplasms (e.g., melanoma or retinoblastoma), diseases of blood or vessels (e.g., leukemia, hemophilia, scurvy, lymphoma), rubeosis iridis, severe iritis, fibrovascular membranes, juvenile xanthogranuloma, occult trauma or delayed bleeding after trauma, hydro-ophthalmos, malignant exophthalmos, histiocytosis X, and postsclerotomy with cautery (Kosmorsky, 1985). Intermittent angle closure glaucoma may also cause brief episodes of monocular TVL that are usually, but not always, associated with ipsilateral eye pain and occasionally simultaneous dilation of the pupil (Chandler, 1954; Miller, 1991; Ravits, 1984; Sarkies, 1985). Finally, TVL may also be associated with the congenital anomalies, peripapillary staphyloma and morning glory syndrome (Ebner, 1995; Gass, 1997; Graether, 1963; Longfellow, 1962a; Seybold, 1977; Zarnegar, 1995). Episodes of TVL with these anomalies may last 15 to 20 seconds (obscurations of vision) or up to 20 minutes, the latter mimicking TVL with thromboembolic disease. The episodes of TVL in patients with peripapillary staphyloma may be associated with intermittent dilation of the retinal veins and may be orthostatic.

Patients with monocular TVL lasting minutes associated with visible retinal emboli need to be evaluated for carotid and aortic vascular disease and cardiac valvular disease. Stroke risk factors (smoking, hypertension, diabetes mellitus, hyperlipidemia, etc.) should be evaluated and controlled. Studies to evaluate the carotid arteries include carotid Doppler and ultrasound, MR angiography, and conventional angiography. Cardiac investigations include transthoracic and trans-esophageal echocardiography and cardiac MR imaging.

Hurwitz et al. performed a prospective clinical and arteriographic study comparing patients with monocular TVL and patients with other transient hemispheral cerebral ischemic attacks (Hurwitz, 1985). In their 93 patients with monocular TVL, a potentially operable atherosclerotic carotid lesion (defined as 50% or greater stenosis or ulceration on the side of TVL) was found in 66% of the patients and the 7 year cumulative rate of cerebral infarction in these patients was 14%. In 212 patients with other hemispheral transient ischemic attacks, an operable carotid lesion was found in 51% of patients with the 7 year cumulative rate of infarction 27%. Therefore, in approximately two-thirds of patients with monocular TVL, a potentially operable carotid lesion is likely to be found.

In patients with monocular TVL and ipsilateral carotid stenosis of 70 to 99%, carotid endarterectomy is indicated if the patient is a good surgical candidate and the perioperative morbidity and mortality of the surgeon is in the 2% or less range (North American SCETC, 1991). Carotid endarterectomy in this group reduces the two year ipsilateral stroke rate from 26 to 9%, and decreases the major or fatal ipsilateral stroke rate from 13.1 to 2.5%. In the patient with less than 30 percent carotid stenosis, a cardiac or aortic embolic source should be sought and, if none is found, the treatment is aspirin plus control of stroke risk factors. In a patient with 30 to 69% stenosis, it remains to be seen whether endarterectomy would be beneficial. In patients with emboli from a cardiac valvular source, especially those with cardiac dysrhythmias such as atrial fibrillation, anticoagulation is warranted if the patient is an appropriate medical candidate.

Patients older than 55 years with a history of monocular TVL lasting minutes without visible retinal emboli should have an urgent erythrocyte sedimentation rate. If this is significantly elevated or the patient has other symptoms of giant cell arteritis, such as recent headaches, jaw claudications, or polymyalgia rheumatic-like symptoms, the patient should undergo temporal artery biopsy. If the sedimentation rate is negative and there are no clinical symptoms suggestive of giant cell arteritis, then evaluation for carotid or cardiac thromboembolic disease is warranted.

Patients with evidence of monocular TVL resulting from ocular hypoperfusion (venous stasis retinopathy and the ocular ischemic syndrome) will have decreased retinal artery pressure documented by ophthalmodynamometry. The patient should be investigated for carotid stenosis and, if this is insignificant, ophthalmic artery stenosis or occlusion is inferred. When carotid stenosis is severe, endarterectomy may be used to reestablish flow; when the internal carotid artery is totally occluded, a superficial temporal artery to middle cerebral artery bypass procedure may be considered if the external carotid is patent (Edwards, 1980; Johnston, 1988; Kearns, 1980; Kiser, 1983; Neupert, 1976; Ros, 1987; Rosenberg, 1984; Shaw, 1981). With early treatment, resolution of the hypoperfusion syndrome may occur; unfortunately, no therapy is clearly effective. Reestablishment of flow in a previously stenotic internal carotid artery may actually produce further visual difficulties by increasing perfusion to the ciliary arteries and causing dramatic increase in intraocular pressure (Bullock, 1972; Coppeto, 1985; Hart, 1971; Huckman, 1972; Rosenberg, 1984). Carotid endarterectomy or superficial temporal artery to middle cerebral artery bypass procedure have been combined with laser panretinal photocoagulation, peripheral retinal cryotherapy, or both (Carter, 1984; Johnston, 1988; Kiser, 1983; Ros, 1988). These latter procedures are thought to decrease the oxygen requirement of the eye and thus reduce the drive for neovascularization. Rarely, the ocular ischemic syndrome may be improved by the calcium channel blocker, verapamil (Winterkorn, 1995).

If no thromboembolic source for the episodes of TVL is documented, then further studies should be performed. These include MR imaging of the brain with MR angiography to investigate for possible vascular malformation, and laboratory studies, including sedimentation rate, complete blood count, antiphospholipid antibodies, antinuclear antibodies, collagen vascular disease profile, and studies to investigate the presence of dysproteinemia. Young patients ($<$ 45 years old) with monocular TVL are unlikely to have significant carotid disease. A cardiac embolic source as well as a vasculitis or coagulopathy must be sought. As noted above, monocular TVL in younger patients has a more benign clinical course than that found in an older population and migraine is a likely cause for many episodes. Calcium channel blockers (e.g., verapamil or nifedipine), if not otherwise contraindicated, may be considered in some of these patients to reduce the frequency of episodes of TVL (Teman, 1995; Winterkorn, 1993).

Finally, all patients with monocular TVL lasting minutes should have a complete ophthalmoscopic examination to investigate for such conditions as intermittent angle closure glaucoma, morning glory syndrome, and peripapillary staphyloma. Spontaneous anterior chamber hemorrhage (hyphema) should also be considered, especially in patients with associated erythropsia and in those who have undergone cataract extraction.

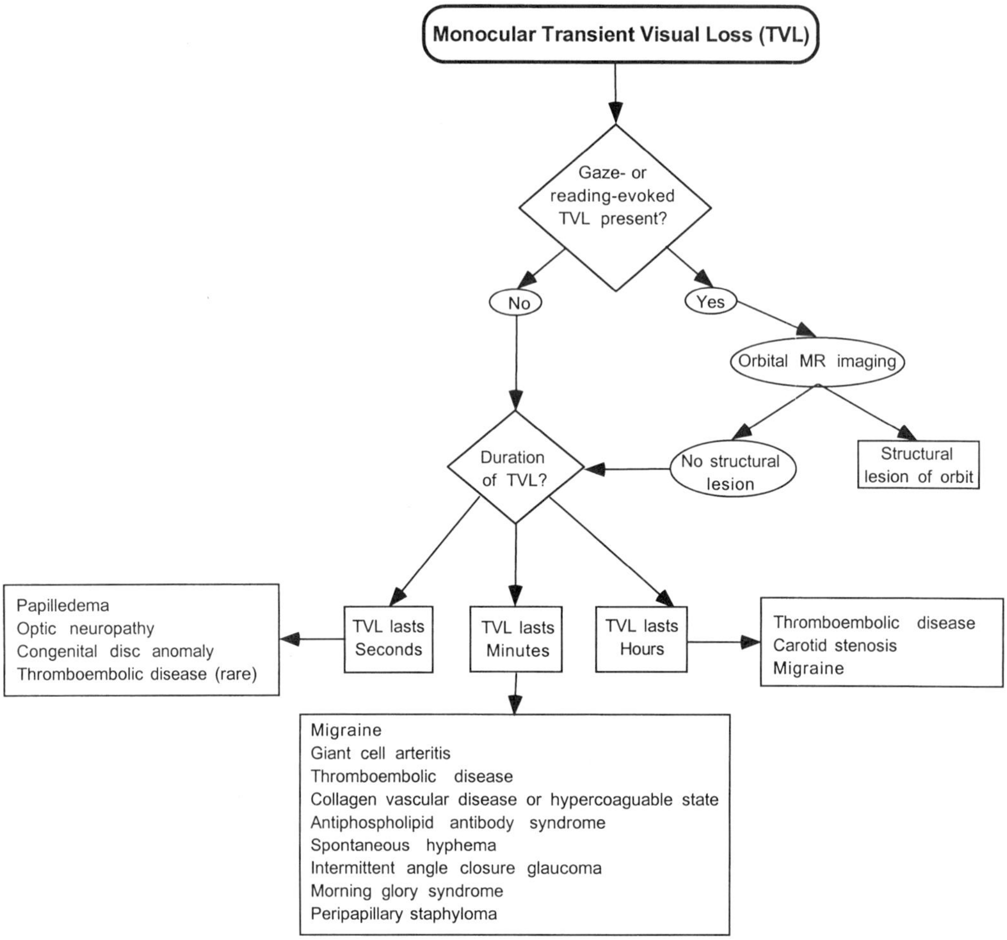

Figure 8–1. Mononuclear transient visual loss (TVL).

Episodes of monocular TVL lasting hours are rare. However, such spells may occur with thromboembolic disease, as a postprandial phenomenon associated with critical carotid stenosis, and with migraine.

An approach to the evaluation of patients with monocular TVL is presented in Figure 8–1.

Are the Episodes of TVL Binocular?

As noted above, transient visual obscurations lasting seconds may occur in one or both eyes in patients with increased intracranial pressure and papilledema. Also, patients with bilateral severe carotid occlusive disease may rarely have bilateral visual loss on exposure to bright light. Otherwise, episodes of bilateral simultaneous visual loss are usually due to migraine, bilateral occipital lobe ischemia, or other occipital lesions.

The presence of a small area of visual loss or a mild disturbance of vision that progressively increases over 15 or more minutes is highly characteristic of migraine (Russell, 1996). This visual abnormality is usually bilateral and homonymous. The patient need not have headache for this diagnosis to be made. Most patients have some abnormal positive visual symptoms associated with the episodes, most commonly fortification spectra around an area of scotoma, scintillations, or distortions within the area of visual disturbance resembling "heat waves" or "water running down a glass." The typical visual aura starts as a flickering, uncolored, zig-zag line in the center of visual field that gradually progresses and expands toward the periphery of one hemifield and often leaves a temporary scotoma. Similar abnormal visual disturbances, often associated with headache, may rarely occur with cerebral structural lesions, such as arteriovenous malformations of the occipital lobe or brain tumors, but these usually do not have the characteristic buildup and resolution of visual symptoms. Instead these lesions usually produce symptoms that steadily increase in frequency and duration until they are present daily.

Occipital lobe tumors may rarely produce scintillating scotomas that mimic migraine (Donin, 1981; Miller, 1991; Pepin, 1990; Riaz, 1991; Selhorst, 1981). In most of these cases, the tumors were diagnosed only after the patients eventually developed papilledema or when a homonymous visual field defect was documented. Riaz et al. described three patients with classical migraine for many years duration that preceded the diagnosis of meningioma (Riaz, 1991). In two patients, the tumors were occipital and in one frontotemporal. Visual symptoms in two of these patients were exceptional by their constant localization to the same hemianopic field while in the third patient they involved either hemianopic field. The visual phenomena sometimes occurred independent of headache.

Arteriovenous malformations (AVMs) of the occipital lobes may also produce visual symptoms and headache that may simulate migraine (Haas, 1991; Kattah, 1980; Kupersmith, 1996; Troost, 1975, 1979; Weiskrantz, 1974). Visual symptoms with occipital AVMs are usually brief, episodic, unformed, and not associated with the angular, scintillating figures that occur with migraine (Troost, 1975). They also tend to occur consistently in the same visual field. However, the clinical symptoms classically noted with migraine may occasionally occur with occipital AVMs. Kupersmith et al. described the clinical presentations of 70 patients with occipital AVMs (Kupersmith, 1996). At the time of presentation, headache was present in 39 (56%); the headache was throbbing in 19 cases (27%) with preceding homonymous positive visual phenomena with migraine-like features in the field contralateral to the AVM in 15 cases. A visual disturbance in the opposite field, not necessarily associated with headache, occurred in 39 patients (56%). Patients often described episodes of scintillating scotomas, jagged flickering fortification images, transient and permanent homonymous hemianopia, blurred vision in a hemifield, hemifield spots, tunnel vision, and diplopia. Three patients had transient field loss as a prodrome to grand mal seizures and two others had episodes of flickering vision associated with seizure activity on electroencephalography. Only 5 of the 23 patients with visual symptoms who had a homonymous field defect did not have recurrent headaches. Fifteen additional patients without visual symptoms, 8 of whom had no recurrent headaches, had homonymous visual field defects. The authors concluded that when either "migraine" headache or visual symptoms are restricted to one side of the head (even if the visual field exam is normal), a neuroimaging study should be performed to investigate the possibility of an occipital AVM and that migraine is a diagnosis of exclusion. Whereas some features of headache and visual symptoms are similar for occipital AVMs and migraine, the two disorders are usually distinguishable. Positive visual phenomena resembling migraine have also been described with cerebral venous sinus thrombosis (Montiero, 1984; Newman, 1989). Finally, scintillating scotomas occasionally occur in patients with systemic lupus erythematosus, but it is not clear if they are a manifestation of a cerebrovascular disorder related with lupus or simply the coexistence of two separate disease processes (Atkinson, 1975; Brandt, 1978; Friedman, 1976; Isenberg, 1982; Lessell, 1979; Miller, 1991).

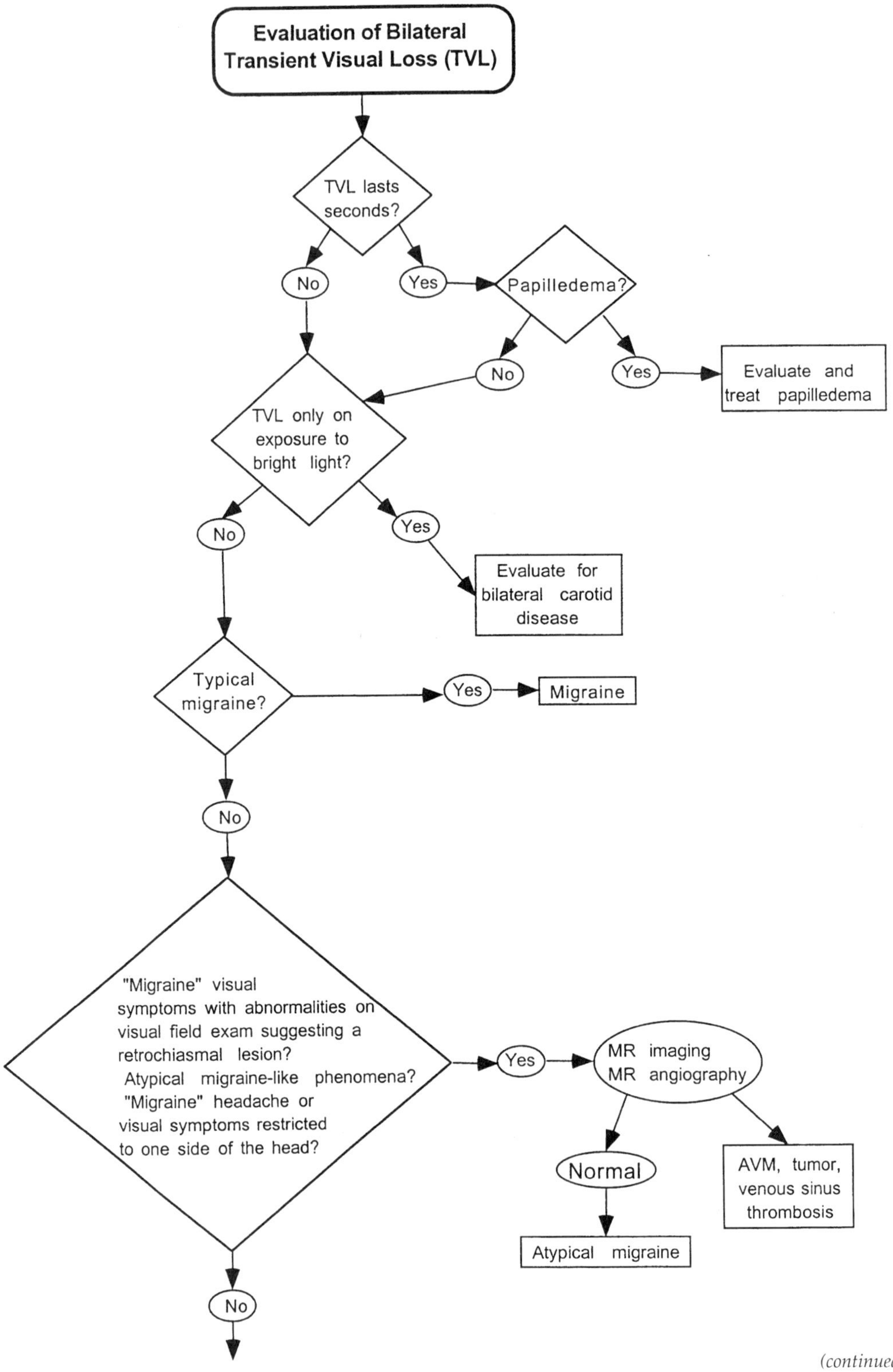

(continued)

Figure 8–2. The evaluation of bilateral transient visual loss (TVL).

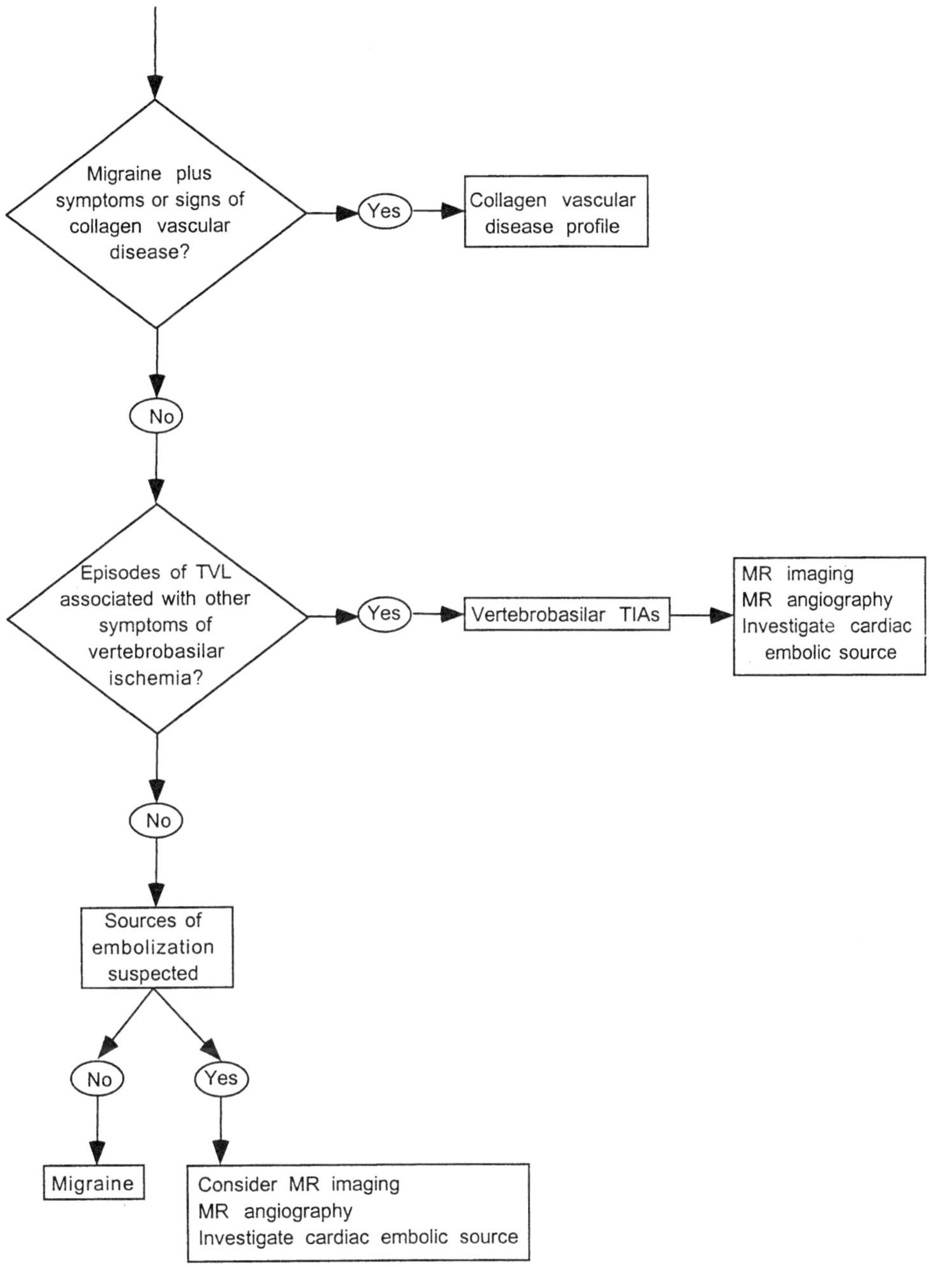

Symptoms similar to the scintillating scotomas of migraine may also occur with acute vitreous or retinal detachment (Miller, 1991f). In these patients, the visual symptoms are clearly monocular, last longer than typical migrainous visual aura, and occur without any associated headache. Scintillating scotomas, as well as monocular TVL, have also been described associated with internal carotid artery dissection (Ramadan, 1991). The first of the three patients described developed sudden severe right occipital headache followed minutes later by nausea and bright dots in both visual fields that spread centrifugally during a 10-minute period and persisted for several hours. The second perceived scintillating and nonmarching "snowflakes" in the entire visual field of the right eye that lasted 10 minutes, during which time the right eye lost vision. This was followed by right frontotemporal sharp pain that lasted for another hour. The third patient noted the abrupt onset of seeing stationary, sharp-edged gray shapes (triangles, squares, and zig-zagged lines), outlined in bright red and blue and superimposed on a glaring background. These positive visual phenomena were perceived in the left eye and lasted for three days. She later developed another episode of visual phenomena in the left eye associated with left supraorbital and temporal throbbing headache. The first patient's episode was binocular but atypical for classic migraine in that the positive visual phenomena lasted for hours; in the other two patients the symptoms were monocular and in one of these the positive symptoms lasted for days, again atypical features for classic migraine.

Binocular episodes of TVL are often due to bilateral occipital ischemia secondary to disease of the vertebrobasilar circulation (rarely bilateral retinal ischemia from systemic hypotension or bilateral carotid disease). Episodes of visual loss or blurring in patients with vertebrobasilar transient ischemic attacks (TIAs) usually occur in association with other symptoms of transient brainstem, cerebellar, or posterior cerebral ischemia, including vertigo, dysarthria, dysphagia, diplopia, weakness, sensory disturbances (especially perioral numbness), coordination difficulties, and gait instability. Visual loss or blurring of vision in these patients is bilateral and symmetric, may be hemianopic or diffuse, and usually lasts several minutes or, occasionally, less than a minute (but not seconds, as noted with obscurations of vision noted with papilledema and increased intracranial pressure). The scintillating and expanding scotomas of migraine rarely occur with vertebrobasilar TIAs, and migrainous visual phenomena usually last 20 to 30 minutes, somewhat longer than visual loss noted with vertebrobasilar TIAs. Also, Hilton-Jones et al. described a patient with a large frontal lobe tumor who experienced frequent, stereotyped episodes of bilateral, simultaneous visual loss lasting 5 to 30 minutes (Hilton-Jones, 1982). This patient did not have papilledema. Thus, intracranial mass lesions without papilledema may rarely cause episodes of transient bilateral visual loss lasting minutes.

The evaluation of patients with bilateral TVL depends on a thorough history, especially directed to the characteristics and temporal course of the episodes of TVL and any associated symptoms, and a complete neuro-ophthalmologic examination, including visual field testing. If the episodes last seconds and papilledema is present, then MR imaging is indicated. If MR imaging is negative, then a spinal tap is warranted. If episodes of bilateral visual loss occur only on exposure to bright light, then evaluation of the carotid arteries for thrombotic disease is indicated. Patients with typical expanding migraine scintillations and positive phenomena lasting 20 to 30 minutes that have been noted to occur on different sides at different times and headaches that have been documented to occur on different sides at different times usually do not require further work-up. However, any patient with abnormalities on visual field examination suggesting a retrochiasmal lesion or any patient with atypical migraine-like phenomena, especially patients with visual symptoms that are brief, episodic, unformed, and not associated with the angular, scintillating figures that occur with migraine, requires MR imaging and MR angiography to investigate the possibility of occipital AVM, venous sinus thrombosis, or tumor. When either "migraine" headache or visual symptoms are restricted to one side of the head (even if the visual field exam is normal), a neuroimaging study should be performed to investigate the possibility of an occipital AVM. Patients with migraine and symptoms or signs of collagen vascular disease require a collagen vascular disease profile.

The evaluation and treatment of patients with vertebrobasilar TIAs is controversial. MR imaging and MR angiography are usually suggested, especially to evaluate the vertebrobasilar circulation, and intra-arterial angiography may be considered. A cardiac embolic source should always be considered and, if warranted, transthoracic or trans-esophageal echocardiography may be performed. Treatment includes control of stroke risk factors and antiplatelet drugs or anticoagulation.

An approach to the evaluation of patients with bilateral TVL is presented in Figure 8–2.

References

Ashby M, Oakley N, Lorentz I, Scott D. (1963). Recurrent transient monocular blindness. *Br Med J 2:*894–897.

Atkinson RA, Appenzeller O. (1975). Headache in small vessel disease of the brain: A study of patients with systemic lupus erythematosus. *Headache 15:*198–201.

Beck RW, Corbett JJ, Thompson HS, et al. (1985). Decreased visual acuity from optic disc drusen. *Arch Ophthalmol 103:*1155–1159.

Boghen DR, Glaser JS. (1975). Ischaemic optic neuropathy. *Brain 98:*689–708.

Booy R. (1990). Amaurosis fugax in young women. (1990). *Lancet 335:*1538.

Borruat, F-X, Bogousslavsky, J, Uffer, S, et al. (1993). Orbital infarction syndrome. *Ophthalmology 100:*562–568.

Bougousslavsky J, Vinuela F, Barnet HJM, Drake CG. (1985). Amaurosis fugax as the presenting manifestation of dural arteriovenous malformation. *Stroke 16:*891–893.

Bradbury PG, Levy IS, McDonald WI. (1987). Transient uniocular visual loss on deviation of the eye in association with intraorbital tumours. *J Neurol Neurosurg Psychiatry 50:*615–619.

Brandt KD, Lessell S. (1978). Migrainous phenomena in systemic lupus erythematosus. *Arthr Rheum 21:*7–16.

Briley DP, Coull BM, Goodnight SH Jr. (1989). Neurological disease associated with antiphospholipid antibodies. *Ann Neurol 25:*221–227.

Brown G, Shields JA. (1981). Amaurosis fugax secondary to presumed cavernous hemangioma of the orbit. *Ann Ophthalmol 13:*1205–1209.

Brown GC, Magargal LE. (1988). The ocular ischemic syndrome. Clinical, fluorescein angiographic and carotid angiographic features. *Int Ophthalmol 11:*239–251.

Bruno A, Corbett JJ, Boller J, et al. (1990). Transient monocular visual loss patterns and associated vascular abnormalities. *Stroke 21:*34–39.

Bullock JD, Falter RT, Downing JE, Snyder HE. (1972). Ischemic ophthalmia secondary to an ophthalmic artery occlusion. *Am J Ophthalmol 74:*486–493.

Burger, SK, Saul RF, Selhorst, JB, Thurston SE. (1991). Transient monocular blindness caused by vasospasm. *New Eng J Med 325:*870–873.

Carter JE. (1985). Chronic ocular ischemia and carotid vascular disease. *Stroke 16:*721–728.

Carter JE. (1984). Panretinal photocoagulation for progressive ocular neovascularization secondary to occlusion of the common carotid artery. *Ann Ophthalmol 16:*572–576.

Chandler PA, Trotter RT. (1954). Angle-closure glaucoma: Subacute types. *Trans Am Ophthalmol Soc 52:*265–290.

Cogan DG. (1961). Blackouts not obviously due to carotid occlusion. *Arch Ophthalmol 66:*180–187.

Cohen GR, Harbison JW, Blair CJ, Ochs AL. (1984). Clinical significance of transient visual phenomena in the elderly. *Ophthalmology 91:*436–442.

Coppeto JR, Wand M, Bear L, Sciarra R. (1985). Neovascular glaucoma and carotid artery obstructive disease. *Am J Ophthalmol 99:*567–570.

Dhooge M, De Laey JJ. (1989). The ocular ischemic syndrome. *Bull Soc Belge Ophthalmol 231:*1–13.

Digre KB, Durcan FJ, Branch DW, et al. (1989). Amaurosis fugax associated with antiphospholipid antibodies. *Ann Neurol 25:*228–232.

Donin JF, Keane JR. (1981). Migraine, pseudotumor cerebri, blindness and death. Presented at the 13th Annual Frank B Walsh Society Meeting, Houston, February 27–28.

Donnan GA, Sharbrough FW, Whisnant JP. (1982). Carotid occlusive disease. Effect of bright light on visual evoked response. *Arch Neurol 39:*687–689.

Ducker JS, Belmont JB. (1988). Ocular ischemic syndrome secondary to carotid artery dissection. *Am J Ophthalmol 106:*750–752.

Ebner R. (1995). Morning glory syndrome, amaurosis fugax, and cortical laser tomography. Presented at the North American Neuro-Ophthalmology Society Annual Meeting, Tucson, AZ.

Edwards MS, Chater NL, Stanley JA. (1980). Reversal of chronic ocular ischaemia by extracranial-intracranial bypass. Case report. *Neurosurgery 7:*480–483.

Ehrenfield WK, Hoyt WF, Wylie EJ. (1966). Embolization and transient blindness from carotid atheroma. *Arch Surg 93:*787–794.

Fisher CM. (1952). Transient monocular blindness associated with hemiplegia. *Arch Ophthalmol 47:*167–203.

Fisher CM. (1951). Transient monocular blindness associated with hemiplegia. *Trans Am Neurol Assoc 47:*154–157.

Friedman AP. (1976). Headache. *Clin Neurol 2:*1–28.

Fritz VU, Klein H-J, Schmidt K. (1989). Arteriovenous malformation of the posterior ethmoidal artery as an unusual case of amaurosis fugax. The ophthalmic steal syndrome. *J Clin Neuro-ophthalmol 9:*165–168.

Frohman LP, Rescigno R, Bielory L. (1989). Neuro-ophthalmologic manifestations of the antiphospholipid antibody syndrome. *Ophthalmology 96 (Suppl):*105.

Fujino T, Akiya S, Takagi S, Shiga H. (1983). Amaurosis fugax for a long duration. *J Clin Neuro-ophthalmology 3:*9–12.

Furlan AJ, Whisnant JP, Kearns TP. (1979). Unilateral visual loss in bright light. An unusual symptom of carotid artery occlusive disease. *Arch Neurol 36:*675–676.

Gass JDM. (1997a). *Stereoscopic Atlas of Macular Disease. Diagnosis and Treatment.* 4th edition. St. Louis, Mosby, pp. 464–466.

Gass JDM. (1997b). *Stereoscopic Atlas of Macular Disease. Diagnosis and Treatment.* 4th edition. St. Louis, Mosby, pp. 984–985.

Goodwin JA, Gorelick P, Helgason C. (1984). Transient monocular visual loss: Amaurosis fugax versus migraine. *Neurology 34 (Suppl 1):*46.

Goodwin JA, Gorelick P, Helgason CM. (1987). Symptoms of amaurosis fugax in atherosclerotic carotid artery disease. *Neurology 37:*829–832.

Graether JM. (1963). Transient amaurosis in one eye with simultaneous dilation of retinal veins; in association with a congenital anomaly of the optic nerve head. *Arch Ophthalmol 70:*34–35.

Gupta A, Jalali S, Bansal RK, Grewal SPS. (1990). Anterior ischemic optic neuropathy and branch retinal artery occlusion in cavernous sinus thrombosis. *J Clin Neuro-ophthalmol 10:*193–196.

Haas DC. (1991). Arteriovenous malformations and migraine: Case reports and analysis of the relationship. *Headache 31:*509–513.

Hamed LM, Guy JR, Moster ML, Bosley T. (1992). Giant cell arteritis in the ocular ischemic syndrome. *Am J Ophthalmol 113:*702–705.

Hampton GR, Krohel GB. (1983). Gaze-evoked blindness. *Ann Ophthalmol 15:*73–76.

Hart RG, Haworth S. (1971). Bilateral common carotid occlusion with hypoxic ocular sequelae. *Br J Ophthalmol 55:*383–388.

Hedges TR. (1962). Ophthalmoscopic findings in internal carotid occlusion. *Bull Johns Hopkins Hosp 3:*89–97.

Higgins RA. (1984). Neovascular glaucoma associated with ocular hypoperfusion secondary to carotid artery disease. *Aust J Ophthalmol 12:*155–162.

Hilton-Jones D, Ponsford JR, Graham N. (1982). Transient visual obscurations, without papilloedema. *J Neurol Neurosurg Psychiatry 45:*832–834.

Hollenhorst RW, Brown JR, Wagener HP, Shick RM. (1960). Neurologic aspects of temporal arteritis. *Neurology 10:*490–498.

Huckman MS, Haas J. (1972). Reversed flow through the ophthalmic artery as a cause of rubeosis iridis. *Am J Ophthalmol 74:*1094–1099.

Hurwitz BJ, Heyman A, Wilkinson WE, et al. (1985). Comparison of amaurosis fugax and transient cerebral ischemia. A prospective clinical, arteriographic study. *Ann Neuol 18:*698–704.

Imes RK, Hoyt WF. (1989). Exercise-induced transient visual events in young healthy adults. *J Clin Neuro-ophthalmol 9:*178–180.

Isenberg DA, Meyrick-Thomas D, Snaith ML, et al. (1982). A study of migraine in systemic lupus erythematosus. *Ann Rheum Dis 41:*30–32.

Jacobs NA, Ridgeway AEA. (1985). Syndrome of ischaemic ocular inflammation: Six cases and a review. *Br J Ophthalmol 69:*681–687.

Johnston ME, Gonder JR, Canny CLB. (1988). Successful treatment of the ocular ischemic syndrome with panretinal photocoagulation and cerebrovascular surgery. *Can J Ophthalmol 23:*114–119.

Kahn M, Green WR, Knox DL, Miller NR. (1986). Ocular features of carotid occlusive disease. *Retina 6:*239–252.

Kattah JC, Luessenhop AJ. (1980). Resolution of classic migraine after removal of an occipital lobe AVM. *Ann Neurol 7:*93.

Kearns JR. (1983). Differential diagnosis of central retinal artery vein obstruction. *Ophthalmology 90:*475–480.

Kearns JR. (1979). Ophthalmology and the carotid artery. *Am J Ophthalmol 88:*714–722.

Kearns TP, Hollenhorst RW. (1963). Venous-stasis retinopathy of occlusive disease of the carotid. *Mayo Clin Proc 38:*304–312.

Kearns TP, Younge BR, Piepgras DG. (1980). Resolution of venous stasis retinopathy after carotid artery bypass. *Mayo Clin Proc 55:*342–346.

Kerty E, Eide N. (1989). Chronic ocular ischemia. *Acta Ophthalmologica 67:*386–392.

Kiser WD, Gonder J, Magargal LE, et al. (1983). Recovery of vision following treatment of the ocular ischemic syndrome. *Ann Opththalmol 15:*305–310.

Kline LB, Kelly CL. (1980). Ocular migraine in a patient with cluster headache. *Headache 20:*253–257.

Knapp ME, Flaharty PM, Sergott RC, et al. (1992). Gaze-induced amaurosis from central retinal artery compression. *Ophthalmology* 238–240.

Knox DL. (1965). Ischemic ocular inflammation. *Am J Ophthalmol 60:*995–1002.

Kohmoto H, Oohira A. (1993). Gaze-evoked scotomata in metastatic orbital tumor. *Neuro-ophthalmology 13:*223–226.

Kosary IZ, Treister G, Tadmor R. (1973). Transient monocular amaurosis due to a contralateral cerebrovascular malformation. *Neurochirurgia 16*:127–130.
Kosmorsky GS, Rosenfeld SI, Burde, RM. (1985). Transient monocular obscuration—? Amaurosis fugax: A case report. *Br J Ophthalmol 69*:688–690.
Kupersmith MJ, Vargas ME, Yashar A, et al. (1996). Occipital arteriovenous malformations: Visual disturbances and presentation. *Neurology 46*:953–957.
Lessell S. (1979). The neuro-ophthalmology of systemic lupus erythematosus. *Doc Ophthalmol 47*:13–42.
Levin LA, Mootha VV. (1997). Postprandial transient visual loss. A symptom of critical carotid stenosis. *Ophthalmology 104*:297–401.
Levine SR, Deegan MJ, Futrell N, Welch KMA. (1990). Cerebrovascular and neurologic disease associated with antiphospholipid antibodies. 48 cases. *Neurology 40*:1181–1189.
Levine SR, Welch KMA. (1989). Antiphospholipid antibodies. *Ann Neurol 26*:386–389.
Levy IS, McDonald WI, Bradbury PG. (1986). Gaze evoked amaurosis. Proceeding of the 6th Meeting of the International Neuro-Ophthalmology Society, Hakone, Japan, June 9–14. *Neuro-ophthalmol Jpn 3*:402.
Lewis JR, Glaser JS, Schatz NJ, Hutson DG. (1993). Pulseless (Takayasu) disease with ophthalmic manifestations. *J Clin Neuro-ophthalmol 13*:242–249.
Longfellow DW, Davis FS Jr, Walsh FB. (1962a). Unilateral intermittent blindness with dilation of retinal veins; undetermined etiology. *Arch Ophthalmol 67*:554–555.
Longfellow DW, Davis FS, Walsh FB. (1962b). Unilateral intermittent blindness and dilation of retinal veins. *Arch Ophthalmol 67*:554–555.
Lorentzen SE. (1966). Drusen of the optic disk: A clinical and genetic study. *Acta Ophthalmol Suppl 90*:9–180.
McCrary JA III. (1989). Venous stasis retinopathy of stenotic or occlusive carotid origin. *J Clin Neuro-ophthalmol 9*:195–199.
McLeod D, Oji EO, Kohner EM, Marshall J. (1978). Fundus signs in temporal arteritis. *Br J Ophthalmol 62*:591–594.
Manor RS, Yassur Y, Hoyt WF. (1996). Reading-induced visual dimming. *Am J Ophthalmol 121*:212–213.
Marshall J, Meadows S. (1968). The natural history of amaurosis fugax. *Brain 91*:419–434.
Meire FM, De Laey JJ, van Thienen MN, Schuddinck L. (1991). Retinal manifestations in fibromuscular dysplasia. *Eur J Ophthalmol 1*:63–68.
Miller NR. (1988). *Walsh and Hoyt's Clinical Neuro-ophthalmology*. 4th edition. Baltimore, Williams and Wilkins, p. 1143.
Miller NR. (1991a). *Walsh and Hoyt's Clinical Neuro-ophthalmology*. 4th edition. Baltimore, Williams and Wilkins, pp. 2300–2307.
Miller NR. (1991b). *Walsh and Hoyt's Clinical Neuro-ophthalmology*. 4th edition. Baltimore, Williams and Wilkins, pp. 2305–2306.
Miller NR. (1991c). *Walsh and Hoyt's Clinical Neuro-ophthalmology*. 4th edition. Baltimore, Williams and Wilkins, p. 2304.
Miller NR. (1991d). *Walsh and Hoyt's Clinical Neuro-ophthalmology*. 4th edition. Baltimore, Williams and Wilkins, p. 2527.
Miller NR. (1991e). *Walsh and Hoyt's Clinical Neuro-ophthalmology*. 4th edition. Baltimore, Williams and Wilkins., p. 2528.
Miller NR. (1991f). *Walsh and Hoyt's Clinical Neuro-ophthalmology*. 4th edition. Baltimore, Williams and Wilkins, pp. 2526–2527.
Mills RP. (1989). Anterior segment ischemia secondary to carotid occlusive disease. *J Clin Neuro-ophthalmol 9*:200–204.
Montiero LR, Hoyt WF, Imes RK. (1984). Puerperal cerebral blindness. *Arch Neurol 41*:1300–1301.
Mundall J, Quintero P, von Kaulla K, et al. (1972). Transient monocular blindness and increased platelet aggregability treated with aspirin. A case report. *Neurology 22*:280–285.
Neupert JR, Brubaker RF, Kearns TP, Sundt TM Jr. (1976). Rapid resolution of venous stasis retinopathy after carotid endarterectomy. *Am J Ophthalmol 81*:600–602.
Newman DS, Levine SR, Curtis VL, Welch KMA. (1989). Migraine-like visual phenomena associated with cerebral venous thrombosis. *Headache 29*:82–85.
North American Symptomatic Carotid Endarterectomy Trial Collaborators. (1991). Beneficial effects of carotid endarterectomy in symptomatic patients with high-grade carotid stenosis. *New Eng J Med 325*:445–453.
Orcutt JC, Tucker WM, Mills RP, Smith CH. (1987). Gaze-evoked amaurosis. *Ophthalmology 94*:213–218.
Orcutt JC, Tucker WM, Smith CH, Mills RP. (1986). Gaze-evoked amaurosis, Proceedings of the 6th Meeting of the International Neuro-Ophthalmology Society, Hakone, Japan, June 9–14, 1986. *Neuro-ophthalmol Jpn 3*:401.
O'Sullivan E, Shaunak S, Matthews, T, et al. (1995). Transient monocular blindness. *J. Neurol Neurosurg Psych 59*:559.
O'Sullivan F, Rossor M, Elston JS. (1992). Amaurosis fugax in young people. *Br J Ophthalmol 76*:660–662.
Pascual J, Combarros O, Berciano J. (1988). Gaze-evoked amaurosis in pseudotumor cerebri. *Neurology 38*:1654–1655.
Pepin EP. (1990). Cerebral metastasis presenting as migraine with aura. *Lancet 336*:127-128.
Pessin MS, Duncan GD, Mohr JP, Poskanzer DC. (1977). Clinical and angiographic features of carotid transient ischemic attacks. *New Eng J Med 296*:358–362.

Poole CJM, Ross Russell RW, Harrison P, Savidge GF. (1987). Amaurosis fugax under the age of 40 years. *J Neurol Neurosurg Psychiatry 50:*81–84.

Qingli L, Orcutt JC, Seifter LS. (1989). Orbital mucormycosis with retinal and ciliary artery occlusions. *Br J Ophthalmol 73:*680–683.

Ramadan NM, Tietjen GE, Levine SR, Welch KMA. (1991). Scintillating scotomata associated with internal carotid artery dissection. Report of three cases. *Neurology 41:*1084–1087.

Ravits J, Seybold ME. (1984). Transient monocular visual loss from narrow-angle glaucoma. *Arch Neurol 41:*991–993.

Riaz G, Selhorst JB, Hennessey, JJ. (1991). Meningeal lesions mimicking migraine. *Neuro-ophthalmol. 11:*41–48.

Ros MA, Magargal LE, Hedges TR Jr, Simeone FA. (1987). Ocular ischemic syndrome: Long-term ocular complications. *Ann Ophthalmol 19:*270–272.

Rosenberg PR, Walsh JB, Zimmerman RD. (1984). Neovascular glaucoma and carotid bruits. *J Clin Neuro-ophthalmol 4:*59–67.

Ross Russell RW, Page NGR. (1983). Critical perfusion of brain and retina. *Brain 106:*4119–4434.

Russell MB, Olesen J. (1996). A nosographic analysis of the migraine aura in a general population. *Brain 119:*355–361.

Sarkies NJC, Sanders MD, Gautier-Smith PC. (1985). Episodic unilateral mydriasis and migraine. *Am J Ophthalmol 99:*217–218.

Selhorst JB, Slatkin N, Waybright EA, Saul RF. (1981). Thirty years of visual migraine. Presented at the 13th Annual Frank B Walsh Society Meeting, Houston, February 27–28.

Seybold ME, Rosen PN (1977). Peripapillary staphyloma and amaurosis fugax. *Ann Ophthalmol 9:*1139–1141.

Shaw HE Jr, Holmes MW, Fleisher AS. (1981). Regression of ischemic oculopathy after carotid artery bypass surgery. In Smith JL (ed). *Neuro-ophthalmology Focus.* New York, Masson, pp 171–175.

Shuaib A, Barcley LL. (1989). Migraine-stroke and antiphospholipid antibody. *Ann Neurol 26:*131.

Sibony PA, Krauss HR, Kennerdell JS, et al. (1984). Optic nerve sheath meningiomas. Clinical manifestations. *Ophthalmology 91:*1313–1316.

Sturrock GD, Mueller HR. Chronic ocular ischemia. (1984). *Br J Ophthalmol 68:*716–723.

Teman AJ, Winterkorn JMS, Weiner D. (1995). Transient monocular blindness associated with sexual intercourse. *New Eng J Med 333:*393.

Tippin J, Corbett JJ, Kerber RE, et al. (1989). Amaurosis fugax and ocular infarction in adolescents and young adults. *Ann Neurol 26:*69–77.

Tomsak RL, Jergens PB. (1987). Benign recurrent transient monocular blindness: A possible variant of acephalgic migraine. *Headache 27:*66–69.

Troost BT, Newton TH. (1975). Occipital lobe arteriovenous malformations. Clinical and radiologic features in 26 cases with comment on the differentiation from migraine. *Arch Ophthalmol 93:*250–256.

Troost BT, Mark LE, Maroon JC. (1979). Resolution of classic migraine after removal of an occipital lobe AVM. *Ann Neurol 5:*199–201.

Unsöld R, Hoyt WF. (1979). Blickinduzierte monokulare Obskurationen bei orbitalem Haemangiom. *Klin Monatsbl Augenheilkd 174:*715–721.

Venables GS, Bates D, Cartlidge NEF, Shaw DA. (1984). Prognosis in amaurosis fugax. *J Neurol Neurosurg Psychiatry 47:*1054.

Wall M, George D. (1991). Idiopathic intracranial hypertension: A prospective study of 50 patients. *Brain 114:*155–180.

Weiskrantz L, Warrington EK, Sanders MD, Marshall J. (1974). Visual capacity in the hemianopic field following a restricted occipital ablation. *Brain 97:*709–728.

Wiebers DO, Swanson JW, Cascino TL, Whisnant JP. (1989). Bilateral loss of vision in bright light. *Stroke 20:*554–558.

Wilkes SR, Trautmann JC, De Santo LW, Campbell RJ. (1979). Osteoma: An unusual cause of amaurosis fugax. *Mayo Clin Proc 54:*258–260.

Winterkorn JMS, Beckman RL. (1995). Recovery from ocular ischemic syndrome after treatment with verapamil. *J Neuro-ophthalmol 15:*209–211.

Winterkorn JMS, Kupersmith, MJ, Wirtschafter, JD, Forman, S. (1993). Brief report: Treatment of vasospastic amaurosis fugax with calcium-channel blockers. *New Eng J Med 329:*396–398.

Wright JE. (1977). Primary optic nerve meningiomas: Clinical presentation and management. *Trans Am Acad Ophthalmol Otolaryngol 83:*617–625.

Wykes WN, Adams GGW, Cullen JF. (1984). Temporal arteritis: Visual loss associated with posture. *Neuroophthalmology 4:*107–109.

Zarnegar, SR, Chung, S, Selhorst, JB. (1995). An unusual cause of amaurosis fugax. Presented at the North American Neuro-Ophthalmology Annual Meeting, Tucson, AZ.

Zimmerman CF, Van Patten PD, Golnik KC, et al. (1995). Orbital infarction syndrome after surgery for intracranial aneurysms. *Ophthalmology 102:*594–598.

◆ 9 ◆

Visual Field Defects

What Is the Topographical Diagnosis of Visual Field Defects?

The localization of visual field defects is outlined in Figure 9–1.

Is the Visual Field Defect Unilateral?

Lesions affecting the retina, nerve fiber layer, or optic nerve produce visual field defects in the ipsilateral eye that correspond in position, shape, extent, and intensity to the lesion. The lesion may be inflammatory, ischemic, degenerative, or neoplastic. Since the nerve fiber layer arising from the peripheral retina arches over the fovea, superior or inferior nerve fiber layer damage results in arcuate shaped visual field defects. Rarely, patients with a lesion of the anterior occipital lobe may have a unilateral, contralateral visual field defect.

Is a Retinal Lesion Responsible for the Visual Field Defect?

Almost all retinal lesions resulting in visual field loss are visible ophthalmoscopically. Careful attention should be directed to the retina and retinal nerve fiber layer corresponding to the visual field defect. Patients with macular disease also may complain of metamorphopsia, micropsia, and positive photopsias (e.g., flashing lights) that are unusual in patients with optic neuropathies. Easily visible retinal lesions are not discussed in detail. Table 9–1 lists some common retinal disorders that may be difficult to visualize without careful attention to the macula with high magnification and stereoscopic viewing.

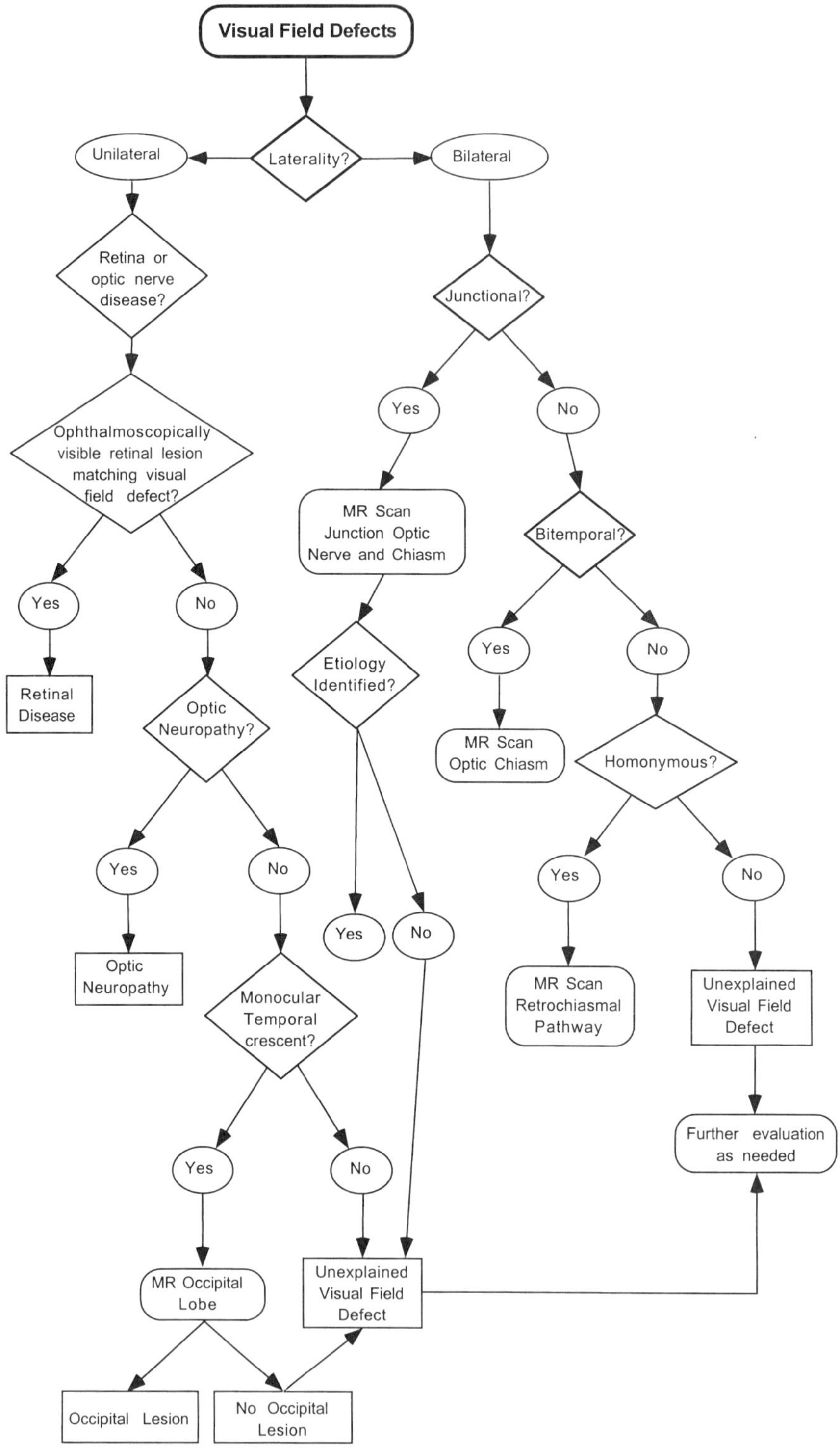

Figure 9–1. Visual field defects.

Table 9–1. Subtle Retinal Diseases That May Cause Visual Field Loss

Cystoid macular edema
Epiretinal membrane
Outer retinal inflammatory diseases
Multiple evanescent white dot syndrome
Acute macular neuroretinitis
Acute retinal pigment epitheliitis
Acute multifocal placoid pigment epitheliopathy
Acute zonal occult outer retinopathy
Serous detachment of the macula
Cone-rod dystrophy
Retinitis pigmentosa sine pigmento
Cancer associated retinopathy
Melanoma associated retinopathy

Is There Evidence for an Optic Neuropathy?

Central visual field defects (unilateral or bilateral) are the result of damage to the papillomacular bundle or optic nerve. Any visual field defect produced by a retinal lesion may be produced by a lesion of the optic nerve (Miller, 1982) and virtually any etiology may be responsible (e.g., glaucomatous, degenerative, ischemic, traumatic, inflammatory, infiltrative, compressive, vascular optic neuropathy). Patients with a unilateral visual field defect and evidence for an optic neuropathy should undergo evaluation for an optic neuropathy (see Chapter 1). Patients with a unilateral hemianopic visual field defect (junctional scotoma of Traquair) may harbor a lesion of the optic nerve at the junction of the optic nerve and chiasm.

Is This the Monocular Temporal Crescent?

Although monocular peripheral temporal visual field defects are most often the result of retinal or optic nerve disease, a lesion of the peripheral nasal fibers in the anterior occipital lobe may also produce a unilateral (monocular) temporal crescent-shaped visual field defect from 60 to 90°. Although retrochiasmal lesions in the visual pathway usually result in homonymous visual field loss, the monocular temporal crescent is the one exception. Homonymous visual field loss with sparing of this temporal crescent or selective involvement of this area localizes the lesion to the occipital lobe and neuroimaging should be directed to the contralateral calcarine cortex (Benton, 1980; Landau, 1995; Meienberg, 1981; Walsh, 1974).

Is the Visual Field Defect Bilateral?

Bilateral lesions of the retina or optic nerve may result in bilateral visual field defects. In the absence of evidence for bilateral retinal disease or bilateral optic neuropathy, bilateral visual field loss results from disease affecting the optic chiasm or retrochiasmal pathways.

Is the Visual Field Defect Junctional in Nature?

Nerve fibers originating in the retina follow a specific topographical arrangement in the optic nerve and chiasm. Compressive lesions at the junction of the intracranial optic nerve and optic chiasm may produce characteristic visual field defects. Optic nerve involvement at the junction of the optic chiasm results in unilateral visual field loss (optic neuropathy). If fibers from the inferonasal retina of the contralateral eye (Wilbrand's knee) are involved, there will also be a superotemporal visual field defect in the contralateral eye (Hoyt, 1969).

The intracranial optic nerves extend posteriorly from the optic foramen and join at the optic chiasm. Within the chiasm, fibers from the nasal retina of each eye cross into the contralateral optic tract, and fibers from the temporal retina pass uncrossed into the ipsilateral optic tract. Within the intracranial optic nerve, the crossed (nasal retinal) and uncrossed (temporal retinal) fibers are anatomically separated at the junction of the optic nerve and chiasm. In addition, inferior nasal crossing fibers may loop anteriorly for a short distance into the contralateral optic nerve. These fibers are often referred to as the anterior knee or Wilbrand's knee.

Lesions at the junction of the optic nerve and chiasm may produce specific types of visual field defects that allow topographical localization. Selective compression of the crossed or uncrossed visual fibers at the junction may result in a unilateral temporal or nasal hemianopic field defect, respectively. In addition, involvement of the inferonasal fibers of the anterior knee (Wilbrand's knee) results in a superotemporal visual field defect contralateral to the lesion.

In 1927, H. M. Traquair used the term "junction scotoma" to refer to a unilateral temporal hemicentral field defect due to compression of the nasal fibers crossing in the intracranial optic nerve at the junction of the optic nerve and chiasm (Scott, 1957). Miller emphasized that the junctional scotoma described by Traquair refers to a strictly unilateral temporal scotoma that is assumed to arise from a lesion at the junction of the optic nerve and chiasm (Miller, 1982). Unfortunately, some confusion has arisen regarding the use of the term junctional scotoma. As opposed to the defect described by Traquair, some authors have used the term to refer to an ipsilateral optic neuropathy with a contralateral superotemporal visual field defect. This superotemporal defect is caused by compression of the inferonasal fibers from the contralateral eye travelling in Wilbrand's knee.

To clarify this distinction, Miller, citing Dr. J. Lawton Smith, recommended that the unilateral temporal visual field defect described by Traquair should be referred to as the "junctional scotoma of Traquair" to differentiate it from the contralateral superotemporal defect more commonly referred to as the "junctional scotoma" (Miller, 1982).

Recently, the existence of Wilbrand's knee has come into question. Wilbrand was restricted to examining human subjects who had undergone enucleation. In the enucleated eye, the nerve fibers atrophied and became distinct from the nerve fibers of the normal eye as seen on myelin staining. Horton (Horton JC, unpublished data presented at the North American Neuro-Ophthalmology Society meeting, February 1995) utilizing axon labeling techniques in non-enucleated monkeys was unable to demonstrate crossing fibers looping into the contralateral optic nerve (Wilbrand's knee). In one monkey that had undergone enucleation four years previously, however, nerve fiber topography similar to that described by Wilbrand was found. Horton hypothesized that Wilbrand's knee may be an artifact of enucleation caused by atrophy of the optic nerve and not a normal anatomic finding. Nevertheless, whether Wilbrand's knee exists anatomically, the localizing value of junctional visual field loss to the junction of the optic nerve and chiasm remains undiminished since chiasmal compression alone may result in the contralateral superotemporal visual field defect (junctional scotoma).

Trobe and Glaser felt that junctional visual field loss would be due to a mass lesion in 98 out of 100 cases (Trobe, 1983). The differential diagnosis of a junctional syndrome includes pituitary tumors, suprasellar meningiomas, supraclinoid aneurysms, craniopharyngiomas, and gliomas (Cullen, 1966; Farris, 1986; Hershenfeld, 1993; Trobe, 1984). Chiasmal neuritis, pachymeningitis and trauma are rare etiologies of the junctional syndrome (Reynolds, 1982; Weinstein, 1987).

Patients with the junctional scotoma of Traquair or the junctional scotoma should be considered to have a compressive lesion at the junction of the optic nerve and chiasm until proven otherwise. Neuroimaging studies (preferably magnetic resonance [MR] imaging) should be directed to this location. Patients with junctional scotoma may be unaware of a small superotemporal visual field defect, and patients presenting with strictly unilateral visual complaints may be misdiagnosed as having an optic neuritis or other unilateral optic neuropathy. Therefore, in any patient with presumed unilateral visual loss, careful visual field testing should be performed in the contralateral asymptomatic eye.

Is a Bitemporal Hemianopsia Present?

Bitemporal hemianopsia may be peripheral, paracentral, or central. The visual field defect may "split" or "spare" the macular central field. The bitemporal defect usually is the result of a compressive mass lesion at the level of the optic chiasm (Miller, 1982; Wybar, 1977). Table 9–2 and Table 9–3 list the possible etiologies of a chiasmal lesion. Neuroimaging (preferably MR imaging) should be directed at the optic chiasm.

Table 9–2. Compressive Chiasmal Syndromes

Most common
- Pituitary apoplexy
- Pituitary tumor (especially pituitary adenoma) (Elkington, 1968; Falconer, 1975; Ikeda, 1995; Kirkham, 1972; Moster, 1986; Peter, 1995; Petruson, 1995; Trobe, 1984; Wilson, 1968)
- Meningioma (Ehlers, 1973; Gregorius, 1975; Kinjo, 1995; Rosenberg, 1984)
- Craniopharyngioma (Bartlett, 1971; Crane, 1982; Mikelberg, 1993)
- Dysgerminoma (Camins, 1974; Isayama, 1980; Kageyama, 1971)
- Suprasellar aneurysm (Berson, 1966; Bird, 1970; Cullen, 1966; Farris, 1986; Krauss, 1982; Norwood, 1986; Rush, 1981)
- Chiasmal glioma (Glaser, 1971; Horwich, 1985; McFadzean, 1983; Rossi, 1994)

Less common
- Abscess (Domingue, 1977; Nelson, 1983)
- Arachnoid cyst (Meyer, 1987; Muraji, 1979; Segall, 1974)
- Aspergillosis (Fuchs, 1985; Larranga, 1989)
- Cavernous hemangioma (Castel, 1989; Corboy, 1989; Hwang, 1993; Manz, 1979; Mohr, 1985; Regli, 1989)
- Chiasmal hematoma (Crowe, 1989; Maitland, 1982; Riishede, 1974)
- Chordoma (Takahashi, 1983; Neetens, 1980)
- Choristomas
- Colloid cyst of the third ventricle
- Dermoid

(continued)

Table 9–2. *(continued)*

Dolichoectatic sclerotic internal carotid arteries (Hilton, 1966; Matsuo, 1980; Slavin, 1990)
Ependymoma (O'Connor, 1979)
Epidermoid
Fibrous dysplasia
Granular cell myoblastoma (Waller, 1972)
Ganglioglioma (Liu, 1996)
Hemangioblastoma (Sawin, 1996)
Histiocytosis X (Smolik, 1968; Goodman, 1979)
Hydrocephalus and distention of the third ventricle
Leukemia and lymphoma (Cantore, 1989; Howard, 1987; McFadzean, 1990)
Lymphocytic hypophysitis (Hungerford, 1982; Stelmach, 1991)
Lymphohistiocytosis (Galetta, 1991)
Melanoma (Aubin, 1997)
Meningeal carcinomatosis
Metastatic disease (Cohen, 1979) to brain or pituitary gland (Buonaguidi, 1983; Duvall, 1982; Leramo, 1981; Max, 1981; Neetens, 1982)
Mucocoele or mucopyocoele (Abla, 1986)
  Intrasellar
  Sphenoid sinus (Goodwin, 1978)
Multiple myeloma (Poon, 1979)
Nasopharyngeal cancer
Non-neoplastic pituitary gland enlargement (Elias, 1987; Yamamoto, 1983)
Plasmacytoma (Poon, 1974)
Rathke cleft cyst (Fischer, 1994; Iraci, 1979; Rao, 1995; Voelker, 1991; Yamamoto, 1993)
Sarcoid granuloma (Godleski, 1984; Tang, 1983; Walsh, 1968)
Septum pellucidum cyst (Kansu, 1980)
Sinus tumors
Syphilitic granuloma
Teratoma (Camins, 1974)
Vascular malformation (Carter, 1982; Hankey, 1987; Lavin, 1984)
Venous angioma (Fermaglich, 1978)

Table 9-3. Other Causes of Chiasmal Syndrome

Cobalamin deficiency (Wilhelm, 1993)
Demyelinating disease (Edwards, 1983; Reynolds, 1982; Sacks, 1975; Spector, 1977, 1980; Wilhelm, 1993)
Empty sella syndrome (primary or secondary) (Berke, 1975; Kansu, 1980; Kaufman, 1989; Kosmorsky, 1997; McFadzean, 1983; Neelon, 1973; Randall, 1984)
Chiasmal ischemia (Ahmadi, 1984; Lee, 1975, 1983)
Optochiasmatic arachnoiditis (Coyle, 1969; Iraci, 1977, 1979)
  Foreign body-induced granuloma (e.g., muslin)
  Idiopathic
  Infection (Krohel, 1981)
    Chronic fungal infection
    Cryptococcus (Takahashi, 1980)
    Encephalitis
    Meningitis

Nasopharyngeal and sinus infections
Syphilis (Oliver, 1968)
Tuberculosis (Navarro, 1981; Scott, 1977)
Inflammatory (Krohel, 1981)
Collagen vascular disease
Rheumatoid pachymeningitis (Weinstein, 1987)
Sarcoid (Ingestad, 1971; Kirkham, 1973)
Multiple sclerosis (Bell, 1975)
Post-hemorrhagic
Post-traumatic (Iraci, 1976)
Radiation necrosis (Hammer, 1983; Harris, 1976; Pasquier, 1989; Schatz, 1975)
Shunt catheter (Coppetto, 1977, 1989; Slavin, 1988)
Toxic (see toxic optic neuropathies)
Ethylclorvynol (Placidyl)
Pheniprazine (Catron)
Trauma including post-surgical (Domingo, 1993; Fisher, 1968; Gilad, 1986; Heinz, 1994; Laursen, 1971; Logan, 1967; Noble, 1987; Obenchain, 1972; Prosperi, 1981; Resnick, 1981; Savino, 1980; Tibbs, 1979; Walsh, 1966)
Vascular occlusion (Hilton, 1966; Lee, 1975; Schneider, 1970)
Vasculitis (Wilhelm, 1993)

Is a Binasal Hemianopsia Present?

Binasal defects are usually due to bilateral intraocular disease of the retina or optic nerve (e.g., chronic papilledema, ischemic optic neuropathy, glaucoma, optic nerve drusen, or retinal disease such as sector retinitis pigmentosa or retinoschisis) (Salinas-Garcia, 1978). Rarely compression of the lateral chiasm may result in a binasal defect (O'Connell, 1976).

Is a Homonymous Hemianopsia Present?

Homonymous visual field impairments appear with lesions of the retrochiasmal pathways. Those affecting the optic tract and lateral geniculate body tend to be incongruous, but the more posteriorly the lesion is located in the optic radiation, the greater the congruity of the defects. In general, tumors produce sloping field defects while vascular lesions produce sharp field defects. The localization of homonymous field defects depends on the nature of the field defect and associated neuro-ophthalmologic and neurologic findings. Homonymous field defects may be caused by lesions affecting the optic tract, lateral geniculate body, optic radiations, or occipital lobe. Rarely, an occipital lesion may cause a monocular field defect (see above).

Where Is the Lesion Causing the Field Defect Localized and What Studies Are Indicated?

Complete unilateral optic tract lesions cause a complete macular splitting homonymous hemianopia, usually without impaired visual acuity, unless the lesion extends to involve the optic chiasm or nerve (Savino, 1978). In general, complete homonymous hemianopias are nonlocalizing and may be seen with any lesions of the retrochiasmal pathway, including lesions of the lateral geniculate body, optic radiations, and striate cortex. Partial optic tract lesions are more common than complete lesions and result in an incongruous field defect that may be scotomatous (Bell, 1978; Bender, 1978; Savino, 1978). Optic tract lesions are often associated with a relative afferent pupillary defect (RAPD) in the eye with the temporal field loss (contralateral to the side of the lesion) (Bell, 1978; Burde, 1967; O'Connor, 1982). An afferent pupillary defect in the contralateral eye in a patient with normal visual acuity bilaterally and a complete homonymous hemianopia are usually indicative of optic tract involvement (Miller, 1982). Recently Wilhelm et al. have described a possible exception to this clinical rule (Wilhelm, 1996). These authors described a RAPD contralateral to the lesions in 16 of 43 patients with congruous homonymous hemianopias (optic tract lesions excluded). Responsible lesions were postgeniculate and closer than 10 mm to lateral geniculate nucleus. A RAPD did not occur in lesions farther than 18 mm from the lateral geniculate nucleus. The authors postulated that the RAPD was probably not caused by a lesion of the visual pathway per se but by a lesion of intercalated neurons between the visual pathways and the pupillomotor centers in the pretectal area of the midbrain. Another abnormality of the pupil that may occur with optic tract lesions is due to concurrent third nerve involvement by the pathologic process causing the tract damage. In these cases, the pupil ipsilateral to the lesion may be large and poorly reactive. Finally, many patients with chronic optic tract lesions develop bilateral optic atrophy with a characteristic "wedge," "band," or "bowtie" pallor in the contralateral eye (identical to that seen in some patients with bitemporal visual field loss from chiasmal lesions), and a more generalized pallor in the ipsilateral optic nerve associated with loss of nerve fiber layer in the superior and inferior arcuate regions corresponding to the bulk of temporal fibers subserving the nasal visual fields (hemianopic optic atrophy) (Savino, 1978; Miller, 1982). Hemianopic optic atrophy indicates postchiasmal, preoptic radiations involvement (i.e., optic tract or lateral geniculate body damage) but has also been rarely described in congenital retrogeniculate lesions (Bajandas, 1976; Hoyt, 1972; Miller, 1982).

Etiologies of optic tract lesions include space-occupying lesions (e.g., glioma, meningioma, craniopharyngioma, metastasis, pituitary adenoma, ectopic pinealoma, abscess), aneurysms, arteriovenous malformations, demyelinating disease, and trauma (e.g., temporal lobectomy) (Anderson, 1989; Bender, 1978; Hoyt, 1972; Miller, 1982; Savino, 1978; Slavin, 1990). A complete neurologic examination and MR imaging, with specific attention to the optic tract region, are warranted in all patients. If MR imaging fails to reveal the responsible lesion, then MR angiography or cerebral angiography is warranted in nontraumatic cases to investigate for the presence of vascular lesions (e.g., aneurysm).

Lateral geniculate body lesions may also cause a complete macular splitting homonymous hemianopia (Gunderson, 1971; Hoyt, 1975; Miller, 1982). Partial lesions result in an incongruous homonymous field defect. Hemianopic optic atrophy may develop and no RAPD is usually evident. Although the study of Wilhelm et al. suggests that a RAPD may occasionally be present with lateral geniculate body or parageniculate optic radiation lesions, this observation has not been confirmed by other investigators (Wilhelm, 1996).

Although lesions of the optic tract or lateral geniculate body often cause incongruous field defects, two relatively specific patterns of congruous homonymous field defects with abruptly sloping borders, associated with sectorial optic atrophy, have been attributed to focal lesions of the lateral geniculate body caused by infarction in the territory of specific arteries. Occlusion of the anterior choroidal artery may cause a homonymous defect in the upper and lower quadrants with sparing of a horizontal sector (quadruple sectoranopia) (Frisen, 1979; Helgason, 1980; Luco, 1992). This defect occurs because the lateral geniculate body is organized in projection columns oriented vertically that represent sectors of the field parallel to the horizontal meridians, and the anterior choroidal artery supplies the hilum and anterolateral part of the nucleus. Bilateral lateral geniculate lesions may therefore cause bilateral hourglass-shaped visual field defects (Donahue, 1995) or bilateral blindness. In three reported cases of isolated bilateral involvement of the lateral geniculate bodies, the pathogenesis included anterior choroidal syphilitic arteritis, methanol toxicity-producing coagulative necrosis of the lateral geniculate body, and geniculate myelinolysis associated with the rapid correction of hyponatremia, respectively (Donahue, 1995; Mackenzie, 1933; Merren, 1972). Interruption of the posterior lateral choroidal artery which perfuses the central portion of the lateral geniculate causes a horizontal homonymous sector defect (wedge shaped) (Borruat, 1995; Frisen, 1978; Luco, 1992; Neau, 1996; Shacklett, 1984). In posterior lateral choroidal territory infarction, the homonymous quadrantanopia may be associated with hemisensory loss and neuropsychological dysfunction (transcortical aphasia, memory disturbances), and delayed contralateral abnormal movements (Neau, 1996). A homonymous horizontal sectoranopia is not diagnostic of a lateral geniculate body lesion, however, as a similar sector defect may occur with lesions affecting the optic radiations (Carter, 1985) or, rarely, affecting the occipital cortex in the region of the calcarine fissure (Grossman, 1990), the temporooccipital junction, the parietotemporal region, or in the distribution of the superficial sylvian artery territory (Growchowicki, 1991). Finally, a patient has been described with bilateral lateral geniculate lesions with bilateral sector defects with preservation of the visual fields in an hourglass distribution (Greenfield, 1996). The patient was a 28-year-old woman who developed incongruous binasal and bitemporal visual field defects one week after having a febrile gastroenteritis, characterized by severe diarrhea, while traveling in Mexico. MR imaging demonstrated bilaterally increased signal intensity within the lateral geniculate bodies. The severe diarrhea was thought to be associated with an aseptic bilateral lateral geniculitis resulting in the hourglass-shaped visual fields.

Patients with lesions of the lateral geniculate body may have no other signs or symptoms of neurologic involvement or may have associated findings related to thalamic or corticospinal tract involvement. Etiologies for lateral geniculate damage include infarction, arteriovenous malformation, trauma, tumor, inflammatory disorders, demyelinating disease, and toxic exposure (e.g., methanol) (Borruat, 1995; Donahue, 1995; Frisen, 1978, 1979; Greenfield, 1996; Gunderson, 1971; Helgason, 1980; Hoyt, 1975; Luco, 1992; Mackenzie, 1933; Merren, 1972; Neau, 1996; Shacklett, 1984). MR imaging, with attention to the lateral geniculate region, is indicated in all cases (Borruat, 1995; Horton, 1990; Neau, 1996).

Lesions of the proximal portion of the optic radiations may result in a complete homonymous hemianopia with macular splitting (Falconer, 1958; Van Buren, 1958). Superior homonymous quadrantic defects ("pie-in-the-sky" field defects) may result from a lesion in the temporal (Meyer's) loop of the optic radiations or in the inferior bank of the calcarine fissure. Large medial occipital lesions are seldom restricted to one bank of the calcarine fissure. Thus, quadrantic defects, especially wedge-shaped defects, more often point to a lesion of the optic radiations. In temporal lobe lesions, the superior quadrantic defect is usually, but not always, incongruous (Miller, 1982) and the inferior margins of the defects may have sloping borders and may cross beyond the horizontal midline (Van Buren, 1958). Also, the ipsilateral nasal field defect is often denser and comes closer to fixation than the defect in the contralateral eye. Macular vision may or may not be involved with the quadrantic defect (Jensen, 1976; Marino, 1968; Miller, 1982).

Although visual field defects may occur in isolation with temporal lobe lesions, other signs of neurologic impairment are often evident (Brazis, 1996). With dominant temporal lobe involvement, aphasic syndromes may occur, whereas nondominant lesions may be associated with impaired recognition of facial emotional expression, sensory amusia (inability to appreciate various characteristics of heard music), and aprosodias (impaired appreciation of emotional overtones of spoken language). Other abnormalities seen with temporal lobe dysfunction include memory impairment and seizures. Etiologies for temporal lobe dysfunction include space-occupying lesions (e.g., tumors, abscesses, hemorrhage), arteriovenous malformations, infarction, infections, congenital malformations, demyelinating disease, and trauma (e.g., temporal lobectomy) (Falconer, 1958; Jensen, 1976; Marino, 1968; Slavin, 1990; Trobe, 1973). MR imaging is required in all patients.

Involvement of the optic radiations in the depth of the parietal lobe gives rise to a congruous homonymous hemianopia, denser below than above. Such defects are usually more congruous than those produced by lesions of the temporal lobe and since the entire optic radiation passes through the parietal lobe, large lesions may produce complete homonymous hemianopia with macular splitting (Miller, 1982). Patients may often be unaware of their visual field defects (Pahwa, 1963; Warrington, 1962). Patients do not have associated pupillary abnormalities and optic atrophy does not occur unless the responsible lesion is congenital (Hoyt, 1972).

Visual field defects may occur in relative isolation, but often parietal lobe lesions betray themselves by other signs of neurologic dysfunction (Brazis, 1996). Parietal lobe lesions may be associated with contralateral somatosensory impairment, including impaired object recognition, impaired position sense, impaired touch and pain sensation, and tactile extinction. Dominant parietal lesions may cause apraxia, finger agnosia, acalculia, right-left disorientation, alexia, and aphasic disturbances, whereas nondominant lesions may be associated with anosognosia (denial of neurologic impairment), autotopagnosia (failure to recognize hemiplegic limbs as belonging to self), spatial disorientation, hemispatial neglect, constructional apraxia (abnormal drawing and copying), and dressing apraxia. Pathologic processes associated with parietal dysfunction are essentially the same as those that may cause temporal lobe dysfunction and are best evaluated by MR imaging (Beck, 1982).

Homonymous quadrantic visual field defects may occur with unilateral occipital lesions (Horton, 1991a). Superior quadrantic defects may be seen with inferior calcarine lesions, and inferior quadrantic defects may occur with superior calcarine lesions. Often these field defects have a sharp horizontal edge that would not be caused by tumors or missile injuries because it is unlikely that they would injure only one bank of the calcarine fissure and leave the fellow calcarine bank untouched. Horton and Hoyt (Horton, 1991b) suggest that a lesion of the extrastriate cortex (areas V2 and V3) would be more likely to explain the sharp horizontal edge of the defect because areas V2 and V3 are divided along the horizontal meridian into separate halves flanking the striate (V1) cortex and, consequently, the upper and lower quadrants in extrastriate cortex are physically isolated on opposite sides of the striate cortex. Although a lesion in this location (e.g., a tumor) may have irregular margins, if it crosses the representation of the horizontal meridian in extrastriate cortex it will produce a quadrantic visual field defect with a sharp horizontal border because of the split layout of the upper and lower quadrants of V2/V3. A congruous inferior quadrantanopia with borders aligned on both the vertical and horizontal meridians, however, has also been described with a lesion of the superior fibers of the optic radiations near the contralateral trigone where the fascicles of visual axons become compact as they approach the calcarine cortex (Borruat, 1993).

Medial occipital lesions cause highly congruous homonymous field defects (Horton, 1994; Pessin, 1987). When both the upper and the lower calcarine cortices are affected, a complete homonymous hemianopia, usually with macular sparing, develops. Sparing of the central five degrees of vision (macular sparing) is common with occipital lesions, probably due to a combination of a large macular representation and dual blood supply (Miller, 1982). The central 10 to 15 degrees of vision fill a majority of the total surface area of the occipital cortex (as much as 50 to 60 percent) (Horton, 1994; McFadzean, 1994). Patients with purely occipital lesions are often aware of the hemianopia, whereas patients with larger or more anterior lesions, affecting parietal regions or associative pathways to the primary or secondary visual association cortex, may be unaware of their deficit (Koehler, 1986).

Lesions of the striate cortex may be classified as anterior, intermediate, or posterior (Benton, 1980; Horton, 1994; Landau, 1995; McAuley, 1979; McFadzean, 1994; Miller, 1982; Walsh, 1974). Anterior lesions lie adjacent to the parietooccipital fissure and affect the monocular temporal crescent of the contralateral visual field (temporal crescent or half-moon syndrome). This area constitutes less than 10% of the total surface area of the striate cortex and the defect begins approximately 60 degrees from fixation. Both upper and lower temporal crescents may be scotomatous in the field of one eye, or only the upper or lower temporal crescent may be involved. Conversely, the temporal crescent may be spared with lesions that destroy the entire calcarine cortex except for the anterior tip (Landau, 1995). Posterior lesions are located in the posterior 50–60% of the striate cortex, including the occipital pole and operculum, affect macular vision (i.e., the central 10 degrees in the contralateral hemifield), and therefore cause scotomatous defects. Intermediate lesions lie between the anterior and posterior confines and affect from 10 to 60 degrees in the contralateral hemifield.

The most common cause of unilateral occipital disease is infarction in the distribution of the posterior cerebral artery (Beal, 1980; Benton, 1980; Fujino, 1986; Gittinger, 1986; Hoyt, 1960; McAuley, 1979; Pessin, 1987; Pessin, 1987; Sato, 1986; Trobe, 1973). Other etiologies include venous infarction, hemorrhage, arteriovenous malformation, tumor, abscess, and trauma (Kupersmith, 1996; Monteiro, 1984; Parkinson, 1951; Troost, 1975). Thus, MR imaging is warranted in all patients.

Bilateral occipital lobe lesions may occur from a single or from consecutive events and may cause bilateral homonymous scotomas, usually with some macular sparing ("ring" scotomas), that respect the vertical midline (Helpern, 1980; Miller, 1982). In some cases there may be "tunnel" or "keyhole" fields with bilateral complete homonymous hemianopias except for macular sparing. Careful testing in these cases reveals that the macular sparing respects the vertical midline. Bilateral lesions affecting the superior or inferior calcarine cortices may produce bilateral altitudinal defects that may mimic the visual field abnormalities seen with bilateral optic nerve or retinal disease (Hansen, 1993; Lakhanpal, 1990; Newman, 1984). Bilateral upper calcarine bank lesions may have associated neurologic findings including Balint's syndrome (apraxia of gaze, optic ataxia, decreased visual attention, and simultanagnosia), abnormal depth perception, defective revisualization of spatial relations, topographic disorientation, and disorientation to place (Brazis, 1996; Caplan, 1990). Bilateral lesions of the inferior banks of the calcarine fissure may be associated with prosopagnosia (inability to identify faces visually), cerebral dyschromatopsia, amnesia, and difficulty revisualizing the morphology and appearance of people and objects (Brazis, 1996; Caplan, 1990). Bilateral lesions of the visual cortices, often due to large bilateral posterior cerebral artery infarcts involving both banks of the calcarine fissure and both temporal lobes, cause cortical blindness often associated with agitated delirium and amnesia (Brazis, 1996; Caplan, 1990).

Cortical blindness implies visual impairment due to discrete involvement of the occipital cortices bilaterally whereas cerebral blindness is a more general term indicating visual loss from any process affecting the retrogeniculate visual pathways. The essential features of cortical and cerebral blindness include (adapted from Miller, 1982) complete loss of all visual sensation including all appreciation of light and dark; loss of reflex lid closure to bright illumination and to threatening gestures; retention of the reflex constriction of the pupils to illumination and to convergence movements; and integrity of the normal structure of the retina as verified by ophthalmoscopy.

There are many etiologies of cerebral and cortical impairment, including hypoxia, infarction, hemorrhage, eclampsia, hypertensive encephalopathy, tentorial herniation from cerebral mass, tumor, arteriovenous malformation, infection (e.g., progressive multifocal leukoencephalopathy, Jacob-Creutzfeldt disease, subacute sclerosing panencephalitis, HIV encephalitis, syphilis, encephalitis, abscess), inflammation (e.g., sarcoidosis), demyelinating disease, trauma, metabolic disorders (e.g., adrenoleukodystrophy, hypoglycemia, porphyria, mitochondrial encephalopathies), toxins (e.g., lead, mercury, ethanol, carbon monoxide), medications (e.g., cyclosporine, tacrolimus, interleukin-2), Alzheimer's disease, postictal after seizures, and complications of cerebral angiography (Aldrich, 1987; Beal, 1980; Coughlin, 1989; Eldridge, 1988; Gibson, 1982; Gittinger, 1986; Greenblatt, 1973; Hinchey, 1996; Horwitz, 1974; Hoyt, 1960; Jaffe, 1988; Karp, 1996; Katafuchi, 1985; Keane, 1980; Kuperschmidt, 1995; Lantos, 1989; Mehler, 1988; Miller, 1982; Monteiro, 1984; Nepple, 1978; Ormerod, 1996; Powers, 1985; Salmon, 1968; Studdard, 1981; Wilson, 1988; Zihl, 1979). Occasionally, patients with cortical blindness deny their visual defect (Anton's syndrome).

As noted from review of this chapter, MR imaging is indicated in all patients with a homonymous visual field defect, except in acute or traumatic cases, in which CT imaging is usually adequate, or in patients in whom MR imaging is contraindicated (e.g., ferromagnetic aneurymal clip, metallic fragments, pacemakers, etc.). There are several clinical situations in which MR imaging may be normal in a patient with a homonymous hemianopia. (1) Homonymous hemianopia or cortical blindness may be an early or initial finding in some patients with the Heidenhain variant of Jacob-Creutzfeldt disease and in most of these patients MR or CT imaging is normal (Aguglia, 1991; Felton, 1996; Kovanen, 1985; Purvin, 1989; Vargas, 1995; Warren, 1992). The EEG is often initially normal in these patients although it usually eventually shows characteristic periodic complexes in most patients. Patients soon also develop mentation impairment, myoclonus, and other signs of Jacob-Creutzfeldt disease but initially the diagnosis may be quite difficult and made only by brain biopsy. (2) Some patients with Alzheimer's disease may develop a homonymous field defect (Trick, 1995). MR imaging may be normal or show only diffuse atrophy and electroencephalograms are normal or show only mild diffuse slowing. This diagnosis is suspected in patients with a slowly progressive dementia without other "focal" neurologic findings and the dementia usually far outweighs the visual field impairment. (3) Most patients with field defects from cerebral infarction or hypoxia demonstrate MR imaging changes compatible with ischemia. However, Moster et al. described two patients, one with bilateral homonymous congruous hemianopic central scotomata after carbon monoxide poisoning and the other with bilateral congruous inferior visual scotomata after global hypoxia, who were initially diagnosed with "functional" visual loss (Moster, 1996). Neither CT nor MR imaging adequately demonstrated the source of the visual dysfunction but SPECT and PET imaging, respectively, confirmed the organic substrate of the visual impairment. Functional imaging techniques, such as SPECT or PET, should thus be considered in patients with suspected cortical visual loss and normal CT or MR studies. Functional MR imaging is also a promising method for the objective detection of abnormalities in the afferent visual system (Miki, 1996). (4) Functional (nonorganic) hemianopias are associated with normal imaging studies (Thompson, 1996). One method of determining if a field defect is nonorganic is to test saccadic eye movements into the supposedly absent portion of the field with the patient assuming that eye movements and not visual fields are being tested (Weller, 1989). Another method is to place a 30 prism diopter Fresnel prism into the upper quadrants of a trial frame (Carlow, 1995). After visual fields are obtained without the prism, the prism is placed first base-out and then base-in and with each change the fields are repeated. Patients with pathologic hemianopsias shift their superior field 15 degrees to the right or to the left of the central vertical meridian with the prism base in or out, respectively, whereas patients with suspected functional hemifield defect do not shift their superior sectors in a similar fashion.

What Should Be Done with an Unexplained Visual Field Defect?

Patients with an unexplained unilateral or bilateral visual field defect should have careful attention paid to the corresponding areas of the retina and optic nerve on ophthalmoscopy. Some patients may have occult retinal and/or choroidal vascular disease that may only be detected by timed and directed (to the location predicted by the visual field defect) fluorescein angiography (Rizzo, 1993). Visual defects respecting the vertical midline with a bitemporal or homonymous "flavor" should undergo a neuroimaging study. Rarely, patients with unilateral or bilateral nasal defects respecting the vertical midline may harbor an underlying compressive lesion (Frisen, 1971; Manor, 1980; Miller, 1982; O'Connell, 1976). In addition, apparently altitudinal (superior or inferior) visual field defects may actually represent bilateral lesions of the optic nerves or retrochiasmal pathway.

Constriction of the visual fields may occur in media opacities, miotic pupils, or uncorrected refractive error; as an artifact of testing; in occult retinal disease (e.g., retinitis pigmentosa, cancer associated retinopathy, etc.); with any optic neuropathy (e.g., optic neuritis, ischemic optic neuropathy, glaucoma, etc.); with bilateral retrochiasmal lesions (e.g., occipital stroke); or in nonorganic patients. In fact, any combination of these entities (e.g., an optic neuropathy and a retrochiasmal homonymous hemianopsia) may produce any number of combinations of associated visual field defects. The simple algorithm presented obviously cannot account for every one of these combinations. Electrophysiologic testing such as electroretinography, visual evoked potentials, and other ancillary testing, such as fluorescein angiography, may disclose an abnormality in the retina or optic nerve even in the absence of an ophthalmoscopically visible lesion.

References

Abla AA, Maroon JC, Wilberger JE, et al. (1986). Intrasellar mucocoele simulating pituitary adenoma: Case report. *Neurosurgery 18*:197–199.

Aguglia U, Gambarelli D, Farnarier G, Quattrone A. (1991). Different susceptibilities of the geniculate and extrageniculate visual pathways to human Creutzfeldt-Jacob disease (a combined neurophysiological-neuropathological study). *Electroencephalogr Clin Neurophysiol 78*:413–423.

Ahmadi J, Keane JR, McCormick GS, et al. (1984). Ischemic chiasmal syndrome and hypopituitarism associated with progressive cerebrovascular occlusive disease. *Am J Neurorad 5*:367.

Aldrich MS, Alessi AG, Beck RW, Gilman S. (1987). Cortical blindness: Etiology, diagnosis, and prognosis. *Ann Neurol 21*:149–158.

Anderson D, Faber P, Marcovitz S, Hardy J, Lorenzetti D. (1983). Pituitary tumors and the ophthalmologist. *Ophthalmology 90*:1265–1270.

Anderson DR, Trobe JD, Hood TW, Gebarski SS. (1989). Optic tract injury after anterior temporal lobectomy. *Ophthalmology 96*:1065–1070.

Aubin MJ, Hardy J, Comtois R. (1997). Primary sellar haemorrhagic melanoma: Case report and review of the literature. *Br J Neurosurg 11*:80–83.

Bajandas FJ, McBeath JB, Smith JL. (1976). Congenital homonymous hemianopia. *Am J Ophthalmol 82*:498–500.

Bartlett JR. (1971). Craniopharyngiomas: A summary of 85 cases. *J Neurol Neurosurg Psych 34*:37–41.

Baskin DS, Wilson CB. (1984). Transsphenoidal treatment of nonneoplastic intrasellar cysts. *J Neurosurg 60*:8.

Beal MF, Chapman PH. (1980). Cortical blindness and homonymous hemianopia in the postpartum period. *JAMA 244*: 2085–2087.

Beck RW, Savino PJ, Schatz NJ, et al. (1982). Plaque causing homonymous hemianopsia in multiple sclerosis identified by computed tomography. *Am J Ophthalmol 94*:229–234.

Bell RA, Thompson HS. (1978). Relative afferent pupillary defect in optic tract hemianopsias. *Am J Ophthalmol 85*:538–540.

Bell RA, Robertson DM, Rosen DA, Kerr AW. (1975). Optochiasmatic arachnoiditis in multiple sclerosis. *Arch Ophthalmol 93*:191–193.

Bender MB, Bodis-Wollner I. (1978). Visual dysfunctions in optic tract lesions. *Ann Neurol 3*:187–193.

Benton S, Levy I, Swash M. (1980). Vision in the temporal crescent in occipital infarction. *Brain 103*:83–97.

Berke JP, Buxton LF, Kokmen E. (1975). The "empty sella." *Neurology 25*:1137–1143.

Berson E, Freeman M, Gay A. (1966). Visual field defects in giant suprasellar aneurysms of the internal carotid artery. *Arch Ophthalmol 76*:52–58.

Bird, AC. (1972). Field loss due to lesions at the anterior angle of the chiasm. *Proc Royal Soc Med 65*:519–520.

Bird AC, Nolan B, Gargano FP, David NJ. (1970). Unruptured aneurysm of the supraclinoid carotid artery: A treatable cause of blindness. *Neurology 20*:445–454.

Borruat F-X, Maeder P. (1995). Sectoranopia after head trauma: Evidence of lateral geniculate body lesion on MRI. *Neurology 45*:590–592.

Borruat F-X, Siatkowski RM, Schatz NJ, Glaser JS. (1993). Congruous quadrantanopia and optic radiation lesion. *Neurology 43*:1430–1432.

Brazis PW, Masdeu JC, Biller J. (1996). *Localization in Clinical Neurology*. Third Edition. Boston, Little Brown, pp. 449–534.

Buonaguidi R, Ferdeghini M, Faggionato F, et al. (1983). Intrasellar metastasis mimicking pituitary adenoma. *Surg Neurol 20*:373.

Burde RM. (1967). The pupil. *Int Ophthalmol Clin 7*:839–855.

Camins MB, Mount LA. (1974). Primary suprasellar atypical teratoma. *Brain 97*:447–456.

Cantore GP, Raco A, Artico M, et al. (1989). Primary chiasmatic lymphoma. *Clin Neurol Neurosurg 91*:71.

Caplan LR. (1990). *Visual perception abnormalities*. Presented at the 42nd Annual Meeting of the American Academy of Neurology, Miami, FL.

Carlow TJ. (1995). *Functional hemianopsia: Identified with fresnel prisms and quantitative perimetry*. Presented at the North American Neuro-Ophthalmology Society Meeting, Tucson, AZ.

Carter JE, O'Connor P, Shacklett D, Rosenberg M. (1985). Lesions of the optic radiations mimicking lateral geniculate nucleus visual field defects. *J Neurol Neurosurg Psychiatry 48*:982–988.

Carter JE, Wymore J, Ansbacher L, et al. (1982). Sudden visual loss and a chiasmal syndrome due to an intrachiasmatic arteriovenous malformation. *J Clin Neuro-ophthalmol 2*:163–167.

Castel JP, Delorge-Kerdiles C, Rivel J. (1989). Cavernous hemangioma of the optic chiasm. *Neurochirurgie 35*:252–256.

Cohen MM, Lessell S. (1979).. Chiasmal syndrome due to metastasis. *Arch Neurol 36*:565–567.

Coppetto JR, Gahm NH. (1977). Bitemporal hemianopic scotomas from intraventricular catheter. *Surg Neurol 8*:361.

Coppetto JR, Monteiro MLR. (1989). Bitemporal hemianopic scotomas form intraventricular catheter: The pinched chiasm syndrome? *Neuro-ophthalmology 9*:343–346.

Corboy JR, Galetta SL. (1989). Familial cavernous angiomas manifesting with an acute chiasmal syndrome. *Am J Ophthalmol 108*:245–250.

Coughlin WF, McMurdo SK, Reeves T. (1989). MR imaging of postpartum cortical blindness. *J Comput Assist Tomogr 13*:572–576.

Coyle JT. (1969). Chiasmatic arachnoiditis. *Am J Ophthalmol 68*:345–349.

Cox TA, Corbett JJ, Thompson HS, Kassell NF. (1981). Unilateral nasal hemianopia as a sign of intracranial optic nerve compression. *Am J Ophthalmol 92*:230–232.

Crane TB, Yee RD, Hepler RS, Hallinan JM. (1982). Clinical manifestations and radiologic findings in craniopharyngiomas in adults. *Am J Ophthalmol 94*:220–228.

Crowe NW, Nickles TP, Troost BT, et al. (1989). Intrachiasmal hemorrhage: A delayed post-traumatic blindness. *Neurology 39*:863.

Cullen AF, Haining WM, Crombie AL. (1966). Cerebral aneurysms presenting with visual field defects. *Br J Ophthalmol 50*:251–256.

Domingo Z, de Villiers JC. (1993). Post-traumatic chiasmatic disruption. *Br J Neurosurg 7*:141–147.

Domingue JN, Wilson CB. (1977). Pituitary abscesses: Report of seven cases and review of the literature. *J Neurosurg 46*:601.

Donahue SP, Kardon RH, Thompson HS. (1995). Hourglass-shaped visual fields as a sign of bilateral lateral geniculate myelinolysis. *Am J Ophthalmol 119*:378–380.

Duvall J, Cullen JF. (1982). Metastatic disease in the pituitary: Clinical features. *Trans Ophthalmol Soc UK 102*:481–486.
Edwards MK, Gilmore RL, Franco JM. (1983). Computed tomography of chiasmal optic neuritis. *Am J Neurorad 4*:816–818.
Ehlers N, Malmros R. (1973). The suprasellar meningioma. *Acta Ophthalmol 121*:52–75.
Eldridge PR, Punt JAG. (1988). Transient traumatic cortical blindness in children. *Lancet 1*:815–816.
Elias Z, Powers SK, Grimson BS. (1987). Chiasmal syndrome caused by pituitary sellar disproportion. *Surg Neurol 28*:395.
Elkington SG. (1968). Pituitary adenoma: preoperative symptomatology in a series of 260 patients. *Br J Ophthalmol 52*:322–328.
Falconer MA, Stafford-Bell MA. (1975). Visual failure from pituitary and parasellar tumours occurring with favorable outcome in pregnant women. *J Neurol Neurosurg Psychiatr 38*:919–930.
Falconer MA, Wilson JL. (1958). Visual field changes following anterior temporal lobectomy: Their significance in relation to "Meyer's Loop" of the optic radiations. *Brain 81*:1–14.
Farris BK, Smith JL, David NJ. (1986). The nasal junction scotoma in giant aneurysms. *Ophthalmology 93*:895–905.
Felton WL. (1996). Presented at the 28th Annual Meeting of the Frank B. Walsh Meeting—Salt Lake City, Utah, February 10–11.
Ferguson GG, Drake CG. (1981). Carotid-ophthalmic aneurysms: Visual abnormalities in 32 patients and the results of treatment. *Surg Neurol 16*:1–8.
Fermaglich J, Kattah J, Manz H. (1978). Venous angioma of the optic chiasm. *Ann Neurol 4*:470–471.
Fischer EG, DeGirolami U, Suojanen JN. (1994). Reversible visual deficit following debulking of a Rathke's cleft cyst: a tethered chiasm? *J Neurosurg 81*:459–462.
Fisher NF, Jampolsky A, Scott AB. (1968). Traumatic bitemporal hemianopsia I. Diagnosis of macular splitting. *Am J Ophthalmol 65*:237–242.
Frisen L. (1971). Genuine, relative binasal hemianopia. *Acta Ophthalmologica 49*:734.
Frisen L. (1979). Quadruple sectoranopia and sectorial optic atrophy: A syndrome of the distal anterior choroidal artery. *J Neurol Neurosurg Psychiatry 42*:590–594.
Frisen L, Holmegaard L, Rosencrantz M. (1978). Sectorial optic atrophy and homonymous, horizontal sectoranopia: A lateral choroidal artery syndrome? *J Neurol Neurosurg Psychiatry 41*:374–380.
Fuchs HA, Evans RM, Gregg CR. (1985). Invasive aspergillosis of the sphenoid sinus manifested as a pituitary tumor. *South Med J 78*:1365.
Fujino T, Kigazawa K, Yamada R. (1986). Homonymous hemianopia: A retrospective study of 140 cases. *Neuro-ophthalmology 6*:17.
Galetta SL, Stadmauer EA, Hicks DA, et al. (1991). Reactive lymphohistiocytosis with recurrence in the optic chiasm. *J Clin Neuro-ophthalmol 11*:25–30.
Gibson JM, Cullen JF. (1982). Blindness and visual field defects following cerebral angiography. *Neuro-ophthalmology 2*:297–303.
Gilad E, Dickerman Z, Laron Z, Cohen S, Manor RS. (1986). Traumatic chiasmal syndrome with panhypopituitarism. *Neuro-ophthalmol 6*:79–83.
Gittinger JW. (1986). Occipital infarction following chiropractic cervical manipulation. *J Clin Neuro-ophthalmol 6*:11–13.
Glaser JS, Hoyt WF, Corbett J. (1971). Visual morbidity with chiasmal glioma: Long-term studies of visual fields in untreated and treated cases. *Arch Ophthalmol 85*:3–12.
Godleski J, Charlin JF, Brasseur G, et al. (1984). Hypothalamic sarcoidosis with involvement of the chiasma. *Rev Otoneuro-ophthalmol 56*:347–355.
Goodman RH, Post KD, Molitch ME, Adelman LS, Altemus LR, Johnston H. (1979). Eosinophilic granuloma mimicking a pituitary tumor. *Neurosurgery 5*:723–725.
Goodwin JA, Glaser JS. (1978). Chiasmal syndrome in sphenoid sinus mucocoele. *Ann Neurol 4*:440–444.
Greenblatt SH. (1973). Posttraumatic transient cerebral blindness: Association with migraine and seizure diatheses. *JAMA 225*:1073–1076.
Greenfield DS, Siatkowski RM, Schatz NJ, Glaser JS. (1996). Bilateral lateral geniculitis associated with severe diarrhea. *Am J Ophthalmol 122*:280–281.
Gregorius FK, Hepler RS, Stern WE. (1975). Loss and recovery of vision with suprasellar meningiomas. *J Neurosurg 42*:69–75.
Grossman M, Galetta SL, Nichols CW, Grossman RI. (1990). Horizontal homonymous sectoral field defect after ischemic infarction of the occipital lobe. *Am J Ophthalmol 109*:234–236.
Growchowicki M, Vighetto A. (1991). Homonymous horizontal sectoranopia: Report of four cases. *Br J Ophthalmol 75*:624.
Gunderson CH, Hoyt WF. (1971). Geniculate hemianopia: Incongruous visual defects in two patients with partial lesions of the lateral geniculate nucleus. *J Neurol Neurosurg Psychiatry 34*:1–6.
Hammer HM. (1983). Optic chiasmal radionecrosis. *Trans Ophthalmol Soc UK 103*:208–211.
Hankey GJ, Khangure MS. (1987). Chiasmal apoplexy due to intrachiasmatic vascular malformation rupture. *Aust N Z J Med 17*:444–446.
Hansen HV. (1993). Bilateral inferior altitudinal hemianopia. *Neuro-ophthalmol 13*:81.
Harris JR, Levene MB. (1976). Visual complications following irradiation for pituitary adenomas and craniopharyngioma. *Radiology 120*:167–171.

Heinz GW, Nunery WR, Grossman CB. (1994). Traumatic chiasmal syndrome associated with midline basilar skull fractures. *Am J Ophthalmol 117:*90–96.

Helgason C, Caplan LR, Goodwin J, Hedges T III. (1980). Anterior choroidal artery territory infarction—Report of cases and review. *Arch Neurol 43:*681–686.

Helpern JL, Sedler RR. (1980). Traumatic bilateral homonymous hemianopic scotomas. *Ann Ophthalmol 12:*1022–1026.

Hershenfeld SA, Sharpe JS. (1993). Monocular temporal hemianopia. *Br J Ophthalmol 77:*422–427.

Hilton GF, Hoyt WF. (1966). An arteriosclerotic chiasmal syndrome. *JAMA 196:*1018–1020.

Hinchey J, Chaves C, Appignani B, et al. (1996). A reversible posterior leukoencephalopathy syndrome. *New Eng J Med 334:*494–500.

Horton JC, Hoyt WF. (1991a). Quadrantic visual field defects. A hallmark of lesions in extrastriate (V2/V3) cortex. *Brain 114:*1703–1718.

Horton JC, Hoyt WF. (1991b). The representation of the visual field in human striate cortex. A revision of the classic Holmes map. *Arch Ophthalmol 109:*816–824.

Horton JC, Landau K, Maeder P, Hoyt WF. (1990). Magnetic resonance imaging of the human lateral geniculate body. *Arch Neurol 47:*1201–1206.

Horwich A, Bloom HG. (1985). Optic gliomas: radiation therapy and prognosis. *Int J Radiat Oncol Biol Phys 11:*1067–1079.

Horwitz NH, Wener L. (1974). Temporary cortical blindness after cerebral angiography. *J Neurosurg 40:*583–586.

Howard RS, Duncombe AS, Owens C, et al. (1987). Compression of the optic chiasm due to lymphoreticular malignancy. *Postgrad Med J 63:*1091.

Hoyt WF. (1969). Correlative functional anatomy of the optic chiasm. *Clin Neurosurg 17:*189–208.

Hoyt WF. (1975). Geniculate hemianopia: Incongruous visual defects from partial involvement of the lateral geniculate nucleus. *Proc Austr Assoc Neurologists 12:*7–16.

Hoyt WF. (1960). Vascular lesions of the visual cortex with brain herniation through the tentorial incisura: Neuro-ophthalmologic considerations. *Arch Ophthalmol 64:*74–78.

Hoyt WF, Rios-Montenegro EN, Behrens MM, Eckelhoff RJ. (1972). Homonymous hemioptic hypoplasia: Funduscopic features in standard and red-free illumination in three patients with congenital hemiplegia. *Br J Ophthalmol 56:*537–545.

Hungerford GD, Biggs PJ, Levine JH, et al. (1982). Lymphoid adenohypophysitis with radiologic and clinical findings resembling a pituitary tumor. *Am J Neurorad 3:*444.

Hwang JF, Yau CW, Huang KI, Tasi CY. (1993). Apoplectic optochiasmal syndrome due to intrinsic cavernous hemangioma. Case report. *J Clin Neuro-ophthalmol 13:*232–236.

Ikeda H, Yoshimoto T. (1995). Visual disturbances in patients with pituitary adenoma. *Acta Neurolog Scand 92:*157–160.

Ingestad R, Stigmar G. (1971). Sarcoidosis with ocular and hypothalamic pituitary manifestations. *Acta Ophthalmol 49:*1–10.

Iraci G, Giordano R, Gerosa M, Rigobello L, Di Stefano E. (1979a). Ocular involvement in recurrent cyst of Rathke's cleft: Case report. *Ann Ophthalmol 11:*94–98.

Iraci G, Giordano R, Gerosa M, Zampieri P, Tomazzoli-Gerosa L. (1979b). Cystic suprasellar and retrosellar arachnoiditis: A clinical and pathologic follow-up case report. *Ann Ophthalmol 11:*1175–1179.

Iraci G, Pellone M, Scuccimarra A. (1977). Optochiasmatic arachnoiditis. Remarks on a case of the cystic form of the disease. *Ann Ophthalmol 9:*147.

Iraci G, Pellone M, Scuccimarra A, Fiore D. (1976). Posttraumatic optochiasmatic arachnoiditis. *Ann Ophthalmol 8:*1313–1328.

Isayama Y, Takahashi T, Inoue M. (1980). Ocular findings of suprasellar germinoma: Long term follow-up after radiotherapy. *Neuro-ophthalmology 1:*53–61.

Jaffe SJ, Roach ES. (1988). Transient cortical blindness with occipital lobe epilepsy. *J Clin Neuro-ophthalmol 8:*221–224.

Jensen I, Seedorf HH. (1976). Temporal lobe epilepsy and neuro-ophthalmology: Ophthalmological findings in 74 temporal lobe resected patients. *Acta Ophthalmol 54:*827–841.

Kageyama N. (1971). Ectopic pinealoma in the region of the optic chiasm. *J Neurosurg 35:*755–759.

Kansu T, Bertan V. (1980). Fifth ventricle with bitemporal hemianopsia. *J Neurosurg 52:*276–278.

Karp BI, Yang JC, Khorsand M, et al. (1996). Multiple cerebral lesions complicating therapy with interleukin-2. *Neurology 47:*417–424.

Katafuchi Y, Nishimi T, Yamaguchi Y, et al. (1985). Cortical blindness in acute carbon monoxide poisoning. *Brain Dev 7:*516–519.

Kaufman B. (1969). The empty sella syndrome—a manifestation of the intrasellar subarachnoid space. *Radiol 90:*931–940.

Kaufman B, Tomsak RL, Kaufmann BA, et al. (1989). Herniation of the suprasellar visual system and third ventricle into empty sellae: Morphologic and clinical considerations. *Am J Neuroradiol 152:*597.

Kayan A, Earl CJ. (1975). Compressive lesions of the optic nerves and chiasm: Pattern of recovery following surgical treatment. *Brain 98:*13.

Keane JR. (1980). Blindness following tentorial herniation. *Ann Neurol 8:*186–190.

Kinjo T, al-Mefty O, Ciric I. (1995). Diaphragma sellae meningiomas. *Neurosurg 36:*1082–1092.

Kirkham TH. (1973). Neuro-ophthalmic presentations of sarcoidosis. *Proc R Soc Med 66:*167–169.
Kirkham TH. (1972). The ocular symptomatology of pituitary tumours. *Proc R Soc Med 65:*517–518.
Knight CL, Hoyt WF, Wilson CB. (1972). Syndrome of incipient prechiasmal optic nerve compression. *Arch Ophthalmol 87:*1–11.
Koehler PJ, Endtz LJ, TeVelde J, Hekster RE. (1986). Aware or non-aware. On the significance of awareness for the localization of the lesion responsible for homonymous hemianopia. *J Neurol Sci 75:*255–262.
Kosmorsky GS, Straga JM. (1997). A descent thing to do for the chiasm. *J Neuro-ophthalmol 17:*53–56.
Kovanen J, Erkinjuntii T, Ilivanainen M, et al. (1985). Cerebral MRI and CT imaging in Creutzfeldt-Jakob disease. *J Comput Assist Tomogr 9:*125–128.
Krauss HR, Slamovits TL, Sibony PA, et al. (1982). Carotid artery aneurysm simulating pituitary adenoma. *J Clin Neuro-ophthalmol 2:*169.
Krohel GB, Charles H, Smith RS. (1981). Granulomatous optic neuropathy. *Arch Ophthalmol 99:*1035–1055.
Kuperschmidt H, Bont A, Schnorf H, et al. (1995). Transient cortical blindness and bioccipital brain lesions in two patients with acute intermittent porphyria. *Ann Intern Med 123:*598–600.
Kupersmith MJ, Vargas ME, Yashar A, et al. (1996). Occipital arteriovenous malformations; Visual disturbances and presentation. *Neurology 46:*953–957.
Lakhanpal A, Selhorst JB. (1990). Bilateral altitudinal visual fields. *Ann Ophthalmol 22:*112–117.
Landau K, Wichmann W, Valavanis A. (1995). The missing temporal crescent. *Am J Ophthalmol 119:*345–349.
Lantos G. (1989). Cortical blindness due to osmotic disruption of the blood-brain barrier by angiographic contrast material: CT and MRI studies. *Neurology 39:*567–571.
Larranaga J, Fanidon J, Gomez-Bueno J, et al. (1989). Aspergillosis of the sphenoid sinus simulating a pituitary tumor. *Neuroradiology 31:*362.
Laursen AB. (1971). Traumatic bitemporal hemianopsia. Survey of the literature and report of a case. *Acta Ophthalmol 49:*134.
Lavin PJM, McCrary JA, Roessmann U, et al. (1984). Chiasmal apoplexy: Hemorrhage from a cryptic vascular malformation in the optic chiasm. *Neurology 34:*1007–1011.
Lee KF. (1983). Ischemic chiasmal syndrome. *Am J Neurorad 4:*777–780.
Lee KF, Schatz NJ. (1975). Ischemic chiasmal syndrome. *Acta Radiol 347:*131–148.
Leramo OB, Booth JD, Zinman B, et al. (1981). Hyperprolactinaemia, hypopituitarism and chiasmal compression due to carcinoma metastatic to the pituitary. *Neurosurgery 8:*477.
Liu GT, Galetta SL, Rorke LB, et al. (1996). Gangliogliomas involving the optic chiasm. *Neurol 46:*1669–1673.
Logan WC, Gordon DS. (1967). Traumatic lesions of the optic chiasma. *Br J Ophthalmol 51:*258–260.
Luco C, Hoppe A, Schweitzer M, et al. (1992). Visual field defects in vascular lesions of the lateral geniculate body. *J Neurol Neurosurg Psychiatry 55:*12–15.
Mackenzie I, Meighan S, Pollock EN. (1933). On the projection of the retinal quadrants on the lateral geniculate bodies, and the relationship of the quadrants to the optic radiations. *Trans Ophthalmol Soc UK 53:*142–169.
Maitland CG, Abiko S, Hoyt WF, Wilson CB, Okamura T. (1979). Chiasmal apoplexy: Report of four cases. *J Neurosurg 56:*118–122.
Manor RS, Ouaknine GE, Matz S, Shalit MN. (1980). Nasal visual field loss with intracranial lesions of the optic pathways. *Am J Ophthalmol 90:*1–10.
Manz HJ, Klein LH, Fermaglich J, Kattah J, Luessenhop AJ. (1979). Cavernous hemangiomas of optic chiasm, optic nerves and right optic tract. *Virchows Arch (Pathol Anat) 383:*225–231.
Marino R Jr, Rasmussen T. (1968). Visual field changes after temporal lobectomy in man. *Neurology 18:*825–835.
Matsuo K, Kobayashi S, Sugita K. (1980). Bitemporal hemianopsia associated with sclerosis of the intracranial internal carotid arteries. *J Neurosurg 53:*566–569.
Max MB, Dick MDF, Rottenberg DA. (1981). Pituitary metastatis. Incidence in cancer patients and clinical differentiation from pituitary adenoma. *Neurology 31:*998–1002.
McAuley DL, Russell RW. (1979). Correlation of CAT scan and visual field defects in vascular lesions of the posterior visual pathways. *J Neurol Neurosurg Psychiatry 42:*298–311.
McFadzean R, Brosnahan D, Hadley D, Mutlukan E. (1994). Representation of the visual field in the occipital striate cortex. *Br J Ophthalmol 78:*185–190.
McFadzean RM, Brewin TB, Doyle D, et al. (1983). Glioma of the optic chiasm and its management. *Trans Ophthalmol Soc UK 103:*199–207.
McFadzean RM, McIlwaine GG, McLellan D. (1990). Hodgkin's disease at the optic chiasm. *J Clin Neuro-ophthalmol 10:*248–254.
Mehler MF. (1988). The neuro-ophthalmologic spectrum of the rostral basilar artery syndrome. *Arch Neurol 45:*966–971.
Meienberg O. (1981). Sparing of the temporal crescent in homonymous hemianopia and its significance for visual orientation. *Neuro-ophthalmol 2:*129–134.
Merren MD. (1972). Bilateral lateral geniculate body necrosis as a cause of amblyopia. *Neurology 22:*263–268.
Meyer FB, Carpenter SM, Laws ER, Jr. (1987). Intrasellar arachnoid cysts. *Surg Neurol 28:*105.
Mikelberg FS, Yidegiligne HM. (1993). Axonal loss in band atrophy of the optic nerve in craniopharyngioma: a quantitative analysis. *Can J Ophthalmol 28:*69–71.
Miki A, Nakajima T, Fujita M, et al. (1996). Functional magnetic resonance imaging in homonymous hemianopsia. *Am J Ophthalmol 121:*258–266.

Miller NR. (1982). Topical diagnosis of lesions in the visual sensory pathway. In Walsh FB, Hoyt WF, (eds). *Clinical Neuro-ophthalmology*. 4th Edition. Baltimore, Williams & Wilkins, pp. 108–152.
Miller NR. (1982). Topical diagnosis of lesions in the visual sensory pathway. In Walsh FB, Hoyt WF, (eds). *Walsh and Hoyt's Clinical Neuro-ophthalmology*. 4th Edition. Baltimore, Williams & Wilkins, pp. 129–152.
Miller NR, Iliff WJ. (1975). Visual loss as the initial symptom in Hodgkin's disease. *Arch Ophthalmol 93:*1158–1161.
Mohr G, Hardy J, Gauvin P. (1985). Chiasmal apoplexy due to ruptured cavernous hemangioma of the optic chiasm. *Surg Neurol 24:*636–640.
Monteiro MLR, Hoyt WF, Imes RK. (1984). Puerperal cerebral blindness: Transient bilateral occipital involvement from presumed cerebral venous thrombosis. *Arch Neurol 41:*1300–1301.
Mojon DS, Odel JG, Rios RJ, Hirano M. (1997). Pituitary adenoma revealed by paracentral junctional scotoma of Traquair. *Ophthalmologica 211:*104–108.
Moster ML, Galetta SI, Schatz NJ. (1996). Physiologic functional imaging in "functional" visual loss. *Survey Ophthalmol 40:*395–399.
Moster ML, Savino PJ, Schatz NJ, Snyder PJ, Sergott RC, Bosley TM. (1986). Visual function in patients with prolactinoma treated with bromocriptine. *Ophthalmology 92:*1332–1341.
Muraji R, Epstein F. (1979). Diagnosis and treatment of suprasellar arachnoid cyst: Report of three cases. *J Neurosurg 50:*515.
Navarro IM, Peralta VHR, Leon JAM, et al. (1981). Tuberculous optochiasmatic arachnoiditis. *Neurosurgery 9:*654.
Neau J-P, Bogousslavsky J. (1996). The syndrome of posterior choroidal artery territory infarction. *Ann Neurol 39:*779–788.
Neelon FA, Goree J, Lebovitz H. (1973). The primary empty sella: Clinical and radiographic characteristics and endocrine function. *Medicine 52:*73–92.
Neetens A, Bultinck J, Martin JJ, Solheid J. (1980). Intrasellar adenoma and chordoma. *Neuro-ophthalmol 2:*123–135.
Neetens A, Mahler K, Bultinck J, Martin JJ. (1982). Sellar metastatic disease. *Neuro-ophthalmology 2:*225–265.
Nelson PB, Haverkos H, Martinez AJ, et al. (1983). Abscess formation within pituitary tumors. *Neurosurgery 12:*331.
Nepple EW, Appen RE, Sackett JF. (1978). Bilateral homonymous hemianopia. *Am J Ophthalmol 86:*536–543.
Newman RP, Kinkel WR, Jacobs L. (1984). Altitudinal hemianopia caused by occipital infarcts: Clinical and computerized topographic correlations. *Arch Neurol 41:*413–418.
Noble MJ, McFadzean R. (1987). Indirect injury to the optic nerves and chiasm. *Neuro-ophthalmology 7:*341.
Norwood EG, Kline LB, Chandra-Sekar B, et al. (1986). Aneurysmal compression of the anterior visual pathways. *Neurology 36:*1035–1041.
Obenchain TG, Killeffer FA, Stern WE. (1972). Indirect injury to the optic nerves and chiasm with closed head injury. *Bull Los Angeles Neurol Soc 37:*13–20.
O'Connell JEA. (1976). The anatomy of the optic chiasma and heteronymous hemianopia. *Mayo Clin Proc 51:*563.
O'Connor PS, Smith JL. (1979). Chiasmal ependymoma. *Ann Ophthalmol 11:*1424–1428.
O'Connor PS, Kasdon D, Tredici TJ, Ivan DJ. (1982). The Marcus Gunn pupil in experimental optic tract lesions. *Ophthalmology 89:*160–164.
Oliver M, Beller AJ, Behar A. (1968). Chiasmal arachnoiditis as a manifestation of generalized arachnoiditis in systemic vascular disease. *Br J Ophthalmol 52:*227–235.
Ormerod LD, Rhodes RH, Gross SA, et al. (1996). Ophthalmologic manifestations of acquired immune deficiency syndrome-associated progressive multifocal leukoencephalopathy. *Ophthalmology 103:*899–906.
Pahwa JM. (1963). Homonymous hemianopias from lesions of parietotemporal lobes. *Mediscope 5:*543–547.
Parkinson D, Craig WM. (1951). Tumours of the brain, occipital lobe: Their signs and symptoms. *Can Med Assoc J 64:*111–125.
Pasquier F, Leys D, Dubois F, et al. (1989). Chiasm and optic nerve necrosis following radiation therapy: Report of two cases. *Neuro-ophthalmol 9:*331.
Pessin MS, Kwan ES, DeWitt LD, et al. (1987). Posterior cerebral artery stenosis. *Ann Neurol 1:*85–89.
Pessin MS, Lathi ES, Cohen MB, et al. (1987). Clinical features and mechanism of occipital infarction. *Ann Neurol 21:*290–299.
Peter M, DeTribolet N. (1995). Visual outcome after transsphenoidal surgery for pituitary adenomas. *Br J Neurosurg 9:*151–157.
Petruson B, Jakobsson KE, Elfverson J, Bengtsson BA. (1995). Five-year follow-up of nonsecreting pituitary adenomas. *Arch Otolaryngol—Head and Neck Surg 121:*317–322.
Poon A, McNeill P, Harper A, O'Day J. (1995). Patterns of visual loss associated with pituitary macroadenomas. *Austr N Z J Ophthalmol 23:*107–115.
Poon M-C, Prehal JT, Murad TM, Galbraith JG. (1979). Multiple myeloma masquerading as chromophobe adenoma. *Cancer 43:*1513–1516.
Powers JM. (1985). Sarcoidosis of the tentorium with cortical blindness. *J Clin Neuro-ophthalmol 5:*112–115.
Prosperi L, Bernasconi S, Cantarelli A, Voccia E. (1978). Traumatic hypopituitarism associated with bitemporal hemianopia in a prepuberal child. *J Pediatr Ophthalmol Strab 15:*376–382.
Purvin V, Bonnin J, Goodman J. (1989). Palinopsia as a presenting manifestation of Creutzfeldt-Jacob disease. *J Clin Neuro-ophthalmol 9:*242–246.
Purvin V, Herr GJ, De Myer W. (1988). Chiasmal neuritis as a complication of Epstein-Barr infection. *Arch Neurol 45:*458.

Randall RV. (1984). Empty sella syndrome. *Compr Ther 10:*57.
Rao GP, Blyth CP, Jeffreys R. (1995). Ophthalmic manifestations of Rathke's cleft cysts. *Am J Ophthalmol 119:*86–91.
Regli L, Tribolet ND, Regli F, Bogousslavsky J. (1989). Chiasmal apoplexy: Hemorrhage from a cavernous malformation in the optic chiasm. *J Neurol Neurosurg Psychiatr 52:*1095–1099.
Resneck JD, Lederman IR. (1981). Traumatic chiasmal syndrome associated with pneumocephalus and sellar fracture. *Am J Ophthalmol 92:*233–237.
Reynolds WD, Smith JL, McCrary JA. (1982). Chiasmal optic neuritis. *J Clin Neuro-ophthalmol 2:*93–110.
Riishede J, Seedorff HH. (1974). Spontaneous hematoma of the optic chiasma. *Acta Ophthalmol 52:*317–322.
Rizzo JF III. (1993). Occult retinal and choroidal vascular disease. The value of timed and directed fluorescein angiography. *Ophthalmol 100:*1407–1416.
Rosenberg LF, Miller NR. (1984). Visual results after microsurgical removal of meningiomas involving the anterior visual system. *Arch Ophthalmol 102:*1019–1023.
Roski RA, Gardner JH, Spetzler RF. (1981). Intrachiasmatic arteriovenous malformation. *J Neurosurg 54:*540–541.
Rossi LN, Pastorino G, Scotti G, et al. (1994). Early diagnosis of optic glioma in children with neurofibromatosis type 1. *Childs Nerv Syst 10:*426–429.
Rush JA, Balis GA, Drake CG. (1981). Bitemporal hemianopsia in basilar artery aneurysm. *J Clin Neuro-ophthalmol 1:*129–133.
Sacks JG, Melen O. (1975). Bitemporal visual field defects in presumed multiple sclerosis. *JAMA 234:*69–72.
Salinas-Garcia RF, Smith JL. (1978). Binasal hemianopia. *Surg Neurol 10:*187–194.
Salmon JH. (1968). Transient postictal hemianopsia. *Arch Ophthalmol 79:*523–525.
Sato M, Tanaka S, Kohama A, Fujii C. (1986). Occipital lobe infarction caused by tentorial herniation. *Neurosurgery 18:*300–305.
Savino PJ, Glaser JS, Schatz NJ. (1980). Traumatic chiasmal syndrome. *Neurology 30:*963–970.
Savino PJ, Paris M, Schatz NJ, et al. (1978). Optic tract syndrome. *Arch Ophthalmol 96:*656–663.
Sawin PD, Follett KA, Wen BC, Laws ER Jr. (1996). Symptomatic intrasellar hemangioblastoma in a child treated with subtotal resection and adjuvant radiosurgery. Case report. *J Neurosurg 84:*1046–1050.
Schatz NJ, Lichtenstein S, Corbett JJ. (1975). Delayed radiation necrosis of the optic nerves and chiasm. In Glaser JS, Smith JL (eds). *Neuro-ophthalmology*. St. Louis, C.V. Mosby, Vol. 8, pp. 131–139.
Schneider RC, Kriss FC, Falls HF. (1970). Prechiasmal infarction associated with intrachiasmal and suprasellar tumors. *J Neurosurg 32:*197–208.
Scott GI. (1957). *Traquair's Clinical Perimetry*. 7th Edition. St. Louis, C.V. Mosby, p. 94.
Scott RM, Sonntag VKH, Wilcox LM, Adelman LS, Rockel TH. (1977). Visual loss from optochiasmatic arachnoiditis after tuberculous meningitis. *J Neurosurg 46:*524–526.
Segall HD, Hassan G, Ling SM, Carton C. (1974). Suprasellar cysts associated with isosexual precocious puberty. *Radiology 111:*607–616.
Shacklett DE, O'Connor PS, Dorwart AH, et al. (1984). Congruous and incongruous sectorial visual field defects with lesions of the lateral geniculate nucleus. *Am J Ophthalmol 98:*283–290.
Slavin ML. (1990). Acute homonymous field loss: Really a diagnostic dilemma. *Surv Ophthalmol 34:*399–407.
Slavin ML. (1990). Bitemporal hemianopia associated with dolichoectasia of the intracranial carotid arteries. *J Clin Neuro-ophthalmol 10:*80–81.
Slavin ML, Rosenthal AD. (1988). Chiasmal compression caused by a catheter in the suprasellar cistern. *Am J Ophthalmol 105:*560.
Smolik LA, Devercerski M, Nelson JS, Smith KR, Jr. (1968). Histiocytosis X in the optic chiasm of an adult with hypopituitarism. *J Neurosurg 29:*290–295.
Spector RH, Glaser JH, Schatz NJ. (1977). Chiasmal neuritis. *Brain 92:*123.
Spector RH, Glaser JH, Schatz NJ. (1980). Demyelinative chiasmal lesions. *Arch Neurol 37:*757–762.
Stelmach M, O'Day J. (1991). Rapid change in visual fields associated wtih suprasellar lymphocytic hypophysitis. *J Clin Neuro-ophthalmol 11:*19–24.
Studdard WE, Davis DO, Young SW. (1981). Cortical blindness after cerebral angiography: Case report. *J Neurosurg 54:*240–242.
Sugita K, Sato O, Hirota T, Tsugane R, Kageyama N. (1975). Scotomatous defects in the central visual field in pituitary adenomas. *Neurochirurgia 18:*155–162.
Takahashi T, Isayama Y. (1980). Chiasmal meningitis. *Neuro-ophthalmology 1:*19.
Takahashi T, Asai T, Isayama Y, Tamaki N, Matsumoto S. (1983). Chordoma. *J Clin Neuro-ophthalmol 3:*251–257.
Tang RA, Grotta JC, Lee KF, Lee YE. (1983). Chiasmal syndrome in sarcoidosis. *Arch Ophthalmol 101:*1069–1073.
Thompson JC, Kosmorsky GS, Ellis BD. (1996). Fields of dreamers and dreamed-up fields. Functional and fake perimetry. *Ophthalmology 103:*117–125.
Tibbs PA, Brooks WH. (1979). Traumatic bitemporal hemianopsia: case report. *J Trauma 19:*129–131.
Trick GL, Trick LR, Morris P, Wolf M. (1995). Visual field loss in senile dementia of the Alzheimer's type. *Neurology 45:*68–74.
Trobe JD, Glaser JS. (1983). *The Visual Fields Manual: A Practical Guide to Testing and Interpretation*. Gainesville, Triad, p. 176.
Trobe JD, Lorber ML, Schlezinger NS. (1973). Isolated homonymous hemianopia. *Arch Ophthalmol 89:*377–381.
Trobe JD, Tao AJ, Schuster JJ. (1984). Pre-chiasmal tumor: Diagnostic and prognostic features. *Neurosurgery 15:*391–399.

Troost BT, Newton TH. (1975). Occipital lobe arteriovenous malformations. Clinical and radiologic features in 26 cases with comments on differentiation from migraine. *Arch Ophthalmol 93:*250–256.

Van Buren JM, Baldwin M. (1958). The architecture of the optic radiations in the temporal lobe of man. *Brain 81:*15–40.

Vargas ME, Kupersmith MJ, Savino PJ, et al. (1995). Homonymous field defect as the first manifestation of Creutzfeldt-Jacob disease. *Am J Ophthalmol 119:*497–504.

Voelker JL, Campbell RL, Muller J. (1991). Clinical, radiographic, and pathological features of symptomatic Rathke's cleft cysts. *J Neurosurg 74:*535–544.

Waller RR, Riley FC, Sundt TM. (1972). A rare cause of the chiasmal syndrome. *Arch Ophthalmol 88:*269–272.

Walsh FB. (1966). Indirect trauma to the optic nerves and chiasm. *Invest Ophthalmol 5:*433–449.

Walsh TJ. (1974). Temporal crescent or half-moon syndrome. *Ann Ophthalmol 6:*501–505.

Walsh TJ, Smith JL. (1968). Sarcoidosis and suprasellar mass. In Smith JL (ed). *Neuro-ophthalmology Symposium.* St. Louis, C.V. Mosby, Vol. 4, pp. 167–177.

Warren FE, Vargas ME, Seidman I, Kupersmith MJ. (1992). *Homonymous field defect in an HIV negative, at risk individual.* Presented at the 24th Annual Frank B. Walsh Society Meeting. Los Angeles, CA, February 28–29.

Warrington BK Jr. (1962). The completion of visual forms across hemianopic field defects. *J Neurol Neurosurg Psychiatry 25:*208–217.

Weinstein GW, Powell SR, Thrush WP. (1987). Chiasmal neuropathy secondary to rheumatoid pachymeningitis. *Am J Ophthalmol 104:*439–440.

Weller M, Wiedemann P. (1989). Hysterical symptoms in ophthalmology. *Doc Ophthalmol 73:*1–33.

Wilhelm H, Grodd W, Schiefer U, Zrenner E. (1993). Uncommon chiasmal lesions: Demyelinating disease, vasculitis, and cobalamin deficiency. *Germ J Ophthalmol 2:*234–240.

Wilhelm H, Wilhelm B, Petersen D, et al. (1996). Relative afferent pupillary defects in patients with geniculate and retrogeniculate lesions. *Neuro-ophthalmology 16:*219–224.

Wilson P, Falconer MA. (1968). Patterns of visual failure with pituitary tumors: Clinical and radiologic correlations. *Br J Ophthalmol 52:*94–110.

Wilson SE, de Groen PC, Aksamit AJ, et al. (1988). Cyclosporine A-induced reversible cortical blindness. *J Clin Neuro-ophthalmol 8:*215–220.

Wybar K. (1977). Chiasmal compression. *Proc R Soc Med 70:*307–317.

Yamamoto M, Jimbo M, Ide M, Umebara Y, Hagiwara S, Kubo O. (1993). Recurrence of symptomatic Rathke's cleft cyst: A case report. *Surg Neurol 39:*263–268.

Yamamoto K, Saito K, Takai T, et al. (1983). Visual field defects and pituitary enlargement in primary hypothyroidism. *J Clin Endocrinol Metab 57:283.*

Zihl J, Von Cramon D. (1979). Restitution of visual function in patients with cerebral blindness. *J Neurol Neurosurg Psychiatry 42:*312–322.

◆ 10 ◆

Diplopia

In this chapter we divide diplopia into several categories (monocular versus binocular, transient versus permanent, horizontal versus vertical). We do not discuss every possible cause of diplopia in detail; instead we have chosen to emphasize certain key factors. Several entities are discussed in detail under specific chapters (e.g., third nerve palsy, myasthenia gravis, etc.). Our general evaluation for diplopia is outlined in Figure 10–1.

Is the Diplopia Monocular?

Monocular diplopia can usually be diagnosed by the history alone. Diplopia that is present monocularly remains present despite covering the fellow eye and then disappears when the involved eye is occluded. It may occur unilaterally or bilaterally. The second image is often described as a less clear and partially superimposed "ghost image" or a "halo" on the first image. A pinhole may dramatically reduce the patient's symptoms. Monocular diplopia usually implies a problem within the eye itself and may respond to refraction, artificial tear trial, or contact lens trial. Table 10–1 lists the ocular causes of monocular diplopia. Monocular diplopia does not require any further neuro-ophthalmologic evaluation.

Table 10–1. Ocular Causes of Monocular Diplopia

Refractive error (Coffeen, 1988; Hirst, 1983; Woods, 1996)
Astigmatism
Poorly fitting contact lens
Corneal
Keratoconus
Corneal surface abnormalities
Tear film disorders including dry eye
Refractive surgery
Corneal transplant
Lid abnormalities
Chalazion

(continued)

Table 10–1. *(continued)*

Iris abnormalities
Iridotomy/iridectomy
Miotic pupils
Lens
Cataract
Subluxation or dislocation
Intraocular lens
Positioning holes (Landry, 1987)
Decentered lens
Retinal abnormalities (Lepore, 1986; Smith, 1986)

Is the Diplopia Binocular?

Binocular diplopia is associated with ocular misalignment. Identification of specific clinical signs and symptoms may allow identification of specific etiologies for the diplopia.

Is the Diplopia Transient or Persistent?

Table 10–2 lists the causes of transient diplopia.

What Are the Causes of Transient or Intermittent Diplopia?

Diplopia may only be noted in certain fields of gaze (e.g., only on looking down in some patients with fourth nerve palsies) and may fluctuate during the day (e.g., the vertical diplopia of thyroid ophthalmopathy may be more apparent in the early morning). Patients with truly intermittent vertical diplopia may be asymptomatic at examination and vertical misalignment may be subtle or not demonstrated. Intermittent diplopia may be due to superior oblique myokymia, paroxysmal superior rectus and levator palpebrae spasm,

Table 10–2. Causes of Transient Diplopia

Transient ischemia (including migraine)
Decompensation of pre-existing phoria
Retinal hemifield slide phenomenon
Myasthenia gravis
Thyroid ophthalmopathy
Increased intraocular pressure
Intermittent phenomena
Neuromyotonia
Intermittent skew deviation
Superior oblique myokymia
Multiple sclerosis (days to weeks)

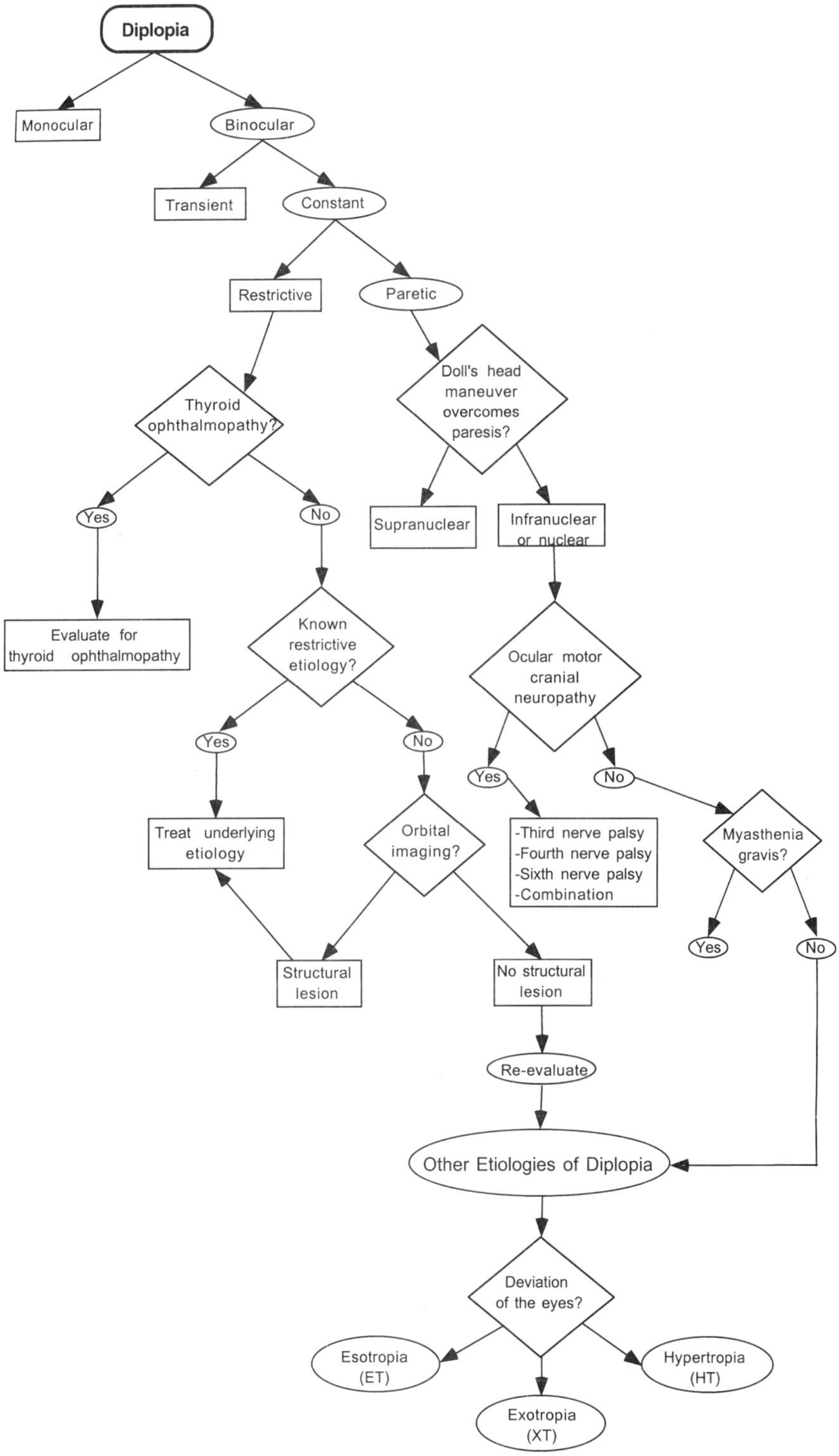

Figure 10–1. Evaluation of diplopia.

neuromyotonia, decompensating hyperphoria (intermittent tropia), ophthalmoplegic migraine, increased intracranial pressure, thyroid eye disease, myasthenia gravis, Brown's syndrome, intermittent or paroxysmal skew deviation, or the hemifield slip phenomena.

Superior oblique myokymia (SOM) is a disorder of unknown etiology characterized symptomatically by oscillopsia, vertical or torsional diplopia, or both. Affected patients show bursts of rotary oscillations of the eye of small amplitude and high frequency, slow frequency large-amplitude intorsional movements, or a combination of these paroxysms. Most patients with SOM complain of brief episodes of rapid vertical or torsional movements of the environment or shimmering sensations, usually lasting only a few seconds. They may also complain of brief episodes of vertical/torsional diplopia. Neuroophthalmologic examination of SOM patients often reveals brief episodes of rapid, fine, torsional movements of one eye that are best seen using either the slit lamp biomicroscope or the direct ophthalmoscope. The abnormal movements can be induced in some patients by having the patient move the affected eye downward and outward, by tilting the patient's head toward the side of the affected eye, by having the patient converge, or by having the patient move the affected eye downward and then moving it back to primary position.

Paroxysmal superior rectus and levator palpebrae spasm is a rare and unique disorder described in a single patient with multiple sclerosis (Ezra, 1996). Paroxysms of vertical diplopia and lid retraction in this patient lasted 3 to 4 seconds and examination revealed intermittent right hypertropia, lid retraction, and restriction of downgaze. MR imaging revealed multiple lesions consistent with multiple sclerosis, including a lesion in the midbrain in the region of the third nerve fascicle. Carbamazepine stopped all of the symptoms which were thought due to spontaneous spasm of the superior rectus/levator complex.

Ocular neuromyotonia is a rare disorder characterized by episodic diplopia, occurring either spontaneously or following sustained eccentric gaze (Ezra, 1996; Frohman, 1995; Morrow, 1996). Most patients have had prior radiation therapy to the sellar or parasellar region. In some cases, however, no responsible structural lesion or history of radiation therapy is noted. One case has been described due to nerve compression by an internal carotid aneurysm and another patient had fourth nerve involvement where spasms of the superior oblique muscle were induced only by alcohol intake (Ezra, 1996). ONM is thought to reflect impaired muscle relaxation due to inappropriate discharges from oculomotor, trochlear, or abducens neurons or axons with unstable cellular membranes. Patients with ONM often benefit from membrane stabilizing agents such as carbamazepine, often at low doses (Ezra, 1996; Frohman, 1995; Morrow, 1996).

Decompensation of a longstanding phoria may cause an intermittent tropia and episodic diplopia (Burde, 1991). Neuroophthalmologic history and examination often reveal supportive evidence for chronic strabismus including a history of childhood strabismus or patching, the presence of a head tilt or turn (old photos), and large vertical fusional amplitude (6–20 prism diopters).

Ophthalmoplegic migraine usually starts in the first decade of life and usually affects the oculomotor nerve, although rare trochlear nerve or multiple ocular motor nerve involvement has been described (Miller, 1991). Clinical criteria essential for the diagnosis of ophthalmoplegic migraine include (1) a history of typical migraine headache (severe, throbbing, unilateral but occasionally bilateral or alternating); headache may last hours to days; (2) ophthalmoplegia that may include one or more nerves and may alternate sides with attacks; extraocular muscle paralysis may occur with the first attack of headache or, rarely, precede it; usually, however, the paralysis appears subsequent to an established migraine pattern; (3) exclusion of other causes, by neuroimaging, surgery, or autopsy

(Walsh, 1960). Friedman et al. studied 5000 patients with migraine and found eight examples (0.16 percent) of ophthalmoplegic migraine (Friedman, 1962). All eight patients had recurrent attacks of headache (usually orbital), usually accompanied by nausea and vomiting, and an ipsilateral third nerve palsy. The third nerve paresis reached a maximum as the headache began to resolve and persisted for one to four weeks. The third nerve paralysis during the attack is often complete or nearly so, but partial third nerve paresis, including superior division third nerve paresis, may occur (Katz, 1989). Most patients have normal neuroophthalmologic examinations between attacks, but some patients may demonstrate partial third nerve paresis or even signs of aberrant regeneration. The differential diagnosis of ophthalmoplegic migraine is that of painful ophthalmoplegia in general; during the initial attack, structural lesions, especially aneurysms, should be suspected and the evaluation is that as described for third nerve palsies (Chapter 11). The diagnosis should thus be made with caution, especially if the first attack occurs in adulthood, and only after other causes of painful ophthalmoplegia have been excluded by appropriate laboratory and neuroimaging studies.

Transient diplopia may rarely occur with increased intracranial pressure (Harrington, 1953). A patient has been described with recurrent attacks of a right third nerve palsy causing diplopia in a setting of headache, papilledema, periodic urinary incontinence, and other neurologic findings. The transient third nerve palsies lasted about five minutes and eventually the patient developed a persistent third nerve palsy. At autopsy, the patient had right frontal and temporal brain metastases with right herniation of the hippocampal gyrus which stretched the right third nerve.

One of the most common causes of intermittent diplopia is myasthenia gravis. The ocular misalignment worsens with fatigue and improves with rest or Tensilon injection. As discussed in Chapter 15, this diagnosis should be considered in any patient with ptosis and/or ocular motor weakness without pupillary involvement. Weakness and fatigue confined to the extraocular muscles or lids combined with orbicularis oculi paresis is especially suggestive of OM. Significant clinical involvement of the pupil, eye pain or headaches, visual loss, or involvement of sensation essentially negate this diagnosis. Brown's syndrome may also cause intermittent vertical diplopia.

Skew deviation refers to vertical eye misalignment resulting from supranuclear derangements. This skew deviation may be constant or transient. It occurs whenever peripheral or central lesions cause an imbalance of graviceptive brainstem pathways and can accompany lesions at different areas of the brainstem (mesencephalon to medulla) or cerebellum. Skew deviation may appear as a comitant or incomitant vertical misalignment that is not associated with the presence of a primary and secondary deviation. Ductional limitations are absent. It rarely occurs in isolation and usually is accompanied by other neurologic signs and symptoms of brainstem involvement. Skew deviation may occasionally be intermittent and cause intermittent vertical diplopia (Allerand, 1962; Hedges, 1982; Straube, 1994). Intermittent skew deviation may be due to vertebrobasilar transient ischemic attacks or brainstem tumors. Thus, the presence of paroxysmal skew deviation requires MR imaging with attention to posterior fossa structures.

The hemifield slip phenomenon is a rare cause of intermittent binocular diplopia noted in some patients with lesions of the optic chiasm (Kirkham, 1972). This phenomenon occurs with complete or nearly complete bitemporal hemianopic visual field defects with disruption of ocular fusion and decompensation of a previous phoria. If the eyes intermittently converge, a blank space is produced between the vertical meridians as the eyes "slip" inwards; ocular divergence causes overlapping of the vertical meridians. Patients complain of intermittent diplopia and difficulty with near work (e.g., threading a needle or sewing). No ocular motor palsy is noted on examination but examination reveals a dense bitemporal hemianopsia. Hemifield slide diplopia may also occur from altitudinal visual field defects (Borchert, 1996). Two cases have been described in which heteronymous altitudinal field defects resulted in loss of fusion and transient overlap of preserved hemifields. This phenomenon resulted in complaints of diplopia similar to that described with bitemporal hemianopsia. The patients had superior altitudinal field defects in one eye and inferior defects in the other. One complained of vertical diplopia and the other had vertical and horizontal diplopia.

Is This an Ocular Motor Cranial Neuropathy?

Ocular motor cranial nerve palsies are discussed in the chapters for third nerve palsy (Chapter 11), fourth nerve palsy (Chapter 12), and sixth nerve palsy (Chapter 13).

Is There Evidence for a Restrictive Ophthalmoplegia Due to Orbital Disease?

Orbital signs, such as proptosis, chemosis, and injection, should be looked for in patients with diplopia. Forced ductions may reveal a restrictive component to the diplopia. Orbital wall fractures, orbital tumors, orbital inflammatory disease or trauma may result in a restrictive strabismus. Orbital imaging is indicated in these patients.

Is This Thyroid Eye Disease?

Although transient or persistent diplopia and ophthalmoplegia may occur without other signs of thyroid eye disease, identification of the distinctive signs of thyroid disease as described in Chapter 16 is essential in the evaluation of any patient with diplopia.

Is This a Supranuclear Process?

In patients with negative forced ductions and no evidence for restrictive ophthalmology, the doll's head maneuver (rapid forced head movements horizontally and vertically to activate the vestibulo-ocular reflex) may overcome a supranuclear ophthalmoplegia (see Chapter 14). Failure of the doll's head maneuver to overcome the ophthalmoplegia suggests an infranuclear etiology.

Is This Myasthenia Gravis?

The evaluation and management of myasthenia gravis is discussed in Chapter 15. Any patient with painless, pupil-spared, nonproptotic ophthalmoplegia or diplopia should be evaluated for the possible diagnosis of myasthenia gravis.

Is the Deviation Vertical or Horizontal?

If there are no distinctive or obvious signs to indicate diagnosis of a specific etiology for the diplopia, then the vertical or horizontal nature of the deviation may allow further classification of the problem.

What Are the Causes of Binocular Vertical Diplopia (Hypertropia/Hyperphoria)?

Patients with vertical diplopia complain of seeing two images, one atop or diagonally displaced from the other. If the patient complains of vertical diplopia in primary gaze, at least one of the vertically acting extraocular muscles is underacting: the right and/or left inferior rectus, superior rectus, inferior oblique, or superior oblique. One then asks if the vertical separation between images is worse on gaze to the left or right. If, for example, vertical separation of images is worse on gaze to the right, then four of the eight extraocular muscles may be underacting (the right superior or inferior rectus or the left inferior or superior oblique). If the separation is worse on gaze to the right and down, the right inferior rectus or left superior oblique must be underacting; if the image separation worsens or improves with left or right head tilt, torsional abnormalities, especially due to oblique muscle involvement, should be suspect.

Patients with binocular vertical diplopia generally adopt a compensatory head, face, or chin position to move their eyes into a gaze angle that achieves binocular single vision. Underaction of the superior or inferior rectus muscles is compensated by chin flexion or extension that seeks to avoid the eye position of maximum image separation. Torsional diplopia is usually caused by underaction of the superior or inferior oblique muscles and may be associated with an angular head tilt. This head tilt is assumed to avoid the vertical and torsional image separation.

The three-step test is a variation of the cover-uncover test that is important in the evaluation of vertical diplopia:

1. Determine whether there is a right or left hypertropia or hyperphoria in primary position. For example, if there is a right hypertropia in primary position, there is paresis of the right eye depressors (right inferior rectus or superior oblique) or left eye elevators (left superior rectus or inferior oblique).
2. Compare the amount of vertical deviation in right and left gaze. For example, if the right hypertropia increases in left gaze, either the right superior oblique or left superior rectus is underacting.
3. Compare the vertical deviation in right head tilt and left head tilt (Bielschowsky maneuver). For example, if the vertical deviation increases with right head tilt, the right superior oblique must be weak; if the hyperdeviation increases on left head tilt, the left superior rectus is weak.

Ocular torsion may be measured with the double Maddox rod test that utilizes a red Maddox rod over the right eye and a white Maddox rod over the left eye in a trial frame. A thin base-down prism may be placed before one eye to separate the horizontal lines induced. The tilt of the retinal image is opposite the tilt of the horizontal line, as seen by the patient. Therefore, when the line is seen slanted toward the nose, an excyclodeviation is present; if the tilt is toward the temple, an incyclodeviation is indicated. A simple mnemonic rule is that the line is always tilted in the direction in which the offending muscle would rotate the eye if it were acting alone (Spector, 1993). For example, a patient with right superior oblique muscle palsy will describe the red line to be lower than the white line and relatively intorted or slanted toward the nose. The Maddox rod is then turned until the two lines are parallel and the magnitude of the cyclotropia can be read off the trial frame. Cyclodeviation may also be noted with indirect ophthalmoscopy (Van Noorden, 1996). Normally, the average location of the fovea in relation to the optic nerve head is 0.3 disc diameters below a horizontal line extending through the geometric center of the optic disc. From this position, an imaginary horizontal line will cross the optic nerve head just below the halfway point between its geometric center and lower pole. Incyclotropia is present when the fovea appears above a line extending horizontally from the center of the optic nerve head and excyclotropia is present when the fovea is below a line extending horizontally from just below the lower pole of the optic disc. Finally, if restrictive ophthalmopathy is thought to be responsible for vertical misalignment, the forced duction test can be used to differentiate whether limitation of ocular movement is due to paresis of extraocular muscle or tethering of the antagonist extraocular muscle. Processes that may cause binocular vertical diplopia and/or hypertropia/hyperphoria are listed in Table 10–3.

Table 10–3. Etiologies of Binocular Vertical Diplopia and Hypertropia/Hyperphoria

- Supranuclear causes
  - Supranuclear monocular elevation paresis (congenital or acquired)
  - Paroxysmal superior rectus and levator palpebrae spasm with multiple sclerosis (see Chapter 17)
  - Skew deviation (see Chapter 14)
  - Vertical one-and-a-half syndrome
  - Wernicke's syndrome
- Ocular motor nerve dysfunction
  - Third nerve palsy (see Chapter 11)
  - Fourth nerve palsy (see Chapter 12)
  - Superior oblique myokymia (see Chapter 17)
  - Ocular neuromyotonia
  - Decompensation of a longstanding phoria
  - Sixth nerve palsy
- Ophthalmoplegic migraine
  - Wernicke's syndrome
  - Fisher's syndrome
  - Guillain-Barré syndrome
- Neuromuscular junction disease
  - Myasthenia gravis (see Chapter 15)
  - Botulism
- Diseases of eye muscle
  - Decompensation of a longstanding phoria
  - Congenital strabismus syndromes
  - Dissociated vertical deviation (DVD)
  - Congenital "double elevator" palsy (monocular elevation deficiency)
  - Double depressor paralysis (unilateral paralysis of the inferior rectus and superior oblique) (congenital or acquired)

- Isolated paresis of a vertical-acting extraocular muscle (e.g., due to congenital causes, myasthenia gravis, Graves' disease, botulism, trauma, post-surgery, trochleitis, orbital metastasis, orbital pseudotumor, muscle ischemia from giant cell arteritis, etc.)
  - Superior oblique muscle
  - Inferior oblique muscle
  - Superior rectus muscle
  - Inferior rectus muscle
- Graves' disease
- Chronic progressive external ophthalmoplegia (CPEO) syndromes
- After surgery (e.g., cataract operation) physiologic hyperdeviation on lateral gaze (asymptomatic)

Mechanical processes causing vertical eye misalignment

- Graves' disease (see Chapter 16)
- Brown's superior oblique tendon sheath syndrome
  - Congenital
  - Acquired (e.g., due to superomedial orbital trauma, tenosynovitis or myositis, adhesions, metastasis to the superior oblique muscle, frontal sinus osteoma, pansinusitis, peribulbar anesthesia, blepharoplasty, maxillo-facial or sinus surgery, and superior oblique tuck)
- Acquired Brown's syndrome associated with underaction of the ipsilateral superior oblique muscle ("canine tooth syndrome")
- Orbital floor blowout fracture
- Direct trauma to the extraocular muscles (e.g., intramuscular hematoma)
- Congenital inferior rectus fibrosis
- Strabismus fixus (generalized fibrosis of extraocular muscles)
- Postoperative sequelae (including retinal detachment surgery, orbital surgery, strabismus surgery, and cataract surgery)
- Orbital inflammation (myositis) and pseudotumor
- Metastatic infiltration of extraocular muscles
- Orbital tumors
- Fallen eye syndrome (longstanding superior oblique muscle paresis in patient who habitually fixate with the paretic eye may develop hypodeviation of the uninvolved eye caused by contracture of the contralateral inferior rectus muscle)
- Rising eye syndrome (longstanding inferior oblique muscle palsy may result in contracture and fibrosis of the contralateral superior rectus muscle

Retinal disease and other processes affecting the visual pathways

- Foveal displacement syndrome (e.g., due to subretinal neovascular membranes)
- Hemifield slip phenomenon from dense bitemporal hemianopsia or heteronymous altitudinal field defects

---

Sources: Allerand, 1962; Alonso-Valdivielso, 1993; Baker, 1991; Bell, 1990; Borchert, 1996; Bogousslavsky, 1984; Brandt, 1987, 1993, 1994; Brazis, 1992; Burde, 1991; Burgess, 1980; Capo, 1996; Deleu, 1991; Engle, 1997; Erie, 1990; Esaki, 1992; Ezra, 1996; Fisher, 1981; Ford, 1984; Friedman, 1962; Frohman, 1985, 1995; Gopal, 1988; Halmagyi, 1990; Hansen, 1968; Harrington, 1953; Hedges, 1982; Helveston, 1980; Hommel, 1990; Hudson, 1992; Hunter, 1995; Hughes, 1992; Hupp, 1990; Jampel, 1968; Katz, 1989; Keane, 1975, 1985, 1992; Kirkham, 1972; Knapp, 1974, 1976; Lessell, 1975; Mazdow, 1979; Merikangas, 1978; Metz, 1976; Miller, 1991; Pearlman, 1972; Rush, 1982; Safran, 1994; Saunders, 1990; Scott, 1980; Slavin, 1988, 1989; Spector, 1993; Straube, 1994; Tatemichi, 1992; Thomke, 1992; Walsh, 1960; Wiest, 1996; Wilson, 1989; von Noorden, 1970, 1986, 1991, 1996; Ziffer, 1992; Zipf, 1973.

Binocular diplopia may result from supranuclear processes, ocular motor nerve dysfunction, neuromuscular junction disease, disease of the eye muscle, mechanical processes, retinal disease, and disease affecting the visual pathways. Etiologies of horizontal diplopia are listed in Table 10–4.

Table 10–4. Etiologies of Acquired Horizontal Diplopia

- Esotropia
  - Acute comitant esotropia
  - Childhood strabismus
    - Infantile esotropia
    - Accommodative esotropia
      - Refractive
      - Nonrefractive
      - Hypoaccommodative
    - Non-accommodative esotropia
    - Partially accommodative esotropia
    - Microtropia
  - Consecutive esotropia (after strabismus surgery)
  - Decompensated esophoria
  - Divergence insufficiency/paralysis
  - Duane's syndrome Type 1
  - Esotropia of myopia
  - Fusional deficiency
  - Myasthenia gravis
  - Myositis (orbital pseudotumor)
  - Nystagmus blockage syndrome
  - Restrictive strabismus
    - Congenital fibrosis
    - Orbital medial wall fracture
    - Postsurgical
    - Esotropia associated with high myopia
  - Sensory esotropia
  - Sixth nerve palsy
  - Spasm of the near reflex
  - Thalamic esotropia
  - Thyroid eye disease
- Exotropia
  - Consecutive exotropia (after strabismus surgery)
  - Convergence insufficiency
  - Decompensated exophoria
  - Fusional deficiency (Pratt-Johnson, 1973, 1979)
  - Internuclear ophthalmoplegia
  - Myasthenia gravis
  - Myositis (orbital pseudotumor)
  - Pontine paralytic exotropia
  - Restrictive strabismus
    - Congenital fibrosis
    - Postsurgical
  - Sensory exotropia
  - Thyroid eye disease (uncommonly exodeviation)

What Are the Causes of Esotropia?

We do not discuss in detail every cause of esotropia. Instead, we focus on the major entities in the differential diagnosis and discuss selected entities of particular neuro-ophthalmologic interest.

Acute comitant esotropia at distance and near in childhood should raise the concern of underlying central nervous system malignancy and these patients should undergo neuroimaging studies (Anderson, 1970; Burian, 1958; Micatavage, 1972; Williams, 1989; Zweifach, 1981).

What Constitutes Convergence Insufficiency?

The clinical features of convergence insufficiency include a remote near point of convergence; decreased fusional convergence at near; and a variable exophoria at near. Convergence insufficiency is associated with stress, fatigue, and anxiety and may follow infection (e.g., diphtheria, mononucleosis, encephalitis) or trauma. Therapy for convergence insufficiency includes orthoptic, prism, or surgical treatment. An associated accommodative insufficiency may accompany the convergence insufficiency (von Noorden, 1973, 1976).

What Is Convergence Paralysis?

Patients with convergence paralysis as opposed to convergence insufficiency often harbor an intracranial lesion (midbrain). There is crossed diplopia at near. Preservation of accommodation or pupillary miosis at near confirms an organic etiology. Other associated neurologic features of the dorsal midbrain syndrome may be present (e.g., light-near dissociation, convergence retraction nystagmus, vertical gaze palsy) (see Chapter 14). A number of conditions may be associated with convergence paralysis including encephalitis, multiple sclerosis, or neurosyphilis.

What Is Convergence Spasm?

Sustained intermittent episodes of maximal convergence that are associated with accommodative spasm, induced myopia, and miosis may result in a variable esotropia. Although frequently nonorganic, convergence spasm has been reported in encephalitis, tabes, labyrinthine fistulas, Chiari malformation, pituitary adenoma, posterior fossa neurofibroma, and trauma (Dagi, 1987; Souders, 1969).

What Constitutes Divergence Insufficiency and Divergence Paralysis?

Divergence insufficiency is characterized by intermittent or constant esotropia at distance with fusion at near (Moore, 1971). There is little change in the deviation in lateral gaze and abduction is relatively full bilaterally. The fusional divergence may be diminished or absent (Cunningham, 1972; Jampolsky, 1970; Moore, 1971). Divergence paralysis is characterized by a complete loss of divergence amplitudes and is felt to be a sign of an underlying organic lesion of the intracranial pathway (e.g., increased intracranial pressure, head trauma, encephalitis, tabes dorsalis, demyelinating disease, vascular disease, and intracranial tumors). Bilateral sixth nerve palsy must be excluded in these patients (Kirkham, 1972; Roper-Hall, 1987; Rutkowski, 1972; Stern, 1986).

What Is Convergence Insufficiency?

Patients with an exodeviation that is greater at near (15 prism diopters) than distance have a convergence insufficiency pattern. It may occur following systemic infections (e.g., diphtheria, mononucleosis, encephalitis, etc.); head trauma; or without definite etiology. Adduction is normal bilaterally. No intracranial lesions are usually associated with convergence insufficiency (Mazow, 1989; von Noorden, 1973).

What Is Convergence Paralysis?

Patients with convergence paralysis, unlike convergence insufficiency, usually harbor an intracranial lesion. The patient is unable to converge, has diplopia at near, and there may or may not be associated accommodation paresis. Etiologies include head trauma, toxins, encephalitis, demyelination, and syphilis (Gilad, 1986).

What Is Acquired Motor Fusion Deficiency?

Loss of both fusional convergence and divergence may occur after head trauma, stroke, brain tumor, or neurosurgery (Pratt-Johnson, 1973, 1979). Despite apparent ocular alignment, patients may develop transient or permanent diplopia. Fusional amplitudes are absent, but sensory fusion and stereopsis are intact during brief episodes of fusion (Harrison, 1987; Hart, 1969; MacLellan, 1974).

References

Allerand CD. (1962). Paroxysmal skew deviation in association with brainstem glioma: Report of an unusual case. *Neurology 12*:520–523.

Alonso-Valdivielso JL, Alvarez Lario B, Alegre Lopez J, et al. (1993). Acquired Brown's syndrome in a patient with systemic lupus erythematosus. *Ann Rheum Dis 52*:63–64.

Anderson WD, Lubow M. (1970). Astrocytoma of the corpus callosum presenting with acute comitant esotropia. *Am J Ophthalmol 69*:594–598.

Baker RS, Epstein AD. (1991). Ocular motor abnormalities from head trauma. *Survey Ophthalmol 35*:245–267.

Bell JA, Fielder AR, Viney S. (1990). Congenital double elevator palsy in identical twins. *J Clin Neuro-ophthalmol 10*:32–34.

Bogousslavsky J, Regli F. (1984). Upgaze palsy and monocular paresis of downward gaze from ipsilateral thalmo-mesencephalic infarction: A vertical "one-and-a-half" syndrome. *J Neurol 231*:43–45.

Borchert MS, Lessell S, Hoyt WF. (1996). Hemifield slide diplopia from altitudinal visual field defect. *J Neuro-ophthalmology 16*:107–109.

Brandt T, Dieterich M. (1987). Pathological eye-head coordination in roll: Tonic ocular tilt reaction in mesencephalic and medullary lesions. *Brain 110*:649–666.

Brandt T, Dieterich M. (1993). Skew deviation with ocular torsion: A vestibular brainstem sign of topographic diagnostic value. *Ann Neurol 33*:528–534.

Brandt T, Dieterich M. (1994). Vestibular syndromes in the roll plane: Topographic diagnosis from brainstem to cortex. *Ann Neurol 36*:337–347.

Brandt T, Dieterich M. (1996). Central vestibular syndromes in the roll, pitch, and yaw planes. *Neuro-ophthalmol 15*:291–303.

Brazis PW. (1992). Ocular motor abnormalities in Wallenberg's lateral medullary syndrome. *Mayo Clin Proc 67*:365–368.

Burde RM, Savino PJ, Trobe JD. (1991). *Clinical Decisions in Neuro-ophthalmology*. 2nd Edition. St Louis, Mosby Yearbook, p. 227.

Burgess D, Roper-Hall G, Burde RM. (1980). Binocular diplopia associated with subretinal neovascular membranes. *Arch Ophthalmol 98*:311–317.

Burian HM, Miller JE. (1958). Comitant convergent strabismus with acute onset. *Am J Ophthalmol 45*:55–64.

Capó H, Guyton DL. (1996). Ipsilateral hypertropia after cataract surgery. *Ophthalmology 103*:721–730.

Capó H, Roth E, Johnson T, et al. (1996). Vertical strabismus after cataract surgery. *Ophthalmology 103*:918–921.

Coffeen P, Guyton DL. (1988). Monocular diplopia accompanying ordinary refractive errors. *Am J Ophthalmol 105*:451.

Cunningham RD. (1972). Divergence paralysis. *Am J Ophthalmol 74*:630.

Dagi LR, Chrousos GA, Cogan DC. (1987). Spasm of the near reflex associated with organic disease. *Am J Ophthalmol 103*:582.

Deleu D, Ebinger G. (1991). Vertical one-and-a-half syndrome. Clinical, oculographic and radiologic findings. *J Neuro-ophthalmol 11*:99.

Dieterich M, Brandt T. (1993). Ocular torsion and tilt of subjective visual are sensitive brainstem signs. *Ann Neurol 33*:292–299.

Engle EC, Goumnerov BC, McKeown CA, et al. (1997). Oculomotor nerve and muscle abnormalities in congenital fibrosis of the extraocular muscles. *Ann Neurol 41*:314–325.

Erie JC. (1990). Acquired Brown's syndrome after peribulbar anesthesia. *Am J Ophthalmol 109*:349–350.

Esaki H, Shinji O. (1992). Skew deviation in Fisher's syndrome. *Neuro-ophthalmol JPN 9:*66.

Ezra E, Plant GT. (1996). Paroxysmal superior rectus and levator palpebrae spasm: A unique presentation of multiple sclerosis. *Br J Ophthalmol 80:*187–188.

Ezra E, Spalton D, Sanders MD, et al. (1996). Ocular neuromyotonia. *Br J Ophthalmol 80:*350–355.

Fisher M. (1981). Ocular skew deviation in hepatic coma. *J Neurol Neurosurg Psychiatry 44:*458.

Ford CS, Schwartze GM, Weaver RG, Troost BT. (1984). Monocular elevation paresis caused by an ipsilateral lesion. *Neurology 34:*1264–1267.

Friedman AP, Harter DH, Merritt HH. (1962). Ophthalmoplegic migraine. *Arch Neurol 7:*320–327.

Frohman EM, Zee DS. (1995). Ocular neuromyotonia: Clinical features, physiological mechanisms, and response to therapy. *Ann Neurol 37:*620–626.

Frohman LP, Kupersmith MJ. (1985). Reversible vertical ocular deviations associated with raised intracranial pressure. *J Clin Neuro-ophthalmol 5:*158–163.

Gilad E, Biger Y. (1986). Paralysis of convergence caused by mushroom poisoning. *Am J Ophthalmol 102:*124.

Gopal KSS. (1988). Acquired double depressor palsy. *Indian J Ophthalmol 36:*35–38.

Halmagyi GM, Brandt T, Dieterich M, et al. (1990). Tonic contraversive ocular tilt reaction due to unilateral mesodiencephalic lesion. *Neurology 40:*1503–1509.

Hansen E. (1968). Congenital general fibrosis of the extraocular muscles. *Acta Ophthalmol 46:*469–476.

Harrington DO, Flocks M. (1953). Ophthalmoplegic migraine. Pathogenesis; report of pathologic findings in a case of recurrent oculomotor paralysis. *Arch Ophthalmol 49:*643–655.

Harrison RL. (1987). Loss of fusional vergence with partial loss of accommodative convergence and accommodation following head injury. *Binoc Vision 2:*93.

Hart CT. (1969). Disturbances of fusion following head injury. *Proc R Soc Med 62:*704.

Hedges TR, Hoyt WF. (1982). Ocular tilt reaction due to an upper brainstem lesion: Paroxysmal skew deviation, torsion, and oscillation of the eyes with head tilt. *Ann Neurol 11:*537–540.

Helveston EM, Bick S, Ellis FD. (1980). Differential intraocular pressure as an indirect measure of generated muscle force. *Ophthalmic Surg 11:*386–391.

Hirst LW, Miller NR, Johnson RT. (1983). Monocular polyopia. *Arch Neurol 40:*756.

Hommel M, Bogousslavsky DC. (1990). The spectrum of vertical gaze palsy following unilateral brainstem stroke. *Neurology 41:*1229–1234.

Hudson HL, Feldon SE. (1992). Late overcorrection of hypotropia in Graves' ophthalmopathy. *Ophthalmology 99:*356–360.

Hughes DS, Beck L, Hill R, Plenty J. (1992). Dysthyroid eye disease presenting as Brown's syndrome. *Acta Ophthalmol 70:*262–265.

Hunter DG, Lam GC, Guyton DL. (1995). Inferior oblique muscle injury from local anesthesia for cataract surgery. *Ophthalmology 102:*501–509.

Hupp SL, Williams JP, Curran JE. (1990). Computerized tomography in the diagnosis of congenital fibrosis syndrome. *J Clin Neuro-ophthalmol 10:*135–139.

Jampel RS, Fells P. (1968). Monocular elevation paresis caused by a central nervous system lesion. *Arch Ophthalmol 80:*45–57.

Jampolsky A. (1970). Ocular divergence mechanisms. *Trans Am Ophthalmol Soc 68:*748.

Katz B, Rimmer S. (1989). Ophthalmoplegic migraine with superior ramus oculomotor paresis. *J Clin Neuro-ophthalmol 9:*181–183.

Keane JR. (1975). Ocular skew deviation. Analysis of 100 cases. *Arch Neurol 32:*185–190.

Keane JR. (1985). Alternating skew deviation: 47 patients. *Neurology 35:*725–728.

Keane JR. (1992). Ocular tilt reaction following lateral pontomedullary infarction. *Neurology 42:*259–260.

Kirkham TH. (1972). The ocular symptomatology of pituitary tumors. *Proc R Soc Med 65:*517–518.

Kirkham TH, Bird AC, Sanders MD. (1972). Divergence paralysis with increased intracranial pressure. *Br J Ophthalmol 56:*776.

Knapp P. (1974). Classification and treatment of superior oblique palsy. *Am Orthopt J 24:*18–22.

Knapp P, Moore S. (1976). Diagnosis and surgical options in superior oblique surgery. *Int Ophthalmol Clin 15:*137.

Landry RA. (1987). Unwanted optical effects caused by intraocular lens positioning holes. *J Cat Refract Surg 13:*421–423.

Lepore FE, Yarian DL. (1986). Monocular diplopia of retinal origin. *J Clin Neuro-ophthalmol 6:*181.

Lessell S. (1975). Supranuclear paralysis of monocular elevation. *Neurology 25:*1134–1143.

MacLellan AV. (1974). A case of recovery from traumatic loss of fusion. *Br Orthoptic J 31:*102.

Mazdow ML. (1979). The 4-step test for the diagnosis of paralytic and/or restrictive strabismus. *Ophthalmology 86:*1297–1400.

Mazdow ML, France TD. (1989). Acute accommodative and convergence insufficiency. *Trans Am Ophthalmol Soc 87:*158.

Merikangas JR. (1978). Skew deviation in pseudotumor cerebri. *Ann Neurol 4:*583.

Metz HS. (1976). Forced duction, active forced generation and saccadic velocity test. In Ellis FD, Helveston EN (eds). *Strabismus Surgery.* Boston, Little Brown.

Mickatavage RC. (1972). Neuro-ophthalmological disease presenting as orthoptic problems. *Am Orthoptic J 22:*44–46.

Miller NR. (1991). *Walsh and Hoyt's Clinical Neuro-ophthalmology.* 4th Edition. Baltimore, Williams & Wilkins, pp. 2533–2538.

Moore S, Harbison JW, Stockbridge L. (1971). Divergence insufficiency. *Am Orthopt J 21:*59.

Morrow MJ, Kao GW, Arnold AC. (1996). Bilateral ocular neuromyotonia: Oculographic correlations. *Neurology 46:*264–266.

Moster ML, Schatz NJ, Savino PJ, et al. (1988). Alternating skew deviation on lateral gaze (bilateral abducting hypertropia). *Ann Neurol 23:*190–192.

Moster ML, Bosley TM, Slavin ML, Rubin SE. (1992). Thyroid ophthalmopathy presenting as superior oblique paresis. *J Clin Neuro-ophthalmol 12:*94–97.

Pearlman JT, Christensen RE. (1972). Motility problems following retinal detachment surgery. *Am Orthopt J 22:*64–67.

Pratt-Johnson JA. (1973). Central disruption of fusional amplitude. *Br J Ophthalmol 57:*347.

Pratt-Johnson JA, Tillson G. (1979). Acquired central disruption of fusional amplitude. *Ophthalmology 86:*2140.

Roper-Hall G, Burde RM. (1987). Diagnosis and management of divergence paresis. *Am Orthoptic J 37:*113–121.

Rush JA, Shafrin F. (1982). Ocular myasthenia presenting as superior oblique weakness. *J Clin Neuro-ophthalmol 2:*125–127.

Rutkowski PC, Burian HM. (1972). Divergence paralysis following head trauma. *Am J Ophthalmol 73:*660.

Safran AB, Vibert D, Issoua D, Hausler A. (1994). Skew deviation after vestibular neuronitis. *Am J Ophthalmol 118:*238–245.

Saunders RA, Stratas BA, Gordon RA, Holgate RC. (1990). Acute-onset Brown's syndrome associated with pansinusitis. *Arch Ophthalmol 108:*58–60.

Scott WE. (1980). Surgical considerations in paretic strabismus based on special diagnostic techniques. *Am Orthopt J 30:*40–43.

Sener EC, Özkan SB, Aribal ME, et al. (1996). Evaluation of congenital Brown's syndrome with magnetic resonance imaging. *Eye 10:*492–496.

Slavin ML. (1989). Hyperdeviation associated with isolated unilateral abducens palsy. *Ophthalmology 96:*512–516.

Slavin ML, Potash SD, Rubin SE. (1988). Asymptomatic physiologic hyperdeviation in peripheral gaze. *Ophthalmology 95:*778–781.

Smith JL. (1986). Monocular diplopia. *J Clin Neuro-ophthalmol 6:*184.

Souders BF. (1969). Functional ocular deviation. *Am Orthopt J 19:*55.

Spector RH. (1993). Vertical diplopia. *Surv Ophthalmol 38:*31–62.

Stern RM, Tomsak RL. (1986). Magnetic resonance images in a case of "divergence paralysis." *Surv Ophthalmol 30:*397–401.

Straube A, Büttner U, Brandt T. (1994). Recurrent attacks with skew deviation, torsional nystagmus, and contraction of the left frontalis muscle. *Neurology 44:*177–178.

Tatemichi TK, Steinke W, Duncan C, et al. (1992). Paramedian thalamopeduncular infarction: Clinical syndromes and magnetic resonance imaging. *Ann Neurol 32:*162–171.

Thomke F, Hopf HC. (1992). Acquired monocular elevation paresis. An asymmetric up-gaze palsy. *Brain 115:*1901–1910.

von Noorden GK. (1970). Congenital hereditary ptosis with inferior rectus fibrosis. *Arch Ophthalmol 83:*378–380.

von Noorden GK. (1976). Resection of both medial rectus muscles in organic convergence insufficiency. *Am J Ophthalmol 81:*223.

von Noorden GK. (1996). *Binocular Vision and Ocular Motility. Theory and Management of Strabismus.* Fifth Edition. St Louis, Mosby-Yearbook.

von Noorden GK, Hansell R. (1991). Clinical characteristics and treatment of isolated inferior rectus paralysis. *Ophthalmology 98:*253–257.

von Noorden GK, Brown DJ, Parks M. (1973). Associated convergence and accommodative insufficiency. *Doc Ophthalmol 34:*393.

von Noorden GK, Murray E, Wong SY. (1986). Superior oblique paralysis. A review of 270 cases. *Arch Ophthalmol 104:*1771–1776.

Walsh JP, O'Doherty DS. (1960). A possible explanation of the mechanism of ophthalmoplegic migraine. *Neurology 10:*1079–1084.

Wiest G, Baumgartner C, Schnider P, et al. (1995). Monocular elevation paresis and contralateral downgaze paresis from unilateral mesodiencephalic infarction. *J Neurol Neurosurg Psychiatry 60:*579–581.

Williams AS, Hoyt CS. (1989). Acute comitant esotropia in children with brain tumors. *Arch Ophthalmol 107:*376–378.

Wilson ME, Eustis HS Jr, Parks MM. (1985). Brown's syndrome. *Survey Ophthalmol 34:*153–172.

Woods RL, Bradley A, Atchison DA. (1996). Monocular diplopia caused by ocular aberrations and hyperopic defocus. *Vision Research 36:*3597–3606.

Ziffer AJ, Rosenbaum AL, Demer JL, Yee RD. (1992). Congenital double elevator palsy: Vertical saccadic velocity utilizing the scleral search coil technique. *J Pediatr Ophthalmol Strabismus 29:*142–149.

Zipf RF, Trokel SL. (1973). Simulated superior oblique tendon sheath syndrome following orbital floor fracture. *Am J Ophthalmol 75:*700–705.

Zweifach PH. (1981). Childhood esotropia with delayed appearance of cerebellar tumor. *Neuro-ophthalmology 1:*291–293.

◆ 11 ◆

Third Nerve Palsies

The oculomotor nerve (third cranial nerve) supplies four extraocular muscles (medial, superior and inferior recti, and inferior oblique) as well as the levator of the lid, and contains parasympathetic fibers that supply the sphincter of the pupil and the ciliary body. A complete peripheral third nerve palsy thus causes ptosis, a fixed and dilated pupil, and a "down and out" resting eye position. Partial third nerve palsies may cause (in combination or isolation) variable ptosis; variable paresis of eye adduction, elevation, and depression; and variable pupillary involvement. In this section, we discuss the localization of third nerve palsies (TNP) associated with other neurologic signs (non-isolated third nerve palsies) (Table 11–1) and third nerve palsies without other associated neurologic or neuro-ophthalmologic deficits (isolated third nerve palsies). We propose a diagnostic approach for non-isolated and isolated third nerve palsies in Figure 11–1. Finally, we examine the phenomena of aberrant regeneration of the third cranial nerve.

Table 11–1. The Localization of Oculomotor Nerve Lesions

Structure Involved	Clinical Manifestation
Lesions affecting the oculomotor nucleus	
Oculomotor nucleus	Ipsilateral complete CN III palsy; contralateral ptosis and superior rectus paresis
Oculomotor subnucleus	Isolated muscle palsy (e.g., inferior rectus)
Isolated levator subnucleus	Isolated bilateral ptosis
Paramedian mesencephalon	Plus-minus syndrome (ipsilateral ptosis and contralateral eyelid retraction)
Lesions affecting the oculomotor fasciculus	
Isolated fascicle	Partial or complete isolated CN III palsy with or without pupil involvement
Fascicle, red nucleus, superior cerebellar peduncle	Ipsilateral CN III palsy with contralateral ataxia and tremor (Claude)

(continued)

Table 11–1. *(continued)*

Structure Involved	Clinical Manifestation
Fascicle and cerebral peduncle	Ipsilateral CN III palsy with contralateral hemiparesis (Weber)
Fascicle and red nucleus/substantia nigra	Ipsilateral CN III palsy with contralateral choreiform movements (Benedikt)
Lesions affecting the oculomotor nerve in the subarachnoid space	
Oculomotor nerve	Complete CN III palsy with or without other cranial nerve involvement; superior or inferior division palsy
Lesions affecting the oculomotor nerve in the cavernous sinus	
Cavernous sinus lesion	Painful or painless CN III palsy; with or without palsies of CN IV, VI, and V1; CN III palsy with small pupil (Horner's syndrome); Primary aberrant CN III regeneration
Lesions affecting the oculomotor nerve in the superior orbital fissure	
Superior orbital fissure lesion	CN III palsy with or without palsies of CN IV, VI, V1; often with proptosis
Lesion affecting the oculomotor nerve in the orbit	
Oculomotor nerve; superior or inferior branch lesion	CN III palsy; superior or inferior CN III branch palsy
Optic nerve; orbital structures	Visual loss; proptosis; swelling of lids; chemosis

Source: From Brazis, PW, Masdeu, JC, and Biller, J. *Localization in Clinical Neurology*. Third Edition. Boston, Little Brown, 1996. With permission.

Is the TNP Isolated or Non-isolated? Can the TNP Be Localized?

Non-isolated TNP should undergo neuroimaging, with attention to areas suggested topographically by the associated neurologic signs and symptoms. Appropriate investigations and neuro-imaging studies are directed at the precise area of interest and this area determined by the "company kept" by the third nerve palsy (Brazis, 1991). In general, magnetic resonance (MR) imaging with and without gadolinium enhancement is the neuro-imaging modality of choice for all these processes (Renowden, 1993). Contrast-enhanced computerized tomography (CT) scanning with narrow (2 mm) collimation is reserved for those cases that cannot tolerate MR scan or in whom MR scan is contraindicated (e.g., pacemaker, claustrophobia, metallic clips in head, etc.) (Renowden, 1993; Teasdale, 1990). CT scanning is also the appropriate first choice neuroimaging study in patients being evaluated for acute head trauma or acute vascular events (infarction or hemorrhage). If there are clinical signs of a meningeal process, lumbar puncture should be performed. The evaluation of a patient with TNP is summarized in Figure 11–1.

Lesions of the third nerve nucleus are rare and often associated with other signs of mesencephalic involvement, especially vertical gaze impairment (Antworth, 1987; Bengel, 1994; Biller, 1984; Bogousslavsky, 1983, 1994; Chee, 1990; Gaymard, 1990; Kömpf, 1987; Reagan, 1978; Tognetti, 1988; Traboulsi, 1985; Zackon 1984). Nuclear lesions may be caused by infarction, hemorrhage, malformations, tumor, trauma, or infection and thus should be investigated by MR scan. Paresis of an isolated muscle innervated by the oculomotor nerve almost always results from a lesion in the orbit or from disease of the muscle or neuromuscular junction; for example, isolated inferior rectus paresis may develop

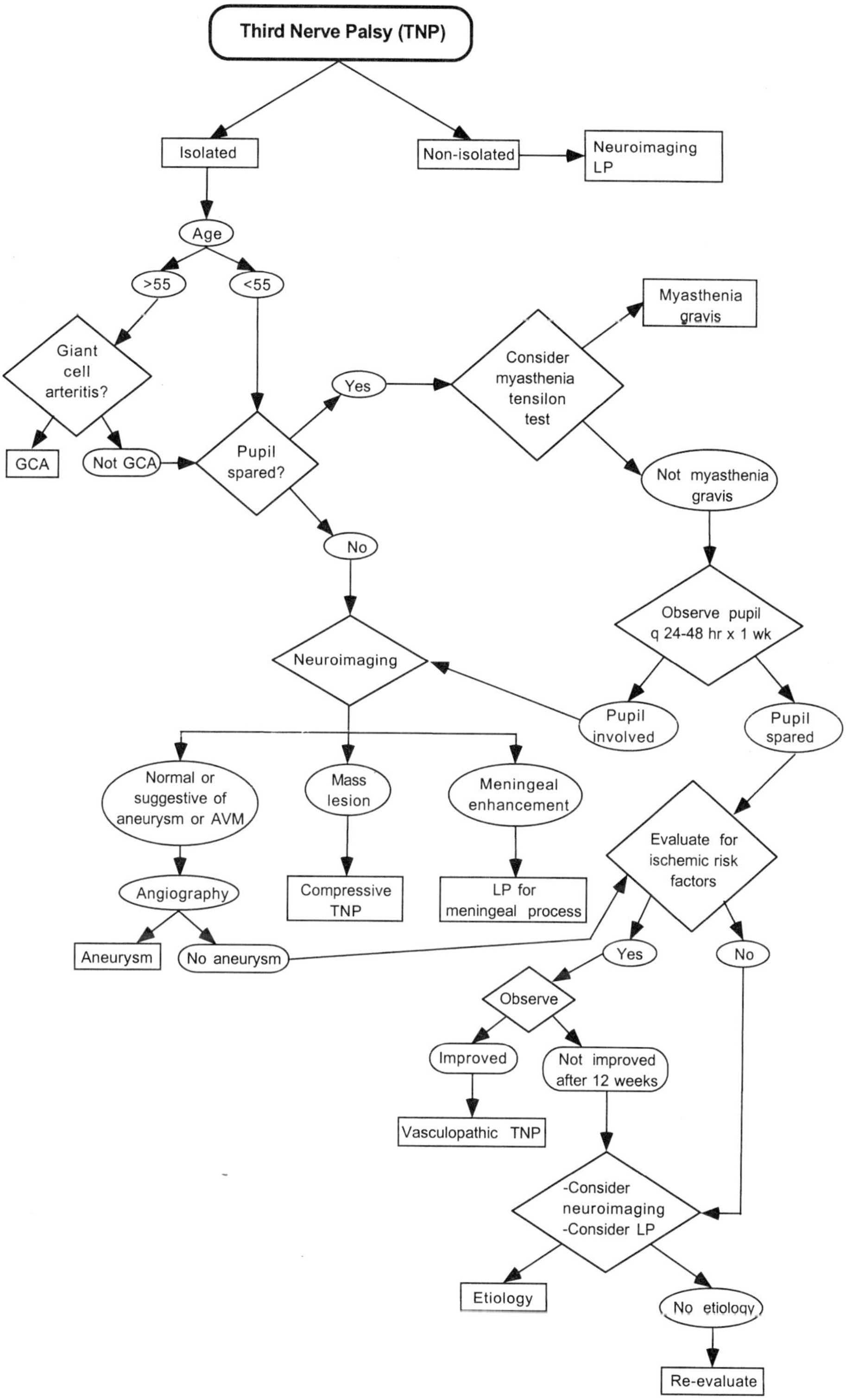

Figure 11–1. Third nerve palsy (TNP).

with trauma, myasthenia gravis, or vascular disease and may also occur on a congenital or idiopathic basis (Von Noorden, 1991). Lesions of the medial rectus subnucleus, however, may also give rise to isolated weakness of the inferior rectus muscle (Pusateri, 1987; Roper-Hall, 1975; Warren, 1982). The levator palpebrae superioris muscles, the superior recti, and the constrictors of the pupils are affected bilaterally with nuclear lesions. Because medial rectus neurons probably lie at three different locations within the oculomotor nucleus, it is unlikely that a medial rectus paralysis (unilateral or bilateral) would be the sole manifestation of a nuclear lesion. Most characteristic of oculomotor nuclear involvement is unilateral third nerve palsy, weakness of the ipsilateral and contralateral superior rectus, and bilateral incomplete ptosis (Kobayashi, 1986; Pratt, 1995). On rare occasions the ipsilateral superior rectus is spared while the contralateral superior rectus is paretic (Dehaene, 1987). Bilateral third nerve palsies with sparing of the lid levators may also be caused by nuclear lesions (the central caudal levator subnucleus is spared) (Bryan, 1992; Elliott, 1969; Keane, 1984) and isolated bilateral ptosis with sparing of the extraocular muscles and pupils may occur with lesions involving the levator subnucleus and sparing more rostral oculomotor subnuclei (Conway, 1983; Growdon, 1974). After surgery for a fourth ventricle ependymoma, bilateral nuclear oculomotor palsies affecting only the levator and superior recti subnuclei have been described, resulting in third nerve paresis affecting only the levators and superior recti bilaterally (Sanli, 1995). Nuclear third nerve palsies may occasionally be associated with ipsilateral ptosis and contralateral eyelid retraction (plus-minus lid syndrome) (Gaymard, 1992). This syndrome occurs with a small lesion located in the paramedian mesencephalon, involving the ipsilateral levator palpebrae fascicles as they emerge from the central caudal nucleus (the central caudal nucleus is spared), and the inhibitory pathways projecting on the levator palpebrae motor neurons immediately before their entrance in the central caudal nucleus.

Lesions of the third nerve fascicle often accompany nuclear lesions because infarction is a common cause of a nuclear third nerve palsy and the paramedian branches near the top of the basilar artery often feed both structures. For example, infarction of the dorsal, paramedian midbrain may cause bilateral ptosis associated with unilateral paresis of all other muscles innervated by the oculomotor nerve (pupil spared) with sparing of the contralateral superior rectus muscle (Liu, 1991). These unique findings suggest a lesion of the proximal third nerve fascicles and the central caudal subnucleus. Third nerve fascicular lesions are most often caused by infarction, hemorrhage, or demyelination. Pure fascicular lesions cause a unilateral peripheral type of oculomotor palsy. Involvement of brainstem structures other than the fascicle of the third nerve identifies the mesencephalic location of the lesion (Liu, 1992). Concomitant damage of the red nucleus and superior cerebellar peduncle will cause contralateral ataxia and outflow tract cerebellar tremor (Claude's syndrome), while a more anterior lesion, affecting the peduncle, gives rise to oculomotor palsy with contralateral hemiparesis (Weber's syndrome). The third nerve palsy with Weber's syndrome may affect or spare the pupillary fibers (Saeki, 1996). Larger lesions that affect the oculomotor fascicle and the red nucleus/substantia nigra region may produce third nerve palsy with contralateral choreiform movements or tremor (Benedikt's syndrome) sometimes associated with contralateral hemiparesis if the cerebral peduncle is also involved. A pupil-sparing third nerve palsy associated with binocular tilts to the contralateral side—thereby indicating a left-sided midbrain lesion that included the fascicle of the third nerve and the supranuclear integration centers for torsional eye movements, the interstitial nucleus of Cajal and the rostral interstitial nucleus of the medial longitudinal fasciculus (MLF)—has been described with a paramedian rostral midbrain infarction in a diabetic with giant cell arteritis (Dichgans, 1995).

Rarely, a unilateral or bilateral fascicular third nerve lesion may occur in isolation without other ocular motor or neurologic signs or symptoms (see below) (Abdollah, 1989; Barbas, 1995; Fleet, 1988; Getenet, 1994; Keane, 1988; Kim, 1993; Newman, 1990; Roper-Hall, 1975; Thömke, 1995; Uitti, 1986). Fascicular lesions, even when bilateral, may occasionally spare the pupil(s) (Wilkens, 1979). Because of the intraaxial topographic arrangement of fibers, fascicular lesions may cause third nerve palsies limited to specific oculomotor-innervated muscles (Ksiazek, 1994). For example, fascicular lesions have resulted in: (1) isolated inferior oblique paresis (Castro, 1990); (2) a unilateral fixed, dilated pupil unassociated with other neurologic dysfunction (Shuaib, 1989); (3) paresis of the superior rectus and inferior oblique without other evidence of oculomotor nerve involvement (Gauntt, 1995); (4) paresis of the inferior oblique, superior rectus, medial rectus, and levator muscle with sparing of the inferior rectus muscle and pupil (Naudea, 1983; Schwartz, 1995; Shuaib, 1987); and (5) paresis of the inferior oblique, superior rectus, medial rectus, levator, and inferior rectus with pupillary sparing (Breen, 1991; Naudea, 1983). Based on these clinical studies, it has been proposed that individual third nerve fascicles in the ventral mesencephalon are arranged topographically from lateral to medial as follows: inferior oblique, superior rectus, medial rectus and levator palpebrae, inferior rectus, and pupillary fibers (Castro, 1990). A rostral-caudal topographic arrangement has also been suggested with pupillary fibers most superior, followed by fibers to the inferior rectus, inferior oblique, medial rectus, superior rectus, and levator, in that order (Schwartz, 1995). This model also serves the description of "superior division" oculomotor palsies (i.e., paresis of the superior rectus and levator muscles without involvement of other groups) (Guy, 1989a; Hriso, 1990; Ksiazek, 1989) and "inferior division" oculomotor palsies (paresis of inferior rectus, inferior oblique, medial rectus, and pupillary fibers with sparing of the superior rectus and levator) (Abdollah, 1990; Eggenberger, 1993; Ksiazek, 1989) associated with intraaxial midbrain lesions. Thus, although superior and inferior divisional third nerve palsies have classically been localized to anterior cavernous sinus or posterior orbital lesions, such reports suggest that a divisional third nerve pattern may occur from damage at any location along the course of the oculomotor nerve, from the fascicle to the orbit (Ksiazek, 1989).

An isolated peripheral third nerve palsy is most often related to an ischemic neuropathy or a lesion affecting its subarachnoid portion. Subarachnoid lesions may distort or injure the brainstem and diffuse processes will show signs of meningeal irritation. Within the subarachnoid space, the third nerve may be compressed by uncal herniation (Fisher, 1969); aneurysms of the internal carotid-posterior communicating, superior cerebellar, basilar, or posterior cerebral arteries (Boccardo, 1986; Branley, 1992; Brodsky, 1988; Cantu, 1969; DiMario, 1992; Feder, 1979; Giombini, 1991; Good, 1990; Greenspan, 1990; Griffiths, 1994; Kwan, 1987; Kyriakides, 1989; Ranganadham, 1992; Renowden, 1993; Richards, 1992; Soni, 1974; Soria, 1989; Striph, 1993; Teasdale, 1990; Tomsak, 1991; Trobe, 1978b; Weinberg, 1996; Wolin, 1992; Zimmer, 1991); ectatic vessels (Nakagawa, 1991; Zingale, 1993); tumors, especially meningiomas, chordomas, or metastases (Cullom, 1993; Eyster, 1972; Kajiya, 1995; Kodsi, 1992; Kwan, 1987; Reifenberger, 1996); infectious or inflammatory processes of the meninges and carcinomatous or lymphomatous meningitis (Balm, 1996; Galetta, 1992; Ing, 1992; Jordan, 1978; Kass, 1972; Keane, 1993; Kwan, 1987; Mark, 1992; Miller, 1976, 1977; Newman, 1995; Olson, 1974; Renowden, 1993; Straube, 1993; Wilkens, 1979); subarachnoid hemorrhage with leukemia (Papke, 1993); pseudotumor cerebri (McCammon, 1981); or hydrocephalus (Rush, 1981). Primary tumors of the third nerve may also occur (Abdul-Rahim, 1989; Hardenack, 1994; Hiscott, 1982; Kadota, 1993; Kansu, 1982; Kaye-Wilson, 1994; Leunda, 1982; Mehta, 1990; Ogilvy, 1993; Platt, 1986;

Schultheiss, 1993; Shuangshoti, 1975; Takano, 1990; Yamada, 1986). The third nerve is also susceptible to trauma in the subarachnoid space, especially during neurosurgical procedures (Elston, 1984; Hedges, 1993; Kruger, 1986; Kudo, 1990; Memon, 1971; Solomons, 1980; Wakai, 1981; Yoss, 1968). Closed head trauma may cause third nerve palsy due to shearing injury resulting in distal fascicular damage or partial root avulsion (Balcar, 1996). Walter et al. (Walter, 1994) described two patients with third nerve palsies precipitated by minor head trauma with negative CT scans who were subsequently discovered to have ipsilateral posterior communicating artery aneurysms.

Compression of the third nerve by an aneurysm characteristically causes dilatation and unresponsiveness of the pupil. Compressive subarachnoid lesions may occasionally spare the pupil, however, perhaps due to the pressure of the lesion being evenly distributed and allowing the relatively pressure resistant, smaller-caliber pupillomotor fibers to escape injury or to the lesion compressing only the inferior portion of the nerve, thus sparing the dorsally situated pupillomotor fibers (Kissel, 1983; Naudea, 1983). With unruptured cerebral aneurysms, third paresis is often incomplete and partial with at least one element of nerve dysfunction (i.e., ptosis, mydriasis, or extraocular muscle weakness) absent (Bartleson, 1986). For example, ptosis has been described in isolation as the sole manifestation of third nerve compression by a posterior communicating artery aneurysm (Good, 1990). Rarely, aneurysmal partial third nerve paresis may even be transient and clear spontaneously (Greenspan, 1990). A normal pupil in the setting of a complete somatic oculomotor paresis, however, essentially excludes a diagnosis of aneurysm (see below), although a single patient has been described in whom a painless, pupil-sparing but otherwise complete oculomotor paresis was the only sign of an aneurysm arising from the basilar artery (Lustbader, 1988). An isolated pupillary paralysis without ptosis or ophthalmoparesis is rarely caused by an aneurysm (Crompton, 1981; Gale, 1982; Payne, 1969) or other subarachnoid lesion (Kaye-Wilson, 1994; Wilhelm, 1995).

Isolated impairment of the third cranial nerve may occur on an ischemic basis, especially associated with diabetes or atherosclerosis, but also occurring with giant cell arteritis (Barricks, 1977; Berlit, 1991; Davies, 1994; Renowden, 1993; Richards, 1992) and systemic lupus erythematosus (Rosenstein, 1989). Significant risk factors for ischemic oculomotor nerve palsies include diabetes, left ventricular hypertrophy, and elevated hematocrit (Jacobson, 1994). Obesity, hypertension, and smoking are also probable risk factors (Teuscher, 1985). Ischemic damage to the trigeminal fibers in the oculomotor nerve may be the source of pain in ischemic-diabetic third nerve palsies (Bortolami, 1993). Ischemic lesions of the oculomotor nerve often spare the pupil because the lesion is confined to the core of the nerve and does not affect peripherally situated pupillomotor fibers. The pupil may, however, be involved in diabetic oculomotor palsies (Grunt, 1976; Naghmi, 1990) and diabetes may even cause a superior branch palsy of the oculomotor nerve (Masucci, 1980). Postmortem examinations in three diabetic patients have demonstrated pathologic changes in the subarachnoid or cavernous sinus portion of the nerves (Asbury, 1970; Dreyfus, 1975; Weber, 1970). Ischemic third nerve palsy with pupillary sparing has, however, also been reported due to fascicular damage with mesencephalic infarcts documented on MR imaging (Breen, 1991; Dichgans, 1995; Hopf, 1990; Murakami, 1994; Thömke, 1995). In a prospective study of 16 patients with ischemic third nerve palsies, 11 (69%) had progression of ophthalmoplegia with a median time between reported onset and peak severity of ophthalmoplegia 10 days (Jacobson, 1995). All patients with an ischemic third nerve palsy will improve within 4 to 12 weeks of onset of symptoms (Capo, 1992).

Lesions of the third nerve in the cavernous sinus often also involve the other ocular motor nerves, the ophthalmic branch of the trigeminal nerve, and sympathetic fibers.

Sensory fibers from the ophthalmic division of the fifth cranial nerve join the oculomotor nerve within the lateral wall of the cavernous sinus. The frontal-orbital pain experienced by patients with enlarging aneurysms could thus be caused by direct irritation of the third nerve (Lanzino, 1993). Compressive cavernous sinus lesions may also spare the pupil because they often preferentially involve only the superior division of the oculomotor nerve that carries no pupillomotor fibers or the superior aspect of the nerve anterior to the point where the pupillomotor fibers descend in their course near the inferior oblique muscle (Trobe, 1978a). The pupillary "sparing" with anterior cavernous sinus lesions may be more apparent than real, resulting from simultaneous injury of nerve fibers to both the pupillary sphincter and dilator, causing a mid-position, fixed pupil (Kissel, 1983) or from aberrant regeneration (see below). Lesions in the neighborhood of the posterior clinoid process may for some time affect only the third nerve as it pierces the dura (e.g., breast and prostatic carcinoma) (Cullom, 1993). Medial lesions in the cavernous sinus, such as a carotid artery aneurysm, may affect only the ocular motor nerves but spare the more laterally located ophthalmic branch of the trigeminal nerve, resulting in painless ophthalmoplegia. Lesions that begin laterally present with retroorbital pain first, and only later does ophthalmoparesis supervene. Third nerve palsy in the cavernous sinus may be due to an aneurysm of the internal carotid artery (Bartleson, 1986; Cogan, 1963; Hepler, 1967; Keane, 1996; Kissel, 1983; O'Connor, 1983); dural carotid–cavernous sinus fistula (Acierno, 1995; Hawke, 1989; Keane, 1996; Keltner, 1987; Kupersmith, 1986; Lee, 1996; Miyachi, 1993; Perez Sempere, 1991); cavernous sinus thrombosis or infection (Archambault, 1988; Marsh, 1977); tumors, including pituitary adenoma, meningioma, neurinoma, nasopharyngeal carcinoma, lymphoma, and metastases (Bixenman, 1982; Hall, 1983; Keane, 1996; Kurokawa, 1992; North, 1993; Petersen, 1985; Renowden, 1993; Robert, 1973; Saul, 1985; Shen, 1993; Sudaresan, 1977; Tao, 1992; Trobe, 1978; Wake, 1993; Walker, 1977; Weisberg, 1977; Wykes, 1985); pituitary infarction or hemorrhage (pituitary apoplexy) (Petersen, 1985; Reid, 1985; Robinson, 1990; Rossitch, 1992; Seyer, 1992; Weisberg, 1977); intraneural hemorrhage (Miyao, 1993); gammopathy (Bogousslavsky, 1986; Lamarca, 1987; Ruggles, 1981); mucocele of the sphenoid sinus (Johnson, 1986); or Tolosa-Hunt syndrome or other granulomatous diseases (Keane, 1996; Mathew, 1970). The clinical findings and etiologies for processes located in the superior orbital fissure are similar to those of the cavernous sinus syndrome.

Lesions within the orbit that produce third nerve dysfunction usually produce other ocular motor dysfunction as well as optic neuropathy and proptosis (Goldberg, 1990a, 1990b). Lesions may extend from the cavernous sinus to the orbital apex and vice versa so that a clear separation between the two syndromes may be impossible. Isolated involvement of the muscles innervated by either the superior or the inferior oculomotor branch has classically been localized to an orbital process—often trauma, tumor, or infection, or a spheno-cavernous lesion (Stefanis, 1993). However, as we noted, the functional division of the third nerve is present probably even at the fascicular level and a divisional pattern may occur from damage anywhere along the course of the nerve. Superior division or inferior division third nerve paresis may occur with subarachnoid lesions (Guy, 1985) and isolated superior division paresis has been described with a superior cerebellar-posterior cerebral artery junction aneurysm that compressed and flattened the interpeduncular third nerve from below (Guy, 1989b). Superior branch palsy has also been described with basilar artery aneurysm, intracavernous carotid aneurysm, diabetes, lymphoma, sphenoidal abscess, frontal sinus mucocele, viral illness, meningitis, and after craniotomy (Chotmongkol, 1992; Derakshan, 1978; Ephrenpries, 1995; Feder, 1979; Guy, 1989b; Masucci, 1980; Stefanis, 1993; Trobe, 1978). Even ophthalmoplegic migraine may cause recurrent paroxysmal superior division oculomotor palsy (Katz, 1989). Isolated superior division-like paresis may be mimicked by myasthenia gravis (Dehaene, 1995). Isolated inferior division involvement has occurred with trauma (Saul, 1986), mesencephalic infarction and tumor (Abdollah, 1990; Eggenberger, 1993; Ksiazek, 1989), basilar artery aneurysm (Kardon, 1991), parasellar tumors (e.g., meningioma, schwannoma) (Carlow, 1990), viral illness (Susac, 1977), or as part of a more generalized vasculitic or demyelinating neuropathy (Cunningham, 1994). Inferior division involvement with tumors may be pupil-sparing, perhaps because of insidious tumor growth sparing pressure-resistant pupillomotor fibers.

Other miscellaneous etiologies for third nerve palsies include congenital (Ing, 1992; Miller, 1977), migraine (Bailey, 1984; Miller, 1977; Woody, 1986), viral infections and immunizations (Chan, 1980; Hertenstein, 1976; Nellhaus, 1966; Sekizawa, 1987), diffuse neuropathic processes (Arroyo, 1995), cervical carotid artery dissection or occlusion (Mokri, 1996; Schievink, 1993; Wilson, 1989), carotid stenosis (Balcar, 1997), subdural hematomas (Berger, 1979; Phookan, 1994), and toxic effects of certain drugs (Pacifici, 1993; Soysal, 1993). For example, partial or complete third nerve palsy may rarely follow dental anesthesia, presumably due to inadvertent injection of an anesthetic agent into the inferior dental artery or superior alveolar artery with subsequent retrograde flow into the maxillary, middle meningeal, and finally the lacrimal branch of the ophthalmic artery (Hyams, 1976; Petrelli, 1980).

What Are Isolated Third Nerve Palsies?

Isolated third nerve palsies may occur with lesions localized anywhere along the coarse of the third nerve from the fascicle to the orbit (Renowden, 1993). For clinical purposes, isolated atraumatic third nerve palsies may be divided into four types (Kwan, 1987; Trobe, 1985):

Type 1. TNP with a normal pupillary sphincter (normal internal function) and completely palsied extraocular muscles (complete external dysfunction).

Type 2. TNP with a normal pupillary sphincter (normal internal function) and incompletely palsied extraocular muscles (incomplete external dysfunction).

Type 3. TNP with a subnormal pupillary sphincter (partial internal dysfunction) and completely palsied extraocular muscles (complete external dysfunction) ("relative pupil-sparing").

Type 4. TNP with complete internal and complete external ophthalmoplegia.

What Investigations Are Warranted for Type 1 TNP?

TNP with a normal pupillary sphincter and completely palsied extraocular muscles is almost never caused by aneurysms. A single patient has, however, been described in whom a painless, pupil-sparing but otherwise complete third nerve paresis was the only sign of an aneurysm arising from the basilar artery (Lustbader, 1988). This type of third nerve palsy is most commonly caused by ischemia, especially related to diabetes (see above). In a retrospective review of 34 consecutive cases of isolated atraumatic third nerve palsies, diabetes was the most common etiology accounting for 46% of the cases (Renowden, 1993). Pupil sparing has been documented in 68 to 86% of palsies resulting from ischemia (Green, 1964; Rucker, 1966). The probable explanation for pupillary sparing in diabetic TNP is the lack of damage to the periphery of the nerve where the majority of pupillomotor fibers are thought to pass (Eames, 1967; Naudea, 1983). This type of third nerve involvement may rarely occur with pituitary adenoma (Bixenman, 1982) or other compressive lesions.

Adults who develop this syndrome do not need angiography. A MR scan need not initially be performed because the yield for a compressive lesion is very low. Neuroimaging should be performed in patients with no vasculopathic risk factors or in those who do not improve by 12 weeks of follow-up. Patients with type 1 TNP should be observed at 24- to 48-hour intervals for one week because some patients with aneurysms may develop delayed pupil involvement (Kissel, 1983). Vasculopathic risk factors, especially diabetes mellitus, hypertension, and increased cholesterol, should be sought and controlled. Patients over the age of 55 years, especially those with other symptoms suggestive of giant cell arteritis (e.g., headache, jaw or tongue claudications, polymyalgia rheumatica symptoms) should have a sedimentation rate. Temporal artery biopsy should be performed if the sedimentation rate is elevated or other systemic symptoms are present. Myasthenia gravis may rarely mimic this type of third nerve palsy so a Tensilon test should be performed, primarily in patients with fluctuating or fatiguing ptosis or ophthalmoplegia (Kwan, 1987).

What Investigations Are Indicated for Type 2 TNP?

Patients with an incomplete motor third nerve palsy with pupillary sparing require an MR scan to rule out a mass lesion. If the MR scan is normal, cerebral angiography should be performed to investigate the presence of an aneurysm, dural-cavernous sinus fistula, or high-grade carotid stensosis. Magnetic resonance angiography may well reveal an aneurysm or other vascular malformation and eventually take the place of arteriography (Kaufman, 1994; Tomsak, 1991; Weinberg, 1996); however, at the time of this writing, cerebral angiography is the "gold standard" for the diagnosis of cerebral aneurysms (Davis, 1996). MR imaging and angiography are especially warranted for superior division third nerve palsies. Myasthenia gravis may rarely mimic a superior division palsy so a Tensilon test should be performed in these cases. If a patient with a partial third nerve palsy has signs of meningeal irritation, other cranial nerve palsies, or signs of more diffuse meningeal involvement (e.g., radiculopathies), then a spinal tap to investigate infectious, inflammatory, or neoplastic meningitis should be performed .

What Investigations Are Warranted for Type 3 Patients?

Patients with a "relative pupil sparing" third nerve palsy should have MR imaging to investigate the possibility of a compressive lesion. Such patients should also have a cerebral angiogram if the MR scan is negative because of the possibility of a cerebral aneurysm. Cullom et al. (Cullom, 1995) published a prospective study of ten patients with "relative pupillary sparing" third nerve palsies and none of the patients demonstrated aneurysms. These authors suggested that the prevalence of aneurysm in patients with palsies of this type may be low enough to preclude routine angiography. This report was, however, based on a very small patient sample. Also, others have reported internal carotid, posterior communicating, and basilar artery aneurysms in isolated third nerve palsies with relative pupillary sparing (Bartleson, 1986; Kasoff, 1975; Kissel, 1983; Trobe, 1985). Thus, cerebral angiography is warranted if MR imaging is negative. Because 10 to 20% of patients with ischemic third nerve palsies have pupillary dysfunction (Capo, 1992; Goldstein, 1960; Green, 1964; Rucker, 1958), there will be a percentage of normal angiograms when using these guidelines.

In evaluating these patients, one must be cautious to avoid mistaking "pseudo" pupil sparing due to aberrant regeneration (below) or coexistent Horner's syndrome with true relative pupil sparing (Naudea, 1983; Trobe, 1985). In both conditions, a compressive lesion is likely, with the latter finding localizing the process to the cavernous sinus. Thus, pupil sparing or "pseudo" pupil sparing third nerve palsies may occur not only with extraaxial ischemic lesions but also in intraaxial (midbrain) lesions in a small proportion of subarachnoid compressive lesions and in a high proportion of cavernous sinus compressive lesions (Naudea, 1983).

What Investigations Are Warranted for Type 4 Patients?

Complete external and internal third nerve palsies occurring in isolation are often the result of compressive lesions or meningeal infiltration (Kwan, 1987); thus, an MR scan is initially warranted. If this study is negative, a cerebral angiogram is necessary to investigate aneurysm or dural-cavernous sinus fistula. If meningeal signs are present, spinal fluid evaluation is warranted.

A suggested evaluation for third nerve palsies is outlined in Figure 11-1. Table 11-2 lists the etiologies of third nerve palsies by their localization.

Table 11–2. Etiologies of Third Nerve Palsies (TNP)

Localization	References
Nuclear TNP	
Infarction or hemorrhage	Antworth, 1987; Bengel, 1994; Biller, 1984; Bogousslavsky, 1983, 1994; Bryan, 1992; Chee, 1990; Gaymard, 1990; Growdon, 1974; Kobayashi, 1986; Kömpf, 1987; Reagan, 1978; Tognetti, 1988; Zackon, 1984
Tumor	Keane, 1984; Pusateri, 1987; Sanli, 1995
Infection	Antworth, 1987; Elliott, 1969; Conway, 1983; Traboulsi, 1985
Trauma	Tognetti, 1988
Fascicular TNP	
Infarction or hemorrhage	Breen, 1991; Castro, 1990; Fleet, 1988; Getenet, 1994; Guy, 1989a; Hopf, 1990; Keane, 1988; Kim, 1993; Ksiazek, 1989, 1994; Liu, 1991; Saeki, 1996; Shuaib, 1987, 1989; Tömke, 1995
Tumor	Barbas, 1995; Eggenberger, 1993; Wilkens, 1979
Multiple sclerosis	Abdollah, 1989; Newman, 1990; Uitti, 1986

Subarachnoid space	
Aneurysms of the internal carotid-posterior communicating, superior cerebellar, basilar, or posterior cerebral arteries	Bartleson, 1986; Boccardo, 1986; Branley, 1992; Brodsky, 1988; Cantu, 1969; Crompton, 1981; DiMario, 1992; Feder, 1979; Gale, 1982; Giombini, 1991; Good, 1990; Greenspan, 1990; Griffiths, 1994; Guy, 1989; Kasoff, 1975; Keane, 1996; Kissel, 1983; Kwan, 1987; Kyriakides, 1989; Lustbader, 1988; Naudea, 1983; Payne, 1969; Ranganadham, 1992; Renowden, 1993; Richards, 1992; Soni, 1974; Soria, 1989; Striph, 1993; Teasdale 1990; Tomsak, 1991; Trobe, 1978b, 1985; Walter, 1994; Weinberg, 1996; Wolin, 1992; Zimmer 1991
Ectatic vessels	Nakagawa, 1991; Zingale, 1993
Tumors, especially meningiomas, chordomas, metastases, or primary tumors of the third nerve	Abdul-Rahim, 1989; Cullom, 1993; Eyster, 1972; Hardenack, 1994; Hiscott, 1982; Kadota, 1993; Kajiya, 1995; Kansu, 1982; Kaye-Wilson, 1994; Kodsi, 1992; Kwan, 1987; Leunda, 1982; Mehta, 1990; Ogilvy, 1993; Platt, 1986; Reifenberger, 1996; Schultheiss, 1993; Shuangshoti, 1975; Takano, 1990; Yamada, 1986
Infectious or inflammatory processes of the meninges and carcinomatous or lymphomatous meningitis	Balm, 1996; Galetta, 1992; Ing, 1992; Jordan, 1978; Kass, 1972; Keane, 1993; Kwan, 1987; Mark, 1992; Miller, 1976, 1977; Newman, 1995; Olson, 1974; Renowden, 1993; Straube, 1993; Traboulsi, 1985; Wilkens, 1979
Subarachnoid hemorrhage with leukemia	Papke, 1993
Pseudotumor cerebri	McCammon, 1981
Trauma, especially during neurosurgical procedures	Balcar, 1996; Elston, 1984; Hedges, 1993; Kruger, 1986; Kudo, 1990; Memon, 1971; Miller, 1977; Solomans, 1980; Wakai, 1981; Yoss, 1968
Nerve infarction from diabetes, atherosclerosis, giant cell arteritis, or systemic lupus erythematosis (nerve infarction may also occur in the cavernous sinus or anywhere along the course of nerve)	Asbury, 1970; Barricks, 1977; Bartolami, 1993; Berlit, 1991; Capo, 1992; Cullom, 1995; Davies, 1994; Dreyfus, 1975; Goldstein, 1960; Grunt, 1976; Jacobson, 1994, 1995; Masucci, 1980; Naghmi, 1990; Renowden, 1993; Richards, 1992; Rosenstein, 1989; Rush, 1981; Teuscher, 1985; Weber, 1970
Uncal herniation	Fisher, 1969
Hydrocephalus	Rush, 1981
Cavernous sinus/superior orbital fissure	
Aneurysm of the internal carotid artery	Bartleson, 1986; Cogan, 1963; Hepler, 1967; Keane, 1996; Kissel, 1983; Lanzino, 1993; O'Connor, 1983; Trobe, 1978a
Dural carotid cavernous sinus fistula	Acierno, 1995; Hawke, 1989; Keane, 1996; Lee, 1996; Miyachi, 1993; Perez Sempere, 1991
Cavernous sinus thrombosis or infection	Archambault, 1988; Marsh, 1977
Tumors, including pituitary adenoma, meningioma, neurinoma, nasopharyngeal carcinoma, myeloma, lymphoma, and metastases	Bixenman, 1982; Cullom, 1993; Hall, 1983; Keane, 1996; Kurokawa, 1992; North, 1993; Petersen, 1985; Reid, 1985; Renowden, 1991; Robert, 1973; Saul, 1985; Shen, 1993; Sudaresan, 1977; Tao, 1992; Trobe, 1978a; Wake, 1993; Walker, 1977; Weisberg, 1977; Wykes, 1986
Pituitary infarction or hemorrhage (pituitary apoplexy)	Petersen, 1985; Reid, 1985; Robinson, 1990; Rossitch, 1992; Seyer, 1992; Weisberg, 1977
Gammopathy	Bogousslavsky, 1986; Lamarca, 1987; Ruggles, 1981
Intraneural hemorrhage	Miyao, 1993

(continued)

Table 11–2. *(continued)*

Localization	References
Mucocele of the sphenoid sinus	Johnson, 1986
Tolosa-Hunt syndrome or other granulomatous diseases	Keane, 1996; Mathew, 1970
Orbit	
Infections, inflammations, and granulomatous processes (e.g., orbital pseudotumor)	Stefanis, 1993
Tumors	Goldberg, 1990a, 1990b
Trauma	Saul, 1986
Unknown localization	
Congenital	Ing, 1992; Miller, 1977
Migraine	Bailey, 1984; Miller, 1977; Woody, 1986
Viral infections and immunizations	Chan, 1980; Hertenstein, 1976; Nellhaus, 1966; Sekizawa, 1987
Diffuse neuropathic processes	Arroyo, 1995
Cervical carotid artery dissection, stenosis, or occlusion	Balcar, 1997; Mokri, 1996; Schievink, 1993; Wilson, 1989
Subdural hematomas	Berger, 1979; Phookan, 1994
Toxic effects of drugs	Pacifici, 1993; Soysal, 1993
Dental anesthesia	Hyams, 1976; Petrelli, 1980

What Are the Characteristics of Aberrant Regeneration?

Months to years after the occurrence of an third nerve lesion, clinical findings of aberrant regeneration of the third nerve may be seen. They include elevation of the lid on downward gaze (pseudo-von Graefe phenomenon) or on adduction, but lid depression during abduction. Other findings with aberrant regeneration include limitation of elevation and depression of the eye with occasional eyeball retraction on attempted vertical gaze, adduction of the eye on attempted elevation or depression, and suppression of the vertical phase of the optico-kinetic response. The pupil may be in a miotic or mid-dilated position; it may be fixed to light but may respond to near (near-light dissociation) or constrict on adduction or down-gaze. Aberrant regeneration to the iris sphincter may be too weak to constrict the pupil on exposure to light but at the slit lamp, clear segmental contraction of the sphincter may be seen when the eye tries to move in any third nerve direction (Czarnecki's sign) (Czarnecki, 1978; Cox, 1986, 1991). This gaze-evoked segmental constriction of the pupil may occur in portions of the sphincter that are unreactive to light, while other segments of the pupil have normal light reaction without Czarnecki's sign (Cox, 1991). Aberrant regeneration within only the inferior division of the third nerve has been described (Spector, 1981).

Aberrant regeneration may be seen after third nerve damage due to congenital causes, trauma, aneurysm, migraine, and syphilis, but is almost never caused by ischemic neuropathy (Elston, 1984; Keane, 1975; Sebag, 1983). Misdirection of regenerating nerve fibers is the likely cause, but it has also been postulated that the syndrome may be due to ephaptic neuron transmission of impulses or from chromatolysis-induced reorganization of oculomotor nuclear synapses. Ephaptic transmission would explain the transient third nerve misdirection described with ophthalmoplegic migraine, temporal arteritis, pituitary apoplexy, and non-Hodgkin's lymphoma (Johnson, 1988; Lee, 1992; Lepore, 1980; Sibony, 1984a, 1984b). Long-standing lesions, such as meningiomas of the cavernous sinus, trigeminal neuromas, or large aneurysms, may present as a primary aberrant regeneration of the third nerve without a history of a previous third nerve palsy (Boghen, 1979; Cox, 1979; Miller, 1985; Sebag, 1983). Primary aberrant regeneration may rarely occur with extracavernous lesions such as neurilemmoma, meningioma, asymmetric mammillary body or intradural aneurysm (Johnson, 1989; Schatz, 1977; Varma, 1994). Bilateral primary aberrant regeneration may also occur with abetalipoproteinemia (Bassen-Kornzweig syndrome) (Cohen, 1985). On rare occasions, the pseudo-von Graefe phenomenon may develop contralateral to a regenerating paretic third nerve (Guy, 1989).

All patients with nontraumatic aberrant third nerve regeneration require MR imaging to investigate the possibility of a compressive lesion. This is especially true if signs of aberrancy develop in a presumed "ischemic" third nerve palsy.

References

Abdollah A, Francis GS. (1989). Demyelinating disease presenting as a partial oculomotor nerve paresis. *Can J Neurol Sci 16:*285.

Abdollah A, Francis GS. (1990). Intraaxial divisional oculomotor nerve paresis suggests intraaxial fascicular organization. *Ann Neurol 28:*589–590.

Abdul-Rahim AS, Savino PJ, Zimmerman RA, et al. (1989). Cryptogenic oculomotor nerve palsy. The need for repeated neuroimaging studies. *Arch Ophthalmol 107:*387–390.

Acierno MD, Trobe JD, Cornblath WT, Gebarski SS. (1995). Painful oculomotor palsy caused by posterior-draining dural carotid cavernous fistulas. *Arch Ophthalmol 113:*1045–1049.

Antworth MV, Beck RW. (1987). Third nerve palsy as a presenting sign of acuired immune deficiency syndrome. *J Clin Neuro-ophthalmol 7:*125–128.

Archambault P, Wise JS, Rosen J, et al. (1988). Herpes zoster ophthalmoplegia. Report of six cases. *J Clin Neuro-ophthalmol 8:*185–191.

Arroyo JG, Horton JC. (1995). Acute, painful, pupil-involving third nerve palsy in chronic inflammatory demyelinating polyneuropathy. *Neurology 45:*846–847.

Asbury AK, Aldridge H, Hersberg R, Fisher CM. (1970). Oculomotor palsy in diabetes mellitus: A clinico-pathological study. *Brain 93:*555–566.

Bailey TD, O'Connor PS, Tredici TJ, Shacklett DE. (1984). Ophthalmoplegic migraine. *J Clin Neuro-ophthalmol 4:*225–228.

Balcar LJ, Galetta SL, Bagley LJ, Pakulo SJ. (1996). Localization of traumatic oculomotor nerve palsy to the midbrain exit site by magnetic resonance imaging. *Am J Ophthalmol 122:*437–439.

Balcar LJ, Galetta SL, Yousem DM, et al. (1997). Pupil-involving third-nerve palsy and carotid stenosis: Rapid recovery following endarterectomy. *Ann Neurol 41:*273–276.

Balm M, Hammack J. (1996). Leptomeningeal carcinomatosis. Presenting features and prognostic factors. *Arch Neurol 53:*626–632.

Barbas NR, Hedges TR, Schwenn M. (1995). Isolated oculomotor nerve palsy due to neoplasm in infancy. *Neuro-ophthalmol 15:*157–160.

Barricks ME, Traviesa DB, Glaser JS, Levy IS. (1977). Ophthalmoplegia in cranial arteritis. *Brain 100:*209–221.

Bartleson JD, Trautmann JC, Sundt TM. (1986). Minimal oculomotor nerve paresis secondary to unruptured intracranial aneurysm. *Arch Neurol 43:*1015–1020.

Bengel D, Huffmann G. (1994). Oculomotor nuclear complex syndrome as a single sign of midbrain hemorrhage. *Neuro-ophthalmology 5:*279–282.

Berger B, Frenkel M. (1979). Complete third nerve paralysis and decreasing vision secondary to subdural hematoma. *Ann Ophthalmol 11:*1817–1819.

Berlit P. (1991). Isolated and combined pareses of cranial nerves III, IV, and VI. A retrospective study of 412 patients. *J Neurol Sci 103:*10–15.

Biller J, Shapiro R, Evans LS, et al. (1984). Oculomotor nuclear complex infarction. Clinical and radiological correlation. *Arch Neurol 41:*985–987.

Bixenman WW. (1982). Atypical clinical presentation of oculomotor (III) nerve palsy. *J Clin Neuro-ophthalmol 2:*249–258.
Boccardo M, Ruelle A, Banchero MA. (1986). Isolated oculomotor palsy caused by aneurysm of the basilar artery bifurcation. *J Neurol 233:*61–62.
Boghen D, Chartrand JP, Laflamme P, et al. (1979). Primary aberrant third nerve regeneration. *Ann Neurol 6:*415–418.
Bogousslavsky J, Maeder P, Regli F, Meuli R. (1994). Pure midbrain infarction: Clinical, MRI, and etiologic patterns. *Neurology 44:*2032–2040.
Bogousslavsky J, Regli F. (1983). Nuclear and prenuclear syndromes of the oculomotor nerve. *Neuro-ophthalmology 3:*211–216.
Bogousslavsky J, Steck AJ. (1986). Bilateral third nerve palsy and anterior ischemic optic neuropathy. *Neuro-ophthalmology 6:*117–120.
Bortolami R, D'Alessandro R, Manni E. (1993). The origin of pain in 'ischemic-diabetic' third-nerve palsy. *Arch Neurol 50:*795.
Branley MG, Wright KW, Borchert MS. (1992). Third nerve palsy due to cerebral artery aneurysm in a child. *Aust NZ J Ophthalmol 20:*137–140.
Brazis PW. (1991). Subject review: Localization of lesions of the oculomotor nerve: Recent concepts. *Mayo Clin Proc 66:*1029–1035.
Breen LA, Hopf HC, Farris RK, Gutman L. (1991). Pupil-sparing oculomotor nerve palsy due to a midbrain infarction. *Arch Neurol 48:*105–106.
Brodsky MC, Frenkel RE, Spoor TC. (1988). Familial intracranial aneurysm presenting as a subtle stable third nerve palsy. *Arch Ophthalmol 106:*173.
Bryan JS, Hamed LM. (1992). Levator-sparing nuclear oculomotor palsy. Clinical and magnetic resonance imaging findings. *J Clin Neuro-ophthalmol 12:*26–30.
Cantu, RC. (1969). Oculomotor palsy with posterior communicating artery aneurysm. Outcome with carotid ligation versus medical therapy. *Int Surg 52:*144–150.
Capo H, Warren F, Kupersmith MJ. (1992). Evolution of oculomotor nerve palsies. *J Clin Neuro-ophthalmol 12:*21–25.
Carlow TJ, Johnson JK. (1990). Parasellar tumors: Isolated pupil-sparing third nerve palsy. *Neurology 40* (Suppl. 1):309.
Castro O, Johnson LN, Mamourian AC. (1990). Isolated inferior oblique paresis from brainstem infarction. Perspective on oculomotor fascicular organization in the ventral midbrain tegmentum. *Arch Neurol 47:*235–237.
Chan CC, Sogg RL, Steinman L. (1980). Isolated oculomotor palsy after measles immunization. *Am J Ophthalmol 89:*446–448.
Chee MW, Tan CB, Tjia HT. (1990). Nuclear third nerve palsy and somnolence due to stroke—a case report. *Ann Acad Med Singapore 19:*382–384.
Chotmongkol V, Techasuknirun A. (1992). Superior division paresis of the oculomotor nerve casued by cryptococcal meningitis. *J Med Assoc Thai 75:*548–550.
Cogan DG, Mount HTJ. (1963). Intracranial aneurysms causing ophthalmoplegia. *Arch Ophthalmol 70:*757–771.
Cohen DA, Bosley TM, Savino PJ, et al. (1985). Primary aberrant regeneration of the oculomotor nerve—occurrence in a patient with abetalipoproteinemia. *Arch Neurol 42:*821–823.
Conway VH, Rozdilsky B, Schneider RJ, Sundaram M. (1983). Isolated bilateral complete ptosis. *Can J Ophthalmol 18:*37–40.
Cox TA. (1986). Czarnecki's sign is the initial finding in acquired oculomotor synkinesis. *Am J Ophthalmol 1986:102:*543.
Cox TA, Goldberg RA, Rootman J. (1991). Tonic pupil and Czarnecki's sign following third nerve palsy. *J Clin Neuro-ophthalmol 11:*55–56.
Cox TA, Wurster JB, Godfrey WA. (1979). Primary aberrant oculomotor regeneration due to intracranial aneurysm. *Arch Neurol 36:*570–571.
Crompton JL, Moore CE. (1981). Painful third nerve palsy: How not to miss an intracranial aneurysm. *Aust J Ophthalmol 9:*113–115.
Cullom ME, Savino PJ. (1993). Adenocarcinoma of the prostate presenting as a third nerve palsy. *Neurology 43:*2146–2147.
Cullom ME, Savino PJ, Sergott RC, Bosley TM. (1995). Relative pupillary sparing third nerve palsies. To angiogram or not? *J Neuro-ophthalmol 15:*136–141.
Cunningham ET, Good WV. (1994). Inferior branch oculomotor nerve palsy: A case report. *J Neuro-ophthalmol 14:*21–23.
Czarnecki JS, Thompson HS. (1978). The iris sphincter in aberrant regeneration of the third nerve. *Arch Ophthalmol 96:*1606–1610.
Davies GE, Shakir RA. (1994). Giant cell arteritis presenting as oculomotor nerve palsy with pupillary dilatation. *Postgrad Med J 70:*298–299.
Davis PC, Newman NJ. (1996). Perspective—Advances in Neuroimagimg of the visual pathways. *Am J Ophthalmol 121:*690–705.
Dehaene I, Marchau M, VanHooren G. (1987). Nuclear oculomotor nerve paralysis. *Neuro-ophthalmol 7:*219–222.

Dehaene I, Van Zandijcke M. (1995). Isolated paralysis of the superior division of the ocular motor nerve mimicked by myasthenia gravis. *Neuro-ophthalmology 5:*257–258.

Derakshan I. (1978). Superior branch palsy of the oculomotor nerve with spontaneous recovery. *Ann Neurol 4:*478–479.

Dichgans M, Dieterich M. (1995). Third nerve palsy with contralateral ocular torsion and binocular tilt of visual vertical, indicating a midbrain lesion. *Neuro-ophthalmology 15:*315–320.

DiMario FJ Jr, Rorke LB. (1992). Transient oculomotor nerve paresis in congenital distal basilar artery aneurysm. *Pediatr Neurol 8:*303–306.

Dreyfus PM, Hakim S, Adams RD. (1975). Diabetic ophthalmoplegia: Report of case with postmortem study and comments on vascular supply of human oculomotor nerve. *Arch Neurol Psychi 77:*337–349.

Eames RA, Lang LS. (1967). Clinical and pathologic study of ischemic neuropathy. *J Neurol Neurosurg Psychiatry 30:*215–226.

Eggenberger ER, Miller NR, Hoffman PN, et al. (1993). Mesencephalic ependymal cyst causing an inferior division paresis of the oculomotor nerve: Case report. *Neurology 43:*2419–2420.

Elliott RL. (1969). Encephalitis and ophthalmoplegia. *Confin Neurol 31:*194–197.

Elston JS. (1984). Traumatic third nerve palsy. *Br J Ophthalmol 68:*538–543.

Ephrenpries SJ, Biedlingmaier JF. (1995). Isolated third-nerve palsy associated with frontal sinus mucocele. *J Neuro-ophthalmology 15:*105.

Eyster EF, Hoyt WF, Wilson CB. (1972). Oculomotor palsy from minor head trauma. An initial sign of basal intracranial tumor. *JAMA 220:*1083–1086.

Feder R, Camp WA. (1979). Superior branch palsy of oculomotor nerve and pupillary constriction caused by intracranial carotid aretery aneurysm. *Ann Neurol 5:*493–495.

Fisher CM. (1969). The neurologic examination of the comatose patient. *Acta Neurol Scand 45:*1–56.

Fleet WS, Rapcsak SZ, Huntley WW, Watson RT. (1988). Pupil-sparing oculomotor palsy from midbrain hemorrhage. *Ann Opthalmol 20:*345–346.

Gale AN, Crockard HA. (1982). Transient unilateral mydriasis with basilar aneurysm. *J Neurol Neurosurg Psychiatry 45:*565–566.

Galetta SL, Sergott RC, Wells GB, et al.. (1992). Spontaneous remission of a third-nerve palsy in meningeal lymphoma. *Ann Neurol 32:*100–102.

Gauntt CD, Kashii S, Nagata I. (1995). Monocular elevation paresis caused by an oculomotor fascicular lesion. *J Neuro-ophthalmol 15:*11–14.

Gaymard B, Lafitte C, Gelot A, de Toffol B. (1992). Plus-minus lid syndrome. *J Neurol Neurosurg Psychiatr 55:*846–848.

Gaymard B, Larmande P, de Toffol B, Autret A. (1990). Reversible nuclear oculomotor nerve paralysis. Caused by a primary mesencephalic hemorrhage. *Eur Neurol 30:*128–131.

Getenet JC, Vighetto A, Nighoghossian N, Trouillas P. (1994). Isolated bilateral third nerve palsy caused by a mesencephalic hematoma. *Neurology 44:*981–982.

Giombini S, Ferraresi S, Pluchino F. (1991). Reversal of oculomotor disorders after intracranial aneurysm surgery. *Acta Neurochir 112:*19–24.

Goldberg RA, Rootman J. (1990a). Clinical characteristics of metastatic orbital tumors. *Ophthalmology 47:*620–624.

Goldberg RA, Rootman J, Kline RA. (1990b). Tumors metastatic to the orbit: A changing picture. *Surv Ophthalmol 35:*1–24.

Goldstein JE, Cogan DG. (1960). Diabetic ophthalmoplegia with special reference to the pupil. *Arch Ophthalmol 64:*592–600.

Good EF. (1990). Ptosis as the sole manifestation of compression of the oculomotor nerve by an aneurysm of the posterior communicating artery. *J Clin Neuro-ophthalmol 10:*59–61.

Green WR, Hackett ER, Schlezinger NS. (1964). Neuro-ophthalmologic evaluation of oculomotor nerve paralysis. *Arch Ophthalmol 72:*154–167.

Greenspan BN, Reeves AG. (1990). Transient partial oculomotor nerve paresis with posterior communicating aneurysm—a case report. *J Clin Neuro-ophthalmol 10:*56–58.

Griffiths PD, Gholkar A, Sengupta RP. (1994). Oculomotor nerve palsy due to thrombosis of a posterior communicating artery eneurysm following diagnostic angiography. *Neuroradiology 36:*614–615.

Growdon JH, Winkler GF, Wray SH. (1974). Midbrain ptosis. A case with clinicopathologic correlation. *Arch Neurol 30:*179–181.

Grunt JA, Destro RL, Hamtil LW, Baska RE. (1976). Ocular palsies in children with diabetes mellitus. *Diabetes 25:*459–462.

Guy JR, Day AL. (1989a). Intracranial aneurysms with superior division paresis of the oculomotor nerve. *Ophthalmology 96:*1071–1076.

Guy J, Engel HM, Lessner AM. (1989b). Acquired contralateral oculomotor synkinesis. *Arch Neurol 46:*1021–1023.

Guy J, Savino PJ, Schatz NJ, et al. (1985). Superior division paresis of the oculomotor nerve. *Ophthalmology 92:*777–784.

Hall S, Carlin L, Roach ES, McLean WT. (1983). Pupillary sparing oculomotor nerve palsy from metastatic carcinoma. *Surg Neurol 19:*363–364.

Hardenack M, Volker A, Schroder JM, et al. (1994). Primary eosinophilic granuloma of the oculomotor nerve. *J Neurosurg 81:*784–787.

Harley RD. (1980). Paralytic strabismus in children. Etiologic incidence and management of the third, fourth, and sixth nerve palsies. *Ophthalmology 87:*24–43.
Hawke SH, Mullie MA, Hoyt WF, et al. (1989). Painful oculomotor nerve palsy due to dural-cavernous sinus shunt. *Arch Neurol 46:*1252–1255.
Hedges TR, Hirsh LF. (1993). Bilateral third nerve palsy from 'minor' head trauma. *Neuro-ophthalmology 13:*219.
Hepler RS, Cantu RC. (1967). Aneurysms and third nerve palsies. *Arch Ophthalmol 77:*604–608.
Hertenstein JR, Sarnat HB, O'Connor DM. (1976). Acute unilateral oculomotor palsy associated with ECHO 9 viral infection. *J Pediatr 89:*79–81.
Hiscott P, Symon L. (1982). An unusual presentation of neurofibroma of the oculomotor nerve. Case report. *J Neurosurg 56:*854–856.
Hopf HC, Gutmann L. (1990). Diabetic third nerve palsy: Evidence for a mesencephalic lesion. *Neurology 40:*1041–1045.
Hriso E, Miller A, Masdeu JC. (1990). Monocular elevation weakness and ptosis. *Neurology 47 (Suppl. 1):*309.
Hyams SW. (1976). Oculomotor palsy following dental anesthesia. *Arch Ophthalmol 94:*1281–1282.
Ing E, Sullivan TJ, Clarke MP, Buncic JR. (1992). Oculomotor nerve palsies in children. *J Pediatr Ophthalmol Strabismus 29:*331–336.
Jacobson DM, Broste SK. (1995). Early progression of ophthalmoplegia in patients with ischemic oculomotor nerve palsies. *Arch Ophthalmol 113:*1535–1537.
Jacobson DM, McCanna TD, Layde PM. (1994). Risk factors for ischemic ocular motor nerve palsies. *Arch Ophthalmol 112:*961–966.
Johnson LN, Hepler SS, Yee RD, Batzdorf U. (1986). Spenoid sinus mucocele (anterior clinoid variant) mimicking diabetic ophthalmoplegia. *Am J Ophthalmol 102:*111–115.
Johnson LN, Kamper CA, Hepler RS, et al. (1989). Primary aberrant regeneration of the oculomotor nerve from presumed extracavernous neurilemmoma, meningioma, and asymmetric mammillary body. *Neuro-ophthalmology 9:*227–232.
Johnson LN, Pack WL. (1988). Transient oculomotor nerve misdirection in a case of pituitary tumor with hemorrhage. Case report. *Arch Ophthalmol 106:*584–585.
Jordan K, Marino J, Damast M. (1978). Bilateral oculomotor paralysis due to neurosyphilis. *Ann Neurol 3:*90–93.
Kadota T, Miyawaki Y, Nakagawa H, et al. (1993). MR imaging of oculomotor nerve neurilemmoma. *Magn Reson Imaging 11:*1071–1075.
Kajiya Y, Nakajo M, Kajiya Y, Miyaji N. (1995). Oculomotor nerve invasion by lymphoma demonstrated by MRI. *J Comput Assist Tomogr 19:*502–504.
Kansu T, Ozcan OE, Ozdirim E, et al. (1982). Neurinoma of the oculomotor nerve. Case report. *J Clin Neuro-ophthalmol 2:*271–272.
Kardon RH, Traynelis VC, Biller J. (1991). Inferior division paresis of the oculomotor nerve caused by basilar artery aneurysm. *Cerebrovasc Dis 1:*171.
Kasoff I, Kelly DL. (1975). Pupillary sparing oculomotor palsies with internal carotid-posterior communicating artery aneurysms. *J Neurosurg 42:*713–717.
Kass MA, Keltner JL, Gay AJ. (1972). Total third nerve paralysis. Recovery in a case of meningococci meningitis. *Arch Ophthalmol 87:*107–109.
Katz B, Rimmer S. (1989). Ophthalmoplegic migraine with superior ramus oculomotor paresis. *J Clin Neuro-ophthalmol 9:*181–183.
Kaufman DI. (1994). Recent advances in neuro-imaging and the impact on neuro-ophthalmology. *Curr Opin Ophthalmol 5:*52–62.
Kaye-Wilson LG, Gibson R, Bell JE, Steers AJW. (1994). Oculomotor nerve neurinoma, early detection by magnetic resonance imaging. *Neuro-ophthalmol 14:*37–41.
Keane JR. (1975). Bilateral aberrant regeneration of the third cranial nerve following trauma. Case report. *J Neurosurg 43:*95–97.
Keane JR. (1988). Isolated brainstem third nerve palsy. *Arch Neurol 45:*813–814.
Keane JR. (1993). Intermittent third nerve palsy with cryptococcal meningitis. *J Clin Neuro-ophthalmol 13:*124–126.
Keane JR. (1996). Cavernous sinus syndrome. Analysis of 151 cases. *Arch Neurol 53:*967–971.
Keane JR, Zaias B, Itabashi HH. (1984). Levator sparing oculomotor nerve palsy caused by a solitary midbrain metastasis. *Arch Neurol 41:*210–212.
Keltner JL, Satterfield D, Dublin AB, Lee BCP. (1987). Dural and carotid cavernous sinus fistulas. Diagnosis, management, and complications. *Ophthalmology 94:*1585–1600.
Kim JS, Kang JK, Lee SA, Lee MC. (1993). Isolated or predominant ocular motor nerve palsy as a manifestation of brain stem stroke. *Stroke 24:*581–586.
Kissel JT, Burde RM, Klingele TG, Zeiger HE. (1983). Pupil-sparing oculomotor palsies with internal carotid-posterior communicating artery aneurysms. *Ann Neurol 15:*149–154.
Kobayashi S, Mukuno K, Tazaki Y, et al.. (1986). Oculomotor nerve nuclear complex syndrome. A case with clinicopathological correlation. *Neuro-ophthalmol 6:*55–59.
Kodsi SR, Younge BR. (1992). Acquired oculomotor, trochlear, and abducent cranial nerve palsies in pediatric patients. *Am J Ophthalmol 114:*568–574.
Kömpf D, Erbguth F, Kreiten K, et al. (1987). Bilateral third nerve palsy in basilar vertebral artery disease. *Neuro-ophthalmology 7:*355–362.

Kruger M, Noel P, Ectors P. (1986). Bilateral primary traumatic oculomotor nerve palsy. *J Trauma, 1986; 26:*1151–1153.

Ksiazek SM, Repka MX, Maguire A, et al. (1989). Divisional oculomotor nerve paresis caused by intrinsic brainstem disease. *Ann Neurol 26:*714–718.

Ksiazek SM, Slamovits TL, Rosen CE, et al. (1994). Fascicular arrangement in partial oculomotor paresis. *Am J Ophthalmol 118:*97–103.

Kudo T. (1990). An operative complication in a patient with a true posterior communicating artery aneurysm: case report and review of the literature. *Neurosurgery 27:*650–653.

Kupersmith MJ, Berenstein A, Flamm E, Ransohoff J. (1986). Neuro-ophthalmologic abnormalities and intravascular therapy of traumatic carotid cavernous fistulas. *Ophthalmology 93:*906–912.

Kurokawa Y, Uede T, Honda O, Honmou O. (1992). Successful removal of intracavernous neurinoma originating from the oculomotor nerve—case report. *Neurol Med Chi 32:*225–228.

Kwan ESK, Laucella M, Hedges III TR, Wolpert SM. (1987). A clinicoenuroradiologic approach to third cranial nerve palsies. *Am J Neuroradiol 8:*459–468.

Kyriakides T, Aziz TZ, Torrens MJ. (1989). Postoperative recovery of third nerve palsy due to posterior communicating aneurysms. *Br J Neurosurg 3:*109–111.

Lamarca J, Casquero P, Pou A. (1987). Mononeuritis multiplex in Waldenstrom's macroglobulinemia. *Ann Neurol 22:*268–272.

Lanzino G, Andreoli A, Tognetti F, et al. (1993). Orbital pain and unruptured carotid-posterior communicating artery aneurysms: The role of sensory fibers of the third cranial nerve. *Acta Neurochir 120:*7–11.

Lee AG. (1996). Third nerve palsy due to a carotid cavernous fistula without external eye signs. *Neuro-ophthalmology 16:*183–187.

Lee SH, Yeow YK, Tan CB, Tjia H. (1992). Transient oculomotor nerve synkinesis in non-Hodgkin's lymphoma. *J Clin Neuro-ophthalmol 12:*203–206.

Lepore FE, Glaser JS. (1980). Misdirection revisited. A critical appraisal of acquired oculomotor nerve synkinesis. *Arch Ophthalmol 98:*2206–2209.

Leunda G, Vaquero J, Cabezydo J, et al. (1982). Schwannoma of the oculomotor nerves. Report of four cases. *J Neurosurg 57:*563–565.

Liu GT, Carrazana EJ, Charness ME. (1991). Unilateral oculomotor palsy and bilateral ptosis from paramedian midbrain infarction. *Arch Neurol 48:*983–986.

Liu GT, Crenner CW, Logigian EL, et al. (1992). Midbrain syndromes of Benedikt, Claude, and Nothnagel: Setting the record straight. *Neurology 42:*1820–1822.

Lustbader JM, Miller NR. (1988). Painless, pupil-sparing but otherwise complete oculomotor paresis caused by basilar artery aneurysm. *Arch Ophthalmol 106:*583–584.

Mark AS, Blake P, Atlas SW, et al. (1992). Gd-DTPA enhancement of the cisternal portion of the oculomotor nerve on MR imaging. *Am J Neuroradiol 13:*1463–1470.

Marsh RJ, Dulley B, Kelly V. (1977). External ocular motor palsies in ophthalmic zoster: A review. *Br J Ophthalmol 61:*677–682.

Masucci EF, Kurtzke JF. (1980). Diabetic superior branch palsy of the oculomotor nerve. *Ann Neurol 7:*493.

Mathew NT, Chandy J. (1970). Painful ophthalmoplegia. *J Neurol Sci 11:*243–256.

McCammon A, Kaufman HH, Sears ES. (1981). Transient oculomotor paralysis in pseudotumor cerebri. *Neurology 31:*182–184.

Mehta VS, Singh RV, Misra NK, Choudry C. (1990). Schwannoma of the oculomotor nerve. *Br J Neurosurg 4:*69–72.

Memon MY, Paine KWE. (1971). Direct injury of the oculomotor nerve in craniocerebral trauma. *J Neurosurg 35:*461–464.

Miller NR. (1976). Isolated oculomotor nerve palsy in childhood from leptomeningeal polymorphic cell sarcoma. *J Pediatr Ophthalmol 13:*211–214.

Miller NR. (1977). Solitary oculomotor nerve palsy in childhood. *Am J Ophthalmol 83:*106–111.

Miller NR. (1985). *Walsh and Hoyt's Clinic Neuro-ophthalmology*. 4th edition. Baltimore, Williams & Wilkins, Vol. 2, p. 680.

Miyachi S, Negoro M, Handa T, Sugita K. (1993). Dural carotid cavernous sinus fistula presenting as isolated oculomotor nerve palsy. *Surg Neurol 39:*105–109.

Miyao S, Takano A, Teramoto J, et al. (1993). Oculomotor nerve palsy due to intraneural hemorrhage in idiopathic thrombocytopenic purpura: a case report. *Eur Neurol 33:*20–22.

Mokri B, Silbert PL, Schievink WI, Piepgras DG. (1996). Cranial nerve palsy in spontaneous dissection of the extracranial internal carotid artery. *Neurology 46:*356–359.

Murakami M, Kitano I, Hitoshi Y, Ushio Y. (1994). Isolated oculomotor nerve palsy following midbrain infarction. *Clin Neurol Neurosurg 96:*188–190.

Nagluni R, Subuhi R. (1990). Diabetic oculomotor mononeuropathy: involvement of pupillomotor fibres with slow resolution. *Horm Metab Res 22:*38–40.

Nakagawa H, Nakajima S, Nakajima Y, et al. (1991). Bilateral oculomotor nerve palsies due to posterior cerbral arterial compression relieved by microvascular decompression—case report. *Neurol Med Chir 31:*45–48.

Naudea SE, Trobe JD. (1983). Pupil sparing in oculomotor palsy: A brief review. *Ann Neurol 13:*143–148.

Nellhaus G. (1966). Isolated oculomotor nerve palsy in infectious mononucleosis. A report of an unusual case and review of the literature. *Neurology 16:*221– 224.

Newman NJ, Lessell S. (1990). Isolated pupil-sparing third-nerve palsy as the preesenting sign of multiple sclerosis. *Arch Neurol 47:*817–818.
Newman NJ, Slamovits TL, Friedland S, Wilson WB. (1995). Neuro-ophthalmic manifestations of meningocerebral inflammation from the limited form of Wegener's granulomatosis. *Am J Ophthalmol 120:*613–621.
North KN, Antony JH, Johnston IH. (1993). Dermoid of cavernous sinus resulting in isolated oculomotor nerve palsy. *Pediatr Neurol 9:*221–223.
O'Connor PS, Tredici TJ, Green RP. (1983). Pupil-sparing third nerve palsies caused by aneurysms. *Am J Ophthalmol 95:*395–397.
Ogilvy CS, Pakzaban P, Lee JM. (1993). Oculomotor nerve cavernous angioma in a patient with Roberts syndrome. *Surg Neurol 40:*39–42.
Olson ME, Chernik NL, Posner JB. (1974). Infiltration of the leptomeninges by systemic cancer. *Arch Neurol 30:*122–137.
Pacifici L, Passarelli F, Papa G, et al. (1993). Acute third cranial nerve ophthalmoplegia: Possible pathogenesis from alpha-II-interferon treatment. *Ital J Neurol Sci 14:*579–580.
Papke K, Masur H, Martinez-Rubio A, et al. (1993). Complete bilateral oculomotor palsy: The only clinical sign of subarachnoid hemorrhage in leukemia. *Acta Neurol Scand 88:*153–156.
Payne JW, Adamkiewicz J Jr. (1969). Unilateral internal ophthalmoplegia with intracranial aneurysm. Report of a case. *Am J Ophthalmol 68:*349–352.
Perez Sempere A, Martinez Menendez B, Cabeza Alvarez C, Calandre Hoenigsfeld L. (1991). Isolated oculomotor nerve palsy due to dural cavernous sinus fistula. *Eur Neurol 31:*186–187.
Petersen P, Lindholm J. (1985). Pituitary apoplexy, the Houssay phenomenon, and accelerated proliferative retinopathy. *Am J Med 79:*385–388.
Petrelli EA, Steller RE. (1980). Medial rectus muscle palsy after dental anesthesia. *Am J Ophthalmol 90:*422–424.
Phookan G, Cameron M. (1994). Bilateral chronic subdural haematoma: an unusual presentation with isolated oculomotor nerve palsy. *J Neurol Neurosurg Psych 57:*1146.
Platt JH, Campbell GA, Oakes WJ. (1986). Papillary meningioma involving the oculomotor nerve in an infant. *J Neurosurg 64:*808–812.
Pratt DV, Orengo-Nania S, Horowitz BL, Oram O. (1995). Magnetic resonance findings in a patient with nuclear oculomotor palsy. *Arch Ophthalmol 113:*141.
Pusateri TJ, Sedwick LA, Margo CE. (1987). Isolated inferior rectus muscle palsy from solitary metastasis to the oculomotor nucleus. *Arch Ophthalmol 105:*675–677.
Ranganadham P, Dinakar I, Mohandas S, Singh AK. (1992). A rare presentation of posterior communicating artery aneurysm. *Clin Neurol Neurosurg 94:*225–227.
Reagan TJ, Trautmann JC. (1978). Combined nuclear and supranuclear defects in ocular motility. A clinicopathologic study. *Arch Neurol 35:*133–137.
Reid RL, Quigley ME, Yen SSC. (1985). Pituitary apoplexy. A review. *Arch Neurol 42:*712–719.
Reifenberger G, Boströmj, Bettag M, et al. (1996). Primary glioblastoma multiforme of the oculomotor nerve. Case report. *J Neurosurg 84:*1062–1066.
Renowden SA, Harris KM, Hourihan MD. (1993). Isolated atraumatic third nerve palsy: Clinical features and imaging techniques. *Br J Radiol 66:*1111–1117.
Richards BW, Jones FR Jr, Younge BR. (1992). Causes and prognosis in 4,278 cases of paralysis of the oculomotor, trochlear, and abducens cranial nerves. *Am J Ophthalmol 113:*489–496.
Robert CM Jr, Feigenbaum JA, Stern EW. (1973). Ocular palsy occurring with pituitary tumors. *J Neurosurg 38:*17–19.
Robinson R, Toland J, Eustace P. (1990). Pituitary apoplexy. A cause for painful third nerve palsy. *Neuro-ophthalmol 10:*257–260.
Roper-Hall G, Burde RM. (1975). Inferior rectus palsies as a manifestation of atypical IIIrd cranial nerve disease. *Am Orthop J 25:*122–130.
Rosenstein ED, Sobelman J, Kramer N. (1989). Isolated, pupil-sparing third nerve palsy as initial manifestation of systemic lupus erythematosis. *J Clin Neuro-ophthalmol 9:*285–288.
Rossitch E Jr, Carrazana EJ, Black PM. (1992). Isolated oculomotor nerve palsy following apoplexy of a pituitary adenoma. *J Neurosurg Sci 36:*103–105.
Rucker CW. (1958). Paralysis of the third, fourth, and sixth cranial nerves. *Am J Ophthalmol 46:*787–794.
Rucker CW. (1966). The causes of paralysis of the third, fourth, and sixth cranial nerves. *Am J Ophthalmol 62:*1293–1298.
Ruggles KH, Massey EW. (1981). Pupil-sparing oculomotor palsy with IgG monoclonal paraproteinemia. *Ann Ophthalmol 13:*875–876.
Rush JA, Younge BR. (1981). Paralysis of cranial nerves III, IV, and VI. Course and prognosis in 1,000 cases. *Arch Ophthalmol 99:*76–79.
Saeki N, Murai N, Sunami K. (1996). Midbrain tegmental lesions affecting or sparing the pupillary fibres. *J Neurol Neurosurg Psychiatry 61:*401–402.
Sanli M, Altinörs N, Bavbek M. (1995). Partial bilateral oculomotor nucleus lesion following surgery of a fourth ventricle ependymoma. *Neuro-ophthalmol 15:*103–105.
Saul RF, Hilliker JK. (1985). Third nerve palsy: The presenting sign of a pituitary adenoma in five patients and the only neurological sign in four patients. *J Clin Neuro-ophthalmol 5:*185–193.
Saul RF, Selhhorst JB. (1986). Traumatic inferior division oculomotor palsy. *Neurology 36 Suppl. 1:*250.

Schatz NJ, Savino PJ, Corbett JJ. (1977). Primary aberrant oculomotor regeneration: A sign of intracavernous meningioma. *Arch Neurol 34:*29–32.

Schievink WI, Mokri B, Garrity JA, et al. (1993). Ocular motor nerve palsies in spontaneous dissections of the cervical internal carotid artery. *Neurology 43:*1938–1941.

Schultheiss R, Kristof R, Schramm J. (1993). Complete removal of an oculomotor nerve neurinoma without permanent functional deficit. *Ger J Ophthalmol 2:*228–233.

Schwartz TH, Lycette CA, Kargman DE. (1995). Clinicoradiographic evidence for oculomotor fascicular anatomy. *J Neurol Neurosurg Psychiatry 59:*338.

Sebag J, Sadun AA. (1983). Aberrant regeneration of the third nerve following orbital trauma. Synkinesis of the iris sphincter. *Arch Neurol 40:*762–764.

Sekizawa T, Nazamura S, Kogure K, et al.. (1987). Idiopathic third cranial nerve palsy associated with herpes simplex virus infection. *Br Med J 295:*813.

Seyer H, Kompf D, Fahlbusch R. (1992). Optomotor palsies in pituitary apoplexy. *Neuro-ophthalmology 12:*217–224.

Shen WC, Yang DY, Ho YJ, Lee SK. (1993). Neurilemmoma of the oculomotor nerve presenting as an orbital mass: MR findings. *Am J Neuroradiol 14:*1253–1254.

Shuaib A, Murphy W. (1987). Mesencephalic hemorrhage and third nerve palsy. *J Comput Tomogr 11:*385–388.

Shuaib A, Israelian G, Lee MA. (1989). Mesencephalic hemorrhage and unilateral pupillary deficit. *J Clin Neuro-ophthalmol 9:*47–49.

Shuangshoti S. (1975). Neurilemmoma of the oculomotor nerve. *Br J Ophthalmol 59:*64–66.

Sibony PA, Lessel S. (1984a). Transient oculomotor synkinesis in temporal arteritis. *Arch Neurol 41:*87–88.

Sibony PA, Lessell S, Gittinger JW Jr. (1984b). Acquired oculomotor synkinesis. *Surv Ophthalmol 28:*382–390.

Solomons NB, Solomon DJ, de Villiers JC. (1980). Direct traumatic third nerve palsy. *S Afr Med J 58:*109–111.

Soni SR. (1974). Aneurysms of the posterior communicating artery and oculomotor nerve paresis. *J Neurol Neurosurg Psychiatry 37:*1803–1808.

Soria E, Camell H, Dang E. (1989). Pupil-sparing oculomotor palsy caused by fusiform arteriosclerotic aneurysm of the basilar artery—a case report. *Angiology 40:*921–927.

Soysal T, Ferhanoglu B, Bilir M, Akman N. (1993). Oculomotor nerve palsy associated with vincristine treatment. *Acta Haematol 90:*209–210.

Spector RH, Faria MA. (1981). Aberrant regeneration of the inferior division of the oculomotor nerve. *Arch Neurol 38:*460–461.

Stefanis L, Przedborski S. (1993). Isolated palsy of the superior branch of the oculomotor nerve due to chronic erosive sphenoid sinusitis. *J Clin Neuro-ophthalmol 13:*229–231.

Straube A, Bandmann O, Buttner U, Schmidt H. (1993). A contrast enhanced lesion of the III nerve on MR of a patient with ophthalmoplegic migraine as evidence for a Tolosa-Hunt syndrome. *Headache 33:*446–448.

Striph GG. (1993). Consecutive oculomotor nerve palsy from a de novo cerebral aneurysm. *J Clin Neuro-ophthalmol 13:*181–187.

Sudaresan N, Noronha A, Hirschauer J, Siqueira EB. (1977). Oculomotor palsy as initial manifestation of myeloma *JAMA 238:*2052–2053.

Susac JO, Hoyt WF. (1977). Inferior branch palsy of the oculomotor nerve. *Ann Neurol 2:*336–339.

Takano S, Endo M, Miyasaka Y, et al. (1990). Neurinoma of the oculomotor nerve—case report. *Neurol Med Chir 30:*132–136.

Tao ZD. (1992). Oculomotor neuropathy syndrome. A diagnostic challenge in nasopharyngeal carcinoma. *Chin Med J 105:*567–571.

Teasdale E, Stratham P, Straiton J, MacPherson P. (1990). Non-invasive radiological investigation for oculomotor palsy. *J Neurol Neurosurg Psychiatry 53:*549–553.

Teuscher AU, Meienberg O. (1985). Ischaemic oculomotor nerve palsy. Clinical features and vascular risk factors in 23 patients. *J Neurol 232:*144–149.

Thömke F, Tettenborn B, Hopf HC. (1995). Third nerve palsy as the sole manifestation of midbrain ischemia. *Neuro-ophthalmology 15:*327–335.

Tognetti F, Godano U, Galassi E. (1988). Bilateral traumatic third nerve palsy. *Surg Neurol 29:*120–124.

Tomsak RL, Masaryk TJ, Bates JH. (1991).Magnetic resonance angiography (MRA) of isolated aneurysmal third nerve palsy. *J Clin Neuro-ophthalmol 11:*16–18.

Traboulsi EI, Azar DT, Achram M, Fares B. (1985). Brainstem tuberculoma and isolated third nerve palsy. *Neuro-ophthalmology 5:*43–45.

Trobe JD. (1985). Isolated pupil-sparing third nerve palsy. *Ophthalmology 92:*58–61.

Trobe JD, Glaser JS, Post JD. (1978a). Meningiomas and aneurysms of the cavernous sinuses: Neuro-ophthalmologic features. *Arch Ophthalmol 96:*457–467.

Trobe JD, Glaser JS, Quencer RC. (1978b). The product of saccular and fusiform aneurysms of the basilar artery. *Arch Ophthalmol 96:*1236–1240.

Uitti RJ, Rajput AH. (1986). Multiple sclerosis presenting as isolated oculomotor nerve palsy. *Can J Neurol Sci 13:*270–272.

Varma R, Miller NR. (1994). Primary oculomotor nerve sykinesis caused by an extracavernous intradural aneurysm. *Am J Ophthalmol 118:*83–87.

Von Noorden GK, Hansell R. (1991). Clinical characteristics and treatment of isolated inferior rectus paralysis. *Ophthalmology 98:*253–257.

Wakai S, Eguchi T, Asano T, Takahura K. (1981). Oculomotor palsy caused by aneurysmal clip: Report of two cases. *Neurosurgery 9:*429–432.

Wake A, Kakinuma A, Mori N, et al. (1993). Angiotropic lymphoma of paranasal sinuses with initial symptoms of oculomotor nerve palsy. *Intern Med 32:*237–242.

Walker JR, Hall CSD. (1977). Pituitary adenoma presenting as recurring painful ophthalmoplegia. *Surg Neurol 8:*319–322.

Walter KA, Newman NJ, Lessell S. (1994). Oculomotor palsy from minor head trauma : Initial sign of intracranial aneurysm. *Neurology 44:*148–150.

Warren W, Burde RM, Klingele TG, Roper-Hall G. (1982). Atypical oculomotor paresis. *J Clin Neuro-ophthalmol 2:*13–18.

Weber RB, Daroff RB, MacKey EA. (1970). Pathology of oculomotor nerve palsy in diabetics. *Neurology 20:*835–838.

Weinberg DA, Kaufman DI, Siebert JD, Pernicone JR. (1996). Negative MRI versus real disease. *Survey Ophthalmol 40:*312–319.

Weisberg LA. (1977). Pituitary apoplexy. Association of degenerative change in pituitary adenoma with radiotherapy and detection by cerebral computed tomography. *Am J Med 63:*1109–115.

Wilhelm H, Klier R, Tóth B, Wilhelm B. (1995). Oculomotor nerve paresis starting as isolated internal ophthalmoplegia. *Neuro-ophthalmology 15:*211–215.

Wilkens DE, Samhouri AM. (1979). Isolated bilateral oculomotor paresis due to lymphoma. *Neurology 29:*1425–1428.

Wilson WB, Leavengood JM, Ringel SP, Bott AD. (1989). Transient ocular motor paresis associated with acute internal carotid artery occlusion. *Ann Neurol 25:*286–290.

Wolin MJ, Saunders RA. (1992). Aneurysmal oculomotor nerve palsy in an 11-year-old boy. *J Clin Neuro-ophthalmol 12:*178–180.

Woody, RC, Blaw ME. (1986). Ophthalmoplegic migraine in infancy. *Clin Pediatrics 25:*82–84.

Wykes WN. (1986). Prolactinoma presenting with intermittent third nerve palsy. *Br J Ophthalmol 70:*706–707.

Yamada T, Nishio S, Matsunaga M, et al. (1986). Cavernous hemangioma in the oculomotor nerve. A case. *J Neurol 233:*63–64.

Yoss RE, Rucker CW, Miller RH. (1968). Neurosurgical complications affecting oculomotor, trochlear, and abducent nerves. *Neurology 18:*594–600.

Zackon DH, Sharpe JA. (1984). Midbrain paresis of horizontal gaze. *Ann Neurol 16:*495–504.

Zimmer DV. (1991). Oculomotor nerve palsy from posterior communicating artery aneurysm. *J LA State Med Soc 143:*22–25.

Zingale A, Chiarmonte I, Mancuso P, et al. (1993). Craniofacial pain and incomplete oculomotor palsy associated with ipsilateral primitive trigeminal artery. *J Neurosurg Sci 37:*251–255.

◆ 12 ◆

Fourth Nerve Palsies

What Is the Topographical Anatomy of the Fourth Nerve?

The topographical anatomy of the fourth cranial nerve is detailed in other reference sources (Miller, 1982). In summary, the fourth nerve nucleus is located in the midbrain beneath the inferior colliculus. It is the only cranial nerve with a dorsal exit from the brainstem. The fourth nerve has the longest intracranial course and crosses in the anterior medullary velum. It passes between the superior cerebellar artery and the posterior cerebellar artery, runs in the subarachnoid space, travels within the lateral wall of the cavernous sinus, and enters the orbit via the superior orbital fissure to innervate the superior oblique muscle.

Fourth cranial nerve palsies may cause (Von Noorden, et al. 1986):

1. Incomitant hypertropia demonstrated with the three-step maneuver. The hypertropia increases on head tilt toward the paralyzed side (positive Bielschowsky's test). Hypotropia may occur in the normal eye if the affected eye is fixating; if the unaffected eye is fixating, hypertropia occurs in the involved eye. This hypertropia is usually most prominent in the field of gaze of the involved superior oblique muscle, especially in cases of acute or recent onset. The hypertropia may also be most prominent in the field of gaze of the ipsilateral overacting inferior oblique muscle in subacute or chronic cases or evident in the entire paretic field (spread of comitance). Duction testing may variably reveal underaction of the ipsilateral superior oblique muscle, overaction of the ipsilateral inferior oblique muscle, or overaction of the contralateral superior oblique muscle. Pseudo-overaction of the superior oblique in the uninvolved eye occurs with spread of comitance and secondary contracture of the superior rectus muscle in the involved eye with the hypertropia involving the entire lower field of gaze. In a patient with a superior oblique muscle paralysis who habitually fixates with the paretic eye and in whom overaction of the ipsilateral inferior oblique muscle has developed, less than the normal

Table 12–1. Criteria for the Diagnosis of Fourth Nerve Palsy

Binocular vertical and/or torsional diplopia
Ipsilateral hyperdeviation in primary position, worsened by contralateral gaze and ipsilateral head tilt
Variable ipsilateral excyclotorsion
Anomalous compensatory head or face position
Weakness of the involved superior oblique muscle on motility examination

amount of innervation will be required when the patient looks up and to the contralateral side. Since the innervation flowing to the opposite superior rectus is "determined" by the overacting ipsilateral inferior oblique (Hering's law), the opposite superior rectus muscle will seem paretic (inhibitional palsy of the contralateral antagonist). In these cases, the head tilt test will correctly determine which of the two eyes is paretic.

2. Excyclotropia, which is usually evident on fundus exam and double Maddox rod testing. This cyclotropia is symptomatic only in acquired (vs. congenital) cases.
3. Head tilt, which is incorporated to eliminate the hypertropia and rarely the cyclotropia. This head tilt is present in approximately 70% of patients and is usually away from the involved side but may be paradoxical (toward the involved side) in about 3%.

It is important to differentiate patients with decompensation of a congenital fourth nerve palsy from those with an acquired fourth nerve palsy. In patients with congenital fourth nerve palsies:

1. Old photos may show head tilt.
2. Patients usually are noted to have cyclotropia on examination but do not complain of cyclotropia (subjective image tilting) as do some patients with acquired fourth nerve palsies.
3. Large vertical fusional amplitudes (> 6 to 8 prism diopters) in primary gaze are characteristic of congenital cases.
4. Facial asymmetry (hypoplasia on side of head turn) suggests a congenital lesion.

Bilateral fourth nerve palsies are suggested by:

1. A right hypertropia in left gaze and left hypertropia in right gaze.
2. A positive Bielschowsky test on tilt to either shoulder ("double Bielschowsky test").
3. Large excyclotropia (>10 degrees).
4. V-pattern esotropia (15 prism diopters or more difference in esotropia between upwards and downward gaze). The "V" pattern is caused by a decrease of the abducting effect of the superior oblique(s) in depression and overaction of the superior oblique muscle(s).
5. Underaction of both superior oblique muscles and/or overaction of both inferior oblique muscles.
6. In general, bilateral fourth nerve palsies tend to have a smaller hypertropia in primary position than do unilateral fourth nerve palsies.

The criteria for the diagnosis of fourth nerve palsies (FNP) are listed in Table 12–1.

FNP may be divided into isolated FNP and non-isolated FNP. For diagnostic classification based on topographic localization, non-isolated FNP may be grouped into the following four syndromes:

1. Midbrain (nucleus/fascicle syndrome) FNP
2. Subarachnoid space FNP

Table 12–2. Etiologies for a Fourth Nerve Palsy Based on Clinical Topographical Localization

- Midbrain (nuclear/fascicular) (Coppeto, 1983; Elliot, 1991; Guy, 1989; Keane, 1986; Krohel, 1982; Mansour, 1986)
  - Aplasia of the nucleus (Mellinger, 1977)
  - Arteriovenous malformation (Gonyea, 1990; Guy, 1989; Kim, 1992)
  - Demyelination (Younge, 1977)
  - Hemorrhage (Tachibana, 1990)
  - Ischemia or Infarction (Kim, 1993)
  - Trauma (including surgical) (Yoss, 1968)
- Subarachnoid space
  - Aneurysm (McKinna, 1983)
    - Superior cerebellar artery (Agostinis, 1992; Collins, 1992)
      - Hydrocephalus (Guy, 1989; Rush, 1981a)
  - Infections
    - Mastoiditis (Khawam, 1967)
    - Meningitis
  - Post-lumbar puncture or spinal anesthesia (King, 1987)
  - Pseudotumor cerebri (Lee, 1995)
  - Trauma (Baker, 1991; Jacobson, 1988; Keane, 1989; Lavin, 1984; Sabates, 1991; Snydor, 1982; Teller, 1988) including surgical (Yoss, 1969; Younge, 1977)
  - Neoplasm (Murray, 1985)
    - Carcinomatous meningitis (Olson, 1974)
    - Cerebellar hemangioblastoma (Sawle, 1989)
    - Ependymoma
    - Meningioma
    - Metastasis
    - Neurilemmoma (Boggan, 1979; Garen, 1987; Gentry, 1991; Ho, 1981; Leunda, 1982; Yamamoto, 1987)
      - Pineal tumors
    - Trochlear nerve sheath tumor (King, 1976)
  - Cavernous sinus
    - Neoplasm
      - Meningioma (Slavin, 1987)
    - Infectious
      - Herpes zoster (Archambault, 1988; Grimson, 1978; Keane, 1975; Lavin, 1984; Marsh, 1977; Rehsef, 1985; Scharf, 1979; Womack, 1983)
    - Inflammation
      - Tolosa-Hunt syndrome
    - Internal carotid artery aneurysm (Arruga, 1991; Maurice-Williams, 1989; Rush, 1981a)
  - Orbit
    - Neoplasm
    - Infection
    - Infiltration
      - Waldenstrom's macroglobulinemia (Moulis, 1989)
    - Inflammation
      - Progressive systemic sclerosis (Rush, 1981b)
    - Trauma
      - Orbital floor fracture (Cantillo, 1978; Keane, 1981)

3. Cavernous sinus FNP
4. Orbital FNP

Non–isolated FNP (Type 1—see below) with findings that localize to the brainstem, subarachnoid space, cavernous sinus, or orbit should undergo a neuroimaging study directed at the particular area of suspected involvement (Berlit, 1991; Brazis, 1993; Burde, 1992; Burger, 1970; Celli, 1992; Cobbs, 1980; Coppeto, 1983; Elliot, 1991; Gacs, 1983; Guy, 1989; Keane, 1989; Kim, 1992; McKinna, 1983; Miller, 1989; Olson, 1974; Richards, 1992; Robert, 1973; Rucker, 1956, 1966; Rush, 1981a; Sawle, 1989; Suzuki, 1962; Vanooteghem, 1992; Wray, 1977; Yoss, 1968; Younge, 1977).

Table 12–2 lists the etiologies for a fourth nerve palsy based on clinical topographical localization.

Is the FNP due to a Midbrain Lesion?

A midbrain (i.e., nuclear/fascicular) FNP is "defined by the company it keeps"; other brainstem signs usually present, including hemisensory loss, hemiparesis, a central Horner's syndrome, or other brainstem cranial neuropathies (e.g., third nerve palsy). The differential diagnosis includes midbrain ischemia, hemorrhage, demyelination, and neoplasm. Neuroimaging (preferably magnetic resonance [MR] imaging) should be directed to the midbrain.

Is the FNP the Result of a Subarachnoid Space Lesion?

Although lesions of the subarachnoid space may be associated with an isolated FNP, as with brainstem lesions, patients with subarachnoid space lesions usually have associated signs and symptoms including headache, stiff neck, and other cranial neuropathies. Neuroimaging (usually MR imaging) should be directed to the brainstem and subarachnoid space. Computed tomographic (CT) imaging should be considered in cases of acute trauma, to evaluate bone lesions, or in the evaluation of acute vascular processes (e.g., subarachnoid hemorrhage). Lumbar puncture following negative neuroimaging should be considered in these cases.

Is the FNP due to a Cavernous Sinus Lesion?

Cavernous sinus lesions are usually associated with other cranial nerve signs (e.g., third, fifth, or sixth nerve paresis) or a Horner's syndrome. Neuroimaging (preferably MR imaging) should be directed to the cavernous sinus.

Is the FNP Caused by an Orbital Lesion?

Orbital lesions usually produce signs such as proptosis, chemosis, and orbital or conjunctival edema. Neuroimaging (preferably MR imaging) should be directed to the orbit.

We define six types of FNP, shown in Table 12–3.

Table 12–3. Definitions of the Six Types of Fourth Nerve Palsy

Type 1: Non-isolated
FNP are considered non-isolated in the presence of the following features:
Other neurologic or neuro-ophthalmological signs
Evidence to suggest myasthenia gravis such as ptosis, or fatiguability of the motility deficit
Evidence for systemic inflammatory disorders such as giant cell arteritis
Type 2: Traumatic
Isolated, unilateral, or bilateral FNP, which have a clearly established temporal relationship to previous head trauma and do not progress, are considered traumatic in origin. Patients have no other neurologic deficits other than those associated with the initial traumatic event.
Type 3: Congenital
Congenital FNP, in addition to the features described above for FNP in general, may show the following:
Large vertical fusional amplitudes (greater than 6 to 8 prism diopters)
Facial asymmetry or sternocleidomastoid muscle hypertrophy
Long-standing anomalous head position that may be present in old photographs
Type 4: Vasculopathic
Vasculopathic FNP occur in patients greater than 50 years of age with or without known hypertension or diabetes, or in younger patients with known vasculopathic risk factors.
Type 5: Nonvasculopathic
Patients without vasculopathic risk factors are considered to have nonvasculopathic, idiopathic FNP.
Type 6: Progressive or unresolved
FNP that worsen after the acute stage (greater than 1 week) as defined by a significant increase in the measured ocular vertical deviation are considered to be progressive, and patients without improvement in the measured ocular vertical deviation after 6 to 8 weeks are considered unresolved.

FNP, fourth nerve palsies.

Is the FNP due to Trauma?

At least 23 retrospective studies of traumatic (Type 2) FNP have recommended that isolated, traumatic, unilateral, or bilateral FNP do not require additional neuroimaging or further evaluation (Baker, 1991; Berlit, 1991; Burde, 1992; Burger, 1970; Cantillo, 1978; Harley, 1980; Jacobson, 1988; Keane, 1981, 1989; Khawam, 1967; King, 1987; Lavin, 1984; Lee, 1985; Miller, 1970, 1989; Neetens, 1981; Pollard, 1985; Richards, 1992; Sabates, 1991; Snydor, 1982; Teller, 1988; Urist, 1953; Yoss, 1968). FNP after mild head trauma and out of proportion to the deficit have been observed in association with an underlying asymptomatic basal intracranial tumor in at least three reports (Jacobson, 1988; Miller, 1989; Neetens, 1981). Neetens reported three such cases, but two cases had other neuro-ophthalmologic signs as well (Neetens, 1981). Although uncommon, neuroimaging may be warranted in patients with FNP after minimal or trivial head trauma to exclude a mass lesion.

Is the FNP Congenital?

Clearly congenital unilateral or bilateral FNP (Type 3) are not associated with intracranial lesions in isolation and therefore do not require further diagnostic evaluation such as neuroimaging studies (Bagolini, 1982; Burde, 1992; Harley, 1980; Miller, 1970; Reynolds, 1984; Robb, 1990; Scott, 1986; Urist, 1953; Von Noorden, 1986, 1994).

Is the FNP Vasculopathic?

Vasculopathic FNP (Type 4) do not require any initial neuroimaging studies, and observation for improvement over the next six to eight weeks is recommended (Burde, 1992; Kennerdell, 1973; Nemet, 1980). Patients with vasculopathic FNP (Type 4), often resolve spontaneously within four to six months. Rush reported a recovery rate for FNP of 53.5% in 172 nonselected cases, and a higher recovery rate of 71% in 166 patients with diabetes mellitus, hypertension, or atherosclerosis (Rush, 1981a). Another report by Ksiazek et al. described improvement in 90% of 39 patients with microvascular and idiopathic FNP within six months (Ksiazek, 1988). Vasculopathic FNP usually improve within a few months (Burde, 1992; Green, 1964; Miller, 1989; Rush, 1981; Shrader, 1960; Von Noorden, 1986; Younge, 1977), and patients with progressive or unresolved FNP, or with new neurological signs or symptoms, should have neuroimaging (Agostinis, 1992; Arruga, 1991; Boggan, 1979; Burde, 1992; Gentry, 1991; King, 1976; Miller, 1989; Rush, 1981; Slavin, 1987; Wise, 1965; Yamamoto, 1987). Patients with spontaneously resolving palsies do not require any further neuroimaging. It is recommended that elderly patients who present with headache, scalp tenderness, jaw claudication, or visual loss undergo an appropriate evaluation for giant cell arteritis, including an erythrocyte sedimentation rate and a temporal artery biopsy (Burde, 1992; Miller, 1989; Reich, 1990).

What is the Evaluation of Nonvasculopathic FNP?

Nonvasculopathic FNP (Type 5) may be observed for improvement over the next six to eight weeks. Patients with resolution of symptoms and signs do not require further evaluation. Patients with progression or lack of resolution should undergo neuroimaging (preferably MR imaging). Myasthenia gravis may mimic FNP, and patients with variable or fatiguable motility findings and/or ptosis should be evaluated for myasthenia gravis (see Chapter 15) (Burde, 1992; Miller, 1989; Rush, 1982).

Testing for vasculopathic risk factors in Type 4 or Type 5 FNP should be performed, even in the absence of a history of previous diabetes or hypertension. Green, et al. reported an isolated third nerve palsy as the initial clinical manifestation of diabetes in almost half of 25 patients (Green, 1964). Shrader and Schlezinger reported that almost 50% of diabetic sixth nerve palsies were the presenting clinical manifestation of the disease (Shrader, 1960). The results of these studies concerning vasculopathic third and sixth nerve palsies may well be applicable to vasculopathic FNP.

Table 12–4 lists a summary of the etiologies of FNP in 11 large retrospective series (Ellis, 1976; Harley, 1980; Keane, 1993; Ksiazek, 1988; Mittleman, 1976; Richards, 1992; Rucker, 1956; Rucker, 1958, 1966; Von Noorden, 1986; Wright, 1977). Traumatic FNP occurred in 35%, idiopathic FNP in 34%, vasculopathic FNP in 16%, neoplasm was reported in 3%, aneurysm in 0.5%, and a wide variety of miscellaneous conditions including myasthenia gravis, infections, thyroid disease, and inflammation in 11% of patients.

Younger patients, or those without vasculopathic risk factors (Type 5), may require initial neuroimaging, but the data suggest that observation for spontaneous improvement may be sufficient. Isolated, idiopathic FNP very rarely have been found to have an underlying etiology after prolonged follow-up, and most resolve spontaneously within several weeks to months (Coppeto, 1978; Ksiazek, 1988; Nemet, 1980). Two retrospective case series with follow-up greater than six months described the prognosis of isolated, idiopathic FNP. Coppeto, et al. reported that 12 of 15 cases had resolved by four months after

Table 12-4. Etiology for Acquired Isolated Fourth Nerve Palsy

Author	Cases	Trauma	Tumor	Vascular	Aneurysm	Unknown	Other
Rucker, 1956	40	12	1	8	1	15	3
Rucker, 1958	67	24	3	24	0	9	7
Rucker, 1966	84	34	7	13	0	28	13
Mittleman, 1975	64	22	—	—	—	42	—
Ellis, 1976	104	32	0	—	1	63	8
Wright, 1977	23	9	0	8	0	3	3
Harley, 1980	18	5	0	0	0	12	1
Richards, 1992	578	169	28	103	5	186	87
Von Noorden, 1986	141	73			0	62	6*
Ksiazek, 1991	88	24	2	39	—	23	—
Keane, 1993	81	64	0	8	—	—	9
TOTAL	1288	457	41	203	7	443	137
	100%	35%	3%	16%	0.5%	34%	11%

*Other in this study included "tumor, vascular, and myasthenia gravis."

a mean follow-up of 5.5 years (Coppeto, 1978). Nemet et al. described 13 cases, with a follow-up ranging from four to seven years, and all had resolved by 10 weeks (Nemet, 1980). None of the patients in either series developed new neurological disease over an extensive follow-up period. Although Type 5 patients who improve may not require neuroimaging, the clinical certainty of such a recommendation is not sufficiently strong in our opinion to obviate the need for neuroimaging in these nonvasculopathic patients. Patients without improvement after two months, however, should undergo neuroimaging. Some reports have described aneurysm as an extremely rare cause for isolated FNP (Agostinis, 1992; Arruga, 1991; Burger, 1970; Collins, 1992; Ellis, 1976; Gacs, 1983; Maurice-Williams, 1989; McKinna, 1983; Richards, 1992; Rucker, 1956; Rush, 1981a), and cerebral angiography is not recommended unless an aneurysm is suggested by other neuroimaging studies. Collins et al. and Agostinis et al. reported isolated FNP due to superior cerebellar aneurysms, but both patients described headaches (Agostinis, 1992; Collins, 1992). In these cases, neuroimaging studies confirmed the presence of the aneurysm before angiography. There is insufficient data to make a comment on the usefulness of MR angiography in FNP.

Although MR scans are generally felt to be a more sensitive and specific than CT in the evaluation of cranial neuropathies, no conclusive evidence demonstrates an increased yield from performing an MR scan rather than a CT scan for the specific evaluation of FNP. Richards et al. reported an etiologic diagnosis in 69 of 144 (48%) FNP using MR imaging and in 289 of 684 (42%) cases using CT. These authors felt that "multiplanar CT may be a sufficient noninvasive study, especially when clinical suspicion is high . . . (or) in patients with other neurologic findings . . . " (Richards, 1992). Nevertheless, we feel that MR imaging is the study of choice for patients with FNP.

A number of cases have been reported in the literature documenting intracranial lesions in patients with FNP. Table 12–5 summarizes 85 cases of "isolated" FNP due to an intracranial lesion. Of these 85 patients, only 4 (4.7%) did not have other neurologic signs or symptoms and thus would be considered truly isolated by our criteria. One developed other neurologic signs after a short follow-up period, and in the remaining three patients, persistence or progression of symptoms would have eventually resulted in a neuroimaging study. Of the remaining 81 patients, six had headache or pain (7.0%), 31 had other neuro-

Table 12–5. "Isolated" Fourth Nerve Palsy due to Intracranial Lesion

Author	Cases	Pathology	Other Neurologic Signs
Suzuki, 1962	4	Pinealomas	Yes
Rucker, 1956	2	Frontal lobe glioma	Unknown
		Aneurysm of circle of Willis	Unknown
Rucker, 1958	3	1 primary brain tumor	Unknown
		2 metastatic	Unknown
Wise, 1965	1	Persistent trigeminal artery	Headache
Rucker, 1966	7	2 midbrain gliomas	Unknown
		1 meningioma	Unknown
		3 primary brain tumors	Unknown
Khawam, 1967	1	"brain tumor"	Unknown
Burger, 1970	8	4 cerebellopontine angle tumors	Yes
		1 cerebellar tumor	Yes
		1 nasopharyngeal cancer	Yes
		1 metastatic lung cancer	Yes
		1 aneurysm	Yes
Robert, 1973	2	Pituitary tumors	Yes
Ellis, 1976	1	"Intracranial aneurysm"	Unknown
King, 1976	1	Schwannoma	No
Scully, 1976	1	Medulloblastoma	Yes
Younge, 1977	4	2 gliomas	Unknown
		1 metastatic breast cancer	Unknown
		1 metastatic ovarian cancer	Unknown
Wray, 1976	2	Pituitary tumors	Yes
Coppetto, 1978	3	1 ependymoma	Yes
		1 medulloblastoma	Yes
		1 acoustic neuroma	Yes
Boggan, 1979	1	Schwannoma	Yes
Rush, 1981a, 1981b	10	2 meningiomas	Unknown
		1 primary brain tumor	Unknown
		4 metastatic tumors	Unknown
		1 intracavernous aneurysm	Yes
		1 basilar aneurysm	Unknown
		1 aneurysm/sub-arachnoid hemorrhage	Yes
Ho, 1981	1	Schwannoma	No
Neetens, 1981	3	Skull base tumors	Yes
Krohel, 1982	w1	Juvenile pilocytic astrocytoma	Yes
Leunda, 1982	1	Schwannoma	Yes
McKinna, 1983	3	Aneurysms	Unknown
Reinecke, 1986	1	Reported in Krohel, 1982	Yes
Jacobson, 1988	1	Vascular malformation	Yes
Slavin, 1987	1	Cavernous meningioma	*
Yamamoto, 1987	1	Schwannoma	Headache
Ksiazek, 1988	2	"Compressive etiologies"	Unknown
Maurice-Williams, 1989	1	Intracavernous carotid aneurysm	Headache
Gonyea, 1990	1	Brainstem vascular malformation	Headache
Arruga, 1991	1	Intracavernous carotid aneurysm	No
Agostinis, 1992	1	Superior cerebellar aneurysm	Headache
Collins, 1992	1	Superior cerebellar aneurysm	Headache
Richards, 1992	14	7 meningioma	Unknown
		1 metastatic	Unknown
		4 glioma	Unknown
		1 acoustic neuroma	Unknown
		1 other primary	Unknown
Kim, 1993	1	Brainstem stroke	Yes

* Patient developed progression of deviation after two years.

logic signs (36%), and the clinical information was insufficient to determine if the FNP was truly isolated in 44 patients (52%). Keane reported intracranial tumor as an etiology in 12 of 95 unilateral cases, but all 12 (100%) had other neuro-ophthalmic signs; and none of 81 isolated FNP later reported by Keane had an intracranial tumor (Keane, 1993).

All patients with progressive FNP (Type 6) should undergo neuroimaging (preferably MR imaging). Lumbar puncture should be considered if neuroimaging is nornal or if there are signs or symptoms of meningeal irritation.

An approach to FNP is outlined in Figure 12–1.

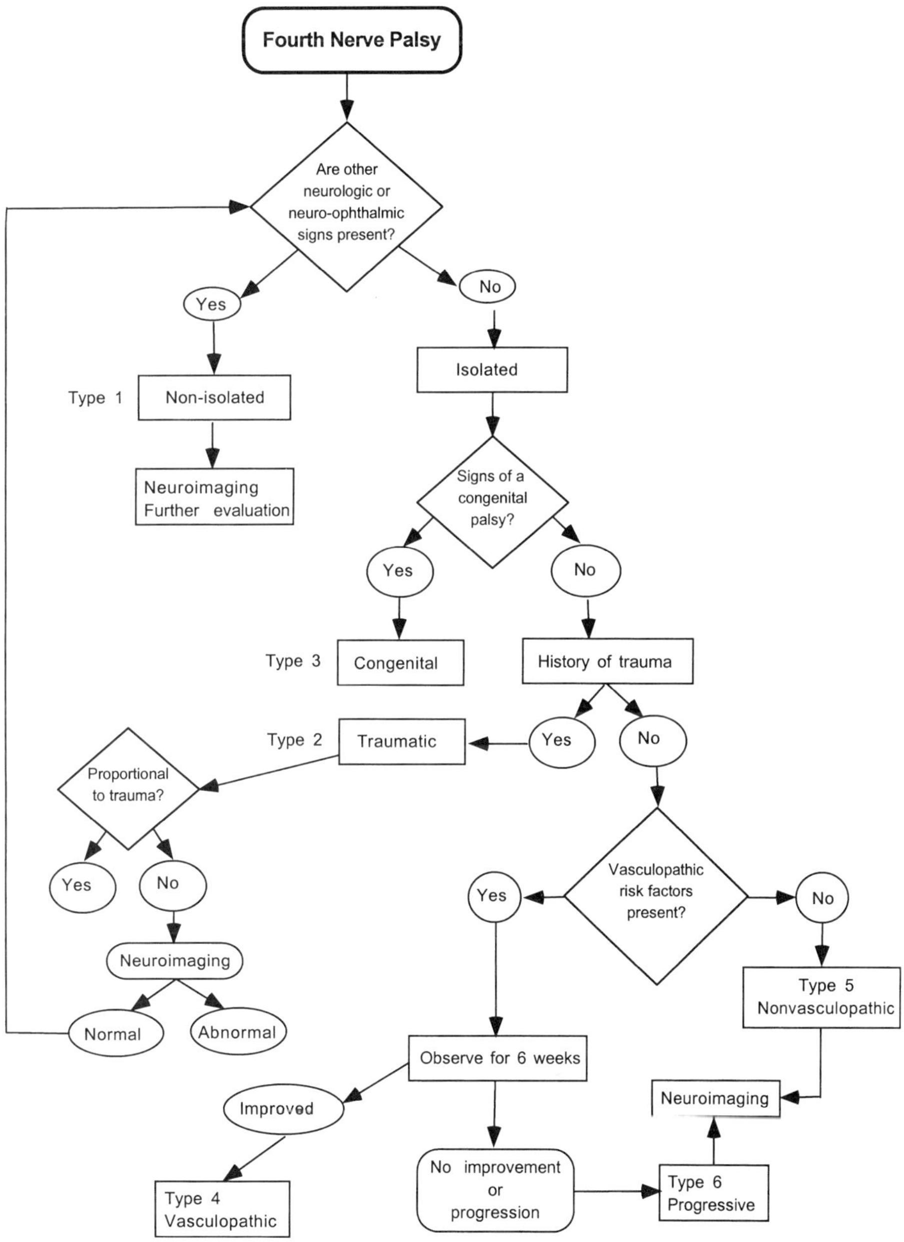

Figure 12–1. Fourth nerve palsy.

References

Agostinis C, Caverni L, Moschini L, et al. (1992). Paralysis of fourth cranial nerve due to superior cerebellar artery. *Neurology 42:*457–458.

Archambault P, Wise JS, Rosen J, et al. (1988). Herpes zoster ophthalmoplegia: Report of six cases. *J Clin Neuro-ophthalmol 8:*185–193.

Arruga J, De Rivas P, Espinet HL, et al. (1991). Chronic isolated trochlear nerve palsy produced by intracavernous internal carotid artery aneurysm: Report of a case. *J Clin Neuro-ophthalmol 11:*104–108.

Bagolini B, Campos EC, Chiesi C. (1982). Plagiocephaly causing superior oblique deficiency and ocular torticollis: A new clinical entity. *Arch Ophthalmol 100:*1093–1096.

Baker RS, Epstein AD. (1991). Ocular motor abnormalities from head trauma. *Surv Ophthalmol 35:*245–267.

Berlit P. (1991). Isolated and combined pareses of cranial nerves III, IV, and VI: A retrospective study of 412 patients. *J Neurol Sci 103:*10–15.

Boggan JE, Rosenblum ML, Wilson CB. (1979). Neurilemmoma of the fourth cranial nerve. *J Neurosurg 50:*519–521.

Brazis PW. (1993). Palsies of the trochlear nerve: Diagnosis and localization-recent concepts. *Mayo Clin Proc 68:*501.

Burde RM, Savino PJ, Trobe JD. (1992). *Clinical Decisions in Neuro-ophthalmology.* 2nd Edition. St. Louis, Mosby Year Book, pp. 289–311.

Burger LJ, Kalvin NH, Smith JL. (1970). Acquired lesions of the fourth cranial nerve. *Brain 93:*567–574.

Cantillo N. (1978). A case of superior oblique palsy in an orbital floor fracture. *Am Orthop J 28:*124–126.

Celli P, Ferrante L, Acqui M, et al. (1992). Neurinoma of the third, fourth, and sixth cranial nerves: A survey and report of a new fourth nerve case. *Surg Neurol 38:*216–224.

Cobbs WH, Schatz NJ, Savino PJ. (1980). Nontraumatic bilateral fourth nerve palsies: A dorsal midbrain sign [abstract]. *Ann Neurol 8:*107–108.

Collins TE, Mehalic TF, White TK, et al. (1992). Trochlear nerve palsy as the sole initial sign of an aneurysm of the superior cerebellar artery. *Neurosurgery 30:*258–261.

Coppeto JM, Lessell S. (1978). Cryptogenic unilateral paralysis of the superior oblique muscle. *Arch Ophthalmol 96:*275–277.

Coppeto JR. (1983). Superior oblique paresis and contralateral Horner's syndrome. *Ann Ophthalmol 15:*681–683.

Elliot D, Cunningham Jr ET, Miller NR. (1991). Fourth nerve paresis and ipsilateral relative afferent pupillary defect without visual sensory disturbance: A sign of contralateral dorsal midbrain disease. *J Clin Neuro-ophthalmol 11:*169–172.

Ellis FD, Helveston EM. (1976). Superior oblique palsy: Diagnosis and classification. *Int Ophthalmol Clin 16:*127–135.

Gacs G, Vinuela F, Fox AJ, et al. (1983). Peripheral aneurysms of the cerebellar arteries: Review of 16 cases. *J Neurosurg 58:*63–68.

Garen PD, Harper CG, Teo C, et al. (1987). Cystic schwannoma of the trochlear nerve mimicking a brain-stem tumor. *J Neurosurg 67:*928–930.

Gentry LR, Mehta RC, Appen RE, et al. (1991). MR imaging of primary trochlear nerve neoplasms. *Am J Neuroradiol 12:*707–713.

Gonyea EF. (1990). Superior oblique palsy due to a midbrain vascular malformation. *Neurology 40:*554–555.

Green WR, Hackett ER, Schlezinger NS. (1964). Neuro-ophthalmic evaluation of oculomotor nerve paralysis. *Arch Ophthalmol 72:*154–167.

Grimson BS, Glaser JS. (1978). Isolated trochlear nerve palsies in herpes zoster ophthalmicus. *Arch Ophthalmol 96:*1233–1235.

Guy J, Day AL, Mickle JP, et al. (1989). Contralateral trochlear nerve paresis and ipsilateral Horner's syndrome. *Am J Ophthalmol 107:*73–76.

Harley RD. Paralytic strabismus in children. (1980). Etiologic incidence and management of the third, fourth, and sixth nerve palsies. *Ophthalmology 87:*24–43.

Ho KL. (1981). Schwannoma of the trochlear nerve. *J Neurosurg 55:*132–135.

Jacobson DM, Warner JJ, Choucair AK, et al. (1988). Trochlear nerve palsy following minor head trauma: A sign of structural disorder. *J Clin Neuro-ophthalmol 8:*263–268.

Keane JR. (1975). Delayed trochlear nerve palsy in a case of zoster oticus. *Arch Ophthalmol 93:*382–383.

Keane JR. (1981). Fourth nerve palsy opposite a black eye. Two patients simulating orbital blow-out fractures. *J Clin Neuro-ophthalmol 1:*209–211.

Keane JR. (1993). Fourth nerve palsy: Historical review and study of 215 patients. *Neurology 43:*2439–2443.

Keane JR. (1989). Neurologic eye signs following motorcycle accidents. *Arch Neurol 46:*761–762.

Keane JR. (1986). Trochlear nerve pareses with brainstem lesions. *J Clin Neuro-ophthalmol 6:*242–246.

Kennerdell JS. (1973). Odds on the etiologies of the third, fourth, and sixth cranial nerve palsies. *Trans Pa Acad Ophthalmol Otolaryngol 26:*27–31.

Khawam E, Scott AB, Jampolsky A. (1967). Acquired superior oblique palsy. *Arch Ophthalmol 77:*761–768.

Kim JS, Kang JK, Lee SA, et al. (1993). Isolated or predominant ocular motor nerve palsy as a manifestation of brain stem stroke. *Stroke 24*:581–586.

Kim JS, Kang JK. (1992). Contralateral trochlear nerve palsy and facial sensory change due to a probable brainstem vascular malformation. *Neuro-ophthalmology 12*:59–62.

King JS. (1976). Trochlear nerve sheath tumor. *J Neurosurg 44*:245–247.

King RA, Calhoun JH. (1987). Fourth cranial nerve palsy following spinal anesthesia: A case report. *J Clin Neuro-ophthalmol 7*:20–22.

Krohel GB, Mansour AM, Petersen WL, et al. (1982). Isolated trochlear nerve palsy secondary to a juvenile pilocytic astrocytoma. *J Clin Neuro-ophthalmol 2*:119–123.

Ksiazek S, Behar R, Savino PJ, et al. (1988). Isolated acquired fourth nerve palsies. *Neurology 38(suppl 1)*:246.

Lavin PJM, Troost BT. (1984). Traumatic fourth nerve palsy. Clinico-anatomic correlations with computed tomographic scan. *Arch Neurol 41*:679–680.

Lavin PJM, Younkin SG, Kori SH. (1984). The pathology of ophthalmoplegia in herpes zoster ophthalmicus. *Neuro-ophthalmology 4*:75–80.

Lee AG. (1995). Fourth nerve palsy in pseudotumor cerebri. *Strabismus 3*:57–59.

Lee J, Flynn JT. (1985). Bilateral superior oblique palsies. *Br J Ophthalmol 69*:508–513.

Leunda G, Vaquero J, Cabezudo J, et al. (1982). Schwannoma of the oculomotor nerves: Report of four cases. *J Neurosurg 57*:563–565.

McKinna AJ. (1983). Eye signs in 611 cases of posterior fossa aneurysms: Their diagnostic and prognostic value. *Can J Ophthalmol 18*:3–6.

Mansour AM, Reinecke RD. (1986). Central trochlear palsy. *Surv Ophthalmol 30*:279–296.

Marsh RJ, Dulley B, Kelly V. (1977). External ocular motor palsies in ophthalmic zoster: A review. *Br J Ophthalmol 61*:677–682.

Maurice-Williams RS, Harvey PK. (1989). Isolated palsy of the fourth cranial nerve caused by an intracavernous aneurysm. *J Neurol Neurosurg Psychiatry 52*:679.

Mellinger JF, Gomez MR. (1977). Agenesis of the cranial nerves. In Vinken PJ, Bruyn GW (eds). *Handbook of Clinical Neurology, Congenital Malformations of the Brain and Skull,* Part 1. Amsterdam, Elsevier, pp. 395–414.

Miller MT, Urist MJ, Folk ER, et al. (1970). Superior oblique palsy presenting in late childhood. *Am J Ophthalmol 70*:212–214.

Miller NR, Morris JE, Maguire M. (1982). Combined use of neostigmine and ocular motility measurements in the diagnosis of myasthenia gravis. *Arch Ophthalmol 100*:761–763.

Miller NR. (1989). *Walsh and Hoyt's Clinical Neuro-ophthalmology*. 4th Edition. Baltimore, Williams & Wilkins, p. 686.

Mittleman D, Folk E. (1976). The evaluation and treatment of superior oblique muscle palsy. *Trans Am Acad Ophthalmol Otolaryngol 81*:893–898.

Moulis H, Mamus SW. (1989). Isolated trochlear nerve palsy in a patient with Waldenstrom's macroglobulinemia: Complete recovery with combination therapy. *Neurology 39*:1399.

Murray RS, Ajax ET. (1985). Bilateral trochlear nerve palsies. *Neurology 5*:57–58.

Neetens A, Van Aerde F. (1981). Extra-ocular muscle palsy from minor head trauma. Initial sign of intracranial tumor. *Bull Soc Belge Ophthalmol 193*:161–167.

Nemet P, Godel V, Baruch E, et al. (1980). Benign palsy of the superior oblique. *J Pediatr Ophthalmol Strabismus 17*:320–322.

Olson ME, Chernik NL, Posner JB. (1974). Infiltration of the leptomeninges by systemic cancer. *Arch Neurol 30*:122–137.

Pollard ZF. (1985). Classification and treatment of bilateral superior oblique palsy. *Ann Ophthalmol 17*:127–131.

Reich KA, Giansiracusa DR, Strongwater SL. (1990). Neurologic manifestations of giant cell arteritis. *Am J Med 89*:67–72.

Reynolds JD, Biglan AW, Hiles DA. (1984). Congenital superior oblique palsy in infants. *Arch Ophthalmol 102*:1503–1505.

Richards BW, Jones Jr FR, Younge BR. (1992). Causes and prognosis in 4,278 cases of paralysis of the oculomotor, trochlear, and abducens cranial nerves. *Am J Ophthalmol 113*:489–496.

Robb RM. (1990). Idiopathic superior oblique palsies in children. *J Pediatr Ophthalmol Strabismus 27*:66–69.

Robert CM, Geigenbaum JA, Stern WE. (1973). Ocular palsy occurring with pituitary tumors. *J Neurosurg 38*:17–19.

Rucker C, Dyer J, Smith D, et al. (1956). The causes of acquired paralysis of the ocular muscles. *Am J Ophthalmol 41*:951–955.

Rucker CW. (1958). Paralysis of the third, fourth and sixth cranial nerves. *Am J Ophthalmol 46*:787–794.

Rucker CW. (1966). The causes of paralysis of the third, fourth, and sixth cranial nerves. *Am J Ophthalmol 61*:1293–1298.

Rush JA. (1981b). Isolated superior oblique paralysis in progressive systemic sclerosis. *Ann Ophthalmol 13*:217–220.

Rush JA, Shafrin F. (1982). Ocular myasthenia presenting as superior oblique weakness. *J Clin Neuro-ophthalmol 2*:125–127.

Rush JA, Younge BR. (1981a). Paralysis of cranial nerves III, IV, and VI. *Arch Ophthalmol 99*:76–79.

Sabates NR, Gonce MA, Farris BK. (1991). Neuro-ophthalmological findings in closed head trauma. *J Clin Neuro-ophthalmol 11:*273–277.
Sawle GV, Sarkies NJC. (1989). Bilateral fourth nerve palsy due to cerebellar haemangioblastoma. *J R Soc Med 82:*111–112.
Scharf J, Meyer E, Zonis S. (1979). Trochlear nerve palsy in a case of herpes zoster ophthalmicus. *Ann Ophthalmol 11:*568–570.
Scott WE, Kraft SP. (1986). Classification and treatment of superior oblique palsies: II. Bilateral superior oblique palsies. *Trans New Orleans Acad Ophthalmol,* 265–292.
Scully RE, Galdabini JJ, McNeely BU. (1976). Case records of the Massachusetts General Hospital-weekly clinicopathological exercises. Case 36-1976. *N Engl J Med 295:*553–561.
Shrader EC, Schlezinger NS. (1960). Neuro-ophthalmologic evaluation of abducens nerve paralysis. *Arch Ophthalmol 63:*84–91.
Slavin ML. (1987). Isolated trochlear nerve palsy secondary to cavernous sinus meningioma. *Am J Ophthalmol 104:*433–434.
Snydor CF, Seaber JH, Buckley EG. (1982). Traumatic superior oblique palsies. *Ophthalmology 89:*134–138.
Suzuki J, Wada T, Kowada M. (1962). Clinical observations on tumors of the pineal region. *J Neurosurg 19:*441–445.
Tachibana H, Mimura O, Shiomi M, et al. (1990). Bilateral trochlear nerve palsies from a brainstem hematoma. *J Clin Neuro-ophthalmol 10:*35–37.
Teller J, Karmon G, Savir H. (1988). Long-term follow-up of traumatic unilateral superior oblique palsy. *Ann Ophthalmol 20:*424–425.
Urist M. (1953). Bilateral superior oblique paralysis. *Arch Ophthalmol 49:*382–391.
Vanooteghem P, Dehaene I, Van Zandycke M, et al. (1992). Combined trochlear nerve palsy and internuclear ophthalmoplegia. *Arch Neurol 49:*108–109.
Von Noorden GK, Helveston EM. (1994). *Strabismus: A Decision Making Approach.* St. Louis, Mosby, pp. 162–169.
Von Noorden GK, Murray E, Wong SY. (1986). Superior oblique paralysis. A review of 270 cases. *Arch Ophthalmol 104:*1771–1776.
Wise BL, Palubinskas AJ. (1965). Persistent trigeminal artery (carotid-basilar anastomosis). *J Neurosurg 21:*199–206.
Womack LW, Liesgang TJ. (1983). Complications of herpes zoster ophthalmicus. *Arch Ophthalmol 101:*42–45.
Wray SH. (1977). Neuro-ophthalmologic manifestations of pituitary and parasellar lesions. *Clin Neurosurg 24:*86–117.
Wright HG, Hansotia P. (1977). Isolated fourth cranial nerve palsies: Etiology and prognosis. *Wis Med J 76:*26–28.
Yamamoto M, Jimbo M, Ide M, et al. (1987). Trochlear neurinoma. *Surg Neurol 28:*287–290.
Yoss RE, Rucker CW, Miller RH. (1968). Neurosurgical complications affecting the oculomotor, trochlear, and abducens nerves. *Neurology 18:*594–600.
Younge BR, Sutula F. (1977). Analysis of trochlear nerve palsies. *Mayo Clin Proc 52:*11–18.

◆ 13 ◆

Sixth Nerve Palsies

What Is the Anatomy of the Sixth Nerve?

The sixth nerve nucleus is located lower pons. The nucleus contains motor neurons for the lateral rectus muscle and interneurons traveling via the medial longitudinal fasciculus (MLF) to the contralateral medial rectus subnucleus of the third nerve. The sixth nerve nucleus thus contains all the neurons responsible for horizontal conjugate gaze. The nerve fascicle leaves the nucleus and travels within the substance of the pontine tegmentum, adjacent to the medial leminiscus and the corticospinal tract. The sixth nerve leaves the brainstem, enters the subarachnoid space (prepontine cistern), courses nearly vertically along the clivus, and travels over the petrous apex of the temporal bone where it is tethered at the petroclinoid ligament in Dorello's canal. It enters the substance of the cavernous sinus lateral to the internal carotid artery and medial to the ophthalmic division of the trigeminal nerve (V1) to enter the orbit via the superior orbital fissure.

Sixth nerve palsies (SNP) may be divided into isolated SNP and non-isolated SNP. The criteria for the diagnosis of an isolated SNP are listed in Table 13–1.

Table 13–1. Criteria for the Diagnosis of Unilateral Isolated Sixth Nerve Palsy

- Ipsilateral abduction deficit with an incomitant esodeviation that is worsened with gaze into the field of the weak lateral rectus muscle
- Exclusion of Duane's retraction syndrome, spasm of the near reflex, and other causes of abduction deficits that can mimic a SNP, and exclusion of patients with signs of the following:
  - Orbital disease (e.g., chemosis, proptosis, lid swelling, injection, and positive forced ductions)
  - Myasthenia gravis (e.g., ptosis, Cogan's lid twitch sign, orbicularis oculi weakness, muscle fatigue or variability)
  - Multiple cranial nerve palsies (including bilateral SNP) or radiculopathy
  - Brainstem signs (e.g., Horner's syndrome, hemiplegia, cerebellar signs)
  - Systemic, infectious, or inflammatory risk factors for an SNP (e.g., history of previous malignancy, giant cell arteritis, collagen vascular disease)
  - Severe headache

Table 13–2. Definitions of the Six Types of Sixth Nerve Palsy

Type 1: Non-isolated
SNP are considered non-isolated in the presence of the exclusionary conditions outlined in Table 13–1.

Type 2: Traumatic SNP
Isolated unilateral SNP, which have a clearly established temporal relationship to significant previous head trauma and do not progress, are considered traumatic in origin. Patients with SNP following minor head trauma were excluded.

Type 3: Congenital SNP
Patients born with a SNP or noted to have a SNP within the first 3 months of life.

Type 4: Vasculopathic SNP
Vasculopathic SNP occur in patients older than age 55 or those with known vasculopathic risk factors (e.g., hypertension or diabetes).

Type 5: Nonvasculopathic SNP
Patients without vasculopathic risk factors defined above are considered to have nonvasculopathic SNP.

Type 6: Progressive or Unresolved SNP
SNP that worsen after the acute stage (greater than 2 weeks) as defined by a significant increase in the measured ocular deviation or who develop new neurologic findings, are considered progressive. Patients without resolution in the measured horizontal deviation after 12 to 16 weeks are considered unresolved.

We define six types of SNP in Table 13–2.

Is the Non-isolated SNP due to a Pontine (Lower Pons) Lesion?

Sixth nerve nuclear lesions cause a horizontal gaze palsy, rather than an isolated abduction deficit. An ipsilateral facial palsy may occur because of the close proximity of the facial and abducens nerve in the pons. Nuclear lesions are usually associated with other brainstem signs (e.g., hemiparesis, hemisensory loss, a central Horner's syndrome). Likewise, lesions of the sixth nerve fascicle involve adjacent structures (e.g., cranial nerves V, VII, and VIII; cerebellar ataxia; a central Horner's syndrome; or contralateral hemiplegia). Patients with a presumed nuclear or fascicular SNP should undergo neuroimaging (usually magnetic resonance [MR] imaging) directed to the pons.

The etiology of nuclear or fascicular lesions in pons are listed in Table 13–3.

Table 13–3. Etiology of a Sixth Nerve Palsy by Topographical Localization

- Nuclear (horizontal gaze palsy)
  - Congenital (Carr, 1997; Harley, 1980)
    - Mobius syndrome (Carr, 1997)
  - Demyelinating
  - Infarction or ischemia
  - Neoplasm (pontine and cerebellar)
    - Histiocytosis X (Pierrot-Deseilligny, 1984)
  - Trauma
  - Wernicke-Korsakoff syndrome

- Fascicular (Keane, 1976)
  - Demyelination (Keane, 1976; Moster, 1984)
  - Infarction (Donaldson, 1988; Keane, 1976; Kellen, 1988)
  - Neoplasm (Robertson, 1970)
  - Trauma
- Subarachnoid space
  - Aneurysm or vascular abnormality
    - Persistent primitive trigeminal artery (Ikezaki, 1989)
    - Posterior inferior cerebellar aneurysm
  - Carcinomatous meningitis
  - Following procedures
    - Cervical traction
    - Lumbar puncture
    - Myelography (Bell, 1990; Miller, 1982; Seyfert, 1978)
    - Post vaccination (Patil, 1977; Werner, 1983)
    - Radiculography (Dinakaran, 1995; Lloyd, 1995)
    - Shunting for hydrocephalus
    - Spinal or epidural anesthesia (De Veuster, 1994; Richer, 1989)
    - Ventriculoatrial shunt
  - Inflammatory
    - Retropharyngeal space inflammation (Fanous, 1992)
    - Necrotizing vasculitis (Sedwick, 1989)
    - Sarcoidosis (Sachs, 1990)
    - Systemic lupus erythematosus (Sedwick, 1983)
  - Infectious
    - Lyme (Lesser, 1990; Mastrianni, 1994)
    - Syphilis (Slavin, 1992)
    - Tuberculosis
    - Cryptococcal meningitis
    - Cysticercosis
    - HIV-CMV encephalitis (Fuller, 1989)
  - Neoplasm (Galetta, 1989; Keane, 1976; Savino, 1982)
    - Abducens nerve tumor (Ginsberg, 1988; Nehls, 1985; Tung, 1991)
    - Cerebellopontine angle tumor
  - Clivus tumor (Bagan, 1980; Handa, 1987; Quencer, 1981; Takahashi, 1983)
    - Leukemia (Averbuch-Heller, 1994)
    - Metastatic (O'Boyle, 1992)
    - Skull base tumors (Volpe, 1993)
    - Trigeminal nerve tumor (Del Priore, 1989)
  - Nonlocalizing sign of increased intracranial pressure (Aroichane, 1995)
    - Pseudotumor cerebri
    - Meningitis of any type
    - Intracranial tumor
  - Subarachnoid hemorrhage (Keane, 1976)
  - Trauma (including surgical)
- Petrous apex
  - Neoplasm (e.g., nasopharyngeal carcinoma)

(continued)

Table 13–3. *(continued)*

- Infection
  - Complicated otitis media (Homer, 1996)
  - Mastoiditis (Gradenigo's syndrome)
- Thrombosis of inferior petrosal sinus (Robertson, 1970)
- Trauma (Antoniades, 1993; Mutyala, 1996)
  - Basilar skull fracture
- Inflammatory

Cavernous sinus (Gurinsky, 1983)

- Cavernous sinus thrombosis (DiNubile, 1988)
- Cavernous sinus fistula (Hawke, 1989; Leonard, 1984)
- Neoplasm
  - Nasopharyngeal cancer
  - Pituitary adenoma
  - Plasmacytoma (Bachmeyer, 1997)
  - Sixth nerve neuroma (Hansman, 1986)
  - Skull base tumors (Currie, 1983)
  - Sphenoid sinus tumors (Suster, 1989)
  - Squamous cell cancer of the pterygopalatine fossa
  - Subarachnoid diverticulum (Kobayashi, 1987)
- Ischemic
- Inflammatory or infectious
  - Herpes zoster (Smith, 1993; Goldsmith, 1968)
  - Tolosa-Hunt syndrome (Kline, 1981)
- Internal carotid artery aneurysms (Abad, 1981) or dissection (Maitland, 1983) or dolichoectasia (Blumenthal, 1997)

Orbital lesions

- Neoplastic
- Inflammation
- Infectious
- Traumatic (Lazow, 1995)

Is the SNP due to a Subarachnoid Space Lesion?

Lesions of the subarachnoid space may result in a unilateral or bilateral sixth nerve palsy. This is a nonlocalizing finding because any cause of increased intracranial pressure may result in a sixth nerve palsy as listed in Table 13–3. Patients with a subarachnoid space lesion should undergo neuroimaging directed to this location followed by a lumbar puncture as needed.

Is the SNP the Result of a Lesion of the Petrous Apex?

Lesions of the petrous apex causing SNP are associated with other neurologic findings, including involvement of other cranial nerves (e.g., fifth, seventh, and eighth) or facial pain. Neuroimaging should be directed toward the petrous apex (MR imaging or computed tomography for bone involvement).

Is the SNP due to a Cavernous Sinus Lesion?

With lesions of the cavernous sinus, SNP usually occur in association with other cranial neuropathies (e.g., third, fourth, or fifth nerves) or a Horner's syndrome. Neuroimaging (usually MR imaging) should be directed to the cavernous sinus. Table 13–3 lists the etiologies of a cavernous sinus lesion causing a SNP.

Is the SNP due to an Orbital Lesion?

Lesions of the orbit causing SNP are usually associated with other orbital signs such as proptosis or chemosis. Neuroimaging (preferably MR imaging) should be directed to the orbit.

A recommendation for management of each type of SNP is made based on the available evidence from the literature.

What Are Some Recommendations for the Evaluation of SNP?

1. Nonisolated SNP (Type 1) should undergo neuroimaging and further evaluation, with attention to areas suggested topographically by the associated neurologic signs or symptoms (see above) (Bagan, 1980; Dumas, 1982; Gailbraith, 1994; Golding, 1980; Harley, 1980; Nemzek, 1995; O'Boyle, 1992; Rush, 1981; Steel, 1994; Volpe, 1993).
2. Traumatic SNP (Type 2) should undergo the appropriate acute neuroimaging (CT scanning) as indicated by the trauma associated neurologic signs and symptoms.
3. Congenital SNP (Type 3) are rare and there is insufficient data to make a strong recommendation for the management of congenital isolated SNP from our review of the literature. Nevertheless, if the SNP can be clearly demonstrated to be congenital in origin, additional neuroimaging is not generally required. Transient SNP may occur following birth trauma in newborns. Galbraith reported the incidence of SNP in a group of 6886 neonates as being 0.4% (Leung, 1987). All of these SNP (Type 3) resolved within 6 weeks, and we recommend that imaging may be deferred in these patients. The incidence of SNP increased with "complexity of instrumentation" with a 0% prevalence for cesarean section, 0.1% prevalence for spontaneous vaginal delivery, 2.4% prevalence for forceps delivery, and a 3.2% for vacuum extraction (Leung, 1987). Leung (Galetta, 1989) reported three cases of right SNP after vaginal delivery that all resolved after four to 12 weeks.
4. Vasculopathic SNP (Type 4) may be observed (without neuroimaging) for improvement for four to twelve weeks (Moster, 1984; Savino, 1982, 1986). Rush and Younge (Steel, 1994) reported a recovery rate of 49.6% in 419 nonselected SNP cases, and a higher rate of 71% in 419 patients with diabetes mellitus, hypertension, or atherosclerosis. Some authors have recommended observing vasculopathic isolated SNP beyond a three month interval of recovery if the esotropia and the abduction deficit were

decreasing (Burde, 1992). Elderly patients who present with an isolated SNP and headache, scalp tenderness, jaw claudication, or visual loss should undergo an appropriate evaluation for giant cell arteritis including an erythrocyte sedimentation rate and, when clinically indicated, a temporal artery biopsy (Currie, 1983; Moster, 1984; Reich, 1990; Savino, 1982, 1986). Patients with progression or lack of improvement (Type 6) should undergo neuroimaging.

5. Nonvasculopathic SNP (Type 5) should undergo neuroimaging (Bagan, 1980; Del Priore, 1989; Fanous, 1992; Gailbraith, 1994; Ginsberg, 1988; Golding, 1980; Gurinsky, 1983; Hansman, 1986; Harley, 1980; Kobayashi, 1987; Michael, 1974; Moster, 1984; Nehls, 1985; O'Boyle, 1992; Quencer, 1981; Rush, 1981; Sachs, 1990; Savino, 1986; Slavin, 1989, 1992; Steel, 1994; Sternberg, 1980; Straussberg, 1993; Takahashi, 1983; Tung, 1991). Younger patients, or those without vasculopathic risk factors (Type 5), should undergo a more extensive evaluation including a fasting blood glucose, complete blood cell count, blood pressure evaluation, lumbar puncture, and neuroimaging (MR imaging). Type 5 SNP have a significant (27%) chance of harboring an underlying malignant neoplasm (Savino, 1986). Evaluation for myasthenia gravis should be particularly considered in these patients.
6. Testing for vasculopathic risk factors in Type 4 or Type 5 SNP should be performed, even in the absence of a previous history of diabetes or hypertension (Abad, 1981; Burde, 1992; Savino, 1982; Watanabe, 1990).
7. Patients with progressive or unresolved SNP (Type 6), or patients with new neurological signs or symptoms, should undergo neuroimaging (Burder, 1992; Harley, 1980; Moster, 1984; Savino, 1982, 1986). Progressive, or unresolved SNP, should undergo neuroimaging (Burde, 1992; Moster, 1984). Galetta and Smith described 13 chronic SNP. Of these, four were idiopathic, four due to tumor, two were traumatic, one was postspinal anesthesia, one was temporal arteritis, and one was intracavernous aneurysm. In their study, "chronic" was defined as an SNP lasting 6 months or longer. Savino et al. (Savino, 1982) reviewed 38 patients with chronic SNP; 14 (37%) were discovered to have an intracranial lesion. These authors specifically recommended neuroradiologic investigation at onset in any patient with a history of carcinoma.

Moster et al. commented on the lack of truly isolated SNP reported in the literature. Most reports do not separate unilateral from bilateral SNP, or isolated SNP from those associated with other neurologic or cranial nerve defects (Savino, 1986). Our review of the literature on SNP revealed 29 case reports and case series describing 199 patients with presumed isolated SNP. Of these 199 patients, 31 were traumatic, none were congenital, 42 were vasculopathic, 43 were "idiopathic," and the remainder had a number of miscellaneous etiologies (7 post lumbar puncture, 7 multiple sclerosis, 2 post-immunizations, 5 "infectious," 5 aneurysms, 1 sarcoid, 4 "presumed inflammation," 1 orbital amyloidosis, and 1 diverticulum of the cavernous sinus). Fifty cases were the result of tumors (21 chordomas, 2 chondrosarcomas, 2 chordomas or chondrosarcomas, 6 meningiomas,1 cylindroma, 1 lymphomatous meningitis, 5 schwannomas, 1 nasopharyngeal carcinoma, 5 metastases, 1 trigeminal neurilemona, 1 pontine glioma, 3 pituitary adenomas, and 1 miscellaneous). The remaining SNP in the literature review were associated with other neurological signs or symptoms, such as headache, tinnitus, disc edema, nystagmus, and so on, or there was insufficient clinical data in the report to determine if the SNP was truly isolated by our criteria in Table 13–1 (Abad, 1981; Antoniades, 1993; Averbuch-Heller, 1994; Bagan, 1980; Barry-Kinsella, 1994; Bell, 1990; Bixenman, 1981; Boger, 1984; Burde, 1992; Decaux, 1980; Del Priore, 1989; Depper, 1993; Dinakaran, 1995; Donaldson, 1988;

Dumas, 1982; Fanous, 1992; Fujuoka, 1995; Fuller, 1989; Gailbraith, 1994; Galetta, 1989; Ginsberg, 1988; Golding, 1980; Gurinsky, 1983; Hamilton, 1993; Hansman, 1986; Harley, 1980; Johnston, 1968; Keltner, 1983; Kirkham, 1976; Knox, 1967; Kobayashi, 1987; Lee, 1992, 1994; Lesser, 1990; Leung, 1987; Lewis, 1995; McCammon, 1981; Michael, 1974; Moster, 1984; Nehls, 1985; Nemzek, 1995; O'Boyle, 1992; Patil, 1977; Quencer, 1981; Reinecke, 1981; Reynolds, 1988; Richer, 1989; Rush, 1981; Sachs, 1990; Savino, 1982, 1986; Sedwick, 1983, 1989; Seyfert, 1978; Simcock, 1994; Slavin, 1989, 1992; Slonim, 1985; Steel, 1994; Sternberg, 1980; Straussberg, 1993; Suster, 1989; Takahashi, 1983; Thomas, 1970; Thorsen, 1947; Tung, 1991; Volpe, 1993; Watanabe, 1990; Werner, 1983; Yang, 1991; Yoshizawa, 1984; Zumla, 1988).

SNP that result after lumbar puncture, post myelographic LP, and spinal anesthesia have been reported in the literature (Donalson, 1988; Sedwick, 1989; Simcock, 1994). Thorsen (Rucker, 1958) reported 229 cases of SNP after spinal anesthesia and LP. Most of these SNP occurred at the tenth day following lumbar puncture, were unilateral, associated with headache, and occurred in young patients (Simcock, 1994; Thorsen, 1947). These patients may be followed for resolution without imaging.

Aneurysm is a rare cause of acquired SNP. Rucker (Rush, 1981) reported 924 cases of SNP and only 3.3% or 31 were due to aneurysm. Rush and Younge (Steel, 1994) described 419 cases of SNP and only 3.6% or 15 were due to aneurysm. Dailey et al. (Dumas, 1982; Rucker, 1958; Rush, 1981; Steel, 1994) did not find any cases of aneurysm presenting with an isolated SNP in their series on cerebral aneurysms with ocular involvement and others have reported similar findings.

A suggested approach to the evaluation of SNP is presented in Figure 13–1.

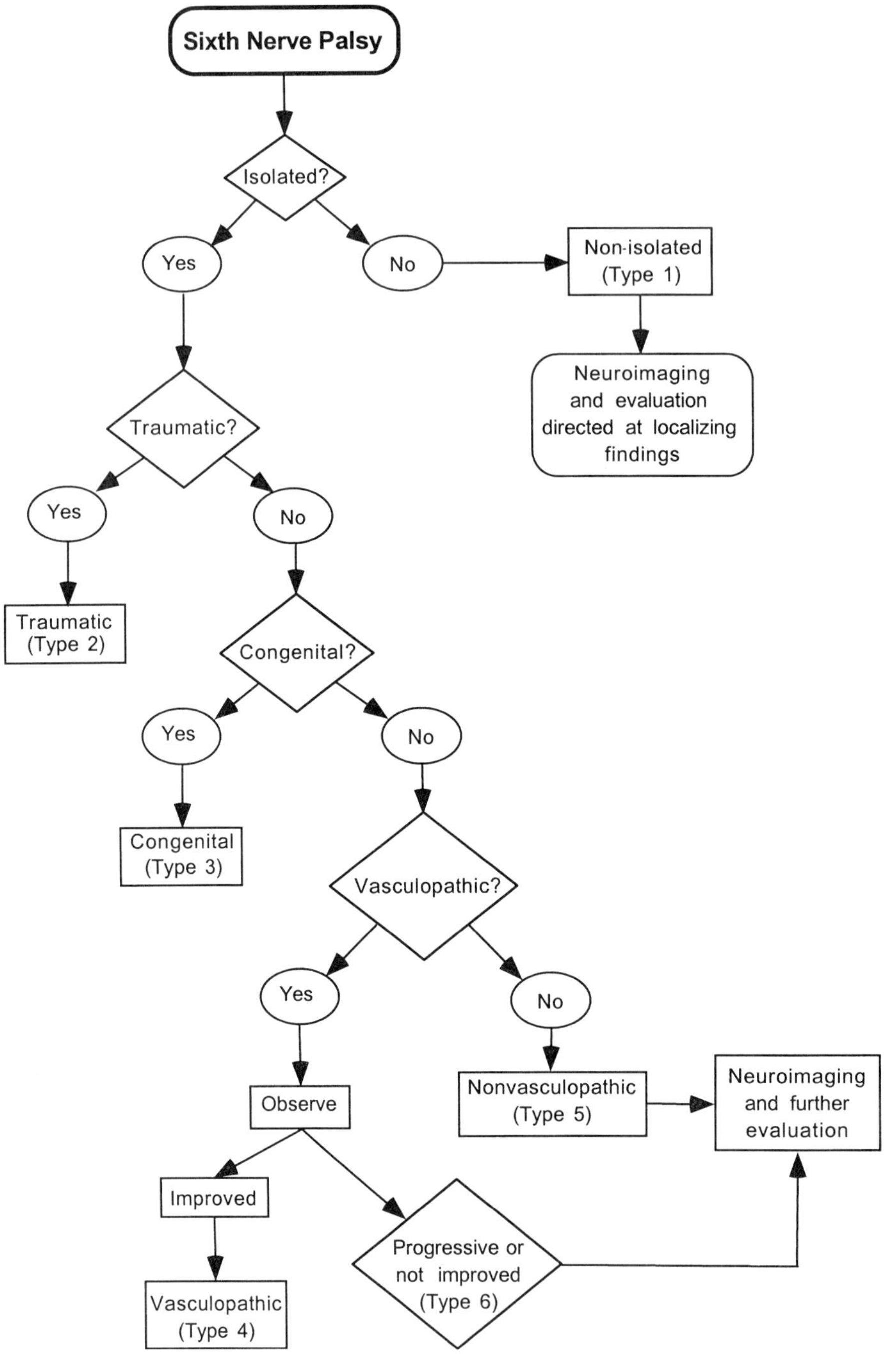

Figure 13–1. Sixth nerve palsy.

References

Abad JM, Alvarez F, Blazquez MG. (1981). An unrecognized neurological syndrome: Sixth-nerve palsy and Horner's syndrome due to traumatic intracavernous carotid aneurysm. *Surg Neurol 16(2):*140–144.

Antoniades K, Karakasis D, Taskos N. (1993). Abducen nerve palsy following transverse fracture of the middle cranial fossa. *J Cranio-Maxillo-Facial Surg 21:*172–175.

Aroichane M, Repka MX. (1995). Outcome of sixth nerve palsy or paresis in young children. *Journal of Pediatric Ophthalmol 32(3):*152–156.

Averbuch-Heller L, Gillis S, Ben-Hur T. (1994). Transient sixth-nerve palsy as the first presentation of acute leukemia. *J Neurol Neurosurg Psychiat 57:*506.

Bachmeyer C, Levy V, Carteret M, et al. (1997). Sphenoid sinus localization of multiple myeloma revealing evolution from benign gammopathy. *Head & Neck 19(4):*347–350.

Bagan SM, Hollenhorst RW. (1980). Ocular manifestations of intracranial chordomas. *Trans Am Ophthal Soc LXXCVIII:*148–155.

Barry-Kinsella C, Milner M, McCarthy N, et al. (1994). Sixth nerve palsy: An unusual manifestation of preeclampsia. *Obstet Gynecol 83(5):*849–850.

Bell JA, Dowd TC, McIlwaine GG, et al. (1990). Postmyelographic abducent nerve palsy in association with the contrast agent iopamidol. *J Clin Neuro-ophthalmol 10(2):*115–117.

Bixenman WW, Von Noorden GK. (1981). Benign recurrent VI nerve palsy in childhood. *J Ped Ophthalmol Strabis 18(3):*29–34.

Blumenthal EZ, Gomori JM, Dotan S. (1997). Recurrent abducens nerve palsy caused by dolichoectasia of the cavernous internal carotid artery. *J Ophthalmol 124(2):*255–257.

Boger WP, Puliafito CA, Magoon EH, et al. (1984). Recurrent isolated sixth nerve palsy in children. *Ann Ophthalmol 16(3):*237–244.

Burde RM, Savino PJ, Trobe JD. (1992). *Clinical Decisions in Neuro-ophthalmology.* 2nd edition. St. Louis, Mosby Year Book, pp. 289–311.

Carr MM, Ross DA, Zuker RM. (1997). Cranial nerve defects in congenital facial palsy [Review]. *J Otolaryngol 26(2):*80–87.

Currie J, Lubin JH, Lessell S. (1983). Chronic isolated abducens paresis from tumors at the base of the brain. *Arch Neurol 40:*226–229.

Decaux G, Szyper M, Extors M, et al. (1980). Central nervous system complications of mycoplasma pneumoniae. *J Neurol Neurosurg Psychiat 43:*883–887.

Del Priore LV, Miller NR. (1989). Trigeminal Schwannoma as a cause of chronic, isolated sixth nerve palsy. *Am J Ophthalmol 108:*726–729.

Depper MH, Truwit CL, Dreisbach JN, et al. (1993). Isolated abducens nerve palsy: MR imaging findings. *AJR 160:*837–841.

De Veuster I, Smet H, Vercauteren M, Tassignon MJ. (1994). The time course of a sixth nerve paresis following epidural anesthesia. *Bull Societe Bel Ophthalmol 252:*45–47.

Dinakaran S, Desai SP, Corney CE. (1995). Case report: Sixth nerve palsy following radiculography. *Br J Radiol 68:*424.

Donaldson D, Rosenberg NL. (1988). Infarction of abducens nerve fascicle as cause of isolated sixth nerve palsy related to hypertension. *Neurology 38:*1654.

Dumas S, Shults WT. (1982). Abducens paresis. *J Clin Neuro-ophthalmol 2:*55–60.

Fanous MM, Margo CE, Hamed LM. (1992). Chronic idiopathic inflammation of the retropharyngeal space presenting with sequential abducens palsies. *J Clin Neuro-ophthalmol 12(3):*154–157.

Fujuoka T, Segawa F, Ogawa K, et al. (1995). Ischemic and hemorrhagic brain stem lesions mimicking diabetic ophthalmoplegia. *Clin Neurol Neurosurg 97:*167–171.

Fuller GN, Guiloff RJ, Scaravilli F, et al. (1989). Combined HIV-CMV encephalitis presenting with brainstem signs. *J Neurol Neurosurg Psych 52:*975–979.

Gailbraith RS. (1994). Incidence of neonatal sixth nerve palsy in relation to mode of delivery. *Am J Obstet 170(4):*1158.

Galetta SL, Lawton-Smith J. (1989). Chronic isolated sixth nerve palsies. *Arch Neurol 46:*79–82.

Ginsberg F, Peyster RG, Rose WS, et al. (1988). Sixth nerve Schwannoma: MR and CT demonstration. *J Comput Assist Tomogr 12(3):*482–484.

Golding R, Peatfield RC, Shawdon HH, et al. (1980). Computer tomographic features of giant intracranial aneurysms. *Clin Radiol 31:*41–48.

Goldsmith MO. (1968). Herpes zoster ophthalmicus with sixth nerve palsy. *Can J Ophthalmol 3(3):*279–283.

Gurinsky JS, Quencer RM, Post MJD. (1983). Sixth nerve ophthalmoplegia secondary to a cavernous sinus lesion. *J Clin Neuro-ophthalmol 3:*277–281.

Gutman I, Levartovski S, Goldhammer Y, et al. (1986). Sixth nerve palsy and unilateral Horner's syndrome. *Ophthalmology 93(7):*913–916.

Hamilton SR, Smith CH, Lessell S. (1993). Idiopathic hypertrophic cranial pachymeningitis. *J Clin Neuro-ophthalmol 13(2):*127–134.

Handa J, Suzuki F, Nioka H, Koyama T. (1987). Clivus chordoma in childhood. *Surg Neurol 28(1):*58–62.

Hansman ML, Hoover ED, Peyster RG. (1986). Sixth nerve neuroma in the cavernous sinus: CT features. *J Comput Assist Tomogr 10(6):*1030–1032.

Harley RD. (1980). Paralytic strabismus in children: Etiologic incidence and management of the third, fourth, and sixth nerve palsies. *Ophthalmology 87:*24–43.

Homer JJ, Johnson IJ, Jones NS. (1996). Middle ear infection and sixth nerve palsy. *J Laryngol & Otol 110(9):*872–874.

Ikezaki K, Fujii K, Kishikawa T. (1989). Persistent primitive trigeminal artery: A possible cause of trigeminal and abducens nerve palsy [letter]. *J Neurol, Neurosurg & Psychiatr 52(12):*1449–1450.

Johnston AC. (1968). Etiology and treatment of abducens paralysis. *Pacific Coast Otolaryngol Ophthal Sci Trans 49:*259–277.

Keane JR. (1976). Bilateral sixth nerve palsy. Analysis of 125 cases. *Arch Neurol 33(10):*681–683.

Kellen RI, Burde RM, Hodges FD 3d, Roper-Hall G. (1988). Central bilateral sixth nerve palsy associated with a unilateral preganglionic Horner's syndrome. *J Clin Neuro-ophthalmol 8(3):*179–184.

Keltner JL. (1983). Neuro-ophthalmology for the pediatrician. *Pediat Ann 12(8):*586–602.

Kirkham TH. (1976). *Sixth Nerve Palsies in Children. Orthoptics: Past, Present, and Future.* New York, Stratton, pp. 359–366.

Kline LB, Galbraith JG. (1981). Parasellar epidermoid tumor presenting as painful ophthalmoplegia. *J Neurosurg 54(1):*113–117.

Knox DL, Clark DB, Schuster FF. (1967). Benign VI nerve palsies in children. *Pediatrics 40(4):*560–564.

Kobayashi T, Negoro M, Awaya S. (1987). Cavernous sinus subarachnoid diverticulum and sixth nerve palsy. *Neuroradiology 29:*306–307.

Lazow SK, Izzo SR, Feinberg ME, Berger JR. (1995). Bilateral abducens nerve palsy secondary to maxillofacial trauma: Report of case with proposed mechanism of injury. *J Oral & Maxillofacial Surg 53(10):*1197–1199.

Lee J, Harris S, Cohen J, et al. (1994). Results of a prospective randomized trial of botulinum toxin therapy in acute unilateral sixth nerve palsy. *J Ped Ophthalmol Strabis 31:*283–286.

Lee J. (1992). Modern management of sixth nerve palsy. *Australian New Zealand J Ophthalmol 20(1):*41–46.

Leonard TJ, Moseley IF, Sanders MD. (1984). Ophthalmoplegia in carotid cavernous sinus fistula. *Brit J Ophthalmol 68(2):*128–134.

Lesser RL, Kornmehl EW, Pachner AR, et al. (1990). Neuro-ophthalmologic manifestations of Lyme disease. *Ophthalmology 97(6):*699–706.

Leung AKC. (1987). Transient sixth cranial nerve palsy in newborn infants. *Br J Clin Prac 41(4):*717–718.

Lewis AI, Tomsick TA, Tew JM. (1995). Management of 100 consecutive direct carotid-cavernous fistulas: Results of treatment with detachable balloons. *Neurosurgery 36(2):*239–245.

Lloyd MN. (1995). Sixth nerve palsy following radiculography [letter; comment]. *Brit J Radiol 68(813):*1039–1040.

Maitland CG, Black JL, Smith WA. (1983). Abducens nerve palsy due to spontaneous dissection of the internal carotid artery. *Arch Neurol 40(7):*448–449.

Mastrianni JA, Galetta SL, Raps EC, Liu GT, Volpe NJ. (1994). Isolated fascicular abducens nerve palsy and Lyme disease. *J Neuro-ophthalmol 14(1):*2–5.

McCammon A, Kaufman HH, Sears SS. (1981). Transient oculomotor paralysis in pseudotumor cerebri. *Neurology 31:*182–184.

Michael WF. (1974). Posterior fossa aneurysms simulating tumors. *J Neurol Neurosurg Psychiat 37:*218–223.

Miller EA, Savino PJ, Schatz NJ. (1982). Bilateral sixth-nerve palsy. A rare complication of water-soluble contrast myelography. *Arch Ophthalmol 100(4):*603–604.

Moster ML, Savino PJ, Sergott RC, et al. (1984). Isolated sixth-nerve palsies in younger adults. *Arch Ophthalmol 102:*1328–1330.

Mutyala S, Holmes JM, Hodge DO, Younge BR. (1996). Spontaneous recovery rate in traumatic sixth-nerve palsy. *Am J Ophthalmol 122(6):*898–899.

Nehls DG, Sonntag VKH, Murphy AR, et al. (1985). Fibroblastic tumor of the abducens nerve. *J Neurosurg 62:*296–299.

Nemzek W, Postma G, Poirier V, et al. (1995). MR features of pachymeningitis presenting with sixth-nerve-palsy secondary to sphenoid sinusitis. *AJNR 16:*960–963.

O'Boyle JE, Gardner TA, Oliva A, et al. (1992). Sixth nerve palsy as the initial presenting sign of metastatic prostate cancer. *J Clin Neuro-ophthalmol 12(3):*149–153.

Patil SN, Padmawar BU, Chandra I. (1977). Sixth nerve paralysis following cholera innoculation. *Ind J Ophthalmol 24(IV):*37.

Pierrot-Deseilligny C, Goasguen J. (1984). Isolated abducens nucleus damage due to histiocytosis X. Electro-oculographic analysis and physiological deductions. *Brain 107(Pt 4):*1019–1032.

Quencer RM. (1981). Unilateral sixth nerve paresis. *J Clin Neuro-ophthalmol 1:*57–62.

Reich KA, Giansiracusa DR, Strongwater SL. (1990). Neurologic manifestations of giant cell arteritis. *Am J Med 89:*67–72.

Reinecke RD, Thompson WE. (1981). Childhood recurrent idiopathic paralysis of the lateral rectus. *Ann Ophthalmol 13(9):*1037–1039.

Reynolds DJM, Aylward GW. (1988). Acute sixth nerve palsy following vaccination. *J Infect 17(1):*84–85.

Richer S, Ritacca D. (1989). Sixth nerve palsy after lumbar anesthesia. *Optomet Vis Sci 66(5):*320–321.

Robertson DM, Hines JD, Rucker CW. (1970). Acquired sixth-nerve paresis in children. *Arch Ophthalmol 83:*574–579.

Rucker CW. (1958). Paralysis of the third, fourth and sixth cranial nerves. *Am J Ophthalmol 46:*787–794.

Rucker CW. (1966). The causes of paralysis of the third, fourth, and sixth cranial nerves. *Am J Ophthalmol 61:*1293–1298.

Rush JA, Younge BR. (1981). Paralysis of cranial nerves III, IV, and VI. *Arch Ophthalmol 99:*76–79.

Sachs R, Kashii S, Burde RM. (1990). Sixth nerve palsy as the initial manifestation of sarcoidosis. *Am J Ophthalmol 110(4):*438–440.

Sakalas R, Harbison JW, Vines FS, Becker DP. (1975). Chronic sixth nerve palsy. An initial sign of basisphenoid tumors. *Arch Ophthalmol 93(3):*186–190.

Savino PJ, Hilliker JK, Casell GH, et al. (1982). Chronic sixth nerve palsies: Are they really harbingers of serious intracranial disease? *Arch Ophthalmol 100:*1442–1444.

Savino PJ. (1986). Diplopia and sixth nerve palsies. *Semin Neurol 6(2):*142–146.

Sedwick LA, Burde RM. (1983). Isolated sixth nerve palsy as initial manifestation of systemic lupus erythematosus: A case report. *J Clin Neuro-ophthalmol 3:*109–110.

Sedwick LA, Margo CE. (1989). Sixth nerve palsies, temporal artery biopsy, and necrotizing vasculitis. *J Clin Neuro-ophthalmol 9(2):*119–121.

Seyfert S, Mager J. (1978). Abducens palsy after lumbar myelography with water soluble contrast media. *J Neurol 219:*213–220.

Simcock PR, Kelleher S, Dunne JA. (1994). Neuro-ophthalmic findings in Botulism Type B. *Eye 8:*646–648.

Slavin M, Haimovic I, Mahendra P. (1992). Sixth nerve palsy and pontocerebellar mass due to Luetic Meningoencephalitis. *Arch Ophthalmol 110:*322.

Slavin ML. (1989). Hyperdeviation associated with isolated unilateral abducens palsy. *Ophthalmology 96(4):*512–516.

Slonim R, McLarty B. (1985). Sixth cranial nerve palsy—unusual presenting symptom of lithium toxicity? *Can J Psychiat 30(6):*443–444.

Smith EF, Santamarina L, Wolintz AH. (1993). Herpes zoster ophthalmicus as a cause of Horner syndrome. *J Clin Neuro-ophthalmol 13(4):*250–253.

Steel TR, Bentivoglio PB, Garrick R. (1994). Vascular neurofibromatosis affecting the internal carotid artery: A case report. *Br J Neurosurg 8:*233–237.

Sternberg I, Ronen S, Arnon N. (1980). Recurrent, isolated, post-febrile abducens palsy. *J Pediat Ophthalmol Strabis 17(5):*323–324.

Straussberg R, Cohen AH, Amir J, et al. (1993). Benign abducens palsy associated with EBV infection. *J Pediat Ophthalmol Strabis 30:*60.

Suster S, Porges R, Tobias J, et al. (1989). Giant-cell neoplasm of the sphenoid sinus. *Mount Sinai J Med 56(2):*118–122.

Takahashi T, Asai T, Isayama Y, et al. (1983). Chordoma. *J Clin Neuro-ophthalmol 3:*251–257.

Thomas JE, Reagan TJ. (1970). Nonhemorrhagic complications of intracranial aneurysms of the internal carotid artery. *Neurology 20(11):*1043–1051.

Thorsen G. (1947). Neurological complications after spinal anesthesia. *Acta Chir Scand 5(Suppl 121):*1–272.

Tung H, Chen T, Weiss MH. (1991). Sixth nerve schwannomas. *J Neurosurg 75:*638–641.

Volpe NJ, Lessell S. (1993). Remitting sixth nerve palsy in skull base tumors. *Arch Ophthalmol 111:*1391–1395.

Watanabe K, Hagura R, Akanuma Y, et al. (1990). Characteristics of cranial nerve palsies in diabetic patients. *Diab Res Clin Prac 10:*19–27.

Werner DB, Savino PJ, Schatz NJ. (1983). Benign recurrent sixth nerve palsies in childhood: Secondary to immunization or viral illness. *Arch Ophthalmol 101:*607–608.

Yang MC, Bateman JB, Yee RD, et al. (1991). Electrooculography an discriminant analysis in Duane's syndrome and sixth-cranial-nerve palsy. *Graefe's Arch Clin Exp Ophthalmol 229:*52–56.

Yoshizawa T, Tomon Y, Nose T, et al. (1984). Juxtasellar mycotic abscess. *Surg Neurol 21:*49–52.

Zumla A, Lipscomb G, Lewis D. (1988). Sixth cranial nerve palsy complicating psittacosis. *J Neurol Neurosurg Psych 51:*1462.

◆ 14 ◆

Supranuclear Palsy

What Is the Anatomy of Horizontal Conjugate Gaze?

Supranuclear structures coordinate the action of muscle groups and control two types of eye movements: conjugate movements, in which both eyes move in the same direction, and vergence movements, in which both eyes either turn in (converge) or turn out (diverge). The final common pathway for horizontal conjugate gaze starts in the abducens nucleus that contains two types of intermingled neurons: motor neurons and internuclear neurons. The axons of the internuclear neurons cross to the contralateral side in the lower pons and, after ascending in the medial longitudinal fasciculus (MLF), synapse in the portion of the oculomotor nucleus that innervates the medial rectus muscle. This final common pathway is controlled by the vestibular system, optokinetic system, smooth pursuit system, and saccadic system. Thus, an excitatory horizontal vestibuloocular impulse originating in the horizontal canal is relayed from the ipsilateral medial vestibular nucleus to the contralateral abducens nucleus, resulting in conjugate horizontal deviation of the eyes to the contralateral side (Johnston, 1992; Pierrot-Deseilligny, 1995; Sharpe, 1989; Tusa, 1988).

Where Are Lesions that Cause Horizontal Gaze Palsies Located?

A lesion anywhere along the pathways that control horizontal eye movements may cause a horizontal gaze palsy. Depending on the location of the lesion, horizontal pursuit, saccades, or both may be impaired.

Lesions causing defects in horizontal smooth pursuit eye movements are summarized in Table 14–1.

Table 14–1. Localization of Lesions Impairing Horizontal Pursuit Eye Movements

Frontal lobe lesions may impair ipsilateral horizontal smooth pursuit and lesions of the posterior parietal cortex or temporal-occipito-parietal region can decrease the amplitude and velocity of smooth pursuit eye movements toward the side of the lesion (Leigh, 1985; Morrow, 1995).

Lesions occurring in a band extending from the occipito-temporal areas posteriorly, through the internal sagittal stratum, the posterior and anterior limbs of the internal capsule with adjacent striatum, to the dorsomedial frontal cortex anteriorly cause predominantly ipsilesional pursuit deficits (Lekwuwa, 1996).

Posterior thalamic hemorrhage may cause a deficit in smooth pursuit toward the side of the lesion by interrupting corticofugal fibers passing to the pontine nuclei near the posterior thalamus or the adjacent retrolenticular portion of the internal capsule (Brigell, 1984).

Unilateral midbrain lesions may result in ipsilateral pursuit defects (Kato, 1990; Zackon, 1984) as may basal pontine lesions that damage the pontine nuclei (Gaymard, 1993; Kato, 1990; Thier, 1991; Waespe, 1992). Because of the double decussation in the brainstem of the motor pursuit pathways, patients with posterior fossa lesions may have impaired ocular smooth pursuit either contralaterally or ipsilaterally (Furman, 1991; Johnston, 1992).

The cerebellar flocculus and vermis play an important role in the production of smooth pursuit (Waterston, 1992); unilateral cerebellar damage results in transient impairment of pursuit in the direction of the involved side (Waespe, 1992), while bilateral damage causes permanent impairment of smooth pursuit eye movements. A posterior vermal lesion may impair pursuit (Pierrot-Deseilligny, 1990) and middle cerebellar peduncle lesions or floccular lesions may cause an ipsilateral pursuit defect (Kato, 1990; Waespe, 1992).

Many drugs or disseminated disease processes may slow down or even abolish smooth pursuit eye movements. For example, pursuit eye movements are often impaired with progressive supranuclear palsy (PSP) (Friedman, 1992; Malessa, 1994), Huntington's disease, Gerstmann-Straussler-Scheinker disease (Yee, 1992), and HIV-related illnesses (Merrill, 1991).

Lesions causing defects in horizontal saccadic eye movements are summarized in Table 14–2.

Table 14–2. Localization of Lesions Causing Impaired Horizontal Conjugate Saccadic Eye Movements

Frontal lobe lesions
- Transient neglect contralaterally
- Defect in generating voluntary saccades
- Transient horizontal gaze deviation ipsilaterally acutely
- Gaze palsy overcome with the oculocephalic maneuver or caloric stimulation
- Late disorders of saccades (contralateral more than ipsilateral) (Tijssen, 1993, 1994)
- Prolonged eye deviation after stroke implies preexisting damage to the contralateral frontal region (Steiner, 1984).

Epileptogenic lesions in the frontal eye fields
- Transient deviation of the eyes and head to the contralateral side (Godoy, 1990).
- Ipsiversive head and eye movements during a seizure may also occur (McLachlan, 1987; Robillard, 1983; Rosenbaum, 1986).
- Initial forced turning (versive) head and eye movements usually correspond to a contralateral epileptiform focus, but these initial contraversive movements may be followed by late ipsiversive or contraversive nonforced movements during the secondary generalization (Kernan, 1993; Wyllie, 1986a, 1986b).

Unilateral parietal lesions
- Unilateral or bilateral increased saccade latencies
- Hypometria for contralateral saccades

- Saccadic slowing
- Bilateral parietal lesions
  - Acquired ocular motor apraxia (Aicardi, 1988; Dehaene, 1991; Harris, 1996; Pierrot-Deseilligny, 1986a, 1986b; Prasad, 1994; Shawkat, 1996).
- Lesions in the corona radiata adjacent to the genu of the internal capsule
  - Contralateral selective saccadic palsy (Fukutake, 1993).
- Hemorrhages deep in a cerebral hemisphere, particularly the thalamus
  - Eye deviation to the side of the hemiparesis ("wrong way eyes") (Tijssen, 1987).
- Mesencephalic
  - Paresis of contralateral saccades (Zackon, 1984)
  - Supranuclear contralateral gaze palsies associated with ipsilateral oculomotor palsies (Masdeu, 1987).
- Pontine lesions affecting the abducens nucleus and/or the PPRF
  - Ipsilateral conjugate gaze palsy
  - Doll's eye maneuver or cold caloric stimulation usually does not overcome gaze palsy (Deleu, 1988).
  - Bilateral horizontal gaze palsies with bilateral lesions
- Selective saccadic palsy (Hanson, 1986)
  - Voluntary saccades in both horizontal and vertical planes slow
  - Smooth pursuit, the vestibuloocular reflex, the ability to hold steady eccentric gaze, and vergence eye movements preserved
- Paraneoplastic loss of horizontal voluntary eye movements (Baloh, 1993)
  - Associated with persistent muscle spasms of the face, jaw, and pharynx
  - Associated prostate carcinoma
- Congenital and familial bilateral horizontal gaze palsy (Ehrenberg, 1980; Granat, 1979; Riley, 1979; Sharpe, 1975; Zweifach, 1969)
  - May occur in isolation
  - May be associated with kyphoscoliosis and facial contraction with myokymia (Ehrenberg, 1980; Granat, 1979; Riley, 1979; Sharpe, 1975; Zweifach, 1969)
- Pseudo-horizontal gaze palsy with pontine lesions
  - Damaging the medial longitudinal fasciculus on one side and the contralateral abducens nerve fascicle

What Studies Are Indicated in a Patient with a Horizontal Gaze Palsy?

In general, unilateral restriction of voluntary horizontal conjugate gaze to one side is usually due to contralateral frontal or ipsilateral pontine damage. At the bedside, pontine lesions can usually be differentiated from supranuclear lesions by associated neurologic findings and by the oculocephalic (doll's eyes) maneuver or caloric stimulation. These latter procedures will overcome gaze deviations induced by supranuclear lesions, but not those caused by pontine lesions. Structural lesions, such as infarction, hemorrhage, vascular malformations, tumors, demyelination, trauma, or infections, are the usual causes of horizontal gaze palsies. Because all processes causing horizontal gaze palsies directly or indirectly damage intraparenchymal brain pathways, neuroimaging studies are necessary in all patients. In the acute setting, in patients with altered levels of consciousness, or those in whom MR imaging is contraindicated (e.g., patients with pacemakers), computed tomography is appropriate. Otherwise, MR imaging is the procedure of choice in evaluating patients with horizontal gaze palsies. In patients with evidence of clinical seizure activity as well as intermittent conjugate gaze deviation, or in obtunded or comatose patients with horizontal gaze palsies and evidence for possible contralateral cortical lesions, an electroencephalogram is indicated to evaluate the possibility a seizure disorder (e.g., status epilepticus). The evaluation of patients with horizontal gaze palsies is outlined in Figure 14–1.

What Is the Anatomy of the Abducens Nucleus and Medial Longitudinal Fasciculus (MLF)?

The abducens nucleus has two types of intermingled neurons: motor neurons and internuclear neurons. The axons of the internuclear neurons cross to the contralateral side in

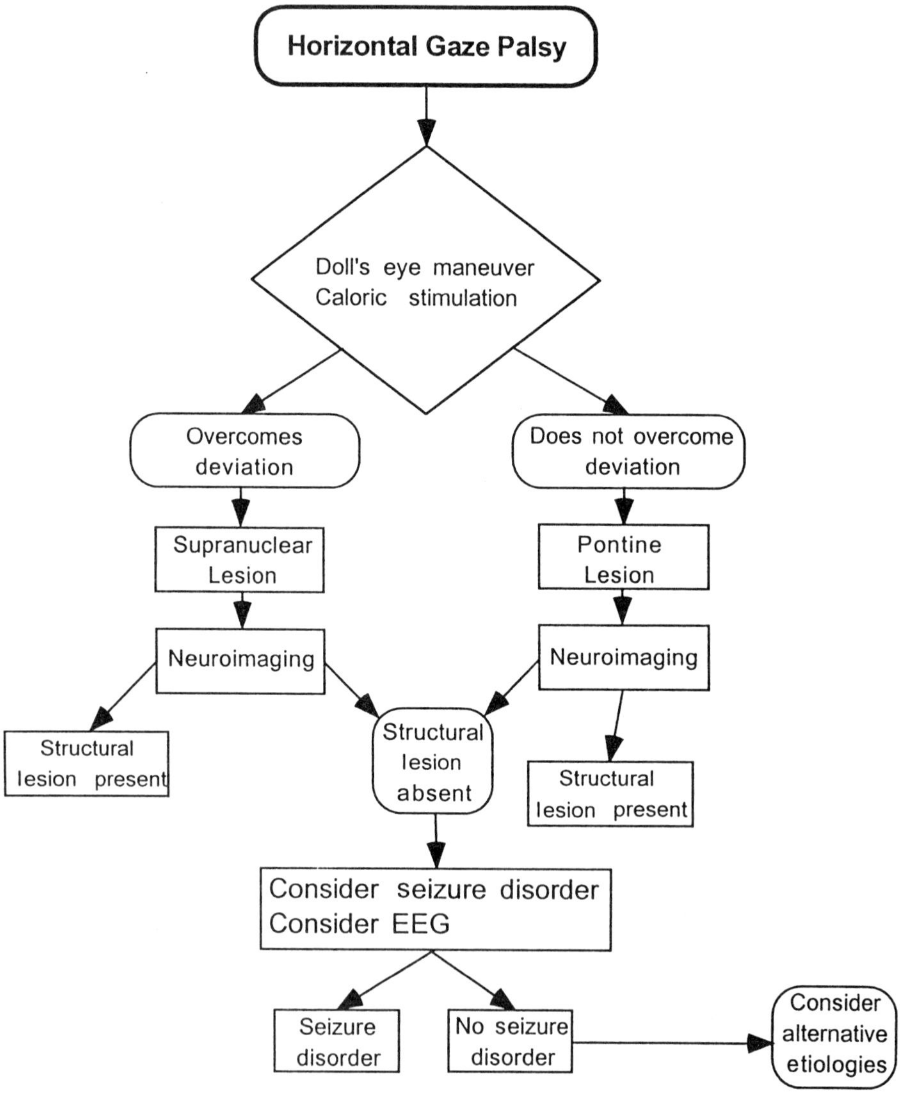

Figure 14–1. Horizontal gaze palsy.

the lower pons and ascend in the MLF to synapse in the portion of the oculomotor nucleus that innervates the medial rectus muscle (Leigh, 1991). In pontine lesions affecting the abducens nucleus and/or the PPRF, a conjugate horizontal gaze palsy to the ipsilateral side occurs. Lesions of the MLF result in internuclear ophthalmoplegia (INO), while lesions of the MLF plus the ipsilateral abducens nucleus and/or PPRF result in the one-and-a-half syndrome. The clinical characteristics of these latter two syndromes and their evaluation are reviewed here.

What Are the Clinical Features of INO?

Clinically, INO is characterized by adduction weakness on the side of the MLF lesion and monocular nystagmus of the opposite abducting eye. Convergence is usually preserved unless the responsible lesion is high in the midbrain. Often patients with INO have no visual symptoms but some complain of diplopia (due to skew deviation) or oscillopsia. INO is most evident during saccadic eye movements and the "adduction lag" is best brought out during optokinetic testing using a tape or drum (Smith, 1964). For example, with a right INO when the drum is rotated to the right the amplitude and velocity of the adducting quick phase of the right eye are smaller and slower than that of the abducting saccades of the left eye. The pathogenesis of the nystagmus in the abducting eye is unclear but is likely a normal adaptive process that helps overcome the adducting weakness of the fellow eye (Getenet, 1993; Thoke, 1996; Zee, 1987).

Other clinical findings noted with unilateral and bilateral INO are outlined in Table 14–3.

What used to be called Lutz posterior internuclear ophthalmoplegia is now known as internuclear ophthalmoplegia of abduction (Bogousslavsky, 1985; Kommerell, 1975; Thomke, 1992; Topilow, 1981). In this rare syndrome, abduction is restricted on volition but can be fully effected by reflex maneuvers, such as cold caloric stimulation. Unilateral or bilateral internuclear ophthalmoplegia of abduction, occasionally associated with adduction nystagmus of the contralateral eye, has been described with ipsilateral rostral pontine or mesencephalic lesions (Thomke, 1992).

Table 14–3. Clinical Findings Noted with INO

Unilateral INO
Skew deviation with the higher eye on the side of the lesion
Vertical gaze-evoked nystagmus and impaired vestibular and pursuit vertical eye movements (Leigh, 1991)
Ipsilateral downbeat nystagmus and contralateral incyclorotatory (torsional) nystagmus (Marshall, 1991)
Transient (disappearing within three days) torsional nystagmus which is clockwise (examiner's view) in cases of left INO and counterclockwise in right INO (Fantin, 1995)
Normal vertical saccades
Rare exotropia (wall-eyed monocular internuclear ophthalmoplegia or WEMINO syndrome) (Johnston, 1994)
Bilateral INO
Bilateral adduction paresis or lag with the eyes generally aligned in primary gaze
Exotropia, with both eyes deviated laterally (WEBINO syndrome) (Strominger, 1986)
Vertical gaze-evoked nystagmus and impaired vestibular and pursuit vertical eye movements (Leigh, 1991)
Impaired vertical gaze holding (Kirkham, 1977).

What Is the Cause of the INO?

INO is due to pathologic processes affecting the medial pontine or midbrain parenchyma. Often there are associated brainstem symptoms and signs, although occasionally unilateral or bilateral INO may occur in isolation. The nature of the responsible pathologic process is suggested by the temporal mode of onset of the INO, the general clinical circumstances, and associated signs on neurologic and neuro-ophthalmologic examination. Etiologies for INO are listed in Table 14–4.

Table 14–4. Etiologies of Internuclear Ophthalmoplegia

Etiology	References
Multiple sclerosis	Atlas, 1987; Baloh, 1978; Bogousslavsky, 1986a; Herishanu, 1983; Hopf, 1991; Muri, 1985; Smith, 1959; Strominger, 1986
Brainstem infarction	Alexander, 1991; Baloh, 1978; Bogousslavsky, 1983; Cogan, 1970; Getenet, 1993; Gonyea, 1974; Herishanu, 1969; Hopf, 1991; Kommerell, 1981; Marshall, 1991; Nozaki, 1983; Okuda, 1993; Smith, 1959
Giant cell arteritis	Askari, 1993; Crompton, 1989; Hughes, 1994; Johnston, 1990; Thomson, 1989; Trend, 1990
Systemic lupus erythematosus	Cogan, 1987; Jackson, 1986; Meyer, 1975
Neuro-Behçet's disease	Masai, 1995
Sickle cell trait	Leavitt, 1994
Polyarteritis nodosa	Kirkali, 1991
Eales' disease	Ataby, 1992
Pyoderma gangrenosum	Lana, 1990
Complication of angiography	Cahill, 1981; Goodman, 1983; Kupfer, 1966; Rennie, 1986
D-penicillamine-induced cerebral vasculitis	Pless, 1997
Brainstem hemorrhage, including hemorrhage due to "crack" cocaine use	Caplan, 1982; Diaz-Calderon, 1991
Brainstem and fourth ventricular tumors	Arnold, 1990; Cogan, 1970; Schraeder, 1981; Tekkok, 1989; Troost, 1980
Infections	
Cryptococcal meningitis	Gonyea, 1972; Sung, 1991
Tuberculosis (granuloma or infectious vasculitis)	Inocencio, 1985; Sandyk, 1984; Teoh, 1989
Viral and bacterial meningoencephalitis	Bodziner, 1983; Gonyea, 1974; Ross, 1966
Syphilis	Cogan, 1970
AIDS	Hamed, 1988; Pfister, 1989; Sherman, 1989
Head trauma	Baker, 1979; Beck, 1981; Catalano, 1986; Doslak, 1980; Haller, 1990; Keane, 1987; Mueller, 1993; Rich, 1974; Rosati, 1981; Strauss, 1995
Cervical injury by hyperextension or manipulation	Jammes, 1989; Zauel, 1977
Cancer-related	
Carcinomatous meningitis	Ford, 1983
Remote effect of cancer	Pillay, 1984
Brainstem demyelination due to chemotherapy/radiation therapy	Lepore, 1981

Etiology	References
Nutritional and metabolic disorders	
Wernicke's encephalopathy	Cogan, 1954; De la Paz, 1992
Pernicious anemia	Kandler, 1988; Reynolds, 1989
Hepatic encephalopathy	Caplan, 1980
Maple syrup urine disease	Zee, 1974
Abetalipoproteinemia	Yee, 1976
Fabry's disease	Ho, 1981
Hexosamiminidase A deficiency	Barnes, 1991
Degenerative diseases	
Progressive supranuclear palsy	Friedman, 1992; Mastaglia, 1975
Familial spinocerebellar degeneration	Senanayake, 1992
Arnold Chiari malformation and associated hydrocephalus or syringobulbia	Arnold, 1990; Cogan, 1970; De la Monte, 1986; Lewis, 1996; Nishizaki, 1985; Samples, 1983; Woody, 1985
Drug intoxications	
Narcotics	El-Mallakh, 1986; Gilman, 1984; Rizzo, 1983
Phenothiazines	Cook, 1981
Tricyclic antidepressants	Donhowe, 1984; Hotson, 1982; Snyder, 1974
Propranolol	Cunningham, 1983
Barbiturates	Barret, 1983
Lithium	Deleu, 1989
Antiobesity treatments	Lledo Carreres, 1992
Miscellaneous causes	
Hydrocephalus	Nishizaki, 1985
Mesencephalic midline clefts	Lagreze, 1996
Subdural hematoma	Devereaux, 1979
Subdural hygroma with an arachnoid cyst in the middle cranial fossa	Minamori, 1992
Supratentorial arteriovenous malformations	Coppeto, 1987
Partial seizures	Glaser, 1966

Although bilateral INO is more common with multiple sclerosis than with vascular insults, bilateral INO may occur with strokes as well as many other pathological processes and the presence of a unilateral or bilateral INO thus cannot be used as a differential feature for etiological diagnosis. For example, in a series of 100 patients with multiple sclerosis, 34 had INO that was bilateral in 14 and unilateral in 20 (Muri, 1985). In another study of 51 patients with INO, 28 had multiple sclerosis and 23 had infarction; INO was bilateral in 33 patients and unilateral in 28 (Hopf, 1991). Most patients with nutritional, metabolic, degenerative, and drug-induced intoxication have bilateral INOs.

The pattern of extraocular muscle weakness with myasthenia gravis (including penicillamine-induced myasthenia) can mimic INO (pseudo-INO) (Acers, 1979; George, 1984; Glaser, 1966; Jay, 1987; Metz, 1977). Myasthenic pseudo-INO is not uncommon and may be associated with downshoot in the adducting eye (Jay, 1987). Pseudo-INO has also been described with Fisher's syndrome (Swick, 1974), Guillain-Barré syndrome (Atwal, 1976; Diamond, 1975), and after surgical paresis of the medial rectus muscle (Wilson, 1985).

What Studies Should Be Ordered in a Patient with INO?

In general, the investigation of a patient with INO depends on clinical circumstances. For example, in a patient with known multiple sclerosis, the appearance of INO as part of an exacerbation of the disease probably does not require neuroimaging, while INO in isolation or with associated unexplained brainstem signs and symptoms does. If there is variability of the adduction deficit, associated fluctuating ptosis, or other variable ocular motor signs suggestive of myasthenia gravis, a myasthenic pseudo-INO should be considered and the first step is a Tensilon test. If the Tensilon test is normal or the clinical situation does not suggest myasthenia and there are no signs of an associated degenerative process (e.g., progressive supranuclear palsy) on clinical examination, neuroimaging is usually warranted. Because brainstem structures are involved in the etiological processes, along with the small volume affected by many of these processes and the nature of common etiologies of INO (e.g., multiple sclerosis, stroke, etc.), MR is superior to CT in evaluating patients with INO (Alexander, 1991; Atlas, 1987; Bogousslavsky, 1986a; Haller, 1990; Hopf, 1991; Strauss, 1995). For example, in a study of 11 patients with INO (9 with multiple sclerosis and 2 with infarct), CT in all 9 tested failed to show a responsible lesion while appropriate MR abnormalities were documented in 10 of the 11 patients (Atlas, 1987). In another study, CT did not detect abnormalities of the MLF in two patients with INO who had abnormal brainstem hypersignals on MR imaging (Awerbach, 1990). CT imaging in a patient with INO is reserved only for acute situations (e.g., brainstem hemorrhage) or for those in whom MR imaging is contraindicated (e.g., patients with pacemakers, etc.). MR imaging may give useful diagnostic data by also supplying information about supratentorial processes likely to be involved in the etiology of the INO, such as multiple sclerosis, multiple cerebral infarcts, and so on. If an infarct is detected as the cause of INO in a patient older than 50 years, giant cell arteritis should be considered as an etiology, especially if other stroke risk factors are not evident. A sedimentation rate is thus warranted, and if it is elevated or the patient has other systemic symptoms of giant cell arteritis (e.g., jaw claudications, headache, polymyalgia rheumatic symptoms, etc.), a temporal artery biopsy should be obtained.

If MR imaging in nontraumatic cases is normal, then rarer etiologies for the INO should be considered. If the INO is bilateral, drug intoxication should be suspected. As pernicious anemia has rarely been reported to cause INO, a B_{12} level is also indicated but of low yield. Syphilis may rarely cause INO so serology for syphilis is also suggested. If MR imaging reveals meningeal enhancement or if meningeal signs or symptoms are present, spinal fluid examination is warranted to investigate for infectious or carcinomatous meningitis. The suggested evaluation of a patient with INO is outlined in Figure 14–2.

What Is the "One and a Half" Syndrome?

In the one and a half syndrome, there is a conjugate gaze palsy to one side ("one") and impaired adduction on looking to the other side ("and a half") (Bronstein, 1990; Celebisoy, 1996; Deleu, 1988; Pierrot-Deseilligny, 1981; Sharpe, 1974; Wall, 1983). As a result, the only horizontal movement remaining is abduction of one eye, which may exhibit nystagmus in abduction. The responsible lesion involves the PPRF or abducens nucleus and the adjacent MLF on the side of the complete gaze palsy. Patients with the one and a half syndrome often have exotropia of the eye opposite the side of the lesion (paralytic pontine exotropia) because, due to the gaze palsy, the eyes tend to drift to the side opposite the lesion, but adduction in this direction is limited by the MLF lesion (Sharpe, 1974).

A somewhat similar syndrome may result from two separate lesions involving both MLFs and the fascicles of the abducens nerve on the side of the unilateral horizontal "gaze" palsy. However, in this case, if the "gaze" palsy is incomplete, the eyes would move disconjugately in the direction of the gaze palsy (Pierrot-Deseilligny, 1981). A true gaze palsy resulting from unilateral PPRF damage causes concomitant paresis of both eyes. Another form of one and a half syndrome consists of a horizontal conjugate gaze

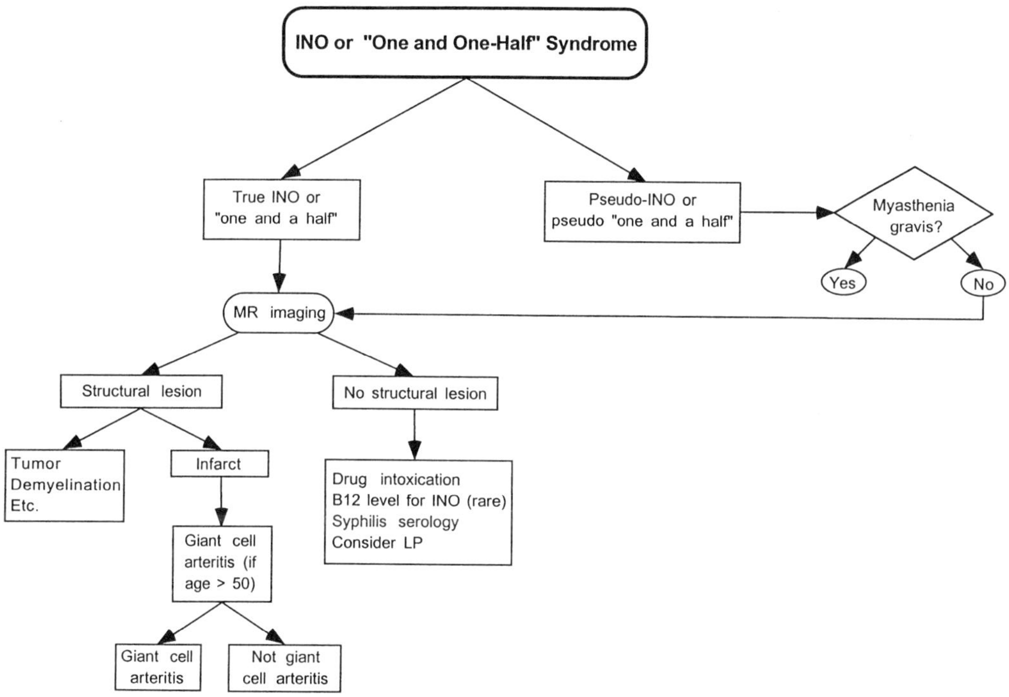

Figure 14–2. Internuclear ophthalmoplegia or one and one-half syndrome.

palsy to one side (e.g., to the left) associated with abduction paralysis of the eye on the side opposite the gaze palsy (e.g., the right eye) with adduction nystagmus in the eye on the side of the gaze palsy (e.g., the left eye) (Celebisoy, 1996). This form of the one and a half syndrome may be seen with rostral brain stem infarction. A fourth type has been described in a patient with mucormycosis of the cavernous sinus (Carter, 1994). The patient had an ipsilateral sixth nerve palsy due to cavernous sinus involvement and a contralateral horizontal gaze palsy from simultaneous carotid artery occlusion with infarction of the frontal lobe. Contrary to the pontine one and a half syndrome, in which abduction in one eye is the preserved horizontal movement, this patient had only preserved adduction in one eye (contralateral to the sixth nerve palsy). Finally, a pseudo one and a half syndrome may be caused by myasthenia gravis (Davis, 1989).

What Etiologies Should Be Considered as a Cause of the One and a Half Syndrome and What Evaluation Is Indicated?

Etiologies of the one and a half syndrome are listed in Table 14–5. Brainstem infarction is the most common cause of this syndrome in the elderly, while multiple sclerosis is the usual cause in young adults. In fact, the one and a half syndrome may be the presenting sign of multiple sclerosis (Martyn, 1988).

Most patients with a one and a half syndrome have other signs and symptoms of brainstem involvement. A patient with an "isolated" one and a half syndrome, especially if other signs of variable ocular motor paresis or ptosis are evident, should have a Tensilon test to investigate for the presence of myasthenia gravis. All others should have MR imaging, with attention to posterior fossa structures, to investigate structural etiologies (Hirose, 1993; Hommel, 1987; Martyn, 1988; Ohta, 1994). The evaluation of patients with the one and a half syndrome is outlined in Table 14–2.

Table 14–5. Etiologies of the One and a Half Syndrome

Etiology	References
Brainstem infarction	Bogousslavsky, 1984; Celebisoy, 1996; Hommel, 1987; Lousa, 1983; Ohta, 1994; Wall, 1983; Yi, 1996
Brainstem hemorrhage	Caplan, 1982; Kase, 1981; Oommen, 1982; Sharpe, 1974
Multiple sclerosis	Martyn, 1988; Wall, 1983
Tumors (primary or metastatic of the brainstem, fourth ventricle, or cerebellum)	Crisostomo, 1985; Jackel, 1986; Newton, 1991; Sharpe, 1974
Postoperatively after the removal of tumors of the posterior fossa	Newton, 1991
Basilar artery aneurysms or brainstem arteriovenous malformations	Wall, 1983
Trauma	Smith, 1980
Mucormycosis of the cavernous sinus	Carter, 1994

What Is the Anatomy of Vertical Gaze?

The ocular motor neurons concerned with vertical gaze and torsional eye movements lie in the oculomotor and trochlear nuclei. These nuclei receive afferents from the vestibular, smooth pursuit, optokinetic, and saccadic systems (Ford, 1984; Leigh, 1991; Tusa, 1988).

Where Are the Lesions Responsible for Vertical Gaze Palsies Localized and What Etiologies Should Be Considered?

The localization of lesions causing vertical gaze palsies is outlined in Table 14–6.

The constellation of neuro-ophthalmologic findings seen with pretectal lesions has been variously designated as Parinaud's syndrome, the Sylvian aqueduct syndrome, the pretectal syndrome, the dorsal midbrain syndrome, and the Koerber-Salus-Elschnig syndrome (Keane, 1990; Leigh, 1991). Ophthalmic findings of this syndrome are outlined in Table 14–7.

Table 14–6. The Localization of Lesions Causing Vertical Gaze Palsies

Bilateral lesions of the rostral interstitial nuclei of the MLF (Auerbach, 1982; Bender, 1980; Cogan, 1974; Ford, 1984; Green, 1993; Hommel, 1990; Jacobs, 1973; Trajanowski, 1981)
Down-gaze saccadic palsy
Paralysis of upward and downward saccades
Bilateral pretectal lesions or midline lesions of the posterior commissure (Auerbach, 1982; Bender, 1980; Cogan, 1974; Ford, 1984; Green, 1993; Hommel, 1990; Jacobs, 1973; Trajanowski, 1981)
Paresis of upward gaze
Unilateral lesions of the riMLF
Mild defects in vertical saccades
Combined up and down gaze palsies (Bogousslavsky, 1990; Leigh, 1991)
Unilateral mesencephalic lesions
Bilateral upgaze palsy (Hommel, 1990)
Palsy of upward and downward saccades (Hommel, 1990; Ranalli, 1988)
Palsy of upward and downward pursuit and vestibular movements

Table 14–7. Ophthalmic Findings with the Dorsal Midbrain Syndrome

Vertical gaze abnormalities, especially upgaze limitation with or without associated limitation of downgaze
Downward gaze preference or a tonic downward deviation of the eyes ("setting sun sign")
Primary position upbeat or downbeat nystagmus
Impaired convergence and divergence. The patient may, thus, be exotropic or esotropic with "A" or "V" patterns
Excessive convergence tone may result in slow or restricted abduction ("midbrain pseudo-sixth palsy") during horizontal refixations

(continued)

Table 14–7. *(continued)*

Convergence-retraction nystagmus, with quick adducting-retraction jerks predominantly on upgaze
Skew deviation often with the higher eye on the side of the lesion
Alternating adduction hypertropia or alternating adduction hypotropia
Bilateral upper eyelid retraction, baring the sclera above the cornea (Collier's "tucked lid" sign)
Bilateral ptosis
Pupillary abnormalities (large with light-near dissociation)

Upgaze palsy, associated with bilateral ptosis, has also been described with unilateral right hemispheral lesions (Averbuch-Heller, 1996). This lateralization of ocular motor function may reflect the special contribution that the nondominant hemisphere makes to attention.

Selective downgaze palsy has been reported after bilateral lesions in the midbrain-diencephalic junction, involving the area that lies ventral to the Sylvian aqueduct and dorsomedial to the red nucleus (Jacobs, 1973). Pseudoptosis on attempted downward gaze may be noted as the levators relax. Bilateral damage to the rostral interstitial nuclei of the medial longitudinal fasciculus and their projections to the third nerve nuclear group is probably critical (Hommel, 1990). Selective downgaze palsy has also been described with bilateral lesions of the dorsolateral mesencephalic periaqueductal grey involving the caudal portions of the nuclei of the posterior commissure from which one of the commissural systems used by the rostral interstitial nucleus of the medial longitudinal fasciculus originates (Jacobs, 1985).

Impaired upward gaze often occurs as a "physiological" finding in the elderly. Etiologies causing impaired vertical gaze are outlined in Table 14–8.

Table 14–8. Etiologies of Vertical Gaze Impairment

Etiology	References
Primary and secondary tumors of the pineal, thalamus, midbrain, aqueduct of Sylvius, or third ventricle	Auerbach, 1982; Baloh, 1985; Büttner-Ennever, 1989; Chang, 1995; Christoff, 1974; Keane, 1990; Moffie, 1983; Peiris, 1975; Poisson, 1980; Posner, 1946
Midbrain or thalamic infarction or hemorrhage	Biller, 1985; Bogousslavsky, 1984, 1986b, 1988, 1990; Büttner-Ennever, 1982; Caplan, 1980; Christoff, 1974; Fisher, 1959, 1985; Gomez, 1988a, 1988b; Green, 1993; Halmagyi, 1978; Hommel, 1990; Kawahara, 1986; Keane, 1976, 1990; Kobari, 1987; Kompf, 1986; Lee, 1996; Mehler, 1988a, 1988b; Mills, 1978; Nagaratnam, 1989; Ranalli, 1988; Reagan, 1978; Sand, 1986; Segarra, 1970; Smith, 1981; Sullivan, 1976; Swanson, 1985; Tatemichi, 1992; Thames, 1984; Trojanowski, 1980; Wall, 1986; Weisberg, 1986a, 1986b; Yijssen, 1996
Hydrocephalus, especially when dilatation of the third ventricle and aqueduct or enlargement of the suprapineal recess cause pressure on and deformity of the posterior commissure	Azar-Kia, 1975; Barrer, 1980; Bleasel, 1992; Chattha, 1975; Frohman, 1985; Katz, 1994; Keane, 1990; Koga, 1983; Lerner, 1969; Osher, 1978; Sandyk, 1982; Shallat, 1973; Swash, 1974
Infectious or inflammatory etiologies	
Encephalitis	Baloh, 1985; Green, 1993; Keane, 1990; Slavin, 1985
Syphilis	Page, 1982

Etiology	References
Sarcoidosis	Schlegel, 1989
Toxoplasmosis	Keane, 1990
Tuberculosis	Keane, 1990
Whipple's disease	Adams, 1987; Finelli, 1977; Fleming, 1988; Grotta, 1987; Knox, 1976; Schwartz, 1986
Multiple sclerosis	Costantino, 1986; Quint, 1993; Slyman, 1981
Degenerative diseases	
Progressive supranuclear palsy	Collins, 1995; David, 1968; Duvoisin, 1987; Friedman, 1989; Jackson, 1983; Kristensen, 1985; Maher, 1986; Steele, 1972
Huntington's disease	Avanzini, 1979; Beenen, 1986; Bollen, 1986; Cogan, 1974; Collewijn, 1988; Leigh, 1983; Starr, 1967
Diffuse Lewy body disease	Fearnley, 1991; Lewis, 1990
Olivopontocerebellar degeneration	Supranuclear, 1976
Motor neuron disease	Okuda, 1992
Idiopathic striopallidodentate calcifications syndrome	Saver, 1994
Lytico-Bodig (amyotrophic lateral sclerosis/parkinsonism-dementia complex of Guam)	Lepore, 1988
Arteriovenous malformations and posterior fossa aneur	Coppeto, 1983; Keane, 1990; Koga, 1983; Stark, 1979
Metabolic diseases	
Bassen-Kornzweig syndrome	Keane, 1990
Niemann-Pick C disease and variants, including sea-blue histiocytosis syndrome, juvenile dystonic lipidoses, and the DAF (downgaze paralysis, ataxia/athetosis, and foam cells) syndrome	Breen, 1981; Cogan, 1981a, 1981b; Coleman, 1988; Fink, 1989; Gartner, 1986; Grover, 1971; Kornfeld, 1975; Neville, 1973; Yan-go, 1984
Tay-Sachs disease	Jampel, 1964
Gaucher's disease	Cogan, 1981a, 1981b; Tripp, 1977
Maple syrup urine disease	MacDonald, 1977; Zee, 1974
Hyperglycinuria	Nightingale, 1991
Hexosaminidase A deficiency	Harding, 1987
Wilson's disease	Kirkham, 1974
Kernicterus	Hoyt, 1978; Keane, 1990
Wernicke's syndrome	Keane, 1990
Vitamin B_{12} deficiency	Sandyk, 1984
Trauma, including neurosurgical procedures and from catheter compression	Keane, 1990; Nittner, 1974; Seaber, 1980; Shults, 1993
Drugs	
Barbiturates	Edis, 1977
Neuroleptics	Doroevitch, 1984; Leigh, 1987
Carbamazepine	Berchou, 1979
(Drugs most often affect vertical gaze by causing oculogyric crisis, an episodic, spasmodic, conjugate ocular deviation that usually occurs in an upward and lateral direction)	Leigh, 1987

(continued)

Table 14–8. *(continued)*

Etiology	References
Miscellaneous causes	
Subdural hematoma	Sandyk, 1982
Tentorial herniation	Keane, 1986, 1990
Paraneoplastic encephalomyelitis	Crino, 1996; Schiff, 1996
Congenital defects	Keane, 1990; Magli, 1991
Wolfram's syndrome (hereditary diabetes mellitus with brainstem and optic atrophy, diabetes insipidus, and deafness)	Scolding, 1996
Benign transient form in childhood (benign paroxysmal tonic upgaze of neonates and children)	Ahn, 1989; Hoyt, 1980; Ouvrier, 1988
Migraine	Chay, 1977
Subdural fluid collection over the cerebellar hemisphere	Rismondo, 1992

What Studies Are Indicated for the Evaluation of a Patient with Impaired Vertical Gaze?

Occasionally, peripheral eye movement abnormalities, such as myasthenia gravis, Lambert-Eaton myasthenic syndrome, thyroid eye disease, or the Miller Fisher variant of Guillain-Barré syndrome may simulate upgaze palsy or even convergence nystagmus (Cruciger, 1981; Keane, 1982, 1990). Retractory nystagmus, for example, may be mimicked by bilateral dysthyroid orbitopathy with bilateral involvement of both medial recti and inferior recti; saccadic upgaze attempts may cause convergence and retraction due to limitation of eye movements (Burde, 1985). Most of these peripheral processes are associated with other peripheral neurological findings suggesting the appropriate localization. If vertical gaze paresis fluctuates and there are no other signs of neurological or systemic disease, a Tensilon test is warranted. The evaluation of patients with vertical gaze impairments due to supranuclear etiologies depends on the clinical situation, especially if signs or symptoms of neurological or systemic disease are present. For example, the presence of isolated impaired upward gaze in an elderly individual is a common "physiological" finding and requires no further evaluation. Vertical gaze disorders in the setting of other clinical manifestations of metabolic diseases of childhood or adolescence require appropriate biochemical investigation of the metabolic derangement. Also, if a vertical gaze impairment occurs as part of degenerative process (e.g., progressive supranuclear palsy), no studies directed at the gaze impairment per se are required. If there is no evidence of a generalized metabolic or degenerative process on clinical evaluation and the vertical gaze impairment occurs in isolation or in association with neurologic findings localized to the meso-diencephalon, MR imaging with attention to the mesencephalon, thalamus, and ventricular system is required to discover a structural lesion. If a pretectal syndrome develops in a patient with shunted hydrocephalus and neuroimaging reveals no ventricular dilitation, shunt dysfunction should still be suspected and neurosurgical consultation for shunt revision is mandatory. If MR imaging is normal and there are signs suggestive of infection, especially meningeal irritation, or if MR imaging reveals diffuse meningeal enhancement by contrast agent, then a lumbar puncture should be performed to investigate for infectious etiologies. Finally, if MR imaging is normal and no other etiologies are evident, a B_{12} level should be obtained and thiamine supplementation instituted. Evaluation for Whipple's disease (e.g., biopsy of intestine for histology and PCR for Tropheryma whippelii) or syphilis should also be considered. A proposed evaluation of the patient with vertical gaze impairment is outlined in Figure 14–3.

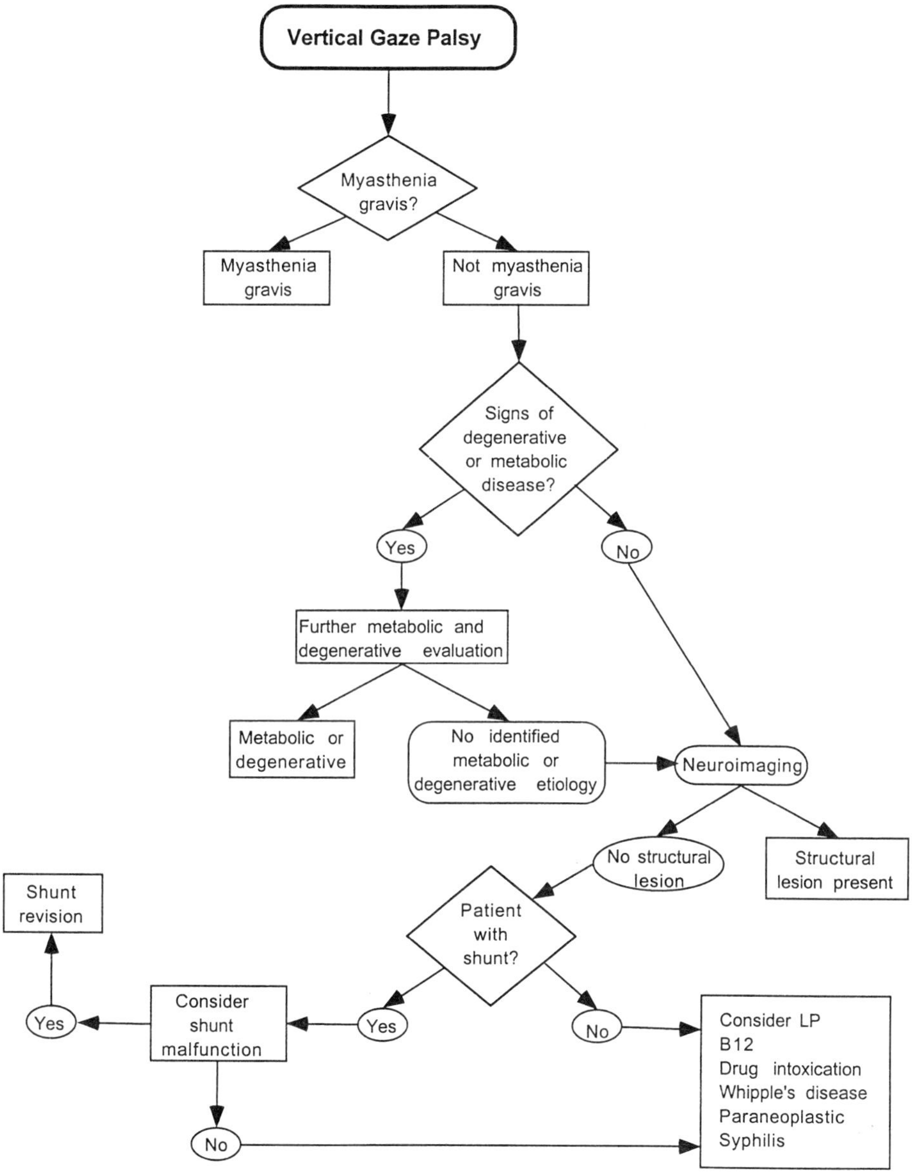

Figure 14–3. Vertical gaze palsy.

What Are the Characteristics of Supranuclear Monocular Elevation Paresis, the Vertical One and a Half Syndrome, and Skew Deviation?

Monocular elevation paresis ("double elevator palsy") may occur on a peripheral basis (e.g., due to primary inferior rectus restriction, primary superior rectus palsy, myasthenia gravis, or a fascicular third nerve lesion) or with pretectal supranuclear lesions. Supranuclear monocular elevation paresis may be congenital (Bell, 1990; Ziffer, 1992) or acquired, with the latter due to a lesion contralateral to the paretic eye or ipsilateral to the paretic eye that interrupt efferents from the rostral interstitial nucleus of the MLF to the superior rectus and inferior oblique subnuclei (often Bell's phenomenon is intact) (Ford, 1984; Hommel, 1990; Jampel, 1968; Lessell, 1975; Thomke, 1992). Double elevator palsy may simply be an asymmetric upgaze palsy that clinically presents as monocular elevation paresis in the more severely affected eye (Thomke, 1992).

A vertical one and a half syndrome, with vertical upgaze palsy and monocular paresis of downgaze on the side of the lesion or contralateral to the lesion, has been described with thalamo-mesencephalic infarction, best explained by selective damage to supranuclear pathways or partial nuclear involvement (Bogousslavsky, 1984; Hommel, 1990; Tatemichi, 1992). Another vertical one and a half syndrome, resulting from bilateral mesodiancephalic infarcts, has been described consisting of impairment of all downward rapid eye movements (including the vestibuloocular reflex) and downward smooth pursuit (nondissociated downgaze paralysis) associated with monocular paralysis of elevation (Deleu, 1991). Finally, monocular elevation paresis of the right eye with contralateral paresis of downward gaze ("crossed vertical gaze paresis") has been described with an infarct involving the left mesodiencephalic junction and medial thalamus (Wiest, 1996).

Although vertical misalignment of the eyes may be caused by lesions of the ocular motor nerves or muscles (e.g., with myasthenia gravis), the term skew deviation is reserved for vertical misalignment resulting from supranuclear derangements. This skew deviation may be constant or transient. It occurs whenever peripheral or central lesions cause an imbalance of graviceptive brainstem pathways and can accompany lesions at different areas of the brainstem (mesencephalon to medulla) or cerebellum (Brandt, 1987, 1993, 1994, 1996; Halmagyi, 1990; Keane, 1975, 1985; Moster, 1988). In a study of patients with unilateral brainstem infarcts presenting with skew deviation and ocular torsion, all skew deviations were ipsiversive (ipsilateral eye was undermost) with caudal pontomedullary lesions and contraversive (contralateral eye was lowermost) with rostral pontomesencephalic lesions (Brandt, 1993). Otolith inputs to the interstitial nucleus of Cajal (INC) from the contralateral vestibular (especially lateral vestibular) nuclei and motor outputs from the INC to cervical and ocular motoneurons are likely involved. In some patients, skew deviation may be associated with ocular torsion and head tilt (the ocular tilt reaction or OTR) (Brandt, 1993, 1994, 1996; Halmagyi, 1990). In the OTR, the head tilt, conjugate eye torsion, and hypotropia are all to the same side—suggesting that this reaction is a motor compensation of a lesion-induced apparent eye-head tilt; the contralateral head tilt represents a compensatory response to the perceived tilt of the subjective visual vertical.

A left OTR could be due to a lesion of the left labyrinth, left vestibular nerve, left vestibular nucleus (e.g., Wallenberg syndrome), or right meso-diencephalon suggesting the existence of a crossed graviceptive pathway (possibly the MLF) between the vestibular nucleus and the contralateral INC (Brazis, 1992; Halmagyi, 1990; Keane, 1992). Thus, cases of OTR have been reported in vestibular nerve injury, auditory trauma, Wallenberg syndrome, lateral medullary compression, pontomedullary ischemia, and mesodiencephalic lesions (Averbuch-Heller, 1997; Brandt, 1987, 1993, 1994, 1996; Brazis, 1992; Dieterich, 1993; Halmagyi, 1990; Hedges, 1982; Keane, 1992; Riordan-Eva, 1997; Safran, 1994). The absence of brainstem signs in peripheral OTR helps to exclude a central cause for the vertical diplopia. Occasionally, increased intracranial pressure (e.g., from benign intracranial hypertension or pseudotumor cerebri) (Frohman, 1985; Merikangas, 1978), Fisher's syndrome (Esaki, 1992) or hepatic coma (Fisher, 1981) may cause skew deviation.

References

Acers TE. (1979). Ocular myasthenia gravis mimicking pseudointernuclear ophthalmoplegia and variable esotropia. *Am J Ophthalmol 88:*319–321.

Adams M, Rhyner PA, Day J, et al. (1987). Whipple's disease confined to the central nervous system. *Ann Neurol 21:*104–108.

Ahn JC, Hoyt WF, Hoyt CS. (1989). Tonic upgaze in infancy. A report of three cases. *Arch Ophthalmol 107:*57–58.

Aicardi J, Barbosa C, Andermann E, et al. (1988). Ataxia-ocular motor apraxia: A syndrome mimicking ataxia-telangiectasia. *Ann Neurol 24:*497–502.

Alexander JA, Castillo M, Hoffman JC Jr. (1991). Magnetic resonance findings in a patient with internuclear ophthalmoplegia. Neuroradiological-clinical correlation. *J Clin Neuro-ophthalmol 11:*58–61.

Arnold AC. (1990). Internuclear ophthalmoplegia from intracranial tumor. *J Clin Neuro-ophthalmol 10:*278–286.

Arnold AC, Baloh RW, Yee RD, Hepler RS. (1990). Internuclear ophthalmoplegia in the Chiari type 2 malformation. *Neurology 40:*1850–1854.

Askari A, Jolobe OM, Sheperd DI. (1993). Internuclear ophthalmoplegia and Horner's syndrome due to presumed giant cell arteritis. *J Roy Soc Med 86:*362.

Ataby C, Erdem E, Kansu T, Eldem B. (1992). Eales' disease with internuclear ophthalmoplegia. *Ann Ophthalmol 24:*267–269.

Atlas SW, Grossman RI, Savino PJ, et al. (1987). Internuclear ophthalmoplegia: MR-anatomic correlation. *Am J Neuroradiol 8:*243–247.

Atwal AJS, Smith BH, Dickenson ES. (1976). Pseudo-internuclear ophthalmoplegia in polyneuritis. *Arch Neurol 33:*457.

Auerbach SH, De Piero TJ, Romanul F. (1982). Sylvian aqueduct syndrome caused by unilateral midbrain lesion. *Ann Neurol 11:*91–94.

Avanzini G, Girotti F, Caraceni T, Spreafico R. (1979). Oculomotor disorders in Huntington's chorea. *J Neurol Neurosurg Psych 42:*581–589.

Averbuch-Heller L, Rottach KG, Zivotofsky AZ, et al. (1997). Torsional eye movements in patients with skew deviation and spasmodic torticollis: Responses to static and dynamic head roll. *Neurology 48:*506–514.

Averbuch-Heller L, Stahl JS, Remler BF, Leigh RJ. (1996). Bilateral ptosis and upgaze palsy with right hemispheric lesions. *Ann Neurol 49:*465–468.

Awerbach G, Brown M, Levin JR. (1990). Magnetic resonance imaging of internuclear ophthalmoplegia. *Int J Neurosci 52:*39–43.

Azar-Kia B, Palacios E, Churchill R. (1975). Aqueductal stenosis and Parinaud's syndrome. *Ill Med J 148:*532–533.

Baker RS. (1979). Internuclear ophthalmoplegia following head injury. Case report. *J Neurosurg 51:*552–555.

Baloh RW, DeRossett SE, Cloughesy TF, et al. (1993). Novel brainstem syndrome associated with prostate carcinoma. *Neurology 43:*2591–2596.

Baloh RW, Furman JM, Yee RD. (1985). Dorsal midbrain syndrome: Clinical and oculographic findings. *Neurology 35:*54–60.

Baloh RW, Yee RD, Honrubia V. (1978). Internuclear ophthalmoplegia. I. Saccades and dissociated nystagmus. *Arch Neurol 35:*484–489.

Barnes D, Misra VP, Young EP, et al. (1991). An adult onset hexosaminidase syndrome with sensory neuropathy and internuclear ophthalmoplegia. *J Neurol Neurosurg Psych 54:*1112–1113.

Barrer SJ, Schut L, Bruce D. (1980). Global rostral midbrain dysfunction secondary to shunt malfunction in hydrocephalus. *Neurosurg 7:*322–325.

Barret LG, Vincent FM, Arsac PL, et al. (1983). Internuclear ophthalmoplegia in patients with toxic coma. Frequency, prognostic value, diagnostic significance. *J Toxicol Clin Toxicol 20:*373–379.

Beck RW, Meckler RJ. (1981). Internuclear ophthalmoplegia after head trauma. *Ann Ophthalmol 13:*671–675.

Beenen N, Büttner U, Lange HW. (1986). The diagnostic value of eye movement recordings in patients with Huntington's disease and their offspring. *Electroencephalography Clin Neurophysiol 63:*119–127.

Bell JA, Fielder AR, Viney S. (1990). Congenital double elevator palsy in identical twins. *J Clin Neuro-ophthalmol 10:*32–34.

Bender MB. (1980). Brain control of conjugate horizontal and vertical eye movements. *Brain 103:*23–69.

Berchou RC. (1979). Carbamazepine-induced oculogyric crisis. *Arch Neurol 36:*522–523.

Biller J, Sand JJ, Corbett JJ, et al. (1985). Syndrome of the paramedian thalamic arteries: Clinical and neuroimaging correlation. *J Clin Neuro-ophthalmol 5:*217–223.

Bleasel AF, Ell JJ, Johnston I. (1992). Pretectal syndrome and shunt dysfunction. *Neuro-ophthalmol 12:*193–196.

Bodziner RA, Singer W, Hedges TR. (1983). Bilateral internuclear ophthalmoplegia in meningoencephalitis. *Dev Med Child Neurol 25:*819–820.

Bogousslavsky J, Fox AJ, Carey LS, et al. (1986a). Correlates of brain-stem oculomotor disorders in multiple sclerosis. Magnetic resonance imaging. *Arch Neurol 43:*1986.

Bogousslavsky J, Miklossy J, Deruaz JP, et al. (1986b). Unilateral left paramedian infarction of thalamus and midbrain: A clinicopathological study. *J Neurol Neurosurg Psych 49:*686–694.

Bogousslavsky J, Miklossy J, Regli F, Janzer R. (1990). Vertical gaze palsy and selective unilateral infarction of the rostral interstitial nucleus of the medial longitudinal fasciculus (riMLF). *J Neurol Neurosurg Psych 53:*67–71.

Bogousslavsky J, Miklossy J, Regli F, et al. (1984). One-and-a-half syndrome in ischaemic locked-in state: A clinicopathological study. *J Neurol Neurosurg Psych 47:*927–935.

Bogousslavsky J, Regli F. (1984). Upgaze palsy and monocular paresis of downward gaze from ipsilateral thalmo-mesencephalic infarction: A vertical "one-and-a-half" syndrome. *J Neurol 231:*43–45.

Bogousslavsky J, Regli F, Uske A. (1988). Thalamic infarcts: Clinical syndromes, etiology, and prognosis. *Neurology 38:*837–848.

Bogousslavsky J, Regli F, Ghika J, Hungerbuhler JP. (1983). Internuclear ophthalmoplegia, prenuclear paresis of contralateral superior rectus, and bilateral ptosis. *J Neurol 230:*197–203.

Bogousslavsky J, Regli F, Ostinelli B, Rabinowicz T. (1985). Paresis of lateral gaze alternating with so-called posterior internuclear ophthalmoplegia. A partial paramedian pontine reticular formation-abducens nucleus syndrome. *J Neurol 232:*38–42.

Bollen E, Reulen JPH, Den Heyer JC, et al. (1986). Horizontal and vertical saccadic eye movement abnormalities in Huntington's chorea. *J Neurol Sci 74:*11–22.

Brandt T, Dieterich M. (1996). Central vestibular syndromes in the roll, pitch, and yaw planes. *Neuro-ophthalmol 15:*291–303.

Brandt T, Dieterich M. (1987). Pathological eye-head coordination in roll: Tonic ocular tilt reaction in mesencephalic and medullary lesions. *Brain 110:*649–666.

Brandt T, Dieterich M. (1993). Skew deviation with ocular torsion: A vestibular brainstem sign of topographic diagnostic value. *Ann Neurol 33:*528–534.

Brandt T, Dieterich M. (1994). Vestibular syndromes in the roll plane: Topographic diagnosis from brainstem to cortex. *Ann Neurol 36:*337–347.

Brazis PW. (1992). Ocular motor abnormalities in Wallenberg's lateral medullary syndrome. *Mayo Clin Proc 67:*365–368.

Breen L, Morris HH, Alperin JB, Schochet SS Jr. (1981). Juvenile Niemann-Pick disease with vertical supranuclear ophthalmoplegia. *Arch Neurol 38:*388–390.

Brigell M, Babikian V, Goodwin JA. (1984). Hypometric saccades and low-gain pursuit resulting from a thalamic hemorrhage. *Ann Neurol 15:*374–378.

Bronstein AM, Rudge P, Gresty MA, et al. (1990). Abnormalities of horizontal gaze. Clinical, oculographic and magnetic resonance imaging findings. II. Gaze palsy and internuclear ophthalmoplegia. *J Neurol Neurosurg Psych 53:*200–207.

Burde RM, Savino PJ, Trobe JD. (1985). *Clinical Decisions in Neuro-ophthalmology*. 2nd edition. St Louis, Mosby, pp. 204–205.

Büttner-Ennever JA, Acheson JF, Büttner U, et al. (1989). Ptosis and supranuclear downgaze paralysis. *Neurology 39:*385–389.

Büttner-Ennever JA, Büttner U, Cohen B, Baumgartner G. (1982). Vertical gaze paresis and the rostral interstitial nucleus of the medial longitudinal fasciculus. *Brain 105:*125–149.

Cahill DW, Salcman M, Hirsch D, Rao CVGK. (1981). Unilateral internuclear ophthalmoplegia due to angiographic embolism through a primitive trigemninal artery. *Neurology 31:*751–753.

Caplan LR. (1980). "Top of the basilar" syndrome. *Neurology 30:*72–79.

Caplan LR, Goodwin JA. (1982). Lateral tegmental brainstem hemorrhages. *Neurology 32:*252–260.

Caplan LR, Scheiner D. (1980). Dysconjugate gaze in hepatic coma. *Ann Neurol 8:*328–329.

Carter JE, Rauch RA. (1994). One-and-a-half syndrome, type II. *Arch Neurol 51:*87–89.

Catalano RA, Sax RD, Krohel GB. (1986). Unilateral internuclear ophthalmoplegia after head injury. *Am J Ophthalmol 101:*491–493.

Çelebisoy N, Akyürekli Ö. (1996). One-and-a-half syndrome, type II: A case with rostral brain stem infarction. *Neuro-ophthalmology 16:*373–377.

Chang SM, Lillis-Hearne PK, Larson DA, et al. (1995). Pinealblastoma in adults. *Neurosurgery 37:*383–391.

Chattha AS, Delong GR. (1975). Sylvian aqueduct syndrome as a sign of acute obstructive hydrocephalus in children. *J Neurol Neurosurg Psych 38:*288–296.

Chay OM, Tong HI, Wong PK. (1977). Parinaud's syndrome complicating migraine—A case report. *Singapore Med J 18:*151–152.

Christoff N. (1974). A clinicopathologic study of vertical eye movements. *Arch Neurol 31:*1–8.

Cogan DG. (1970). Internuclear ophthalmoplegia. Typical and atypical. *Arch Ophthalmol 84:*583–589.

Cogan DG. (1974). Paralysis of down-gaze. *Arch Ophthalmol 91:*192–199.

Cogan DG, Victor M. (1954). Ocular signs of Wernicke's disease. *Arch Ophthalmol 51:*204–211.

Cogan DG, Wray SH. (1970). Internuclear ophthalmoplegia as an early sign of brainstem tumors. *Neurology 20:*629–633.

Cogan DG, Chu FC, Bachman DM, Barranger J. (1981a). The DAF syndrome. *Neuro-ophthalmol 2:*7–16.

Cogan DG, Chu FC, Reingold D, Barranger J. (1981b). Ocular motor signs in some metabolic disease. *Arch Ophthalmol 99:*1802–1808.

Cogen MS, Kline LB, Duvall ER. (1987). Bilateral internuclear ophthalmoplegia in systemic lupus erythematosus. *J Clin Neuro-ophthalmol 7:*69–73.

Coleman RJ, Robb SA, Lake BD, et al. (1988). The diverse neurological features of Neimann-Pick disease type C: A report of two cases. *Mov Disorder 3:*295–299.

Collewijn H, Went LN, Tamminga EP, Vegter-Van der Vlis M. (1988). Oculomotor defects in patients with Huntington's disease and their offspring. *J Neurol Sci 86:*307–320.

Collins SJ, Ahlskog JE, Parisi JE, Maraganore DM. (1995). Progressive supranuclear palsy: Neuropathologically based diagnostic clinical criteria. *J Neurol Neurosurg Psych 58:*167–173.

Cook FF, Davis RG, Russo LS Jr. (1981). Internuclear ophthalmoplegia caused by phenothiazine intoxication. *Arch Neurol 38:*465–466.

Coppeto JR, Greco P. (1987). Unilateral internuclear ophthalmoplegia, migraine, and supratentorial arteriovenous malformation. *Am J Ophthalmol 104:*191–192.

Coppeto JR, Lessell S. (1983). Dorsal midbrain syndrome from giant aneurysm of the posterior fossa: Report of two cases. *Neurology 33:*732–736.

Costantino A, Black SE, Carr T, et al. (1986). Dorsal midbrain syndrome in multiple sclerosis with magnetic resonance imaging correlation. *Can J Neurol Sci 13:*62–65.

Crino PB, Galetta SL, Sater RA, et al. (1996). Clinicopathologic study of paraneoplastic brainstem encephalitis and ophthalmoparesis. *J Neuro-ophthalmol 16:*44–48.

Crisostomo EA. (1985). One-and-a-half syndrome in a patient with metastatic breast disease. *J Clin Neuro-ophthalmol 5:*270–272.

Crompton JL, Burrow DJ, Iyer PV. (1989). Bilateral internuclear ophthalmoplegia—an unusual initial presenting sign of giant cell arteritis. *Australian New Zealand J Ophthalmol 17:*71–74.

Cruciger MP, Brown B, Magoon E, et al. (1981). Pseudo-sylvian aqueduct syndrome. *JAMA 246:*2324.

Cunningham GM. (1983). Drug-induced internuclear ophthalmoplegia. *Can Med Assoc J 128:*892–893.

David NJ, Mackey EA, Smith JL. (1968). Further observations in progressive supranuclear palsy. *Neurology 18:*349–356.

Davis TL, Lavin PJ. (1989). Pseudo one-and-a-half syndrome with ocular myasthenia. *Neurology 39:*1553.

De la Monte SM, Horowitz SA, Larocque AA, Richardson EP Jr. (1986). Keyhole aqueduct syndrome. *Arch Neurol 43:*926–929.

De la Paz MA, Chung SM, McCrary JA 3rd. (1992). Bilateral internuclear ophthalmoplegia in a patient with Wernicke's encephalopathy. *J Clin Neuro-ophthalmol 12:*116–120.

Dehaene I, Lammens M. (1991). Acquired ocular motor apraxia. A clinicopathologic study. *Neuro-ophthalmol 11:*117–122.

Deleu D, Ebinger G. (1989). Lithium-induced internuclear ophthalmoplegia. *Clin Neuropharmacology 12:*224–226.

Deleu D, Ebinger G. (1991). Vertical one-and-a-half syndrome. Clinical, oculographic and radiologic findings. *Neuro-ophthalmol 11:*99–101.

Deleu D, Solheid C, Michotte A, Ebinger G. (1988). Dissociated ipsilateral horizontal gaze palsy in one-and-a-half syndrome: A clinicopathologic study. *Neurology 38:*1278–1280.

Devereaux MW, Brust JCM, Keane JR. (1979). Internuclear ophthalmoplegia caused by subdural hematoma. *Neurology 29:*251–255.

Diamond S, Schear HE, Leeds MF. (1975). Pseudo-internuclear oculomotor ophthalmoplegia secondary to Guillain-Barré polyneuritis simulating myasthenia gravis in an air transport pilot. *Aviat Space Environ Med 46:*204–207.

Diaz-Calderon E, Del Brutto OH, Aguire R, Alarcon TA. (1991). Bilateral internuclear ophthalmoplegia after smoking "crack" cocaine. *J Clin Neuro-ophthalmol 11:*297–299.

Dieterich M, Brandt T. (1993). Ocular torsion and tilt of subjective visual are sensitive brainstem signs. *Ann Neurol 33:*292–299.

Donhowe SP. (1984). Bilateral internuclear ophthalmoplegia from doxipin overdose. *Neurology 34:*259.

Dorevitch A. (1984). Neuroleptic as a cause of oculogyric crisis. *Arch Neurol 41:*15–16.

Doslak MJ, Kline LB, Dell'Osso LF, Daroff RB. (1980). Internuclear ophthalmoplegia: Recovery and plasticity. *Invest Ophthalmol Vis Sci 19:*1506–1511.

Duvoisin RC, Golbe LI, Lepore FE. (1987). Progressive supranuclear palsy. *Can J Neurol Sci 14:*547–554.

Edis R, Mastaglia F. (1977). Vertical gaze palsy in barbiturate intoxication. *Br Med J 1:*144.

Ehrenberg M, Sidrys LA, Fritz KJ. (1980). Congenital bilateral horizontal gaze palsy in a brother and sister. *J Pediatr Ophthalmol Strabismus 17:*224–226.

El-Mallakh RS. (1986). Internuclear ophthalmoplegia with narcotic overdosage. *Ann Neurol 20:*107.

Esaki H, Shinji O. (1992). Skew deviation in Fisher's syndrome. *Neuro-ophthalmol JPN 9:*66.

Fantin A. (1995). Torsional nystagmus in unilateral internuclear ophthalmoplegia. Presented at the Annual Meeting of the North American Neuro-Ophthalmology Society, Tucson, Arizona.

Fearnley JM, Revesz T, Brooks DJ, et al. (1991). Diffuse Lewy body disease presenting with a supranuclear gaze palsy. *J Neurol Neurosurg Psych 54:*159–161.

Finelli PF, McEntee WJ, Lessell S, et al. (1977). Whipple's disease with predominantly neuro-ophthalmic manifestations. *Ann Neurol 1*:247–252.
Fink JK, Filling-Katz MR, Sokol J, et al. (1989). Clinical spectrum of Neimann-Pick disease type C. *Neurology 39*:1040–1049.
Fisher A, Knezevic W. (1985). Ocular and ocular motor aspects of primary thalamic haemorrhage. *Clin Exp Neurol 21*:129–139.
Fisher CM. (1959). The pathologic and clinical aspects of thalamic hemorrhage. *Trans Am Neurol Assoc 84*:56–59.
Fisher M. (1981). Ocular skew deviation in hepatic coma. *J Neurol Neurosurg Psych 44*:458.
Fleming JL, Weisner RH, Shorter RG. (1988). Whipple's disease: Clinical, biochemical, and histopathologic features and assessment of treatment in 29 patients. *Mayo Clin Proc 63*:539–551.
Ford CS, Cruz J, Biller J, et al. (1983). Bilateral internuclear ophthalmoplegia in carcinomatous meningitis. *J Clin Neuro-ophthalmol 3*:127–130.
Ford CS, Schwartze GM, Weaver RG, Troost BT. (1984). Monocular elevation paresis caused by an ipsilateral lesion. *Neurology 34*:1264–1267.
Friedman DI, Jankovic J. (1989). Progressive supranuclear palsy: A quarter century of progress. In SH Appel (ed). *Current Neurology*. Chicago, Yearbook, Vol. 9, pp. 191–218.
Friedman DI, Jankovic J, McCrary JA. (1992). Neuro-ophthalmic findings in progressive supranuclear palsy. *J Clin Neuro-ophthalmol 12*:104–109.
Frohman LP, Kupersmith MJ. (1985). Reversible vertical ocular deviations associated with raised intracranial pressure. *J Clin Neuro-ophthalmol 5*:158–163.
Fukutake T, Hirayama K, Sakakibara R. (1993). Contralateral selective saccadic palsy after a small haematoma in the corona radiata adjacent to the genu of the internal capsule. *J Neurol Neurosurg Psych 56*:221.
Furman JMR, Hurtt MR, Hirsch WL. (1991). Asymmetrical ocular pursuit with posterior fossa tumors. *Ann Neurol 30*:208–211.
Gartner JC Jr, Bergman I, Malatack JJ, et al. (1986). Progression of neurovisceral storage disease with supranuclear ophthalmoplegia following orthotopic liver transplantation. *Pediatrics 77*:104–106.
Gaymard B, Pierrot-Deseilligny C, Rivaud S, Velut S. (1993). Smooth pursuit eye movement deficits after pontine nuclei lesions in man. *J Neurol Neurosurg Psych 56*:799–807.
George J, Spokes EG. (1984). Myasthenia pseudo-internuclear ophthalmoplegia due to penicillamine. *J Neurol Neurosurg Psych 47*:1044.
Getenet JC, Ventre J, Vighetto A, Tadary B. (1993). Saccades in internuclear ophthalmoplegia: Are abduction disorders related to interocular disconjugacy? *J Neurol Sci 114*:160–164.
Gibb WRG, Luthert PJ, Marsden CD. (1989). Corticobasal degeneration. *Brain 112*:1171–1192.
Gillman MA, Sandyk R. (1984). Bilateral internuclear ophthalmoplegia reversed by naloxone. *Arch Neurol 41*:703.
Glaser JS. (1966). Myasthenic pseudo-internuclear ophthalmoplegia. *Arch Ophthalmol 75*:363–366.
Godoy J, Lüders H, Dinner DS, et al. (1990). Versive eye movements elicited by cortical stimulation of the human brain. *Neurology 40*:296–299.
Gomez CR, Gomez SM, Selhorst JB. (1988a). Acute thalamic esotropia. *Neurology 38*:1759–1762.
Gomez CR, Hogan PA, Cruz-Rodriguez RF, Jumao-AS AP. (1988b). Altered sensorium, confusion, and vertical gaze paresis: The top of the basilar syndrome. *South Med J 81*:842–845.
Gonyea EF. (1974). Bilateral internuclear ophthalmoplegia. *Arch Neurol 31*:168–174.
Gonyea EF, Heilman KM. (1972). Neuro-ophthalmic aspects of central nervous system cryptococcosis. Internuclear and supranuclear ophthalmoplegia. *Arch Ophthalmol 87*:164–168.
Goodman GK, Crawford KH. (1983). Internuclear ophthalmoplegia following arch aortography. Occurrence in association with an occult vertebral artery aneurysm. *Neuroradiology 25*:171–172.
Granat M, Friedman Z, Aloni T. (1979). Familial infantile scoliosis associated with bilateral paralysis of conjugate gaze. *J Med Genet 16*:448–452.
Green JP, Newman NJ, Winterkorn JS. (1993). Paralysis of down gaze in two patients with clinical-radiologic correlation. *Arch Ophthalmol 111*:219–222.
Grotta JC, Pettigrew LC, Schmidt WA, et al. (1987). Oculomasticatory myorhythmia. *Ann Neurol 22*:395–396.
Grover W, Naiman JL. (1971). Progressive paresis of vertical gaze in lipid storage disease. *Neurology 21*:896–899.
Haller KA, Miller-Meeks M, Kardon R. (1990). Early magnetic resonance imaging in acute traumatic internuclear ophthalmoplegia. *Ophthalmology 97*:1162–1165.
Halmagyi GM, Brandt T, Dieterich M, et al. (1990). Tonic contraversive ocular tilt reaction due to unilateral mesodiencephalic lesion. *Neurology 40*:1503–1509.
Halmagyi GM, Evans WA, Hallinan JM. (1978). Failure of downward gaze. The site and nature of the lesion. *Arch Neurol 35*:22–26.
Hamed LM, Schatz NJ, Galetta SL. (1988). Brainstem ocular motility defects and AIDS. *Am J Ophthalmol 106*:437–442.
Hanson MR, Hamid MA, Tomsak RL, et al. (1986). Selective saccadic palsy caused by pontine lesions: Clinical, physiological, and pathological correlations. *Ann Neurol 20*:209–217.
Harding AE, Young EP, Schon F. (1987). Adult-onset supranuclear ophthalmoplegia, cerebellar ataxia and neurogenic proximal muscle weakness in a brother and sister: Another hexosaminidase A deficiency syndrome. *J Neurol Neurosurg Psych 50*:687–690.

Harris CM, Shawkat F, Russell-Eggitt I, et al. (1996). Intermittent horizontal saccade failure ('ocular motor apraxia') in children. *Br J Ophthalmol 80:*151–158.

Hedges TR, Hoyt WF. (1982). Ocular tilt reaction due to an upper brainstem lesion: Paroxysmal skew deviation, torsion, and oscillation of the eyes with head tilt. *Ann Neurol 11:*537–540.

Herishanu Y, Lavy S. (1969). Transient bilateral internuclear ophthalmoplegia of vascular origin. *Ophthalmologica 159:*324–327.

Herishanu YO, Sharpe JA. (1983). Saccadic intrusions in internuclear ophthalmoplegia. *Ann Neurol 14:*67–72.

Hirose G, Furui K, Yoshioka A, Sakai K. (1993). Unilateral conjugate gaze palsy due to a lesion of the abducens nucleus. Clinical and neuroradiological correlation. *J Clin Neuro-ophthalmol 13:*54–58.

Ho PC, Feman SS. (1981). Internuclear ophthalmoplegia in Fabry's disease. *Ann Ophthalmol 13:*949–951.

Hommel M, Bogousslavsky DC. (1990). The spectrum of vertical gaze palsy following unilateral brainstem stroke. *Neurology 41:*1229–1234.

Hommel M, Gato JM, Pollack P, et al. (1987). Magnetic resonance imaging and the "one-and-a-half syndrome": A case report. *J Clin Neuro-ophthalmol 7:*161–164.

Hopf HC, Thomke F, Gutmann L. (1991). Midbrain vs. pontine medial longitudinal fasciculus lesions: the utilization of masseter and blink reflexes. *Muscle Nerve 14:*326–330.

Hotson JR, Sachdev HS. (1982). Amitriptyline: Another cause of internuclear ophthalmoplegia with coma. *Ann Neurol 12:*62.

Hoyt CS, Billson FA, Alpins N. (1978). The supranuclear disturbances of gaze in kernicterus. *Ann Ophthalmol 10:*1487–1492.

Hoyt CS, Mousel DK, Weber AA. (1980). Transient supranuclear disturbances of gaze in healthy neonates. *Am J Ophthalmol 89:*708–713.

Hughes TA, Wiles CM, Hourihan M. (1994). Cervical radiculopathy and bilateral internuclear ophthalmoplegia caused by temporal arteritis. *J Neurol Neurosurg Psych 57:*764–765.

Inocencio FP, Ballecer R. (1985). Tuberculosis granuloma in the midbrain causing wall-eyed bilateral internuclear ophthalmoplegia (Webino). *J Clin Neuro-ophthalmol 5:*31–35.

Jackel RA, Gittinger JW Jr, Smith TW, Passarelli CB. (1986). Metastatic adenocarcinoma presenting as a one-and-a-half syndrome. *J Clin Neuro-ophthalmol 6:*116–119.

Jackson G, Miller M, Littlejohn G, et al. (1986). Bilateral internuclear ophthalmoplegia in systemic lupus erythematosus. *J Reumatol 13:*1161–1162.

Jackson JA, Jankovic J, Ford J. (1983). Progressive supranuclear palsy: Clinical features and response to treatment in 16 patients. *Ann Neurol 13:*273–278.

Jacobs L, Anderson PJ, Bender MB. (1973). The lesions producing paralysis of downward but not upward gaze. *Arch Neurol 28:*319–323.

Jacobs L, Heffner RR, Newman RP. (1985). Selective paralysis of downward gaze caused by bilateral lesions of the mesencephalic periaqueductal gray matter. *Neurology 35:*516–521.

Jammes JL. (1989). Bilateral internuclear ophthalmoplegia due to acute cervical hyperextension without head trauma. *J Clin Neuro-ophthalmol 9:*112–115.

Jampel RS, Fells P. (1968). Monocular elevation paresis caused by a central nervous system lesion. *Arch Ophthalmol 80:*45–57.

Jampel RS, Quaglio ND. (1964). Eye movements in Tay-Sachs disease. *Neurology 14:*1013–1019.

Jay WM, Nazarian SM, Underwood DW. (1987). Pseudo-internuclear ophthalmoplegia with downshoot in myasthenia gravis. *J Clin Neuro-ophthalmol 7:*74–76.

Johnston JI, Sharpe JA. (1994). The WEMINO syndrome—Wall-eyed monocular internuclear ophthalmoplegia: An oculographic and neuropathologic characterization. *Neurology (Suppl. 2) 44:*A311.

Johnston JL, Sharpe JA, Morrow MJ. (1992). Paresis of contralateral smooth pursuit and normal vestibular smooth eye movements after unilateral brainstem lesions. *Ann Neurol 31:*495–502.

Johnston JL, Thomson GT, Sharpe JA, Inman RD. (1990). Internuclear ophthalmoplegia in giant cell arteritis. *J Neurol Neurosurg Psych 55:*84–85.

Kandler RH, Davies-Jones GAB. (1988). Internuclear ophthalmoplegia in pernicious anemia. *Br Med J 297:*1583.

Kase C, Maulsby G, Mohr J. (1981). Partial pontine hematomas. *Neurology 30:*652–655.

Kato I, Watanabe J, Nakamura T, et al. (1990). Mapping of brainstem lesions by the combined use of tests of visually-induced eye movements. *Brain 113:*921–935.

Katz DM, Trobe JD, Muraszko KM, Dauser RC. (1994). Shunt failure without ventriculomegaly proclaimed by ophthalmic findings. *J Neurosurg 81:*721–725.

Kawahara Y, Sato K, Muraki M, et al. (1986). CT classification of small thalamic hemorrhages and their clinical implications. *Neurology 36:*165–172.

Keane J. (1986). Bilateral ocular motor signs after tentorial herniation in 25 patients. *Arch Neurol 43:*806–807.

Keane JE, Finstead BA. (1982). Upward gaze paralysis as the initial sign of Fisher's syndrome. *Arch Neurol 39:*781–782.

Keane JR. (1985). Alternating skew deviation: 47 patients. *Neurology 35:*725–728.

Keane JR. (1975). Ocular skew deviation. Analysis of 100 cases. *Arch Neurol* 185–190.

Keane JR. (1992). Ocular tilt reaction following lateral pontomedullary infarction. *Neurology 42:*259–260.

Keane JR. (1990). The pretectal syndrome: 206 patients. *Neurology 40:*684–690.

Keane JR. (1987). Traumatic internuclear ophthalmoplegia. *J Clin Neuro-ophthalmol 7:*165–166.

Keane JR, Rawlinson DG, Itabashi HH. (1976). Sustained downgaze deviation. Two cases without structural pretectal lesions. *Neurology 26:*594–595.

Kernan JC, Devinsky O, Luciano DJ, et al. (1993). Lateralizing significance of head and eye deviation in secondary generalized tonic-clonic seizures. *Neurology 43:*1308–1310.

Kirkali P, Topaloglu R, Kansu T, Bakkaloglu A. (1991). Third nerve palsy and internuclear ophthalmoplegia in periarteritis nodosa. *J Ped Ophthalmol Strabismus 28:*45–46.

Kirkham TH, Kamin DF. (1974). Slow saccadic eye movements in Wilson's disease. *J Neurol Neurosurg Psych 37:*191–194.

Kirkham TH, Katsarkas A. (1977). An electrooculographic study of internuclear ophthalmoplegia. *Ann Neurol 2:*385–392.

Knox DL, Bayless TM, Pittman FE. (1976). Neurologic disease in patients with treated Whipple's disease. *Medicine 55:*467–476.

Kobari M, Ishihara N, Yinoki K. (1987). Bilateral thalamic infarction associated with selective downward gaze paralysis. *Eur Neurol 26:*246–251.

Koga H, Mori K, Kawano T, et al. (1983). Parinaud's syndrome in hydrocephalus due to a basilar artery aneurysm. *Surg Neurol 19:*548–553.

Kommerell G. (1975). Internuclear ophthalmoplegia of abduction. Isolated impairment of phasic ocular motor activity in supranuclear lesions. *Arch Ophthalmol 93:*531–534.

Kommerell G. (1981). Unilateral internuclear ophthalmoplegia. The lack of inhibitory involvement in medial rectus muscle activity. *Invest Ophthalmol Vis Sci 21:*592–599.

Kömpf D, Oppermann J. (1986). Vertical gaze palsy and thalamic dementia. Syndrome of the posterior thalmo-subthalamic paramedian artery. *Neuro-ophthalmol 6:*121–124.

Kornfeld M, Appenzeller O, Saiki J, Troup GM. (1975). Sea-blue histiocytes and sural nerve in neurovisceral storage disorder with vertical ophthalmoplegia. *J Neurol Sci 25:*291–302.

Kristensen MO. (1985). Progressive supranuclear palsy—20 years later. *Acta Neurol Scand 71:*177–189.

Kupfer C, Cogan DG. (1966). Unilateral internuclear ophthalmoplegia: A clinicopathological case report. *Arch Ophthalmol 75:*484–489.

Lagreze W-D, Warner JEA, Zamani AA, et al. (1996). Mesencephalic clefts associated with eye movement disorders. *Arch Ophthalmol 114:*429–432.

Lana MA, Moreira PR, Nerves LB. (1990). Wall-eyed bilateral internuclear ophthalmoplegia (Webino syndrome) and myelopathy in pyoderma gangrenosum. *Arq Neuropsiquiqtr 48:*497–501.

Leavitt JA, Butrus SI. (1994). Internuclear ophthalmoplegia in sickle cell trait. *J Neuroophthalmol 14:*49–51.

Lee AG, Brown DG, Diaz PJ. (1996). Dorsal midbrain syndrome due to mesencephalic hemorrhage. Case report with serial imaging. *J Neuro-ophthalmol 16:*281–285.

Leigh RJ, Tusa RJ. (1985). Disturbance of smooth pursuit caused by infarction of occipitoparietal cortex. *Ann Neurol 17:*185–187.

Leigh RJ, Zee DS. (1991). *The Neurology of Eye Movements.* 2nd edition. Philadelphia, Davis.

Leigh RJ, Foley JM, Remler BF, Civil RH. (1987). Oculogyric crisis: A syndrome of thought disorder and ocular deviation. *Ann Neurol 22:*13–17.

Leigh RJ, Newman SA, Folstein SE, et al. (1983). Abnormal ocular motor control in Huntington's disease. *Neurology 33:*1268–1275.

Lekwuwa GU, Barnes GR. (1996). Cerebral control of eye movements. I. The relationship between cerebral lesion sites and smooth pursuit deficits. *Brain 119:*473–490.

Lepore FE, Nissenblatt MJ. (1981). Bilateral internuclear ophthalmoplegia after intrathecal chemotherapy and cranial irradiation. *Am J Ophthalmol 92:*851–853.

Lepore FE, Steele JC, Cox TA, et al. (1988). Supranuclear disturbances of ocular motility in Lytico-Bodig. *Neurology 38:*1849–1853.

Lerner MA, Kosary IZ, Cohen BE. (1969). Parinaud's syndrome in aqueduct stenosis: Its mechanism and ventriculographic features. *Br J Radiol 42:*310–312.

Lessell S. (1975). Supranuclear paralysis of monocular elevation. *Neurology 25:*1134–1143.

Lewis AJ, Gawel MJ. (1990). Diffuse Lewy body disease with dementia and oculomotor dysfunction. *Movement Disorders 5:*143–147.

Lewis AR, Kline LB, Sharpe JA. (1996). Acquired esotropia due to Arnold-Chiari I malformation. *J Neuro-ophthalmol 16:*49–54.

Lledo Carreres M, Lajo Garrido JL, Gonzalez Rico M, et al. (1992). Toxic internuclear ophthalmoplegia related to antiobesity treatment. *Ann Pharmacotherapy 26:*1457–1458.

Lousa M, Gobernado JM, Gimeno A. (1983). One-and-a-half syndrome due to polycythemia. *J Neurol Neurosurg Psych 46:*873.

MacDonald JT, Sher PK. (1977). Ophthalmoplegia as a sign of metabolic disease in the newborn. *Neurology 27:*971–973.

McLachlan RS. (1987). The significance of head and eye turning in seizures. *Neurology 37:*1617–1619.

Magli A, DeMarco R, DiMaio S, et al. (1991). A case of Parinaud's syndrome in a boy with delayed puberty. *Ophthalmologica 202:*132–137.

Maher ER, Lee AJ. (1986). The clinical features and natural history of the Steele-Richardson-Olszewski syndrome (progressive supranuclear palsy). *Neurology 36:*1005–1008.

Malessa S, Gaymard GD, Rivaud S, et al. (1994). Role of pontine nuclei damage in smooth pursuit impairment of progressive supranuclear palsy: A clinical-pathological study. *Neurology 44:*716–721.

Marshall RS, Sacco RL, Krueger R, et al. (1991). Dissociated vertical nystagmus and internuclear ophthalmoplegia from a midbrain infarction. *Arch Neurol 48:*1304–1305.

Martyn CN, Keane D. (1988). The one-and-a-half syndrome. Clinical correlation with a pontine lesion demonstrated by nuclear magnetic resonance imaging in a case of multiple sclerosis. *Br J Ophthalmol 72:*515–517.

Masai H, Kashii S, Kimura H, Fukuyama H. (1995). Neuro-Behçet disease presenting with internuclear ophthalmoplegia. *Am J Ophthalmol 122:*897–898.

Masdeu JC, Rosenberg M. (1987). Midbrain-diencephalic horizontal gaze paresis. *J Clin Neuro-ophthalmol 7:*227–234.

Mastaglia FL, Grainger KMR. (1975). Internuclear ophthalmoplegia in progressive supranuclear palsy. *J Neurol Sci 25:*303–308.

Mehler MF. (1988). The neuro-ophthalmologic spectrum of the rostral basilar artery syndrome. *Arch Neurol 45:*966–971.

Mehler MF. (1989). The rostral basilar artery syndrome: Diagnosis, etiology, prognosis. *Neurology 39:*9–16.

Merikangas JR. (1978). Skew deviation in pseudotumor cerebri. *Ann Neurol 4:*583.

Merrill PT, Paige GD, Abrams RA, et al. (1991). Ocular motor abnormalities in human immunodeficiency virus infection. *Ann Neurol 30:*130–138.

Metz HS. (1977). Myasthenia gravis presenting as internuclear ophthalmoplegia. *J Ped Ophthalmol 14:*23–24.

Meyer MW, Wild JH. (1975). Unilateral internuclear ophthalmoplegia in systemic lupus erythematosus. *Arch Neurol 32:*486.

Mills RP, Swanson PD. (1978). Vertical oculomotor apraxia and memory loss. *Ann Neurol 4:*149–153.

Minamori Y, Yamamoto M, Tanaka A, et al. (1992). Medial longitudinal fasciculus syndrome associated with a subdural hygroma and an arachnoid cyst in the middle cranial fossa. *Intern Med 31:*1286–1290.

Moffie D, Ongerboer de Visser BW, Stefanko SZ. (1983). Parinaud's syndrome. *J Neurol Sci 58:*175–183.

Morrow MJ, Sharpe JA. (1995). Deficits in smooth-pursuit eye movements after unilateral frontal lobe lesions. *Ann Neurol 37:*443–451.

Morrow MJ, Sharpe JA. (1993). Retinotopic and directional deficits of smooth pursuit initiation after posterior cerebral hemispheric lesions. *Neurology 43:*595–603.

Moster ML, Schatz NJ, Savino PJ, et al. (1988). Alternating skew deviation on lateral gaze (bilateral abducting hypertropia). *Ann Neurol 23:*190–192.

Mueller C, Koch S, Toifl K. (1993). Transient bilateral internuclear ophthalmoplegia after minor head-trauma. *Dev Med Child Neurol 35:*163–166.

Muri RM, Meienberg O. (1985). The clinical spectrum of internuclear ophthalmoplegia in multiple sclerosis. *Arch Neurol 42:*851–855.

Nagaratnam N, Ghougassian DF, Mugridge V. (1989). Syndrome of downgaze paralysis, amnesia and hypersomnolence. *Postgrad Med J 65:*840–842.

Neville BGR, Lake BD, Stephens R, Sanders MD. (1973). A neurovisceral storage disease with vertical supranuclear ophthalmoplegia, and its relationship to Neimann-Pick disease. *Brain 96:*97–120.

Newton HB, Miner ME. (1991). "One-and-a-half" syndrome after a resection of a midline cerebellar astrocytoma: case report and discussion of the literature. *Neurosurg 29:*768–772.

Nightingale S, Barton ME. (1991). Intermittent vertical supranuclear ophthalmoplegia and ataxia. *Mov Disord 6:*76–78.

Nishizaki T, Tamaki N, Nishida Y, Matsumoto S. (1985). Bilateral internuclear ophthalmoplegia due to hydrocephalus: A case report. *Neurosurgery 17:*822–825.

Nittner K, Petrovici IN. (1974). Contributions to the pathogenesis of Parinaud's syndrome. Vertical gaze paralysis following bilateral stereotactic lesions in the interstitial nucleus region. *Acta Neurochir 21:*57–63.

Nozaki S, Mukuno K, Ishikawa S. (1983). Internuclear ophthalmoplegia associated with ipsilateral downbeat nystagmus and contralateral incyclorotatory nystagmus. *Ophthalmologica 187:*210–216.

Ohta K, Gotoh F, Fukuuchi Y, et al. (1994). Midpontine tegmentum infarction with "one-and-a-half syndrome" demonstrated by magnetic resonance imaging. *Keio J Med 43:*164–165.

Okuda B, Tachibana H, Sugita M, Maeda Y. (1993). Bilateral internuclear ophthalmoplegia, ataxia, and tremor from a midbrain infarction. *Stroke 24:*481–482.

Okuda B, Yamamoto T, Yamasaki M, et al. (1992). Motor neuron disease with slow eye movements and vertical gaze palsy. *Acta Neurol Scand 85:*71–76.

Oommen KJ, Smith MS, Labadie EL. (1982). Pontine hemorrhage causing Fisher one-and-a-half syndrome with facial paralysis. *J Clin Neuro-ophthalmol 2:*129–132.

Osher RH, Corbett JJ, Schatz NJ, et al. (1978). Neuro-ophthalmological complications of enlargement of the third ventricle. *Br J Ophthalmol 62:*536–542.

Ouvrier RA, Billson F. (1988). Benign paroxysmal tonic upgaze of childhood. *J Child Neurol 3:*177–188.

Page NGR, Leans JS, Sanders MD. (1982). Vertical supranuclear gaze palsy with secondary syphilis. *J Neurol Neurosurg Psych 45:*86–88.

Peiris JB, Wickremasinghe HR, Sivayoham IS. (1975). An unusual brain stem astrocytoma producing complicated Parinaud's syndrome. *J Indian Med Assoc 64:*340–341.

Pfister HW, Einhaupl KM, Büttner U, et al. (1989). Dissociated nystagmus as a common sign of ocular motor disorders in HIV-infected patients. *Eur Neurol* 277–280.

Pierrot-Deseilligny C, Rivaud S, Samson Y, Cambon H. (1989). Some instructive cases concerning the circuitry of ocular smooth pursuit in the brainstem. *Neuro-ophthalmology 9:*31–42.

Pierrot-Deseilligny C, Amarenco P, Roullet E, Marteau R. (1990). Vermal infarct with pursuit eye movement disorders. *J Neurol Neurosurg Psych 53:*519–521.

Pierrot-Deseilligny C, Chain F, Serdaru M, et al. (1981). The one and a half syndrome. Electro-oculographic analysis of five cases with deductions about the physiological mechanisms of lateral gaze. *Brain 104:*665–699.

Pierrot-Deseilligny C, Gautier J, Loron P. (1988). Acquired ocular motor apraxia due to bilateral frontoparietal infarcts. *Ann Neurol 23:*199–202.

Pierrot-Deseilligny C, Gray F, Brunet P. (1986). Infarcts of both inferior parietal lobules with impairment of visually guided eye movements, peripheral visual inattention, and optic ataxia. *Brain 109:*81–97.

Pierrot-Deseilligny C, Rivaud S, Gaymard B, et al. (1995). Cortical control of saccades. *Ann Neurol 37:*557–567.

Pillay N, Gilbert JJ, Ebers GC, Brown JD. (1984). Internuclear ophthalmoplegia and "optic neuritis": Paraneoplastic effects of bronchial carcinoma. *Neurology 34:*788–791.

Pless M, Sandson T. (1997). Chronic internuclear ophthalmoplegia. A manifestation of D-penicillamine cerebral vasculitis. *J Neuro-ophthalmol 17:*44–46.

Poisson M, Van Effentere R, Mashaly R. (1980). Pituitary apoplexy with retraction nystagmus. *Ann Neurol 7:*286.

Posner M, Horax G. (1946). Eye signs in pineal tumors. *J Neurosurg 3:*15–24.

Prasad P, Nair S. (1994). Congenital ocular motor apraxia: Sporadic and familial. Support for natural resolution. *J Neuro-ophthalmol 14:*102–104.

Quint DJ, Cornblath WT, Trobe JD. (1993). Multiple sclerosis presenting as Parinaud syndrome. *Am J Neuroradiol 14:*1200–1202.

Ranalli PJ, Sharpe JA, Fletcher WA. (1988). Palsy of upward and downward saccadic, pursuit, and vestibular movements with a unilateral midbrain lesion: Pathophysiologic correlations. *Neurology 38:*114–122.

Reagan TJ, Trautmann JC. (1978). Combined nuclear and supranuclear defects in ocular motility. A clinicopathologic study. *Arch Neurol 35:*133–137.

Rennie IG, Wright JGC, Wilkinson JL. (1986). Iatrogenic internuclear ophthalmoplegia. *J Neurol Neurosurg Psych 49:*842.

Reynolds EH. (1989). Internuclear ophthalmoplegia in pernicious anemia. *Br Med J 298:*460–461.

Rich JR, Gregorius FK, Hepler RS. (1974). Bilateral internuclear ophthalmoplegia after trauma. *Arch Ophthalmol 92:*66–68.

Riley DE, Lang AE, Lewis A, et al. (1990). Cortico-basal ganglionic degeneration. *Neurology 40:*1203–1212.

Riley E, Swift M. (1979). Congenital horizontal gaze palsy and kyphoscoliosis in two brothers. *J Med Genet 16:*314–316.

Rinne JO, Lee MS, Thompson PD, Marsden CD. (1994). Corticobasal degeneration. A clinical study of 36 cases. *Brain 117:*1183–1196.

Riordan-Eva P, Jarcourt JP, Faldon M, et al. (1997). Skew deviation following vestibular nerve surgery. *Ann Neurol 41:*94–99.

Rismondo V, Borchert M. (1992). Position-dependent Parinaud's syndrome. *Am J Ophthalmol 114:*107–108.

Rizzo M, Corbett J. (1983). Bilateral internuclear ophthalmoplegia reversed by naloxone. *Arch Neurol 40:*242–243.

Robillard A, Saint-Hilaire JM, Mercier M, Bouvier G. (1983). The lateralizing and localizing value of adversion in epileptic seizures. *Neurology 33:*1241–1242.

Rosati G, Pinna L, Paolino E, D'Agostini G. (1981). Reversible bilateral internuclear ophthalmoplegia due to head trauma: A case report. *Eur Neurol 20:*81–83.

Rosenbaum DH, Siegel M, Rowan AJ. (1986). Contraversive seizures in occipital epilepsy: Case report and review of the literature. *Neurology 36:*281–284.

Rosenberg ML, Jabbari B. (1991). Miosis and internuclear ophthalmoplegia as a manifestation of partial seizures. *Neurology 41:737–739.*

Ross AT, De Myer WE. (1966). Isolated syndrome of the medial longitudinal fasciculus in man. *Arch Neurol 15:*203–206.

Safran AB, Vibert D, Issoua D, Hausler A. (1994). Skew deviation after vestibular neuronitis. *Am J Ophthalmol 118:*238–245.

Samples JR, Howard FM Jr, Okazaki H. (1983). Syringomesencephalia. Report of a case. *Arch Neurol 40:757–759.*

Sand JJ, Biller J, Corbett JJ, et al. (1986). Partial dorsal mesencephalic hemorrhages: Report of three cases. *Neurology 36:*529–533.

Sandyk R. (1982). Isolated failure of upward gaze as a sign of chronic subdural haematoma. *South Afr Med J 61:*32.

Sandyk R. (1982). Paralysis of conjugate upward gaze in acute decompensating hydrocephalus. *S Afr Med J 61:*261.

Sandyk R. (1984). Paralysis of upward gaze as a presenting symptom of vitamin B_{12} deficiency. *Europ Neurology 23:*198–200.

Sandyk R, Brennan MJW. (1984). Internuclear ophthalmoplegia in tuberculous meningitis. A report of two cases. *Eur Neurol 23:*148–150.

Saver JL, Liu GT, Charness ME. (1994). Idiopathic striopalidodentate calcification with prominent supranuclear abnormality of eye movement. *J Neuro-ophthalmol 14:*29–33.

Schiff ND, Moore DF. (1996). Predominant downgaze ophthalmoparesis in anti-Hu encephalomyelitis. *J Neuro-ophthalmol 16:*302–303.

Schlegel U, Clarenbach P, Cordt A, Steudel A. (1989). Cerebral sarcoidosis presenting as supranuclear gaze palsy with hypokinetic rigid syndrome. *Mov Disord 4:*274–277.

Schraeder PL, Cohen MM, Goldman W. (1981). Bilateral internuclear ophthalmoplegia associated with fourth ventricular epidermoid tumor. *J Neurosurg 54:*403–405.

Schwartz MA, Selhorst JB, Ochs AL, et al. (1986). Oculomasticatory myorhythmia: A unique movement disorder occurring in Whipple's disease. *Ann Neurol 20:*677–683.

Scolding NJ, Kellar-Wood HF, Shaw C, et al. (1996). Wolfram syndrome: Hereditary diabetes mellitus with brainstem and optic atrophy. *Ann Neurol 39:*352–360.

Seaber JH, Nashold BS. (1980). Comparison of ocular motor effects of unilateral stereotactic midbrain lesions in man. *Neuro-ophthalmol 1:*95–99.

Segarra JM. (1970). Cerebral vascular disease and behavior. I. The syndrome of the mesencephalic artery (basilar artery bifurcation). *Arch Neurol 22:*408–418.

Senanayake N. (1992). A syndrome of early onset spinocerebellar ataxia with optic atrophy, internuclear ophthalmoplegia, dementia, and startle myoclonus in a Sri Lanken family. *J Neurol 239:*293–294.

Shallat RF, Pawl RP, Jerva MJ. (1973). Significance of upward gaze palsy (Parinaud's syndrome) in hydrocephalus due to shunt malfunction. *J Neurosurg 38:*717–721.

Sharpe JA, Morrow MJ, Johnston JL. (1989). Smooth pursuit: Anatomy, physiology, and disorders. *Bull Soc Belge Ophthalmol 237:*113–144.

Sharpe JA, Rosenberg MA, Hoyt WF, Daroff RB. (1974). Paralytic pontine exotropia. A sign of acute unilateral pontine gaze palsy and internuclear ophthalmoplegia. *Neurology 24:*1076–1081.

Sharpe JA, Silversides JL, Blair RD. (1975). Familial paralysis of horizontal gaze. Associated with pendular nystagmus, progressive scoliosis, and facial contraction with myokymia. *Neurology 25:*1035–1040.

Shawkat FS, Harris CM, Taylor DSI, Kriss A. (1996). The role of ERG/VEP and eye movement recordings in children with ocular motor apraxia. *Eye 10:*53–60.

Sherman MD, Allinson RW, Obbens EA, et al. (1989). Internuclear ophthalmoplegia in acquired immunodeficiency syndrome. *Ann Ophthalmol 21:*294–295.

Shults WT, Hamby S, Corbett JJ, et al. (1993). Neuro-ophthalmic complications of intracranial catheters. *Neurosurgery 33:*135–138.

Slavin ML. (1985). Gaze palsy associated with viral syndrome. *Am J Ophthalmol 100:*468–473.

Slyman JF, Kline LB. (1981). Dorsal midbrain syndrome in multiple sclerosis. *Neurology 31:*196–198.

Smith JL, Cogan DG. (1959). Internuclear ophthalmoplegia. A review of fifty-eight cases. *Arch Ophthalmol 61:*687–694.

Smith JL, David NJ. (1964). Internuclear ophthalmoplegia: Two new clinical signs. *Neurology 14:*307–309.

Smith MS, Laguna JF. (1981). Upward gaze paralysis following unilateral pretectal infarction. *Arch Neurol 38:*127–129.

Smith MS, Buchsbaum HW, Masland WS. (1980). One and a half syndrome. Occurrence after trauma with computerized tomographic correlation. *Arch Neurol 37:*251.

Snyder BD, Blonde L, McWhirter WR. (1974). Reversal of amitriptyline intoxication by physostigmine. *JAMA 230:*1433–1434.

Stark RJ. (1979). Supranuclear ophthalmoplegia with basilar artery aneurysms. *Surg Neurology 12:*447–452.

Starr A. (1967). A disorder of rapid eye movements in Huntington's chorea. *Brain 90:*545–567.

Steele JC. (1972). Progressive supranuclear palsy. *Brain 95:*693–704.

Steiner I, Melamed E. (1984). Conjugate eye deviation after acute hemispheric stroke: Delayed recovery after previous contralateral frontal lobe damage. *Ann Neurol 16:*509–511.

Strauss C, Ganslandt O, Huk WJ, Jonas JB. (1995). Isolated unilateral internuclear ophthalmoplegia following head injury. Findings in magnetic resonance imaging. *Neuro-ophthalmology 15:*15–19.

Strominger MB, Mincy EJ, Strominger AI, et al. (1986). Bilateral internuclear ophthalmoplegia with absence of convergent eye movements—Clinicopathological correlation. *J Clin Neuro-ophthalmology 6:*57–65.

Sullivan HG, Harbison JW, Becker DP. (1976). Parinaud's syndrome: Cerebrovascular disease as a common etiology: Analysis of 16 cases. *Surg Neurol 6:*301–305.

Sung JY, Cheng PN, Lai KN. (1991). Internuclear ophthalmoplegia in cryptococcal meningitis. *J Trop Med Hygiene 94:*116–117.

Supranuclear ophthalmoplegia in olivopontocerebellar degeneration. *Neurology 26:*764–768.

Swanson RA, Schmidley JW. (1985). Amnestic syndrome and vertical gaze palsy: Early detection of bilateral thalamic infarction by CT and NMR. *Stroke 16:*823–827.

Swash M. (1974). Periaqueductal dysfunction (the Sylvian aqueduct syndrome): A sign of hydrocephalus? *J Neurol Neurosurg Psych 37:*21–26.

Swick HM. (1974). Pseudointernuclear ophthalmoplegia in acute idiopathic polyneuritis (Fisher's syndrome). *Am J Ophthalmol 77:*725–728.

Tatemichi TK, Steinke W, Duncan C, et al. (1992). Paramedian thalamopeduncular infarction: Clinical syndromes and magnetic resonance imaging. *Ann Neurol 32:*162–171.

Tekkok IH, Ayberk G, Kansu T, Saglam S. (1989). Bilateral internuclear ophthalmoplegia associated with fourth ventricular dermoid tumor. *J Clin Neuro-ophthalmol 9:*254–257.

Teoh R, Humphries MJ, Chan JCN, et al. (1989). Internuclear ophthalmoplegia in tuberculous meningitis. *Tubercle 70:*61–64.

Thames PB, Trobe JD, Ballinger WE. (1984). Gaze paralysis caused by lesion of the periaqueductal gray matter. *Arch Neurol 41:*437–440.

Thier P, Bachor A, Faiss J, et al. (1991). Selective impairment of smooth-pursuit eye movements due to an ischemic lesion of the basal pons. *Ann Neurol 29:*443–448.

Thöke F. (1996). Some observations on abduction nystagmus in internuclear ophthalmoplegia. *Neuro-ophthalmology 16:*27–38.

Thomke F, Hopf HC. (1992). Acquired monocular elevation paresis. An asymmetric up-gaze palsy. *Brain 115:*1901–1910.

Thomke F, Hopf HC, Kramer G. (1992). Internuclear ophthalmoplegia of abduction: Clinical and electrophysiological data on the existence of an abduction paresis of prenuclear origin. *J Neurol Neurosurg Psych 55:*105–111.

Thomson GT, Johnston JL, Sharpe JA, Inman RD. (1989). Internuclear ophthalmoplegia in giant cell arteritis. *J Rheumatol 16:*693–695.

Tijssen CC. (1994). Contralateral conjugate eye deviation in acute supratentorial lesions. *Stroke 25:*1516–1519.

Tijssen CC, van Gisbergen JAM. (1993). Conjugate eye deviation after hemispheric stroke. A contralateral saccadic palsy? *Neuro-ophthalmol 13:*107–118.

Topilow HW. (1981). Posterior internuclear ophthalmoplegia of Lutz. *Ann Ophthalmol 13:*221–225.

Trajanowski JQ, Lafontaine MH. (1981). Neuroanatomical correlates of selective downgaze paralysis. *J Neurol Sci 52:*91–101.

Trend P, Graham E. (1990). Internuclear ophthalmoplegia in giant-cell arteritis. *J Neurol Neurosurg Psych 53:*532–533.

Tripp JH, Lake BD, Young E, et al. (1977). Juvenile Gaucher's disease with horizontal gaze palsy in three siblings. *J Neurol Neurosurg Psych 40:*470–478.

Trojanowski JQ, Wray SH. (1980). Vertical gaze ophthalmoplegia: Selective paralysis of downgaze. *Neurology 30:*605–610.

Troost BT, Martinez J, Abel LA, Heros RC. (1980). Upbeat nystagmus and internuclear ophthalmoplegia with brainstem glioma. *Arch Neurol 37:*453–456.

Tusa RJ, Ungerleider LG. (1988). Fiber pathways of cortical areas mediating smooth pursuit eye movements in monkeys. *Ann Neurol 23:*174–183.

Waespe W. (1992). Deficits of smooth-pursuit eye movements in two patients with a lesion in the (para-)floccular or dorsolateral pontine region. *Neuro-ophthalmology 12:*91–96.

Wall M, Slamovits TL, Weisberg LA, Trufant SA. (1986). Vertical gaze ophthalmoplegia from infarction of the posterior thalamo-subthalamic paramedian artery. *Stroke 17:*546–555.

Wall M, Wray SH. (1983). The one-and-a-half syndrome—a unilateral disorder of the pontine tegmentum: A study of 20 cases and review of the literature. *Neurology 33:*971–980.

Wallace TW, Culebras-Fernandez A. (1970). Posterior cerebral artery embolism: Hemianopsia and median longitudinal fasciculus syndrome. Report of a case. *Cleveland Clinic Quart 37:*157–160.

Waterston JA, Barnes GR, Grealy MA. (1992). A quantitative study of eye and head movements during smooth pursuit in patients with cerebellar disease. *Brain 115:*1343–1358.

Weisberg LA. (1986). Mesencephalic hemorrhages: Clinical and computed tomographic correlations. *Neurology 36:*713–716.

Weisberg LA. (1986). Thalamic hemorrhage: Clinical-CT correlations. *Neurology 36:*1382–1386.

Wiest G, Baumgartner C, Schnider P, et al. (1996). Monocular elevation paresis and contralateral downgaze paresis from unilateral mesodiencephalic infarction. *J Neurol Neurosurg Psych 60:*579–581.

Wilson WB. (1985). Pseudo-internuclear ophthalmoplegia after surgical paresis of the medial rectus muscle. *Am J Ophthalmol 99:*737–738.

Woody RC, Reynolds JD. (1985). Association of bilateral internuclear ophthalmoplegia and myelomeningocele with Arnold-Chiari malformation, type II. *J Clin Neuro-ophthalmol 5:*124–126.

Wyllie E, Lüders H, Morris H, et al. (1986a). Ipsilateral forced head and eye turning at the end of the generalized tonic-clonic phase of versive seizures. *Neurology 36:*1212–1217.

Wyllie E, Lüders H, Morris HH, et al. (1986b). The lateralizing significance of versive head and eye movements during epileptic seizures. *Neurology 36:*606–611.

Yan-go FL, Yanigahara T, Puerre RV, Goldstein NP. (1984). A progressive neurologic disorder with supranuclear vertical gaze paresis and distinctive bone marrow cells. *Mayo Clin Proc 59:*404–410.

Yee RD, Cogan DG, Zee DS. (1976). Ophthalmoplegia and dissociated nystagmus in abetalipoproteinemia. *Arch Ophthalmol 94:*571–575.

Yee RD, Farlow MA, Suzuki DA, et al. (1992). Abnormal eye movements in Gerstmann-Straussler-Scheinker disease. *Arch Ophthalmol 110:*68–74.

Yi it A, Bingöl A, Mutluer N, Taçilar N. (1996). The one-and-a-half syndrome in systemic lupus erythematosus. *J Neuro-ophthalmol 16:*274–276.

Yijssen CC, De Letter MACJ, Op de Coul AAW. (1996). Convergence-retraction nystagmus. *Neuro-ophthalmology 16:*215–218.

Zackon DH, Sharpe JA. (1984). Midbrain paresis of horizontal gaze. *Ann Neurol 16:*495–504.

Zauel D, Carlow TJ. (1977). Internuclear ophthalmoplegia following cervical manipulation. *Ann Neurol 1*:308.
Zee DS, Freeman JM, Holtzman NA. (1974). Ophthalmoplegia in maple syrup urine disease. *J Pediatr 84*:113–115.
Zee DS, Hain TC, Carl JR. (1987). Abduction nystagmus in internuclear ophthalmoplegia. *Ann Neurol 21*:383–388.
Ziffer AJ, Rosenbaum AL, Demer JL, Yee RD. (1992). Congenital double elevator palsy: Vertical saccadic velocity utilizing the scleral search coil technique. *J Pediatr Ophthalmol Strabismus 29*:142–149.
Zweifach PH, Walton DS, Brown RH. (1969). Isolated congenital horizontal gaze paralysis. Occurrence of the near reflex and ocular retraction on attempted lateral gaze. *Arch Ophthalmol 81*:345–350.

♦ 15 ♦

Ocular Myasthenia Gravis

What Are the Clinical Findings in Myasthenia Gravis?

Myasthenia gravis (MG) is a chronic disorder of neuromuscular transmission characterized clinically by varying degrees of weakness and fatigue of voluntary muscles. MG is caused by an acquired autoimmunity to the motor endplate and is associated with antibodies that block or cause increased degradation of acetylcholine receptors (AChR). There is abnormal weakness in some or all voluntary muscles. The most commonly affected muscles are the levator palpebrae superioris, the extraocular muscles, the orbicularis oculi, triceps, quadriceps, and the tongue (Simpson, 1981). Other voluntary muscles innervated by cranial nerves (facial, masticatory, pharyngeal, and laryngeal muscles) and cervical, pectoral girdle, and hip flexor muscles are also frequently affected. The weakness increases with repeated or sustained exertion and over the course of the day but is improved by rest; it also may be worsened by elevation of body temperature and is often improved by cold (Engel, 1994; Miller, 1985; Weinberg, 1994).

The levator palpebrae superioris and extraocular muscles are involved initially in approximately 50 to 70% of cases, and these muscles are eventually affected in about 90% of patients (Mattis, 1941; Oosterhuis, 1982; Osserman, 1967). Ocular myasthenia (OM) is a form of MG confined to the extraocular, levator palpebrae superioris, and/or orbicularis oculi muscles. Approximately 50% of patients initially present with OM, but only 12 to 50% of these remain ocular (Bever, 1983; Evoli, 1988; Ferguson, 1955; Garland, 1956; Grob, 1953, 1987; Oosterhuis, 1988, 1989; Perlo, 1966; Schlezinger, 1959; Simpson, 1966). Of the 50 to 80% of patients with purely ocular symptoms and signs at onset that go on to develop generalized MG, most, but not all, develop generalized symptoms within two to three years of onset of the disorder. Bever et al. (Bever, 1983) performed a retrospective study and found that 226 (84%) of 269 myasthenics displayed ocular findings at onset of disease and 142 (53%) demonstrated only ocular involvement. Follow-up (average 14 years, range 1 to 39 years) of 108 patients with MG who had only ocular symptoms and signs at onset showed that 43 (40%) remained ocular and 53 (49%) became generalized. Of the 53 patients who became generalized, 44 (83%) did so within two years of onset of the disease.

Age of onset in their patients was of prognostic significance. Patients older than 50 years at onset had a greater risk of generalized MG and severe complications, while patients who were younger at onset had a more benign outcome. In another study of 1487 myasthenic patients, 53% presented with ocular MG and 202 (15%) continued to demonstrate purely ocular involvement for up to 45 years of follow-up (mean, 17 years) (Oosterhuis, 1982). Of those patients with strictly ocular signs and symptoms during the first month after onset (40% of the 1487 patients), 66% subsequently developed clinically generalized disease; of these, 78% became generalized within one year after onset of symptoms and 94% within three years.

Ptosis in MG may occur as an isolated sign or in association with extraocular muscle involvement. Evoli et al. studied 48 patients with ocular myasthenia (OM) and noted that 10% had ptosis only, 90% had ptosis and extraocular muscle involvement, and 25% had weakness of the orbicularis oculi (Evoli, 1988). The ptosis may be unilateral or bilateral and, when bilateral, is usually asymmetric. The ptosis may be absent when the patient awakens and appear later in the day, becoming more pronounced as the day progresses. Prolonged upward gaze may increase the ptosis. Enhanced or seesaw ptosis may be demonstrated (i.e., a worsening of ptosis on one side when the opposite eyelid is elevated and held in a fixed position) (Gorelick, 1981), but this sign is not specific for MG because it may rarely be seen with senile ptosis, ocular myopathy, Fisher's syndrome, and even third nerve palsy (Averbuch-Heller, 1995; Suzuki, 1989). We have also seen enhanced ptosis with the Lambert-Eaton myasthenic syndrome. During refixation (a vertical saccade) from down to the primary position, the upper eyelid may either slowly begin to droop or else twitch several times before settling in a stable position (Cogan's lid-twitch sign) (Cogan, 1965). This sign is characteristic, but not diagnostic of MG (Moorthy, 1989; Phillips, 1997; Ragge, 1992). MG may also be associated with three types of eyelid retraction (Miller, 1985):

1. Contralateral eyelid retraction due to bilateral excessive innervation (Hering's law) to raise the ptotic lid
2. Brief eyelid retraction lasting only seconds following a saccade from downgaze to primary position (Cogan's lid twitch sign)
3. Transient eyelid retraction lasting seconds or minutes after staring straight ahead or looking upward for several seconds.

Involvement of extraocular muscles with MG usually occurs in association with ptosis; however, cases without clinical involvement of the levator muscles occur. MG should be considered in any case of ocular motor weakness without pupil involvement because MG may mimic any pattern of neurogenic paresis. Any extraocular muscle may be selectively impaired, especially the medial rectus, and weakness characteristically increases with sustained effort (Acers, 1979; Cleary, 1973; George, 1984; Glaser, 1966; Jay, 1987; Miller, 1985; Odel, 1992; Romano, 1973; Rush, 1982; Spooner, 1979; Spoor, 1979; Van Delan, 1984; Weinberg, 1994). Myasthenia can mimic pupil sparing third nerve palsies, superior division third nerve palsies, abducens nerve palsies, or trochlear nerve palsies (Dehaene, 1995; Miller, 1985; Osher, 1979; Spoor, 1979; Wienberg, 1994). Myasthenia may also mimic internuclear ophthalmoplegia (Acers, 1979; George, 1984; Glaser, 1966; Jay, 1987), the one and a half syndrome (Davis, 1989), horizontal or vertical gaze palsy (Glaser, 1978; Miller, 1985), double elevator palsy (McCrary, 1970), and complete external ophthalmoplegia (Brust, 1974). MG may also be associated with abnormalities of saccadic eye movements including (Miller, 1985; Schmidt, 1977, 1980a, 1980b):

1. Hypermetric saccades
2. Hypometric saccades that begin with normal velocity but ultimately show a decrease in velocity (intersaccadic fatigue) and undershoot the target
3. Small, jerky, "quivering" eye movements
4. Gaze-evoked nystagmus.

Patients with MG often have weakness of the orbicularis oculi muscles. In some cases, a "peek sign" may occur. In an attempt to sustain forceful eye closure, the orbicularis oculi may fatigue, resulting in the patient "peeking" through the partially opened palpebral fissure (Osher, 1979). Lower eyelid ectropion may occur in myasthenic patients, and become especially noticeable as the day progresses (Miller, 1985). Finally, although abnormalities of pupillary function and accommodation have been described in myasthenia gravis, this dysfunction is not clinically significant (Miller, 1979, 1985; Weinberg, 1995).

What Studies Are Suggested to Diagnosis Ocular Myasthenia Gravis?

The diagnosis of OM is based on the clinical history, physical findings, pharmacological testing, sleep test, electromyography (EMG) investigations including study of the decremental response, conventional needle EMG, single-fiber recordings, and determination of the serum anti-AChR antibody titers. In some instances, in vitro microelectrode studies of neuromuscular transmission and ultrastructural studies of the neuromuscular junction may be required to establish the diagnosis (Engel, 1994). In general, microelectrode and ultrastructural studies are reserved for patients with generalized MG and will not be discussed further.

The diagnosis of OM should be considered in any patient with ptosis and/or ocular motor weakness without pupillary involvement. Weakness and fatigue confined to the extraocular muscles or lids combined with orbicularis oculi paresis is especially suggestive of OM. Significant clinical involvement of the pupil, eye pain or headaches, proptosis, visual loss, or involvement of trigeminal sensation essentially negate this diagnosis.

A positive Tensilon (edrophonium hydrochloride) or Prostigmin (neostigmine methylsulfate) test is usually, but not always, indicative of ocular myasthenia. The improvement of extraocular muscle function should be quantified with prisms, a Hess screen, or the Lancaster red-green test (Coll, 1992; Kelly, 1982; Retzlaff, 1969). Ptosis tends to respond better to anticholinesterases than does ophthalmoparesis (Evoli, 1988; Miller, 1985). Evoli studied 43 OM patients with both ptosis and diplopia and found that Tensilon relieved only the ptosis in 15 (35%) patients (Evoli, 1988). False-positive responses to anticholinesterases have been described with brainstem and parasellar tumors, aneurysms, metastasis to the orbital apex, multiples sclerosis, Lambert-Eaton myasthenic syndrome, poliomyelitis, Guillain-Barré syndrome, motor neuron disease, botulism, orbital myositis, congenital ptosis, snake bites, diabetic sixth nerve palsy, and dermatomyositis (Campbell, 1970; Dirr, 1989; Hodes, 1948; Mastaglia, 1977; Miller, 1985; Mindel, 1989; Moorthy, 1989; Mulder, 1959, 1983; Ragge, 1992; Rowland, 1955, 1980; Schwab, 1966; Seybold, 1981, 1986; Straube, 1990; Watt, 1986; Weinberg, 1994; Wray, 1971). In most of these reports, the correct diagnosis was evident by associated neurological signs and symptoms. Moorthy et al., however, described eight cases originally diagnosed as having MG in whom an intracranial lesion instead of, or in addition to, MG was later identified (Moorthy, 1989). Four of these patients probably had both MG and an intracranial lesion, but the other four had only intracranial lesions with clinical "pseudo-myasthenic" features, including fatiguable weakness, Cogan's lid twitch sign, and positive Tensilon or Prostigmin tests. Three had pupil sparing third nerve palsies and one had a third nerve palsy associated with a sixth nerve palsy. These authors suggested that patients with clinical features consistent with MG restricted to the ocular or cranial muscles should be carefully evaluated for intracranial lesions using CT or MR imaging. We do not routinely perform neuroimaging on all patients with OM but agree with Miller who suggests that it is advisable to rule out an intracranial lesion by CT or MR imaging in all patients with isolated, unilateral, pupil-sparing ophthalmoparesis, even when the diagnosis of MG seems assured by positive Tensilon or Prostigmin test or other studies (Miller, 1985).

A negative Tensilon or Prostigmin test in no way rules out MG (Binder, 1983; Campbell, 1970; Evoli, 1988; Miller, 1979, 1985; Seybold, 1986; Spector, 1976; Weinberg, 1994). For example, Spector and Daroff noted negative responses to Tensilon in two of 11 (18%) myasthenics with only ocular involvement and in six of 21 (28.5%) of patients with both ocular and generalized disease (Spector, 1976). Paradoxical responses to Tensilon may also occur in OM patients, including paresis of previously nonparetic muscles and increased eye misalignment due to further weakening of paretic muscles (Daroff, 1986; Komiyama, 1988; Retzlaff, 1969). The "sleep test" may also be incorporated to demonstrate objective improvement in myasthenic symptoms after rest (Odel, 1991). The patient is kept in a quiet, darkened room and instructed to close the eyes and rest for 30 minutes; ptosis and ocular motility are quantified before and after the rest period. This study may be positive in some Tensilon-negative myasthenics but may also be negative in Tensilon-positive patients (Weinberg, 1994). Another noninvasive test is the ice pack test that may be useful in the diagnosis of OM in the patient with ptosis (Sethi, 1987). Ice in a surgical glove is placed over one lightly closed eye for two minutes or to the limit of patient tolerance. In cases of bilateral ptosis, the opposite (uncooled) eye serves as control. Improvement of ptosis was noted in 8 of 10 patients with myasthenia gravis (Sethi, 1987).

Fluctuations in the amplitude and duration of motor unit potentials recorded during voluntary activity with needle electromyography, decremental responses of evoked compound muscle action potentials to repetitive supramaximal motor nerve stimulation, and single fiber electromyography (SFEMG) demonstrating impulse blocking and increased "jitter" are all valuable neurophysiological studies demonstrating impaired neuromuscular transmission in MG (Engel, 1994; Hermann, 1996; Miller, 1985; Odel, 1991). Repetitive stimulation studies must include proximal and facial nerves to increase diagnostic yield. The diagnostic yield of these studies in patients with OM is unknown, but Sanders and Howard observed decremental responses in hand or shoulder muscles in only 10% of patients with OM (Sanders, 1986). If repetitive nerve stimulation studies are negative in a patient with suspected MG, SFEMG studies should be considered. SFEMG is positive in 75% of myasthenic patients in remission, 80 to 88% of those with ocular signs and symptoms only, 91 to 100% of patients with generalized symptoms, and 88 to 94% of patients with myasthenia overall (Emeryk, 1990; Sanders, 1979, 1986; Stalberg, 1980; Weinberg, 1994). For example, in one study SFEMG in limb muscles was abnormal in 17 of 20 patients with OM (Emeryk, 1990). SFEMG is quite sensitive for detecting abnormalities of the neuromuscular junction but is not specific for MG.

AChR antibody titers are quite useful in the diagnosis of MG. In one large and representative study, the percentage of positive tests in different clinical forms of MG were as follows: remission, 24%; ocular, 50%; mild generalized, 80%; moderately severe or acutely severe, 100%; chronic severe, 89% (Tindall, 1981). Overall, AChR antibodies are positive in 80 to 95% of patients with generalized MG and 34 to 56% of those with OM (Bartoccioni, 1986; Drachman, 1987; Evoli, 1988; Howard, 1987; Limburg, 1983; Morel, 1988; Newsom-Davis, 1987; Oosterhuis, 1988; Seybold, 1983; Soliven, 1988; Vincent, 1985; Weinberg, 1994). Testing for AChR binding, blocking, and modulating antibodies increases the assay yield in patients with generalized MG and OM (Howard, 1987). In OM, the antibody titer tends to be low and the serum antibody titer correlates poorly with the severity of MG when a group of patients is studied (Engel, 1994).

No test is specific for OM and its diagnosis should not be based exclusively on any single test. Kelly et al. advised that all patients with suspected MG should have serum assays of AChR antibodies, repetitive stimulation studies, and SFEMG, in addition to Tensilon or Prostigmin test (Kelly, 1982). These procedures confirm the diagnosis in at least 95% of patients. Muscle biopsy with receptor assay, in addition to these studies, should diagnose close to 100% of patients, including those with OM (Miller, 1985). Oh et al. studied 20 patients diagnosed with OM and found SFEMG positive in 80%, AChR antibodies present in 70%, and repetitive nerve stimulation studies positive in 35 to 45% (Oh, 1992). These authors advised initial AChR antibody assay and repetitive nerve stimulation studies, and follow-up SFEMG if the first two studies are normal. Evoli et al. studied 48 patients with OM and found Tensilon tests positive in 47, repetitive nerve stimulation of the limb muscles positive in 50% (24 of 48), and elevated AChR antibody titers in 45.5% (20 of 44) (Evoli, 1988). In another study of 19 Tensilon-positive OM patients, Tsujihata et al. found that six of 16 (37%) were seronegative for AChR antibodies, eight of 13 (61%) had normal SFEMG of arm muscles, and 15 of 17 (88%) had normal repetitive nerve stimulation study of the facial nerve to the orbicularis oculi muscles (Tsujihata, 1989).

Because there is an increased risk of thymoma in patients with MG, all patients with the diagnosis of MG should undergo CT or MR imaging of the mediastinum. Thymoma occurs in 5 to 20% of myasthenic patients overall and about one-third to one-half of those with thymoma have myasthenia gravis (Berrih-Aknin, 1987; Castleman, 1966; Compston, 1980; Lewis, 1987; Perlo, 1975). The risk of thymoma in patients with OM is probably lower—4% in patients with OM compared to 12% in those with generalized MG in one series (Papetestas, 1971). Thymoma is more common in older patients and in patients with high AChR antibody titers (Compston, 1980; Oger, 1993). In a large series of patients with MG, striated muscle antibodies were present in 84% of patients with thymoma (Limburg, 1983). In those without thymoma, striational antibodies were found in 5% or 47%, respectively, depending on whether the onset of MG was before or after the age of 40. Because thyroid disease may be associated with MG, all patients should also have sensitive (thyroid stimulating hormone) TSH levels measured.

An approach to the diagnosis and evaluation of patients with possible OM is outlined in Figure 15–1.

What Is the Suggested Management of Ocular Myasthenia Gravis?

Patients with purely OM must be warned of the possibility of generalization of the disease process and should specifically be instructed to inform their physician immediately if symptoms such as dysphagia, respiratory involvement, or extremity weakness develop. Generalized MG may be a life-threatening disease requiring aggressive treatment with

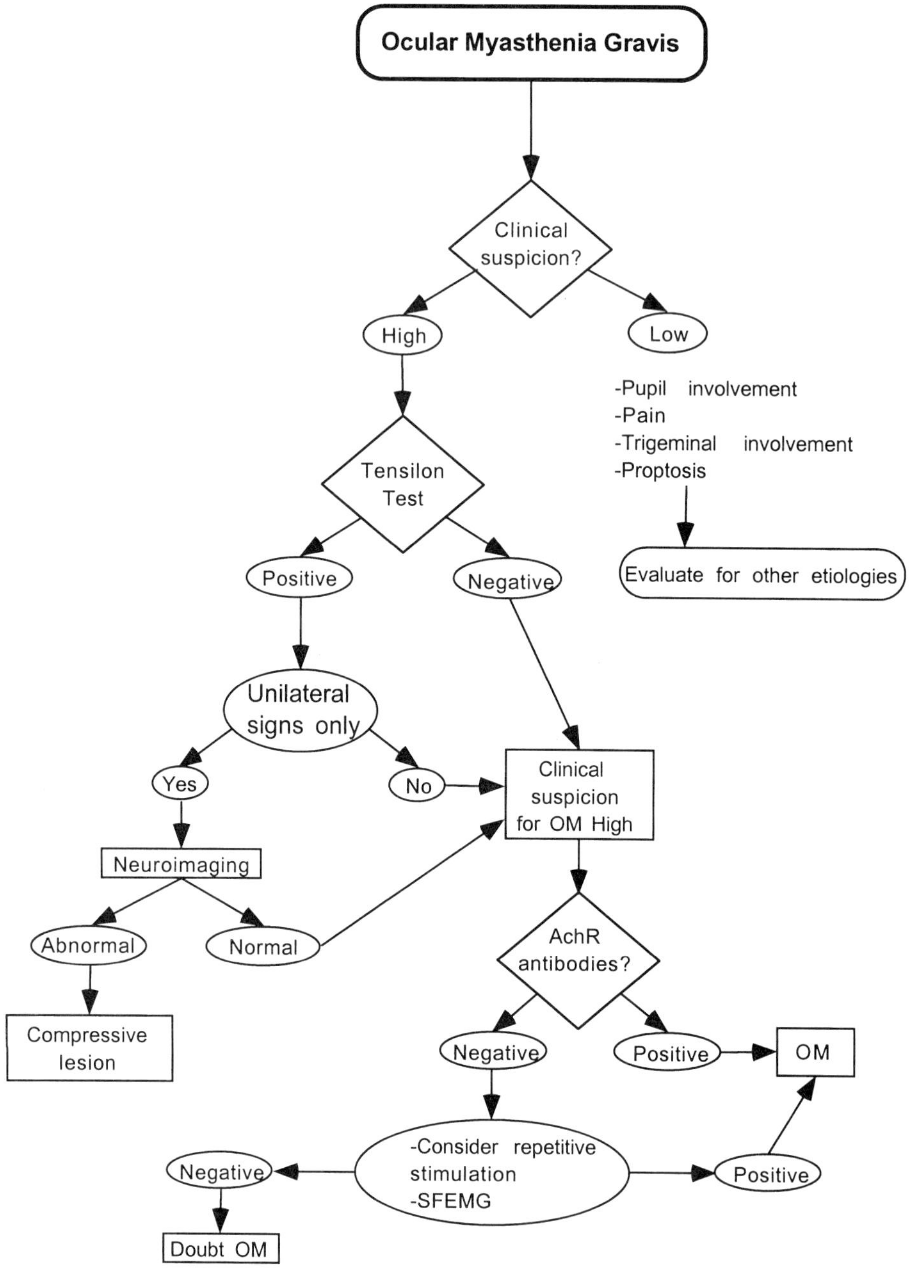

Figure 15–1. Ocular myasthenia gravis.

anticholinesterase drugs, corticosteroids, other immunosuppressive agents, plasmapheresis, intravenous gamma globulin, and possible thymectomy.

For patients with OM, if the diplopia or ptosis is mild, then observation or patching one eye may be sufficient. Ptosis may be eliminated in some patients by having a crutch attachment placed on a spectacle frame for one or both eyes, although this often causes irritation of the eyes from exposure (Miller, 1985). Ptosis surgery may be performed in some patients, particularly those who are refractory to medical therapy or in whom ptosis is a predominant finding (Miller, 1985). In some patients, prisms can alleviate diplopia, particularly when there is a relatively comitant deviation. For more severe ocular motor weakness, anticholinesterase agents, such as pyridostigmine bromide (Mestinon), are warranted, although these agents often do not succeed in correcting the diplopia. Diplopia is often more refractory to treatment than ptosis. If moderate or large doses of anticholinesterase drugs fail or cannot be tolerated and symptoms are troublesome, then corticosteroids, often at relatively low alternate-day doses, are usually effective in correcting the diplopia (Evoli, 1988; Fischer, 1976; Kupersmith, 1996). Although some authors have suggested the use of azathioprine for patients who are inadequately controlled on low-dose steroids or experiencing steroid side effects (Weinberg, 1994), this agent, cyclophosphamide, cyclosporine, intravenous immunoglobulin, and plasmapheresis are not usually used in patient with purely ocular myasthenia because their benefit-risk ratios have not been adequately studied. The presence of a thymoma in any patient with MG is an absolute indication for thymectomy (Engel, 1994) and so all patients with OM should be evaluated with mediastinal CT or MR imaging. Although thymectomy can be effective in ocular myasthenia gravis without thymoma and may prevent generalization of the disease (Schumm, 1985), most clinicians are reluctant to recommend this procedure for purely ocular symptoms (Lanska, 1990).

About 10 to 20% of patients with OM will undergo spontaneous remission that may be temporary or permanent (Simpson, 1966). Although corticosteroid treatment produces a higher incidence of remission and improvement, there is no evidence that anticholinesterase agents affect the course of the disease (Grob, 1987; Kupersmith, 1996).

Kupersmith et al. reported a retrospective review of 32 patients with OM who were treated with corticosteroids and followed for a minimum of two years (Kupersmith, 1996). Diplopia was initially present in the primary position in 29 patients and in downgaze position in 26. Ptosis was present in 24 patients (unilateral in 13 and bilateral in 11). Tensilon test was positive in 31 patients (one patient did not have a Tensilon test but had marked fatigability of the lids and ocular muscles that recovered with rest), SFEMG or repetitive stimulation studies were abnormal in 6 of 19 patients, and AChR antibodies were elevated in 10 of 28 patients. CT scan of the chest revealed no thymomas in any of the 32 patients. Patients were treated with one or more courses of daily prednisone (the highest initial dose, 40 to 80 mg) gradually withdrawn over 4 to 6 weeks. Subsequently, in six patients, 2.5 to 20 mg of prednisone was given on alternate days for more than six months. No patients had major steroid complications. Two years after diagnosis, diplopia was found in primary position in 11 patients and in downward gaze in 11 patients (9 of whom also had diplopia in primary gaze) and 66% of patients had normal ocular function. Ptosis was found in 7 patients. Generalized MG had developed in 3 patients (9.4%) at two years; elevated AChR antibody levels and abnormal electrophysiologic studies were not predictive of worsening. Of the 16 patients who had follow-up for 3 years and the 13 for 4 or more years, ocular motility was normal in 56% at 3 years and 62% at 4 years, with two additional patients developing generalized MG at 4 years. The authors concluded that moderate dose daily prednisone for 4 to 6 weeks, followed by low-dose alternate-day therapy as needed, can control the diplopia of OM and that the frequency of deterioration to generalized MG at 2 years may be reduced.

Sommer et al retrospectively analyzed 78 patients with OM with a mean disease duration of 8.3 years (Sommer, 1997). In 54 patients (69%) symptoms and signs remained confined to the extraocular muscles during the observation period while the remaining 24 patients (31%) developed symptoms of generalized myasthenia (50% of them within two years and 75% within four years after onset). A somewhat reduced risk of generalization was found in those with mild symptoms, normal repetitive stimulation studies, and low or absent AChR antibodies at the time of diagnosis. Patients receiving immunosuppressive treatment (corticosteroids and/or azathioprine) rarely developed generalized myasthenia (6 of 50 or 12%). Those without such treatment, usually due to uncertain diagnosis and late referral, converted into generalized myasthenia significantly more often (18 of 28 or 64%). The authors concluded that short-term corticosteroids and long-term azathioprine seemed adequate for achieving remission in most patients. The proportion of patients developing generalized myasthenia gravis was smaller in this population compared to previously published groups and early immunosuppressive treatment was thought to be at least partially responsible for this finding. Thymectomy (performed in 12 patients with an abnormal chest CT) also correlated with a good outcome, but had no apparent advantage over medical treatment alone (Sommer, 1997).

Until a prospective clinical trial of corticosteroids or other immunosuppressive is performed in patients with OM, the value of these agents in the prevention of the development of generalized MG remains undefined.

References

Acers TE. (1979). Ocular myasthenia mimicking pseudointernuclear ophthalmoplegia and variable esotropia. *Am J Ophthalmol 88:*319–321.

Averbuch-Heller L, Poonyathalang A, von Maydell RD, Remler BF. (1995). Hering's law for eyelids: Still valid. *Neurology 45:*1781–1783.

Bartoccioni E, Scuderi F, Evoli A, et al. (1986). Ocular myasthenia gravis: Two different diseases. *Lancet 1:*1038–1039.

Berrih-Aknin S, Morel E, Raimond F, et al. (1987). The role of the thymus in myasthenia gravis: Immunohistological and immunological studies in 115 cases. *Ann NY Acad Sci 505:*50.

Bever CT Jr, Aquino AV, Penn AS, et al. (1983). Prognosis of ocular myasthenia gravis. *Ann Neurol 14:*516–519.

Binder S, Graf M, Mamoli B, Drobec P. (1983). The value of edrophonium tonography in the diagnosis of myasthenia gravis. *Graefe's Arch Klin Exp Ophthalmol 221:*78–80.

Brust J, List T, Catalano L, Lovelace R. (1974). Ocular myasthenia gravis mimicking progressive external ophthalmoplegia. *Neurology 24:*755–760.

Campbell JJ, Simpson E, Cronbie AL, Walton JN. (1970). Ocular myasthenia: Evaluation of Tensilon tomography and electronystagmography as diagnostic tests. *J Neurol Neurosurg Psych 33:*639–646.

Castleman B. (1966). The pathology of the thymus gland. *Ann NY Acad Sci 135:*496–505.

Cleary PE. (1973). Ocular manifestations of myasthenia gravis. *Br Orthopt J 30:*38–51.

Cogan D. (1965). Myasthenia gravis—a review of the disease and a description of lid twitch as a characteristic sign. *Arch Ophthalmol 74:*217–221.

Coll GE, Demer JL. (1992). The Edrophonium-Hess screen test in the diagnosis of ocular myasthenia gravis. *Am J Ophthalmol 114:*489–493.

Compston DA, Vincent A, Newsom-Davis J, Batchelor JR. (1980). Clinical, pathological, HLA antigen, and immunological evidence for disease heterogeneity in myasthenia gravis. *Brain 103:*579–601.

Daroff R. (1986). The office Tensilon test for ocular myasthenia. *Arch Neurol 43:*843–844.

Davis T, Lavin P. (1989). Pseudo one-and-a-half syndrome with ocular myasthenia. *Neurology 39:*1553.

Dehaene I, van Zandijcke M. (1995). Isolated paralysis of the superior division of the ocular motor nerve mimicked by myasthenia gravis. *Neuro-ophthalmology 15:*257–258.

Dirr LY, Donofrio PD, Patton JF, Troost TB. (1989). A false-positive edrophonium test in patient with a brainstem glioma. *Neurology 39:*865–867.

Drachman D, De Silva S, Ramsay D, Pestronk A. (1987). Humoral pathogenesis of myasthenia gravis. *Ann NY Acad Sci 505:*90–104.

Emeryk B, Rowinska-Marcinska K, Nowak-Michalska T. (1990). Pseudoselectivity of the neuromuscular block in ocular myasthenia: A SFEMG study. *Electromyograph Clin Neurophysiol 30:*53–59.

Engel AG. (1994). Disturbances of neuromuscular transmission. Acquired autoimmune myasthenia gravis. In Engel AG and Franzini-Armstrong C (eds). *Myology. Basic and clinical.* 2nd edition. New York, McGraw-Hill, pp.1769–1797.

Evoli A, Tonali P, Bartoccioni AP, Lo Monaco M. (1988). Ocular myasthenia: Diagnostic and therapeutic problems. *Acta Neurol Scand 77:*31–35.

Ferguson FR, Hutchinson EC, Liversedge LA. (1955). Myasthenia gravis: Results of medical management. *Lancet 2*:636–639.

Fischer KC, Schwartzman RJ. (1976). Oral corticosteroids in the treatment of ocular myasthenia gravis. *Ann NY Acad Sci 274*:652–658.

Garland H, Clark ANG. (1956). Myasthenia gravis: A personal study of 60 cases. *Br Med J 2*:1259–1262.

George J, Spokes EG. (1984). Myasthenic pseudo-internuclear ophthalmoplegia due to penicillamine. *J Neurol Neurosurg Psych 47*:1044.

Glaser JS. (1966). Myasthenic pseudo-internuclear ophthalmoplegia. *Arch Ophthalmol 75*:363–366.

Glaser JS. (1978). *Neuro-ophthalmology*. New York, Harper and Row, p. 270.

Gorelick PB, Rosenberg M, Pagano RJ. (1981). Enhance ptosis in myasthenia gravis. *Arch Neurol 38*:531.

Grob D, Arsura E, Brunner N, Namba T. (1987). The course of myasthenia and therapies affecting outcome. *Ann NY Acad Sci 505*:472–499.

Grob D. (1953). Course and management of myasthenia gravis. *JAMA 153*:529–532.

Hermann RC Jr. (1996). Repetitive stimulation studies. In Daube JR (ed): *Clinical Neurophysiology*. Philadelphia, FA Davis, pp. 237–247.

Hodes R. (1948). Electromyographic study of defects of neuromuscular transmission in human poliomyelitis. *Arch Neurol Psych 60*:457–473.

Howard FM, Lennon VA, Finley J, et al. (1987). Clinical correlations of antibodies that bind, block, or modulate human acetylcholine receptors in myasthenia gravis. *Ann NY Acad Sci 505*:526–538.

Jay W, Nazarian S, Underwood D. (1987). Pseudo-internuclear ophthalmoplegia with downshoot in myasthenia gravis. *J Clin Neuro-ophthalmol 7*:74–76.

Kelly JJ Jr, Daube JR, Lennon VA, et al. (1982). The laboratory diagnosis of mild myasthenia gravis. *Ann Neurol 12*:238–242.

Komiyama A, Hirayama K. (1988). Paradoxical response of ptosis in myasthenia gravis by edrophonium administration. *J Neurol Neurosurg Psych 51*:315.

Kupersmith MJ, Moster M, Bhuiyan S, et al. (1996). Beneficial effects of corticosteroids on ocular myasthenia gravis. *Arch Neurol 53*:802–804.

Lanska DJ. (1990). Indications for thymectomy in myasthenia gravis. *Neurology 40*:1828–1829.

Lewis JE, Wick MRS, Schweithauer BW, et al. (1987). Thymoma: A clinicopathologic review. *Cancer 60*:2727–2743.

Limburg PC, The TH, Hummel-Tappel E, Oosterhuis HJGH. (1983). Anti-acetylcholine receptor antibodies in myasthenia gravis. I. Relation to clinical parameters in 250 patients. *J Neurol Sci 58*:357–370.

Litchy WJ. (1996). Quantitative electromyography and single-fiber electromyography. In Daube JR (ed). *Clinical Neurophysiology*. Philadelphia, FA Davis, pp. 282–300.

McCrary JA III. (1970). Tensilon and the pseudo-double elevator palsy. In Smith JL (ed). *Neuro-ophthalmology Symposium of the University of Miami and the Bascom Palmer Eye Institute*. Huffman Publishing Co, Hallandale, FL, Vol. 5, pp. 119–122.

Mastaglia FI, Black JI, Collins DWK, et al. (1977). Saccadic velocities in the diagnosis of myasthenia gravis. *Lancet 2*:83.

Mattis RD. (1941). Ocular manifestations of myasthenia gravis. *Arch Ophthalmol 26*:969–982.

Miller N. (1979). Myasthenia gravis: Systemic and ocular considerations. *Ophthalmology 86*:2165–2174.

Miller NR. (1985). *Walsh and Hoyt's Clinical Neuro-ophthalmology*. 4th edition. Baltimore, Williams & Wilkins, pp. 841–891.

Mindel JS, Charney JZ. (1989). Bilateral intracavernous carotid aneurysms presenting as pseudo-ocular myasthenia gravis. *Trans Am Ophthalmol Soc 87*:445–457.

Moorthy G, Behrens MM, Drachman DB, et al. (1989). Ocular pseudomyasthenia or ocular myasthenia 'plus': A warning to clinicians. *Neurology 39*:1150–1154.

Morel E, Vernet-der-Garabedian B, Eymard B, et al. (1988). Binding and blocking antibodies to the human acetylcholine receptor: Are they selected in various myasthenia gravis forms? *Immunol Res 7*:212–217.

Mulder DG, Hermann C, Keesey J, Edwards H. (1983). Thymectomy for myasthenia gravis. *Am J Surg 146*:61–66.

Mulder DW, Lambert EH, Eaton LM. (1959). Myasthenic syndrome in patients with amyotrophic lateral sclerosis. *Neurology 9*:627–631.

Newsom-Davis J, Willcox N, Scadding G, et al. (1987). Immunological heterogeneity and cellular mechanisms in myasthenia gravis. *Ann NY Acad Sci 505*:12–26.

Odel J, Winterkorn J, Behrens M. (1991). The sleep test for myasthenia gravis—a safe alternative to Tensilon. *J Clin Neuro-ophthalmol 11*:288–292.

Odel J. (1992). Ocular myasthenia. North American Neuro-Ophthalmology Society Meeting, Rancho Bernardo, CA, February.

Oger JJF. (1993). Thymus histology and acetylcholine receptor antibodies in generalized myasthenia gravis. *Ann NY Acad Sci 681*:110–112.

Oh SJ, Kim DE, Kuruoglu A, et al. (1992). Diagnostic sensitivity of the laboratory tests in myasthenia gravis. *Muscle Nerve 15*:720–724.

Oosterhuis HJGH. (1982). The ocular signs and symptoms of myasthenia gravis. *Doc Ophthalmol 52*:363–378.

Oosterhuis HJGH. (1988). Long-term effects of treatment in 374 patients with myasthenia gravis. *Monogr Allergy 25*:75–85.

Oosterhuis HJGH. (1989). The natural course of myasthenia gravis: A long-term follow up study. *J Neurol Neurosurg Psych 52*:1121–1127.

Osher RH, Griggs RC. (1979). Orbicularis fatigue: The "peak" sign in myasthenia gravis. *Arch Ophthalmol 97:*677–679.
Osher RH. (1979). Myasthenic "oculomotor" palsy. *Ann Ophthalmol 11:*31–34.
Osserman KE. (1967). Ocular myasthenia gravis. *Invest Ophthalmol 6:*277–287.
Papetestas AE, Genkins G, Horowitz SH, Kornfield P. (1971). Studies in myasthenia gravis: Effects of thymectomy. Results in 1985 patients with nonthymomatous and thymomatous myasthenia gravis, 1941–1969. *Am J Med 50:*465–476.
Perlo VP, Arnason B, Castleman B. (1975). The thymus gland in elderly patients with myasthenia gravis. *Neurology 25:*294–295.
Perlo VP, Poskanzer DC, Schwab RS, et al. (1966). Myasthenia gravis: Evaluation of treatment in 1,335 patients. *Neurology 16:*431–439.
Phillips PH, Newman NJ. (1997). Here today . . . Gone tomorrow. *Survey Ophthalmol 41:*354–356.
Ragge NK, Hoyt WF. (1992). Midbrain myasthenia: Fatiguable ptosis, 'lid twitch' sign, and ophthalmoparesis from a dorsal midbrain glioma. *Neurology 42:*917–919.
Retzlaff JA, Kearns TP, Howard FM Jr, Cronin ML. (1969). Lancaster red-green test in evaluation of edrophonium chloride (Tensilon) tonography in the diagnosis of myasthenia gravis. *Am J Ophthalmol 67:*13–21.
Romano PE, Stark WJ. (1973). Pseudomyopia as a presenting sign in ocular myasthenia gravis. *Am J Ophthalmol 75:*872–875.
Rowland LP. (1955). Prostigmine-responsiveness and diagnosis of myasthenia gravis. *Neurology 5:*612–624.
Rowland LP. (1980). Controversies about the treatment of myasthenia gravis. *J Neurol Neurosurg Psych 43:*644–659.
Rush JA, Shafrin F. (1982). Ocular myasthenia presenting as superior oblique weakness. *J Clin Neuro-ophthalmol 2:*125–127.
Sanders DB, Howard JF. (1986). Single fiber EMG in myasthenia gravis. *Muscle Nerve 9:*809–819.
Sanders DB, Howard JF, Johns TR. (1979). Single-fiber electromyography in myasthenia gravis. *Neurology 29:*68–76.
Schlezinger NS, Fairfax WA. (1959). Evaluation of ocular signs and symptoms in myasthenia gravis. *Arch Ophthalmol 62:*985–990.
Schmidt D, Dell'Osso LF, Abel LA, Daroff RB. (1980a). Myasthenia gravis: Saccadic eye movement waveforms. *Exp Neurol 68:*346–364.
Schmidt D, Dell'Osso LF, Abel LA, Daroff RB. (1980b). Myasthenia gravis: Dynamic changes in saccadic waveforms. *Exp Neurol 68:*365–377.
Schmidt D. (1977). Saccadic eye movements in myasthenic ocular muscle paresis. In Glaser JS (ed). *Neuro-ophthalmology*. St. Louis, CV Mosby, Vol. 9, pp. 177–189.
Schumm F, Wiethölter H, Fateh-Moghadam A, et al. (1985). Thymectomy in myasthenia with pure ocular symptoms. *J Neurol Neurosurg Psych 48:*332–337.
Schwab RS, Perlo VP. (1966). Syndromes simulating myasthenia gravis. *Ann NY Acad Sci 135:*350–366.
Sethi KD, Rivner MH, Thomas TR. (1987). Ice pack test for myasthenia gravis. *Neurology 37:*1383–1385.
Seybold ME, Langstrom JM. (1981). Myasthenia gravis in infancy. *Neurology 31:*476.
Seybold ME. (1983). Myasthenia gravis: A clinical and basic science review. *JAMA 250:*2516–2521.
Seybold ME. (1986). The office Tensilon test for ocular myasthenia gravis. *Arch Neurol 43:*842–843.
Simpson JA, Westerberg MR, Magee KR. (1966). Myasthenia gravis: An analysis of 295 cases. *Acta Neurol Scand 42:*1–27.
Simpson JA. (1981). Myasthenia gravis and myasthenic syndromes. In Walton J (ed). *Disorders of Voluntary muscle*. Edinburgh, Churchill Livingstone, pp. 585–624.
Soliven BC, Lange DJ, Penn AS, et al. (1988). Seronegative myasthenia gravis. *Neurology 38:*514–517.
Sommer N, Sigg B, Melms A, et al. (1997). Ocular myasthenia gravis: response to long term immunosuppressive treatment. *J Neurol Neurosurg Psych 62:*156–162.
Spector RH, Daroff RB. (1976). Edrophonium infrared optokinetic nystagmography in the diagnosis of myasthenia gravis. *Ann NY Acad Sci 274:*642–651.
Spooner JW, Baloh RW. (1979). Eye movement fatigue in myasthenia gravis. *Neurology 29:*29–33.
Spoor TC, Shippman S. (1979). Myasthenia gravis presenting as an isolated inferior rectus paresis. *Trans Acad Ophthalmol Otolaryngol 86:*2158–2160.
Stalberg E. (1980). Clinical electrophysiology in myasthenia gravis. *J Neurol Neurosurg Psych 43:*622–633.
Straube A, Witt T. (1990). Oculo-bulbar myasthenic symptoms as the sole sign of tumour involving or compressing the brainstem. *J Neurol 237:*369–371.
Suzuki T, et al. (1989). Three cases of ocular myopathy with enhanced ptosis phenomenon. *Shinkeiganka 6:*434–436.
Tindall RSA. (1981). Humoral immunity in myasthenia gravis: Biochemical characterization of acquired antireceptor antibodies and clinical correlation. *Ann Neurol 10:*437–447.
Tsujihata M, Yoshimura T, Satoh A, et al. (1989). Diagnostic significance of IgG, C3, and C9 at the limb muscle motor end-plate in minimal myasthenia gravis. *Neurology 39:*1359–1363.
Van Delan JTW, Van Mourek-Noordenbos AM. (1984). Isolated inferior rectus paresis: A report of six cases. *Neuro-ophthalmology 4:*89–94.
Vincent A, Newsom-Davis J. (1985). Acetylcholine receptor antibody as a diagnostic test for myasthenia gravis: Results in 153 validated cases and 2967 diagnostic assays. *J Neurol Neurosurg Psych 48:*1246–1252.

Watt G, Theakston RDG, Hayes CG, et al. (1986). Positive response to edrophonium in patients with neurotoxic envenoming by cobras (Naja philippinensis). *New Eng J Med 315:*1444–1448.

Weinberg DA, Lesser RL, Vollmer TL. (1994). Ocular myasthenia: A protean disorder. *Surv Ophthalmol 39:*169–210.

Wray SH, Pavan-Langston D. (1971). A reevaluation of edrophonium chloride (Tensilon) tonography in the diagnosis of myasthenia gravis. *Neurology 21:*586–593.

◆ 16 ◆

Thyroid Eye Disease: Graves' Ophthalmopathy

What Are the Typical Clinical Features of Graves' Ophthalmopathy?

Graves' ophthalmopathy (GO) is characterized clinically by the signs listed in Table 16–1.

Table 16–1. Typical Features of Graves' Ophthalmopathy

Eyelid signs
Lid retraction (the most common clinical feature of GO) (Bartley, 1994, 1995, 1996)
Stare
Lid lag in downgaze
Exophthalmos
Enlargement of extraocular muscles (Feldon, 1982)
Increased orbital fat volume (Hudson, 1991; Peyster, 1986)
Diplopia/ophthalmoplegia secondary to extraocular muscle inflammation or fibrosis (Feldon, 1982; Huber, 1984; Schultz, 1960)
Visual loss due to a compressive optic neuropathy (CON)
Extraocular muscle involvement in the orbital apex (Barrett, 1988; Day, 1962; Feldon, 1984; Hedges, 1955; Henderson, 1958; Igersheimer, 1955; Kennerdell, 1981; Liu, 1992; Mourits, 1990; Neigel, 1988; Trobe, 1978, 1981)
Stretching of the optic nerve due to proptosis (Anderson, 1989; Feldon, 1985; Liu, 1992)
Severe proptosis and secondary exposure keratopathy
Signs and symptoms of orbital congestion
Due to proptosis with or without venous outflow obstruction
Conjunctival injection and chemosis
Eyelid and periorbital edema
Tearing, photophobia, and orbital discomfort (Bahn, 1990; Bartelena, 1989a; Bleeker, 1987; Dresner, 1985; Nunery, 1991; Riddick, 1981a, 1981b; Sergott, 1981; Van Dyk, 1981)

Patients without the typical features of GO should undergo further evaluation for other etiologies of proptosis (e.g., orbital tumor or pseudotumor), strabismus (e.g., myasthenia gravis), lid retraction (see Chapter 19), and so on.

What Are the Imaging Findings in Graves' Ophthalmopathy?

Orbital imaging, such as computed tomography (CT) and magnetic resonance (MR) scans, often demonstrate extraocular muscle (EOM) enlargement typically sparing the tendons (Enzman, 1979; Hallin, 1988a, 1988b; Hosten, 1989; Just, 1991; Trokel, 1979, 1981), increased orbital fat volume (Chang, 1990; Char, 1991; Forbes, 1986; Peyster, 1986), and sometimes engorgement of the superior ophthalmic vein (Peyster, 1984). Some authors have suggested that MR may be superior to CT in differentiating EOM edema (with elevated T2 relaxation times) from fibrosis (Just, 1991). Ultrasonography of the orbit can also demonstrate EOM enlargement consistent with GO (Skalka, 1980). MR imaging, however, is usually more costly than CT imaging. Apical compression of the optic nerve in compression optic neuropathy (CON) may be seen on CT or MR imaging and we recommend an orbital imaging study in patients with clinical evidence of CON (Kennerdell, 1981).

What Is the Relationship Between Graves' Disease and Systemic Thyroid Status?

Although GO is often associated with systemic hyperthyroidism, GO may occur in patients with primary hypothyroidism, Hashimoto's thyroiditis, and sometimes in euthyroid individuals (Gorman, 1983; Kramar, 1974; Ormston, 1973; Salvi, 1990; Sergott, 1981; Soloman, 1977; Teng, 1977).

What Is the Treatment for Graves' Ophthalmopathy?

Treatment of the underlying systemic thyroid abnormalities is the logical first step in the management of thyroid disease. Although the evidence is controversial regarding the effect of the degree of thyroid abnormality or the speed, type (e.g., medical or surgical), or completeness of systemic therapy (Barbosa 1972; Calissendorff, 1986; Feldon, 1990; Gorman, 1983; Gwinup, 1982; Havard, 1972; Huber, 1984; Marushak, 1984; Sergott, 1981; Sjöberg, 1989; Solem, 1979) on the incidence or severity of GO, systemic thyroid control alone may improve the signs and symptoms of GO (Bahn, 1987; Gorman, 1983; Gott, 1980; Ivy, 1972; Jacobson, 1984; Prummel, 1989b, 1990; Schultz, 1960; Tallstedt, 1992; Wiersinga, 1984). Prummel et al. studied 90 patients with GO and hyperthyroidism in whom the severity of GO and thyroid function were assessed. Patients were assigned to four groups with increasingly severe GO. More dysthyroid patients were in the groups with severe GO than in the other groups (Prummel, 1990). Other uncontrolled studies, however, failed to show regression of GO after careful treatment of hyperthyroidism. In addition, we routinely advise our patients to discontinue smoking, because it has been associated with worsening GO (Balazs, 1990; Bartalena et al., 1989a; Hagg, 1987; Nunery, 1993; Shine, 1990; Prummel, 1993; Tallstedt, 1993; Tellez, 1992).

The natural history of the GO is variable and although most GO appears within a few months of the diagnosis of hyperthyroidism, it may develop many months to years before or after the onset of the systemic diagnosis of thyroid abnormality. Some patients never show clinical or laboratory evidence for systemic thyroid abnormalities (euthyroid GO). In many patients GO is a self-limited disease that may not require any therapy and the disease often stabilizes within 1 to 3 years. Therefore, treatment is usually directed at short-term control of the inflammatory component of the disease (usually within the first 6 to 36 months); acute intervention for vision-threatening proptosis or CON; and long-term reconstructive management of lid retraction, strabismus, and proptosis.

Medical and other conservative therapy should generally precede consideration of surgical intervention. Shorr and Seif described a logical stepwise approach to the surgical rehabilitation of GO (Shorr, 1986). These authors proposed the following four stages for GO:

1. Orbital decompression
2. Strabismus surgery
3. Lid margin repositioning surgery
4. Blepharoplasty.

The rationale for this sequential approach to GO is that orbital decompression often results in worsening, new, or changed extraocular muscle dysfunction as well as changes in lid position. Therefore, orbital decompression should precede strabismus and lid surgery.

Patients with CON should undergo treatment to preserve or improve vision. Trobe summarized the natural course of untreated CON in 3 series of 32 eyes. In this report, 21% of these eyes were left with a visual acuity of 20/100 or less, including a final vision of counting fingers to no light perception in five eyes (Trobe, 1978).

What Therapies Are Suggested for Local Ocular and Orbital Inflammatory Signs?

Patients with lid or ocular irritation, mild inflammation, or exposure keratopathy may benefit from conservative treatments, such as topical artificial tears and/or lubricating ointments, tinted or wrap-around glasses, elevation of the head of the bed, or taping the eyelids shut during sleep (Feldon, 1983; Leone, 1984; Liu, 1992). Although some authors have advocated the use of topical, peribulbar, or retrobulbar steroids (Huber, 1984; Kramar, 1974; Leone, 1984; Marcocci, 1987), we do not usually employ these routes of steroid therapy for periorbital swelling. The evidence to support the use of steroids in this manner is anecdotal at best and these treatments may be associated with complications, such as secondary increased intraocular pressure (Kramar, 1974; Leone, 1984).

Patients may experience worsening of GO after systemic treatment procedures (e.g., thyroid surgery, radioiodine [RAI] treatment, and neck radiotherapy for nonthyroidal neoplasms) that may be associated with leakage of thyroid antigens and subsequently increase circulating thyroid autoantibodies (Barbosa, 1972; Fenzi, 1979; Hamilton, 1967; Jackson, 1979; Jones, 1969; Kriss, 1967; Pequegnat, 1967; Pinchera, 1969, 1982; Wasnich, 1973; Werner, 1967). Bartalena et al. studied 26 patients treated with RAI alone and 26 treated with RAI and systemic prednisone for four months (Bartalena, 1989). The initial dose of prednisone was 0.4 to 0.5 mg/kg of body weight for one month with a gradual taper over 3 months. Before RAI, 15 patients had no evidence for GO and none of these developed GO after RAI. Of the patients treated with RAI alone with initial GO, 56%

worsened and 44% were unchanged in soft tissue abnormalities and EOM function. Conversely, there was an improvement in GO in 52% and no change in 48% of RAI patients treated with steroids. These authors and others (Bartalena, 1989) have recommended systemic corticosteroid treatment to prevent exacerbation of GO in patients undergoing RAI who have some degree of ocular involvement before treatment, but there is some disagreement with this recommendation (Beck, 1990).

Should Immunosuppressive Therapy Be Considered in GO?

Although systemic corticosteroids have been employed for GO, there is limited evidence outlining the specific indications for their use or the results of treatment, except in patients with CON (Apers, 1976; Day, 1968; Kramar, 1974; Liu, 1992; Mulherin, 1972; Trobe, 1978; Werner, 1966; Wiersinga, 1988). In addition, although medical therapy usually consists of prednisone, other immunosuppressive agents [e.g., azathioprine (Imuran), cyclophosphamide (Cytoxan) or cyclosporine] have also been recommended, although experience with these agents is limited (Apers, 1976; Bahn, 1987; Bartalena, 1983; Bigos, 1979; Brabant, 1984; Day, 1968; Feldon, 1983; Howlett, 1984; Kahaly, 1986a, 1986b; Prummel, 1989a; Utech, 1987; Weetman, 1983). Perros et al. reported negative results with azathioprine for moderate GO in a matched study of 20 patients (Perros, 1990). Other studies have reported little effect with azathioprine (Burrow, 1970; Wall, 1979) or ciamexone (Kahaly, 1990). Anecdotal success has been reported with plasmapheresis and bromocriptine, but the relative efficacy of these therapies compared with traditional treatment for GO remains to be defined (Dandona, 1979; Glinoer, 1986; Harden, 1967; Kolodziej-Maciejweska, 1985; Lopatynsky, 1989; Sawers, 1981; Utech, 1987).

Prummel et al. reported a single-blind, randomized clinical trial comparing the efficacy of prednisone (60 mg/day with a tapering dose) versus cyclosporine (7.5 mg/kg of body weight/day) (Prummel, 1989a). During the 12-week treatment period, 11 prednisone-treated and 4 cyclosporine-treated patients responded to therapy (61% vs. 22%; $p = 0.018$) as defined by decrease in EOM enlargement and proptosis, improved vision, and subjective eye scores. There were no differences at baseline between the patients who responded later and those who did not, but the prednisone was less well tolerated than the cyclosporine and combination therapy was better tolerated than prednisone alone. These authors concluded that single-drug therapy with prednisone was more effective than cyclosporine in patients with severe GO, but that the combination may be effective in patients who did not respond to either drug alone (Prummel, 1989a).

Corticosteroids have been shown to reduce EOM enlargement in CON (Kennerdell, 1981; Liu, 1992). Many authors recommend relatively high doses of prednisone (1 to 1.5 mg/kg/day) for the treatment of CON (Liu, 1992; Werner, 1966). Kazim et al. reviewed 84 cases of acute GO treated with either high-dose systemic steroids or radiotherapy (RT) and reported that RT (1 of 29 required decompression) was more effective than corticosteroids (6 of 16 patients required decompression) and that RT had fewer complications than steroids (Kazim, 1991). Guy et al. reported the use of high dose pulse intravenous corticosteroids (Guy, 1989). Many authors believe that improvement in CON following prednisone therapy is usually evident within the first few weeks of treatment and that there is no justification for maintaining patients with CON on prolonged corticosteroid regimens (Apers, 1976; Trobe, 1981; Trokel, 1993).

Table 16–2. Treatment of GO with Orbital RT: Summary of Selected Studies

Author	Patient number	Response rate (%)	Comment
Donaldson, 1973	80	67%	> 1 year follow-up
Ravin, 1975	9 patients with optic neuropathy	All 9 improved vision	Little effect on soft tissue abnormalities
Brennan, 1983	14 patients	13/14 (93%) reduced soft tissue inflammation	Myopathy showed the least improvement
Hurbli, 1985	62 patients	34/46 (74%) improved motility and 10/14 (71%) CON improved	Patients with duration < 6 months responded better
Wiersinga, 1988	39 patients (34/39 treated previously with steroids)	25 (64%) improved	Improvement based on NOSPECS system
Sandler, 1989	35	71% improved	
Lloyd, 1992	36	33/36 (92%) improved	
Kazim, 1991	29	28/29 (97%)	1 required decompression

What Is the Role of Radiotherapy in GO?

Low dose radiotherapy (RT) has been reported with good results for the treatment of acute inflammation (soft tissue signs) and/or CON due to GO. The typical cumulative RT dose is 2000 centiGray (cGy), which is well tolerated and generally safe. RT may also be useful in reducing the dosage or eliminating the need for corticosteroid or other immunosuppressive treatments (Bartalena, 1983; Brennan, 1983; Covington, 1977; Donaldson, 1973, 1982; Glaser, 1984; Harnett, 1988; Hermann, 1972; Hurbli, 1985; Kazim, 1991; Marcocci, 1987; Olivotto, 1985; Palmer, 1987; Petersen, 1990; Pigeon, 1987; Ravin, 1975; Sandler, 1989; Teng, 1980; Van Ouwerkerk, 1985; Wiersinga, 1988). Table 16–2 summarizes the reported cases of orbital RT in the treatment of GO.

Most authors do not believe that RT is indicated for patients with mild or long-standing noninflammatory GO (Hurbli, 1985; Teng, 1980). Previous head or orbit RT is probably a contraindication to further RT for GO. No significant morbidity has been reported in patients with appropriate RT dosing for GO, although there is a theoretical risk of RT-induced cataracts or neoplasms, radiation optic neuropathy, or radiation retinopathy (Rubenzik, 1975). Several cases of radiation retinopathy have been described in patients with inappropriate RT dosing (Kinyoun, 1984). We recommend that only centers with considerable experience with RT perform this treatment for GO (Char, 1991).

What Is the Treatment for Lid Retraction in GO?

Lid retraction may be due to Müller's muscle (sympathetic) or levator overaction, levator contraction (degeneration of the muscle or aponeurosis), levator adhesions, or pseudoretraction (Frueh, 1986; Gonnering, 1988; Lemke, 1991). Upper eyelid retraction may be treated surgically by a number of approaches (Harvey, 1981), including levator marginal myotomies (Grove, 1980a, 1980b, 1981), Müller's muscle excision (Chalfin, 1979;

Putterman, 1981), levator stripping (Putterman, 1972, 1980; Stephenson, 1985), and levator spacers placed into the upper eyelid to create length (Dryden, 1977; Flanagan, 1974). Detailed descriptions of these procedures are beyond the scope of this text. Patients with lesser degrees of proptosis may benefit from eyelid procedures more than orbital procedures. Char recommended that patients with exophthalmometry readings of under 23 or 24 with good motility are probably better treated with eyelid procedures (Char, 1989). The use of topical alpha-adrenergic agents, such as guanethidine, have been advocated by some authors (Bouzas, 1980; Cant, 1969), but significant corneal toxicity usually limits the use of these agents. Botulinum toxin injections into the lids may also transiently relieve lid retraction (Biglan, 1989; Ceisler, 1995).

What Treatments Should Be Considered for Strabismus due to GO?

Strabismus in GO may be treated with patching, prism therapy, or strabismus surgery. Patients with difficulty in downgaze and the reading position may benefit from simply occluding the lower segment of their bifocal, raising the bifocal height, or using two pairs of spectacles (one pair of single vision glasses for reading and one pair for distance). The surgical technique to correct strabismus will vary depending on the severity and distribution of extraocular involvement. A detailed description of these procedures is beyond the scope of this text (Day, 1979; Ellis, 1979; Kulla, 1979; Mourits, 1990; Scott, 1981). Limited anecdotal success has been reported with botulinum toxin injections into EOMs (Biglan, 1989; Dunn, 1986). Surgical treatment for strabismus should be deferred until after the acute inflammatory phase of GO has been treated adequately (Dunn, 1986; Kramer, 1974; Schimek, 1972).

What Treatments Are Suggested for Proptosis and/or Compressive Optic Neuropathy due to GO?

The natural history of compressive optic neuropathy (CON) is poorly documented. Carter et al. reviewed the combined reports of 16 untreated patients (26 eyes). There was spontaneous visual improvement to 20/50 acuity or better in 19 eyes (72%), but 6 eyes (22%) did not improve (range, counting fingers to no light perception) (Carter, 1991; Day, 1962; Hedges, 1955; Henderson, 1958; Igerscheimer, 1955). CON may be treated with systemic corticosteroids, orbital radiotherapy, or orbital surgical decompression (Day, 1968; Gorman, 1974; Guy, 1989; Harting, 1986; Kazim, 1991; Linberg, 1981; Panzo, 1983; Ravin, 1975; Riley, 1972; Trobe, 1978). Kazim et al. retrospectively reviewed 84 cases of acute GO and reported that only 1 of 29 patients with CON treated with RT required surgical decompression versus 6 of 16 treated with corticosteroids (Kazim, 1991). Nevertheless, oral or intravenous corticosteroids may be the first line treatment for CON (Guy, 1989). Guy et al. reported the use of pulse intravenous methylprednisolone (1 gram daily for 3 days) in five patients with CON. Oral corticosteroids and orbital RT allowed the treatment response to be maintained in all 5 patients for several months (Guy, 1989). Patients with CON who fail or cannot tolerate steroid treatment and/or RT should be considered for orbital decompression.

A wide variety of surgical approaches for orbital decompression have been advocated, including one, two, three, and even four wall decompressions (Algvere, 1973a, 1973b; Anderson, 1981; Antozyck, 1992; Apers, 1977; Bartalena, 1989; Bayliss, 1980; Buschmann, 1989; Carter, 1991; DeSanto, 1972, 1973; Fatourechi, 1993; Fells, 1987; Garrity, 1989, 1993; Grahne, 1985; Härting, 1986, 1989; Hallin, 1988c; Hamby, 1969; Hecht, 1984; Hurwitz, 1985, 1992; Kennedy, 1990; Kennerdell, 1982; Kulwin, 1990; Lamberg, 1985; Leatherbarrow, 1991; Leone, 1980, 1989; Linberg, 1981; Long, 1966; MacCarty, 1970; Maroon, 1982; McCord, 1981, 1985; Mourits, 1990; Olivari, 1991; Roncevic, 1989; Schimek, 1972; Sessions, 1972; Shorr, 1982, 1986; Small, 1981; Streeten, 1987; Thaller, 1990; Trokel, 1979a; Warren, 1989; Wilson, 1991; Wolfe, 1979). Wulc et al. also advocated lateral wall advancement as an adjunct to orbital decompression to enhance the decompressive effect and provide a potential space for lateral expansion (Wulc, 1990). Table 16–3 summarizes several studies concerning surgical orbital decompression in the treatment of proptosis and/or CON in GO.

Table 16–3. Orbital Decompression (Results in Selected Series)

Author/Year	Number of Eyes/Patients	Surgical Approach	Results
Algevere, 1973	22 eyes	Pteryional decompression	20/22 improved visual acuity
Trobe, 1978	9 eyes (6 patients)	4 temporal decompression 3 temporal and orbital floor 2 transfrontal	66% improved 3/4 steroid failures 3/5 primary surgery
Linberg, 1981	11 eyes	Transorbital	82% improved
Leone, 1981	14 eyes (CON)	Inferior orbital	100% improved
McCord, 1981	11 patients (CON)	Antral ethmoidal	6/11 (55%) improved with surgery alone, 5/11 (45%) improved after RT
Hurwitz, 1985	27 eyes (CON)	Inferomedial approach	22/27 (81%) improved
Lamberg, 1985	27 bilateral and 3 unilateral	Transantral approach	28/30 (93%) improved proptosis
Shorr, 1986	28 patients (CON)	Transantral approach	100% improved
Hallin, 1988	25 patients (48 eyes) (CON)	Transantral approach	77% improved visual acuity
Härting, 1989	28 patients (CON)	Variable techniques over a 14 year period	14/28 (50%) improved
Leone, 1989	2 patients	Medial and lateral wall	2/2 (100%) improved
Warren, 1989	305 patients	Transantral	95% improved or maintained preoperative visual acuity
Kennedy, 1990	4 patients with CON	Endoscopic transnasal	3/4 (75%) improved

(continued)

Table 16–3. *(continued)*

Author/Year	Number of Eyes/Patients	Surgical Approach	Results
Mourits, 1990	25 patients	13 inferomedial 5 inferomedial + lateral 7 coronal	76% improved
Carter, 1991	30 (52 orbits)	Transantral-ethmoidal	92% improved acuity or visual field defects
Leatherbarrow, 1991	4 patients	3 wall coronal	2/4 (50%) improved acuity
Olivari, 1991	10 patients	Intraorbital fat removal	6/10 (60%) improved
Hurwitz, 1992	25 patients (46 orbits) with CON	Ethmoidectomy (medial wall)	19/22 (86%) color vision improved
Antozyck, 1992	5 orbits	Transorbital 3 wall (modified blepharoplasty incision)	4/5 (80%) improved acuity to 20/40 or better
Garrity, 1993	217 patients with CON	Transantral	89% improved visual acuity; 91% improved visual field
Neugenbauer, 1996	21	Endoscopic-endonasal	95% improved vision

What Is the Treatment for Proptosis in GO?

McCord in 1985 reported that more than 60% of orbital decompressions were performed for mild to severe exophthalmos to correct corneal exposure or disfigurement based on a survey of members of the American Society of Ophthalmic Plastic and Reconstructive Surgeons and the Orbital Society. The majority of decompressions were via an antral-ethmoidal decompression and translid or fornix approach (McCord, 1985). Kennerdell et al. suggested that patients with proptosis less than 25 to 26 mm, especially if accompanied by lid retraction but without CON, could be treated with lid lengthening procedures alone to disguise the proptosis (Kennerdell, 1987). Lyons and Rootman reported orbital decompression on 65 orbits (34 patients) for disfiguring exophthalmos and achieved a mean retroplacement of 4 mm (range −1.0 to 10 mm). Diplopia, however, arose de novo in five (18%) previously asymptomatic patients in this series (Lyons, 1994). Fatourechi et al. described 34 patients with GO who underwent transantral orbital decompression primarily for cosmetic reasons (Fatourechi, 1994). There was a mean reduction in proptosis of 5.2 mm. Continuous diplopia developed in 73% of 15 patients who were asymptomatic preoperatively. Other reports have confirmed that although orbital decompression for primarily cosmetic reasons is successful, ocular motility deficits and diplopia may occur post-decompression in a significant number of patients (Bayliss, 1980; Carter, 1991; Fatourechi, 1994; Shorr, 1982; Trokel, 1979). In addition to diplopia, orbital decompression may result in loss of vision, globe or eyelid damage, worsening lid retraction, cerebrospinal fluid leakage, infraorbital anesthesia, or sinus complications. Therefore, patients should be counseled appropriately preoperatively regarding these possible complications.

Trokel et al. performed orbital fat removal on 81 patients (158 decompressions) (Trokel, 1993). These authors reported an average reduction of proptosis of 1.8 mm (range 0 to 6.0 mm). The greatest reduction in proptosis (3.3 mm) was produced in patients with greater than 25 mm of proptosis (Hertel measurements). Trokel et al. reserve decompression with bone removal for patients with CON who are unresponsive to medical therapy or patients with persistent deforming exophthalmos following primary orbital fat removal.

An approach to the patient with thyroid eye disease is outlined in Figure 16–1.

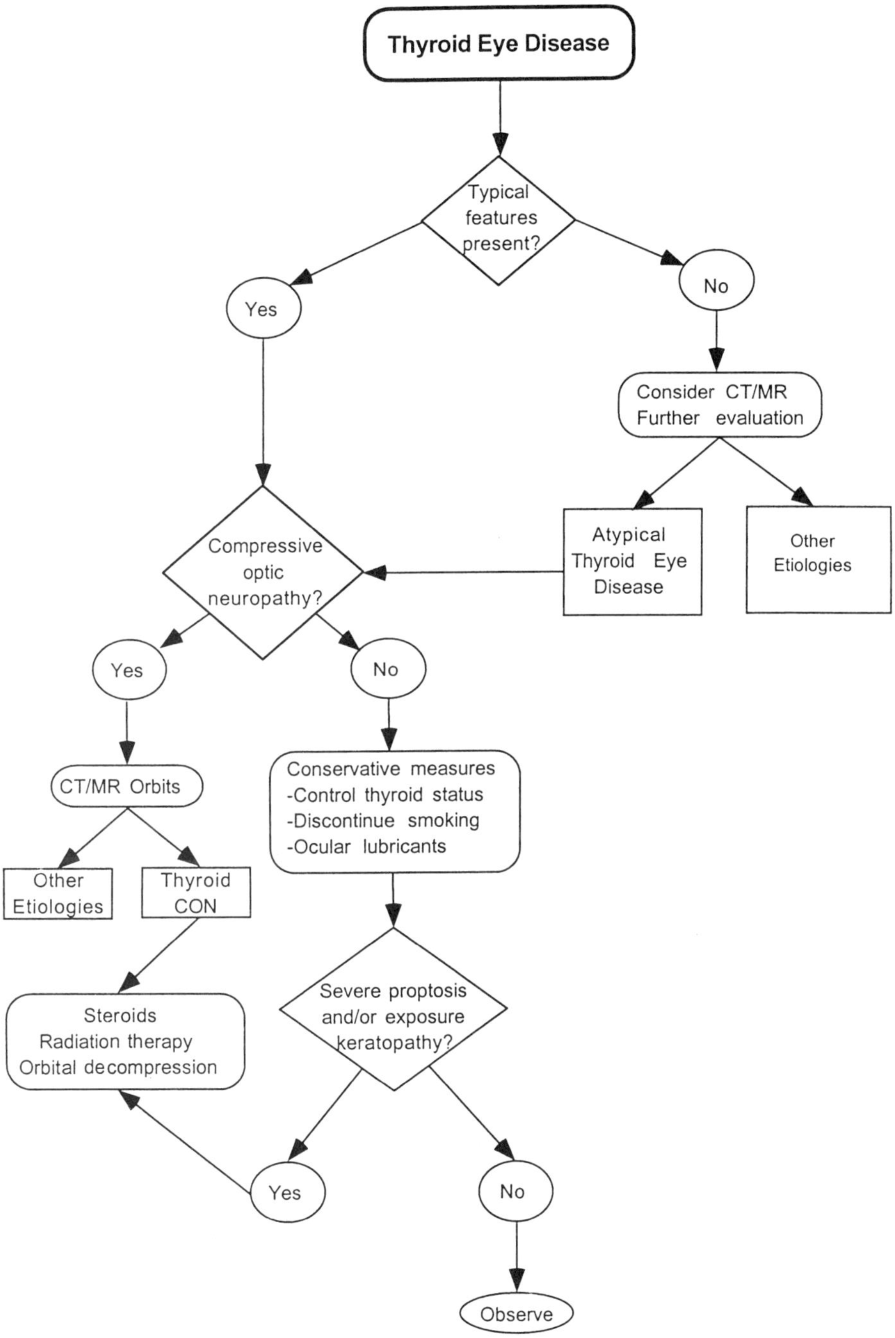

Figure 16–1. Thyroid eye disease.

References

Algvere P, Almquist S, Backlund EO. (1973a). Pterional orbital decompression in progressive ophthalmopathy of Graves' disease: I. Short term effects. *Acta Ophthalmol 51:*461–474.

Algvere P, Almquist S, Backlund EO. (1973b). Pterional orbital decompression in progressive ophthalmopathy of Graves' disease: II. A follow-up study. *Acta Ophthalmol 51:*475–482.

Anderson RL, Linberg JV. (1981). Transorbital approach to decompression of the orbit. *Arch Ophthalmol 99:*120–124.

Anderson RL, Tweeten JP, Patrinely JR, et al. (1989). Dysthyroid optic neuropathy without extraocular muscle involvement. *Ophthalmic Surg 20:*568–574.

Antozyck JH, Tucker N, Codere F. (1992). Orbital decompression for Graves' disease: Exposure through a modified blepharoplasty incision. *Ophthalmic Surg 23:*516–521.

Apers RC, Oosterhuis JA, Bierlaagh JJM. (1976). Indications and results of prednisone treatment in thyroid ophthalmopathy. *Ophthalmologica 173:*163–167.

Apers RC, Ossterhuis JA, Sedee E, Bierlaagh J. (1977). Results of transantral decompression in hyperthyroid exophthalmos. *Doc Ophthalmol 44:*207–214.

Bahn RS, Gorman CA. (1987). Choice of therapy and criteria for assessing treatment outcome in thyroid-associated ophthalmopathy. *Endocrinol Metab Clin North Am 16:*391–407.

Bahn RS, Garrity JA, Gorman CA. (1990). Diagnosis and management of Graves' ophthalmopathy. *J Clin Endocrinol Metab 71:*559–563.

Bahn RS, Heufelder AE. (1993). Pathogenesis of Graves' ophthalmopathy. *N Engl J Med 329:*1468–1475.

Balazs C, Stenszky V, Farid NR. (1990). Association between Graves' ophthalmopathy and smoking. *Lancet 336:*754.

Barbosa J, Wong E, Doe RP. (1972). Ophthalmopathy of Graves' disease: Outcome after treatment with radioactive iodine, surgery, or antithyroid drugs. *Arch Intern Med 130:*111–113.

Barrett L, Glatt HJ, Burde RM, et al. (1988). Optic nerve dysfunction in thyroid eye disease. *Radiology 167:*503–507.

Bartalena L, Marcocci C, Bogazzi F, et al. (1989a). A new ophthalmopathy index for quantitation of eye changes of Graves' disease. *Acta Endocrinol 121(supp2):*190–192.

Bartalena L, Marcocci C, Bogazzi F, et al. (1989b). Orbital decompression for severe Graves' ophthalmopathy. Results of a three-wall operative technique. *J Neurosurg Sci 33:*323.

Bartalena L, Marcocci C, Bogazzi F, Panicucci M, Lepri A, Pinchera A. (1990). Use of corticosteroids to prevent progression of Graves' ophthalmopathy. *Arch Int Med 150:*1098–1101.

Bartalena L, Marcocci C, Bogazzi F, et al. (1989c). Use of corticosteroids to prevent progression of Graves' ophthalmopathy after radioiodine therapy for hyperthyroidism. *N Engl J Med 321:*1349–1352.

Bartalena L, Marcocci C, Chiovato L, et al. (1983). Orbital cobalt irradiation combined with systemic corticosteroids for Graves' ophthalmopathy: Comparison with systemic corticosteroids alone. *J Clin Endocrinol Metab 56:*1139–1144.

Bartalena L, Martino E, Marcocci C, et al. (1989d). More on smoking habits and Graves' ophthalmopathy. *J Endocrinol Invest 12:*733–737.

Bartley GB. (1995). Evolution and classification systems for Graves' ophthalmopathy. *Ophthalm Plast Reconstr Surg 11:*229–237.

Bartley GB. (1994). The epidemiologic characteristics and clinical course of ophthalmopathy associated with autoimmune thyroid disease in Olmstead County, Minnesota. *Trans Am Ophthalmol Soc 92:*477–588.

Bartley GB. (1996). The differential diagnosis and classification of eyelid retraction. *Ophthalmology 103:*168–176.

Bartley GB, Fatourechi V, Kadrmas EF, et al. (1995). The incidence of Graves' ophthalmopathy in Olmsted County, Minnesota. *Am J Ophthalmol 120:*511–517.

Bayliss HS, Call BN, Shibata CS. (1980). The transantral orbital decompression (Ogura technique) as performed by the ophthalmologist. *Ophthalmology 87:*1005–1012.

Beck RW, DiLoreto DA. (1990). Treatment of Graves' ophthalmopathy. *N Engl J Med 322:*1088–1089.

Biglan AW, Bornstine RA, Rogers GC, et al. (1989). Management of strabismus with botulinum A toxin. *Ophthalmology 96:*935.

Bigos ST, Nisula BC, Daniels GH, et al. (1979). Cyclophosphamide in the management of advanced Graves' ophthalmopathy: A preliminary report. *Ann Intern Med 90:*921–923.

Bleeker GM. (1987). Graves' disease. (Editorial). *Orbit 6:*151–152.

Bouzas AG. (1980). Endocrine ophthalmopathy. *Trans Ophthalmol Soc UK 100:*511–526.

Brabant G, Peter H, Becker H, Schwarzrock R, Wonigeit K, Hesch RD. (1984). Cyclosporine in infiltrative eye disease. *Lancet 1:*515–516.

Brennan MW, Leone CR Jr, Janaki L. (1983). Radiation therapy for Graves' disease. *Am J Ophthalmol 96:*195–199.

Burrow GN, Mitchell MS, Howard RO, et al. (1970). Immunosuppressive therapy for the eye changes of Graves' disease. *J Clin Endocrinol Metab 31:*307–311.

Buschmann W, Richter W, Kley W, Brunner FX, Kruse P. (1989). Indications and results of orbital decompression surgery. *Dev Ophthalmol 20:*173–184.

Buschmann W, Richter W, Kruse P, Neumann O. (1986). Functional results in Graves' disease following ophthalmo-rhinosurgical orbital decompression. *Orbit 5:*117–121.

Calcaterra TC. (1977). Paranasal sinus decompression of the orbit in Graves' disease. *Arch Ophthalmol 87:*655.
Calcaterra TC, Thompson JW. (1980). Antral-ethmoidal decompression of the orbit in Graves' disease: Ten-year experience. *Laryngoscope 90:*1941–1949.
Calissendorf BM, Söderström M, Alveryd A. (1986). Ophthalmopathy and hyperthyroidism: a comparison between patients receiving different antithyroid treatments. *Acta Ophthalmol 64:*698–703.
Cant JS, Lewis DRH, Harrison MT. (1969). *Br J Ophthalmol 53:*233.
Carter KD, Frueh BR, Hessburg TP, Musch DC. (1991). Long-term efficacy of orbital decompression for compressive optic neuropathy of Graves' eye disease. *Ophthalmology 98:*1435–1442.
Ceisler EJ, Bilyk JA, Rubin PA, et al. (1995). Results of Mullerectomy and levator aponeurosis transposition for the correction of upper eyelid retraction in Graves' disease. *Ophthalmology 102:*483–492.
Chalfin J, Putterman AM. (1979). Müller's muscle excision and levator palpebrae recession in the treatment of thyroid upper eyelid retraction. *Arch Ophthalmol 97:*1487–1491.
Chang TC, Huang KM, Chang TJ, Lin SL. (1990). Correlation of orbital computed tomography and antibodies in patients with hyperthyroid Graves' disease. *Clin Endocrinol 32:*551–558.
Char DH. (1989). Advances in the management of thyroid related eye disease. *Int Ophthalmol Clin 29:*226–231.
Char DH. (1991). The ophthalmopathy of Graves' disease. *Med Clin No Amer 75:*97–119.
Char DH. (1992). Advances in thyroid orbitopathy. *Neuro-ophthalmology 12:*25–39.
Covington EE, Lobes L, Sudarsanam A. (1977). Radiation therapy for exophthalmos. *Radiology 122:*797.
Dallow RL, Momose KJ, Weber AL, Wray SH. (1976). Comparison of ultrasonography, computerized tomography (EMI scan), and radiographic techniques in evaluation of exophthalmos. *Trans Am Acad Ophth Otol 81:*305–322.
Dandona P, Marshall NJ, Bidey SP, et al. (1979). Successful treatment of exophthalmos and pretibial myxedema with plasmapheresis. *Br Med J 1:*374.
Day RM, Carrol FD. (1962). Optic nerve involvement associated with thyroid dysfunction. *Arch Ophthalmol 67:*289–297.
Day RM, Carrol FD. (1968). Corticosteroids in the treatment of optic nerve involvement associated with thyroid dysfunction. *Arch Ophthalmol 79:*279–282.
Day RM. (1979). Extraocular muscle problems associated with Graves' disease. *Ophthalmology 86:*2051–2087.
DeSanto LW. (1980). The total rehabilitation of Graves' ophthalmopathy. *Laryngoscope 90:*1652.
DeSanto LW. (1972). Surgical palliation of ophthalmopathy of Graves' disease. *Mayo Clin Proc 47:*989–992.
DeSanto LW, Gorman CA. (1973). Selection of patients and choice of operation for orbital decompression in Graves' ophthalmopathy. *Laryngoscope 83:*945–959.
Donaldson SS, Bagshaw MA, Kriss JP. (1973). Supervoltage orbital radiotherapy for Graves' ophthalmopathy. *J Clin Endocr Metab 37:*276–285.
Donaldson SS, Kriss JP, McDougall IR, Bagshaw MA. (1982). Orbital irradiation in the treatment of Graves' ophthalmopathy—results in 141 consecutive patients. *Int J Radiat Oncol Biol Phys 8:*112–113.
Dresner SC, Kennerdell JS. (1985). Dysthyroid orbitopathy. *Neurology 35:*1628–1734.
Dryden RM, Soll DB. (1977). The use of scleral transplantation in cicatricial entropion and eyelid retraction. *Trans Amer Acad Ophthalmol Otolaryngol 83:*669–678.
Dunn WJ, Arnold AC, O'Connor PS. (1986). Botulinum toxin for the treatment of dysthyroid ocular myopathy. *Ophthalmology 93:*470–475.
Ellis FD. (1979). Strabismus surgery for endocrine ophthalmopathy. *Ophthalmology 86:*2059–2063.
Enzman DR, Donaldson SS, Kriss JP. (1979). Appearance of Graves' disease on orbital computed tomography. *J Comput Assist Tomogr 3:*815–819.
Enzmann D, Marshall WH, Rosenthal AR, Kriss JP. (1976). Computed tomography in Graves' ophthalmopathy. *Radiology 118:*615–620.
Fatourechi V, Garrity JA, Bartley GB, Bergstrahl EJ, DeSanto LW, Gorman CA. (1994). Graves' ophthalmopathy: Results of transantral orbital decompression performed primarily for cosmetic indications. *Ophthalmology 101:*1341–1346.
Fatourechi V, Garrity JA, Bartley GB, Bergstrahl EJ, Gorman CA. (1993). Orbital decompression in Graves' ophthalmopathy associated with pretibial myxedema. *J Endocrinol Invest 16:*433–437.
Feldon SE. (1983). Management of thyroid-eye disease. Focal points: Clinical modules for ophthalmologists. *Member benefit module 2:*1–12.
Feldon SE. (1990). Graves' ophthalmopathy: Is it really thyroid disease? *Arch Int Med 150:*948–950.
Feldon S. (1993). Classification of Graves' ophthalmopathy [letter]. *Thyroid 3:*171.
Feldon SE, Lee CP, Muramatsu SK, Weiner JM. (1985). Quantitative computed tomography of Graves' ophthalmopathy. Extraocular muscle and orbital fat in development of optic neuropathy. *Arch Ophthalmol 103:*213–215.
Feldon SE, Muramatsu S, Weiner JM. (1984). Clinical classification of Graves' ophthalmopathy: Identification of risk factors for optic neuropathy. *Arch Ophthalmol 102:*1469–1472.
Feldon SE, Weiner JM. (1982). Clinical significance of extraocular muscle volumes in Graves' ophthalmopathy. A quantitative computed tomography study. *Arch Ophthalmol 100:*1266–1269.
Fells P. (1987). Orbital decompression for severe dysthyroid eye disease. *Br J Ophthalmol 71:*107–111.
Fenzi G, Hashizume K, Roudebush CP, DeGroot LJ. (1979). Changes in thyroid-stimulating immunoglobulins during antithyroid therapy. *J Clin Endocrinol Metab 48:*572–576.

Flanagan JC. (1974). Eye bank sclera in oculoplastic surgery. *Ophthalmic Surg 5:*45–53.
Forbes G, Gorman CA, Brennan MD, Gerhring DG, Ilstrup DM, Earnest F IV. (1986). Ophthalmopathy of Graves' disease: Computerized volume measurements of the orbital fat and muscle. *Am J Neuroradiol 7:*651–656.
Frueh BR. (1992). Why the NOSPECS classification of Graves' eye disease should be abandoned, with suggestions for the characterization of this disease. *Thyroid 2:*85–88.
Frueh BR, Musch DC, Garber FW. (1986). Lid retraction and levator aponeurosis defects in Graves' eye disease. *Ophthalmic Surg 17:*216–220.
Garrity JA, Fatourechi V, Bergstralh EJ, Bartley GB, Beatty CW, DeSanto LW, et al. (1993). Results of transantral orbital decompression in 428 patients with severe Graves' ophthalmopathy. *Am J Ophthalmol 116:*533–547.
Garrity JA, McCaffrey TV, Gorman CA. (1989). Compression and decompression of orbital contents in Graves' ophthalmopathy. *Acta Endocrinol 121:*160.
Glaser JS. (1984). Graves' ophthalmopathy (editorial). *Arch Ophthalmol 102:*1448–1449.
Glinoer D, Etienne-Decerf J, Schrooyen M, et al. (1986). Beneficial effects of intensive plasma exchange followed by immunosuppressive therapy in severe Graves' ophthalmopathy. *Acta Endocrinol 111:*30–38.
Golding-Wood PH. (1969). Transantral ethmoid decompression in malignant exophthalmos. *J Laryngol Otol 83:*683–694.
Gonnering RS. (1988). Pseudoretraction of the eyelid in thyroid-associated orbitopathy. *Arch Ophthalmol 106:*1078–1080.
Gorman CA. (1983). Temporal relationship between onset of Graves' ophthalmopathy and diagnosis of thyrotoxicosis. *Mayo Clin Proc 58:*515–519.
Gorman CA. (1983). Ophthalmopathy of Graves' disease. [Editorial] *N Engl J Med 308:*453–454.
Gorman CA. (1991). Clever is not enough: NOSPECS is form in search of function. *Thyroid 1:*353–355.
Gorman CA, DeSanto LW, MacCarty CS, Riley FC. (1974). Optic neuropathy of Graves' disease. Treatment by transantral or tranfrontal orbital decompression. *N Engl J Med 290:*70–75.
Gott PH. (1980). Treatment of Graves' disease. *JAMA 244:*1558.
Grahne B, Lamberg B-A, Rinne J, et al. (1985). Transantral orbital decompression in the treatment of Graves' disease. *J Laryngol Otolaryngol 99:*865–870.
Grove AS, Jr. (1980a). Eyelid retraction treated by levator marginal myotomy. *Ophthalmology 87:*1013–1018.
Grove AS, Jr. (1980b). Levator lengthening by marginal myotomy. *Arch Ophthalmol 98:*1433–1438.
Grove AS, Jr. (1981). Upper eyelid retraction and Graves' disease. *Ophthalmology 88:*499–506.
Guy JR, Fagien S, Donovan JP, Rubin ML. (1989). Methylprednisolone pulse therapy in severe dysthyroid optic neuropathy. *Ophthalmology 96:*1048–1053.
Gwinup G, Elias AN, Ascher MS. (1982). Effect on exophthalmos of various methods of treatment of Graves' disease. *JAMA 247:*2135–2138.
Hagg E, Asplund K. (1987). Is endocrine ophthalmopathy related to smoking? *BMJ 295:*634–635.
Hallin ES, Feldon SE. (1988a). I. Simple CT estimates of extraocular muscle volume. *Br J Ophthalmol 72:*674–677.
Hallin ES, Feldon SE, Luttrell J. (1988b). Graves' ophthalmopathy: II. Correlation of clinical signs with measures derived from computed tomography. *Br J Ophthalmol 72:*678–682.
Hallin ES, Feldon SE. (1988c). Graves' ophthalmopathy III. Effect of transantral orbital decompression on optic neuropathy. *Br J Ophthalmol 72:*683–687.
Hamby WB. (1970). Orbital decompression for exophthalmos. *Clin Neurosurg 17:*18.
Hamilton RD, Mayberry WE, McConhaey WM, Hanson KC. (1967). Ophthalmopathy of Graves' disease: A comparison between patients treated surgically and patients treated with radioiodide. *Mayo Clin Proc 42:*812–818.
Hanabury MR, Cole TB, Clark CE, et al. (1984). Surgical treatment for malignant exophthalmos of endocrine origin. *Laryngoscope 94:*1193–1197.
Harden RM, Chisholm CJS, Cant JS. (1967). The effect of metronidazole on thyroid function and exophthalmos in man. *Metabolism 16:*890.
Harnett AN, Doughty D, Hirst A, Plowman PN. (1988). Radiotherapy in benign orbital disease. II: Ophthalmic Graves' disease and orbital histiocytosis X. *Br J Ophthalmol 72:*289–292.
Härting R, Koornneef L, Peeters HJF, Gillissen JPA. (1986). Fourteen years of orbital decompression in Graves' disease. *Orbit 5:*123–129.
Härting R, Koornneef L, Peeters HJF, Gillissen JPA. (1989). Decompression surgery in Graves' orbitopathy—A review of 14 years' experience at the Orbita Centrum, Amsterdam. *Dev Ophthalmol 20:*185–198.
Harvey JT, Anderson RL. (1981). The aponeurotic approach to eyelid retraction. *Ophthalmology 88:*513–524.
Havard CWH. (1972). Endocrine exophthalmos. *Br Med J 1:*360–363.
Hecht SD, Guibor P, Wolfley D, Wiggs EO. (1984). Orbital dissection defatting technique for Graves' disease. *Ann Ophthalmol 16:*314–318.
Hedges TR, Scheie HG. (1955). Visual field defects in exophthalmos associated with thyroid disease. *Arch Ophthalmol 54:*885–892.
Henderson JW. (1958). Optic neuropathy of exophthalmic goiter (Graves' disease). *Arch Ophthalmol* 59:471–480.
Hermann JS. (1982). Paretic thyroid myopathy. *Ophthalmology 89:*473–478.
Hermann K. (1972). Pituitary exophthalmos: an assessment of methods of treatment. *Br J Ophthalmol 36:*1–19.
Hosten N, Sander B, Cordes M, Schubert CH, Schorner W, Felix R. (1989). Graves' ophthalmopathy: MR imaging of the orbits. *Radiology 172:*759–762.

Howlett TA, Lawton NF, Fells P, Besser GM. (1984). Deterioration of severe Graves' ophthalmopathy during cyclosporin treatment. *Lancet 2:*1101.

Huber A. (1984). Ocular motility in Graves' disease. *Neuro-ophthalmology 4:*227–236.

Hudson HL, Levin L, Feldon SE. (1991). Graves' exophthalmos unrelated to extraocular muscle enlargement. *Ophthalmology 98:*1495–1499.

Hurbli T, Char DH, Harris J, Weaver K, Greenspan F, Sheline G. (1985). Radiation therapy for thyroid eye diseases. *Am J Ophthalmol 99:*633–637.

Hurwitz J, Derek B. (1985). An individualized approach to orbital decompression in Graves' orbitopathy. *Arch Ophthalmol 103:*660–665.

Hurwitz JJ, Freeman JL, Eplett CJ, Fliss DM, Avram DR. (1992). Ethmoidectomy decompression for the treatment of Graves' optic neuropathy. *Can J Ophthalmol 27:*283–287.

Hurwitz J, Rosenstock T. (1983). Management of inadequate transantral orbital decompression with extended lateral orbitotomy. *Can J Ophthalmol 18:*194–196.

Igerscheimer J. (1955). Visual changes in progressive exophthalmos. *Arch Ophthalmol 53:*94–104.

Ivy HK. (1972). Medical approach to ophthalmopathy of Graves' disease. *Mayo Clin Proc 47:*969–974.

Jackson R, Rosenberg C, Kleinmann R, Vagenakis AG, Baverman LE. (1979). Ophthalmopathy after neck irradiation therapy for Hodgkin's disease. *Cancer Treat Rep 63:*1393–1395.

Jacobson DH, Gorman CA. (1984). Endocrine ophthalmopathy: Current ideas concerning etiology, pathogenesis, and treatment. *Endocrin Rev 5:*200–220.

Jones DI, Munro DS, Wilson GM. (1969). Observations on the course of exophthalmos after I^{131} therapy. *Proc R Soc Med 62:*15–18.

Just M, Kahaly G, Higer HP, et al. (1991). Graves' ophthalmopathy: Role of MR imaging in radiation therapy. *Radiology 179:*187–190.

Kahaly G, Lieb W, Müller-Forell W, et al. (1990). Ciamexone in endocrine orbitopathy. *Acta Endocrinol 122:*13–21.

Kahaly G, Schrezenmeir J, Krause U, et al. (1986a). Cyclosporin and prednisone v. prednisone in treatment of Graves' ophthalmopathy: A controlled, randomized and prospective study. *Eur J Clin Invest 16:*415–422.

Kahaly G, Schrezenmeir J, Schweikert B, et al. (1986b). Remission-maintaining effect of cyclosporin and endocrine ophthalmopathy. *Transplant Proc 18:*844–845.

Kazim M, Trokel S, Moore S. (1991). Treatment of acute Graves' orbitopathy. *Ophthalmology 98:*1443–1448.

Kelly W, Longson D, Smithard D, et al. (1983). An evaluation of plasma exchange for Graves' ophthalmopathy. *Clin Endocrinol 18:*485–493.

Keltner JL, Burde RM, Miller NR, Gittinger JW. (1982). Acquired diplopia. Not always a neurologic problem. *Surv Ophthalmol 26:*345–349.

Kendler DL, Lippa J, Rootman J. (1993). The initial clinical characteristics of Graves' orbitopathy vary with age and sex. *Arch Ophthalmol 111:*197–201.

Kennedy DW, Goldstein ML, Miller NR, Zinreich SJ. (1990). Endoscopic transnasal orbital decompression. *Arch Otolaryngol Head Neck Surg 116:*275–282.

Kennerdell JS, Maroon JC. (1982). An orbital decompression for severe dysthyroid exophthalmos. *Ophthalmology 89:*467–472.

Kennerdell JS, Maroon JC, Buerger GF. (1987). Comprehensive surgical management of proptosis in dysthyroid orbitopathy. *Orbit 6:*153–179.

Kennerdell JS, Rosenbaum AE, El-Hoshy MH. (1981). Apical optic nerve compression of dysthyroid optic neuropathy on computed tomography. *Arch Ophthalmol 99:*807–809.

Kinyoun JL, Kalina RE, Brower SA, Mills RP, Johnson RH. (1984). Radiation retinopathy after orbital irradiation for Graves' ophthalmopathy. *Arch Ophthalmol 102:*1473–1476.

Kolodziej-Maciejweksa H, Reterski Z. (1985). Positive effect of bromocriptine in Graves' disease orbitopathy. *Exp Clin Endocrinol 86:*241.

Kramar P. (1974). Management of eye changes of Graves' disease. *Surv Ophthalmol 18:*369–382.

Kriss JP. (1975). Graves' ophthalmopathy: Etiology and treatment. *Hospital Practice 10:*125.

Kriss JP, Pleshakov V, Rosenbaum AL, Holderness M, Sharp G, Utiger R. (1967). Studies on the pathogenesis of the ophthalmopathy of Graves' disease. *J Clin Endocrinol Metab 27:*582–593.

Kulla S, Moore S. (1974). Orthoptics in Graves' disease. *Ophthalmology 86:*2053–2058.

Kulwin DR, Cotton RT, Kersten RC. (1990). Combined approach to orbital decompression. *Otolaryngol Clin No Am 23:*381–390.

Lamberg BA, Grahne B, Tommila V, et al. (1985). Orbital decompression in endocrine exophthalmos of Graves' disease. *Acta Endocrinol 109:*335–340.

Lanier V, Jr. (1975). The surgical treatment of exophthalmos. *Plast Reconstr Surg 55:*56–64.

Laurberg P, Hansen PEB, Iversen E, Jensen SE, Weeke J. (1986). Goitre size and outcome of medical treatment of Graves' disease. *Acta Endocrinol 111:*39–43.

Leatherbarrow B, Lendrum J, Mahaffey PJ, Noble JL, Kwartz J, Davies H. (1991). Three wall orbital decompression for Graves' ophthalmopathy via a coronal approach. *Eye 5:*456–465.

Lemke BN. (1991). Management of thyroid eyelid retraction. *Focal Point* Vol IX, Module 6, 1–9.

Leone CR, Jr. (1984). The management of ophthalmic Graves' disease. *Ophthalmology 91:*770–779.

Leone CR, Jr., Bajandas FJ. (1980). Inferior orbital decompression for thyroid ophthalmopathy. *Arch Ophthalmol 98:*890–892.

Leone CR, Jr, Bajandas FJ. (1981). Inferior orbital decompression for dysthyroid optic neuropathy. *Ophthalmology 88:*525–532.

Leone CR, Jr, Piest KL, Newman RJ. (1989). Medial and lateral wall decompression for thyroid ophthalmopathy. *Am J Ophthalmol 108:*160–166.

Linberg JV, Anderson RL. (1981). Transorbital decompression. Indications and results. *Arch Ophthalmol 99:*113–119.

Liu D, Feldon SE. (1992). Thyroid ophthalmopathy. *Ophthalmol Clin No Amer 5(3):*597–622.

Lloyd WC, Leone CR. (1992). Supervoltage orbital radiotherapy in 36 cases of Graves' disease. *Am J Ophthalmol 113:*374–380.

Long JC, Ellis GC. (1966). Temporal decompression of the orbit for thyroid exophthalmos. *Am J Ophthalmol 62:*1089–1097.

Lopatynsky MO, Krohel GB. (1989). Bromocriptine therapy for thyroid ophthalmopathy. *Am J Ophthalmol 107:*680–681.

Lyons CJ, Rootman J. (1994). Orbital decompression for disfiguring exophthalmos in thyroid ophthalmopathy. *Ophthalmology 101:*223–230.

MacCarty CS, Kenefick TP, McConahen WM. (1970). Ophthalmopathy of Graves' disease treated by removal of roof, lateral walls, and lateral sphenoid ridge. *Mayo Clin Proc 45:*488–493.

McCord CD, Jr. (1985). Current trends in orbital decompression. *Ophthalmology 92:*21–33.

McCord CD, Jr. (1981). Orbital decompression for Graves' disease: Exposure through lateral canthal and inferior fornix incision. *Ophthalmology 88:*533–541.

Mann W, Kahaly G, Lieb W, Rothoff T, Springborn S. (1993). Orbital decompression for endocrine ophthalmopathy: The endonasal approach. *Dev Ophthalmol 25:*142–150.

Marcocci C, Bartalena L, Bogazzi F, Bruno-Bossio G, Lepri A, Pincrea A. (1991). Orbital radiotherapy combined with high dose systemic glucocorticoids for Graves' ophthalmopathy is more effective than radiotherapy alone: Results of a prospective randomized study. *J Endocrinol Invest 14:*853–860.

Marcocci C, Bartalena L, Panicucci M, et al. (1987). Orbital cobalt irradiation combined with retrobulbar or systemic corticosteroids for Graves' ophthalmopathy: A comparative study. *Clin Endocrinol (Oxford) 27:*33–42.

Maroon JC, Kennerdell JS. (1982). Radical orbital decompression for severe dysthyroid exophthalmos. *J Neurosurg 56:*260–266.

Marushak D, Faurschon S, Blicher-Toft M. (1984). Regression of ophthalmopathy in Graves' disease following thyroidectomy. *Acta Ophthalmol 62:767–779.*

Moran RE, Letterman GS, Schurter MA. (1972). The surgical correction of exophthalmos: History, technique and long-term follow up. *Plast Reconstr Surg 49:*595.

Moses JL, McCord CD, Jr. (1979). Orbital decompression. *Am J Surg 45:*608–611.

Mourits M, Koorneef L, Van Mourik-Noordenbos AM, et al. (1990). Extraocular muscle surgery for Graves' ophthalmopathy: does prior treatment influence surgical outcomes? *Br J Ophthalmol 74:*481–483.

Mourits MP, Koorneef L, Wiersinga WM, Prummell MF, Berghout A, van der Gaag R. (1990). Orbital decompression for Graves' ophthalmopathy by inferomedial plus lateral and coronal approach. *Ophthalmology 97:*636–641.

Mourits M, Suttorp-Schulten MSA, Tijssen RO, Apkarian P. (1990). Contrast sensitivity and the diagnosis of dysthyroid optic neuropathy. *Doc Ophthalmol 74:*329–335.

Mulherin JL, Jr, Temple TE, Jr, Cundey DW. (1972). Glucocorticoid treatment of progressive infiltrative ophthalmopathy. *South Med J 65:*77–80.

Neigel JM, Rootman J, Belkin RI, et al. (1988). Dysthyroid optic neuropathy. The crowded orbital apex syndrome. *Ophthalmology 95:*1515–1521.

Neugenbauer A, Nishino K, Neugebauer P, Konen W, Michel O. (1996). Effects of bilateral orbital decompression by an endoscopic endonasal approach in dysthyroid orbitopathy. *Br J Ophthalmol 80:*58–62.

Nunery WR. (1991). Ophthalmic Graves' disease: A dual theory of pathogenesis. *Ophthalmol Clin No Am 4:*73–87.

Nunery WR, Martin RT, Heinz GW, Gavin TJ. (1993). The association of cigarette smoking with clinical subtypes of ophthalmic Graves' disease. *Ophthalm Plast Reconstr Surg 9:*77–82.

Ogura JH. (1971). Decompression of the orbit. *J Otolaryngol Soc Aust 3:*241–243.

Ogura JH, Lucente FE. (1974). Surgical results of orbital decompression of malignant exophthalmos. *Laryngoscope 84:*637–644.

Ogura JH, Thawley SE. (1980). Orbital decompression of exophthalmos. *Otolaryngol Clin No Amer 13:*39–51.

Ogura JH, Wessler S, Avioli LV. (1971). Surgical approach to the ophthalmopathy of Graves' disease. *JAMA 216:*1627–1631.

Olivari N. (1991). Tranpalpebral decompression of endocrine ophthalmopathy (Graves's disease) by removal of intraorbital fat: Experience with 147 operations over 5 years. *Plast Reconstruct Surg 87:*627–643.

Olivotto IA, Ludgate C, Allen LH, Rootman J. (1985). Supervoltage radiotherapy for Graves' ophthalmopathy. *Int J Radiat Oncol Biol Phys 11:*2085–2090.

Ormston BJ, Alexander L, Evered DC, et al. (1973). Thyrotropin response to thyrotrophin releasing hormone in ophthalmic Graves' disease: Correlation with other aspects of thyroid function, thyroid suppressibility and activity of eye signs. *Clin Endocrinol 2:*369–376.

Palmer D, Greenberg P, Cornell P, Parker RG. (1987). Radiation therapy for Graves' ophthalmopathy: A retrospective analysis. *Int J Radiat Oncol Biol Phys 13:*1815–1820.

Panzo GJ, Tomsak RL. (1983). A retrospective review of 26 cases of dysthyroid optic neuropathy. *Am J Ophthalmol 96:*190–194.

Pequegnat EP, Mayberry WI, McConahey WM, Wyse EP. (1967). Large doses of radioiodide in Graves' disease: Effect on ophthalmopathy and long-acting thyroid stimulator. *Mayo Clin Proc 42:*802–811.

Perros P, Weightman DR, Crombie AL, Kendall-Taylor P. (1990). Azathioprine in the treatment of thyroid-associated ophthalmopathy. *Acta Endocrinol 122:*8–12.

Petersen IA, Kriss JP, McDougall IR, Donaldson SS. (1990). Prognostic factors in the radiotherapy of Graves' ophthalmopathy. *Int J Radiation Oncol Biol Phys 19:*259–264.

Peyster RG, Ginsberg F, Siliber JH, Adler LP. (1986). Exophthalmos caused by excessive fat: CT volumetric analysis and differential diagnosis. *Am J Roentgenol 146:*459–464.

Peyster RG, Savino PJ, Hoover ED, Schatz NJ. (1984). Differential diagnosis of the enlarged superior ophthalmic vein. *J Comput Assist Tomogr 8:*103–107.

Pigeon P, Orgiazzi J, Berthezene F, Gerard JP, Haguenauer JP, Mornex R. (1987). High voltage orbital radiotherapy and surgical orbital decompression in the management of Graves' ophthalmopathy. *Horm Res 26:*172–176.

Pinchera A, Fenzi GF, Macchia E, Bartalena L, Mariotti S, Monzani F. (1982). Thyroid-stimulating immunoglobulins. *Horm Res 16:*317–328.

Pinchera A, Liberti P, Martino E, et al. (1969). Effects of antithyroid therapy on the long-acting thyroid stimulator and the antithyroglobulin and antithyroglobulin antibodies. *J Clin Endocrinol Metab 29:*231–238.

Pinchera A, Marcocci C, Bartalena L, et al. (1987). Orbital cobalt radiotherapy and systemic or retrobulbar corticosteroids for Graves' ophthalmopathy. *Horm Res 26:*177–183.

Prummel MF, Mourits MP, Berghout A, et al. (1989a). Prednisone and cyclosporine in the treatment of severe Graves' ophthalmopathy. *N Engl J Med 321:*1353–1359.

Prummel MF, Wiersinga WM, Mourits MP, Koornneef L, Berghout A, van der Gaag R. (1989b). Amelioration of eye changes of Graves' ophthalmopathy by achieving euthyroidism. *Acta Endocrinol (Copenh) 121:*Supp 2:185–189.

Prummel MF, Wiersinga WM, Mourits MP, Koornneef L, Berghout A, van der Gaag R. (1990). Effect of abnormal thyroid function on the severity of Graves' ophthalmopathy. *Arch Intern Med 150:*1098–1101.

Prummel MF, Wiersinga WM. (1993). Smoking and risk of Graves' disease. *JAMA 269:*479–482.

Putterman AM. (1981). Surgical treatment of thyroid-related upper eyelid retraction; graded Müller's muscle excision and levator recession. *Ophthalmology 99:*507–512.

Putterman AM. (1980). Surgical treatment of dysthyroid eyelid retraction and orbital fat hernia. *Otolaryng Clin North Amer 13:*39–51.

Ravin JG, Sisson JC, Knapp WT. (1975). Orbital radiation for the ocular changes of Graves' disease. *Am J Ophthalmol 79:*285–288.

Riddick FA. (1981a). Update on thyroid diseases. *Ophthalmology 88:*467–470.

Riddick FA. (1981b). Immunologic aspects of thyroid disease. *Ophthalmology 88:*471–475.

Riley FC. (1972). Surgical management of ophthalmopathy in Graves' disease. *Mayo Clin Proc 47:*986.

Roncevic R, Jackson IT. (1989). Surgical treatment of thyrotoxic exophthalmos. *Plast Reconst Surg 84:*754–759.

Rubenzik R. (1975). Orbital radiation in Graves' disease. *Am J Ophthalmol 79:*888.

Salvi M, Zhang ZG, Haegart D, et al. (1990). Patients with endocrine ophthalmopathy not associated with overt thyroid disease have multiple thyroid immunological abnormalities. *J Clin Endocrinol Metab* pp. 89–94.

Sandler HM, Rubensten JH, Fowble BL, Sergott RC, Savino PJ, Bosley TM. (1989). Results of radiotherapy for thyroid ophthalmopathy. *Int J Rad Onc Biol Phys 17:*823–827.

Sawers JS, Irvine WJ, Toft AD, et al. (1981). Plasma exchange in conjunction with immunosuppressive drug therapy in the treatment of endocrine exophthalmos. *J Clin Lab Immunol 6:*245.

Schaeffer SD, Meritt JH, Close LG. (1988). Orbital decompression for optic neuropathy secondary to thyroid eye disease. *Laryngoscope 98:*712.

Schimek RA. (1972). Surgical management of ocular complications of Graves' disease. *Arch Ophthalmol 87:*655–664.

Schultz RO, Van Allen MW, Blodi FC. (1960). Endocrine ophthalmoplegia. *Arch Ophthalmol 63:*217–225.

Scott WE, Thalacker JA. (1981). Diagnosis and treatment of thyroid myopathy. *Ophthalmology 88:*493–498.

Sergott RC, Felberg NT, Savino PJ, et al. (1981). Graves' ophthalmopathy-immunologic parameters related to corticosteroid therapy. *Invest Ophthalmol Vis Sci 20:*173–182.

Sergott RC, Felberg NT, Savino PJ, et al. (1981). The clinical immunology of Graves' ophthalmopathy. *Ophthalmology 88:*484–487.

Sergott RC, Glaser JS. (1981). Graves' ophthalmopathy: A clinical and immunologic review. *Surv Ophthalmol 26:*1–21.

Sessions RB, Wilkins RB, Wyer JS. (1972). Endocrine exophthalmos and surgical management. *Arch Ophthalmol 95:*46–52.

Shine B, Fells P, Edwards OM, Weetman AP. (1990). Association between Graves' ophthalmopathy and smoking. *Lancet 335:*1261–1263.

Shorr N, Seiff SR. (1986). The four stages of surgical rehabilitation of the patient with dysthyroid ophthalmopathy. *Ophthalmology 93:*476–483.

Shorr N, Neuhaus RW, Baylis HI. (1982). Ocular motility problems after orbital decompression for dysthyroid ophthalmopathy. *Ophthalmology 9:*323–328.

Sjöberg HE, Sääf M, Boström L, Lundell G, Tallstedt L. (1989). Observations on progress periods in Graves' ophthalmopathy. *Acta Endocrinol 121:*(supp 2):179–181.

Shulka R, Kurinczuk JJ. (1990). Graves' ophthalmopathy and smoking. *Lancet 336:*184.

Skalka HW. (1980). The use of ultrasonography in the diagnosis of endocrine ophthalmopathy. *Neuro-ophthalmol 1:*109–113.

Small RG, Meiring NL. (1981). A combined orbital and antral approach to surgical decompression of the orbit. *Ophthalmology 88:*542–547.

Solem JH, Segaard E, Ytteborg J. (1979). The course of endocrine ophthalmopathy during antithyroid therapy in a prospective study. *Acta Med Scand 205:*111–114.

Solomon DH, Chopra IJ, Chopra U, Smith FJ. (1977). Identification of subgroups of euthyroid Graves' ophthalmopathy. *N Engl J Med 296:*181–186.

Stephenson CM, Brown BZ. (1985). The use of tarsus as a free autogenous graft in eyelid surgery. *Ophthalmic Plast Reconstr Surg 1:*43–50.

Stranc M, West M. (1988). A four wall orbital decompression for dysthyroid orbitopathy. *J Neurosurg 68:*671.

Streeten SHP, Anderson GH, Jr, Reed GF, Woo P. (1987). Prevalence, natural history and surgical treatment of exophthalmos. *Clin Endocrinol 27:*125–133.

Surks MI. (1981). Assessment of thyroid function. *Ophthalmology 88:*476–478.

Tallstedt L, Lundell G, Taube A. (1993). Graves' ophthalmopathy and tobacco smoking. *Acta Endocrinol 129:*147–150.

Tallstedt L, Lundell G, Tørring O, et al. (1992). Occurrence of ophthalmopathy after treatment for Graves' hyperthyroidism. *N Engl J Med 326:*1733–1738.

Tellez M, Cooper J, Edmonds C. (1992). Graves' ophthalmopathy in relation to cigarette smoking and ethnic origin. *Clin Endocrinol 36:*291–294.

Teng CS, Crombie AL, Hall R, Ross WM. (1980). An evaluation of supervoltage orbital irradiation for Graves' ophthalmopathy. *Clin Endocrinol 13:*545–551.

Teng CS, Yeo PPB. (1977). Ophthalmic Graves' disease: Natural history and detailed thyroid function studies. *BMJ 1:*273–275.

Thaller SR, Kawamoto HK. (1990). Surgical correction of exophthalmos secondary to Graves' disease. *Plastic Reconstr Surg 86:*411–417.

Trobe JD. (1981). Optic nerve involvement in dysthyroidism. *Ophthalmology 88:*488–492.

Trobe JD, Glaser JS, Laflamme P. (1978). Dysthyroid optic neuropathy: Clinical profile and rationale for management. *Arch Ophthalmol 96:*1199–1209.

Trokel SL, Cooper WC. (1979a). Orbital decompression effect on motility and globe position. *Ophthalmology 86:*2064–2070.

Trokel SL, Hilal SK. (1979b). Recognition and differential diagnosis of enlarged extraocular muscles in computed tomography. *Am J Ophthalmol 87:*503–512.

Trokel SL, Jakobiec FA. (1981). Correlation of CT scanning and pathologic features of ophthalmic Graves' disease. *Ophthalmology 88:*553–564.

Trokel S, Kazim M, Moore S. (1993). Orbital fat removal: Decompression for Graves' orbitopathy. *Ophthalmology 100:*674–682.

Utech C, Wulle KG, Pfannensteil P, Adam W. (1987). Ciamexon-treatment in endocrine ophthalmopathy. *Acta Endocrinol (suppl) 281:*342–343.

Van Dyk HJL. (1981). Orbital Graves's disease: A modification of the "NO SPECS" classification. *Ophthalmology 88:*479–487.

Van Ouwerkerk VM, Wijngaarde R, Hennemann G, et al. (1985). Radiotherapy of severe ophthalmic Graves' disease. *J Endocrinol Invest 8:*241.

Wall JR, Strakosch CR, Fang SL, et al. (1979). Thyroid binding antibodies and other immunological abnormalities in patients with Graves' ophthalmopathy: Effect of treatment with cyclophosphamide. *Clin Endocrinol 10:*79–91.

Warren JD, Spector JG, Burde R. (1989). Long-term follow-up and recent observations on 305 cases of orbital decompression for dysthyroid orbitopathy. *Laryngoscope 99:*35–40.

Wasnich RD, Grumet FC, Payne RO, Kriss JP. (1973). Graves' ophthalmopathy following external neck irradiation therapy for nonthyroidal neoplastic disease. *J Clin Endocrinol Metab 37:*703–713.

Weetman AP, McGregor AM, Ludgate M, et al. (1983). Cyclosporine improves Graves' ophthalmopathy. *Lancet 2:*486–489.

Werner SC. (1972). The eye changes of Graves' disease: Overview. *Mayo Clin Proc 47:*969–974.

Werner SC. (1966). Prednisone in emergency treatment of malignant exophthalmos. *Lancet 1:*1004–1007.

Werner SC, Coleman DJ, Franzen LA. (1974). Ultrasonic evidence of a consistent orbital involvement in Graves' disease. *N Engl J Med 290:*1447.

Werner SC, Feind CR, Aida M. (1967). Graves' disease and total thyroidectomy progression of severe eye changes and decrease in serum long-acting thyroid stimulator after operation. *N Engl J Med 276:*132–138.

Wiersinga WM. (1984). Conceptual evolution in the relationship between Graves' ophthalmopathy and thyroidal Graves' disease. *Orbit 3:*213–222.

Wiersinga WM, Smit T, Schuster-Uittenhoeve AL, van der Gaag R, Koorneef L. (1988). Therapeutic outcome of prednisone medication and of orbital irradiation in patients with Graves' ophthalmopathy. *Ophthalmologica 197:*75–84.

Wiersinga WM, Smit T, van der Gaag R, Mourits M, Koorneef L. (1989). Clinical presentation of Graves' ophthalmopathy. *Ophthalmic Res 21:*73–82.

Wilson WB, Manke WF. (1991). Orbital decompression in Graves' disease. 109:343–345.

Wolfe SA. (1979). Modified three-wall orbital expansion to correct persistent exophthalmos or exorbitism. *Plast Reconst Surg 64:*448–455.

Wolfe SA. (1981). Surgical treatment of exophthalmos and enophthalmos. *Ann Ophthalmol 13:*995–1002.

Wolfe SA. (1977). A rationale for the surgical treatment of exophthalmos and exorbitism. *J Maxillofac Surg 5:*249.

Wolfe SA, Hemmy D. (1988). How much does moving the lateral wall help in expanding the orbit? *Ophthalmic Plast Reconstr Surg 4:*111–114.

Wulc AE, Popp JC, Bartlett SP. (1990). Lateral wall advancement in orbital decompression. *Ophthalmology 97:*1358–1369.

Yamamoto K, Saito K, Takai T, Yoshida S. (1982). Treatment of Graves' ophthalmopathy by steroid therapy, orbital radiation, plasmapheresis and thyroxine replacement. *Endocrinol Jpn 29:*495–501.

◆ 17 ◆

Nystagmus and Other Ocular Oscillations

Nystagmus is a repetitive, to-and-fro movement of the eyes that includes smooth sinusoidal oscillations (pendular nystagmus) and alternation of slow drift and corrective quick phase (jerk nystagmus) (Leigh, 1991a). Nystagmus induced by optokinetic or vestibular stimuli is physiologic. Nystagmus in extreme lateral or vertical gaze (end-point nystagmus) can also be found in normal persons. It tends to wane easily and belongs to the variety described below as "gaze-evoked" nystagmus.

An approach to pathologic nystagmus is presented in this chapter. In analyzing the features of the nystagmus, it is important to note that it is almost always the slow phase that reflects the underlying abnormality causing the nystagmus; the slow component may have a uniform velocity or may reduce or gain speed as the eyes move in the direction of the slow component. This slow phase abnormality is usually due to disruption of the mechanisms that normally function to hold gaze steady. Thus, disorders of the vestibular system, the gaze-holding mechanisms (e.g., the neural integrator), and visual stabilization and pursuit systems may lead to nystagmus (Leigh, 1991a).

Vestibular tone imbalance results in an asymmetric input to the horizontal gaze generator; vestibular nystagmus shows linear, constant velocity slow phases reflecting a persistent drive of the eyes toward the damaged vestibular apparatus (labyrinth, nerve, nuclei). An impaired neural integrator ("leaky" integrator) may cause gaze-evoked nystagmus with a negative exponential slow phase. The velocity of the slow component decreases as the eyes move from the periphery of the orbit, where the pull due to the viscosity of the orbital tissues is greatest, toward resting in primary position. The inability of the gaze-holding mechanisms to keep the eyes eccentric in the orbit is often present with central or peripheral lesions causing weakness of eye movements. For this reason, this type of nystagmus is often referred to as "gaze-paretic" nystagmus. High gain instability of slow eye movement subsystems (e.g., the pursuit system) may also cause nystagmus, with the nystagmus slow phase having an exponentially increasing time course ("runaway" movements). Such nystagmus in the horizontal plane is seen in congenital nystagmus and in the vertical plane is seen with cerebellar disease. High gain instability may also result in congenital or acquired pendular nystagmus.

The types of nystagmus and other ocular oscillations are outlined in Figure 17–1.

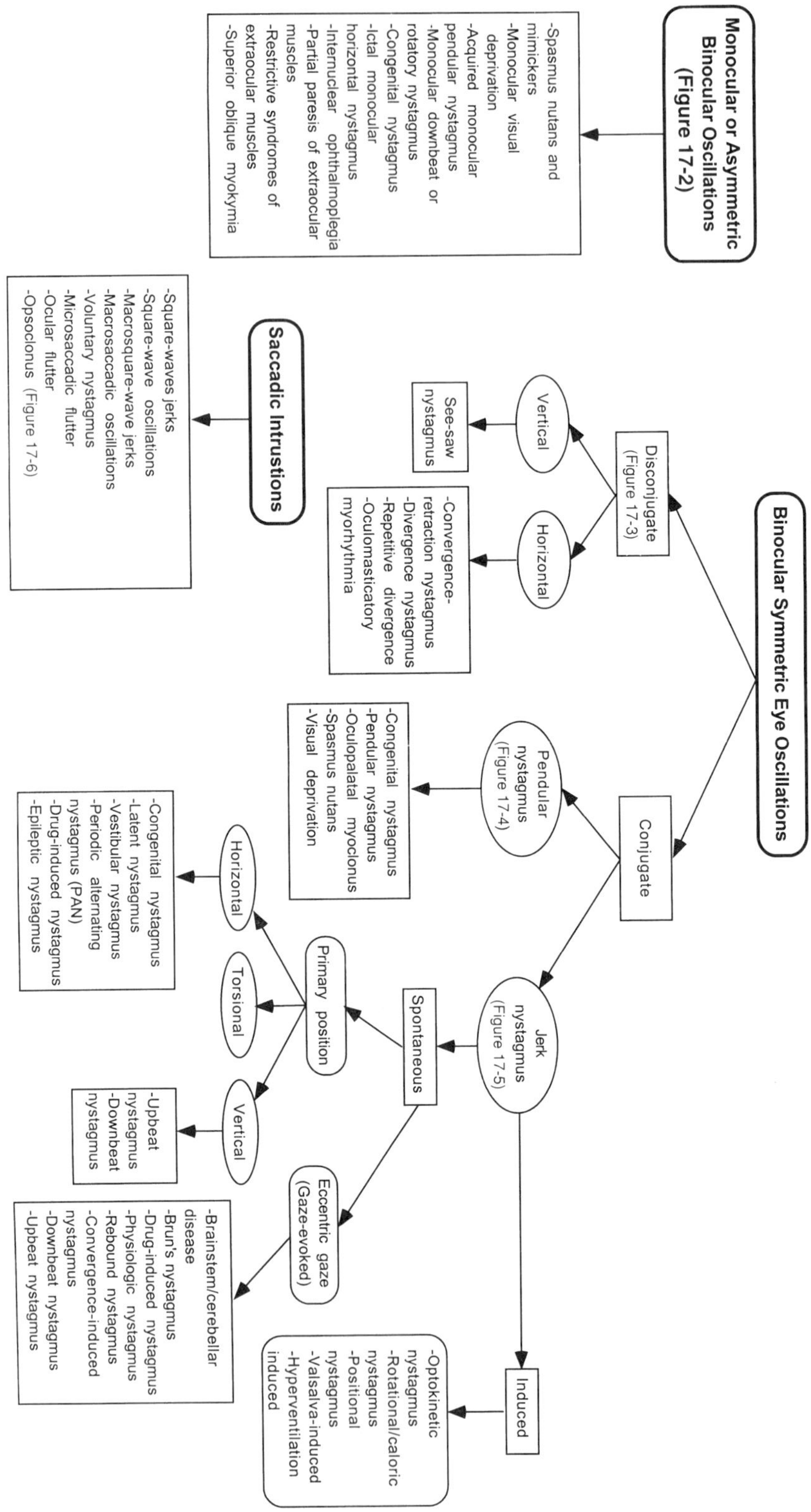

Figure 17–1. Nystagmus and other ocular oscillations.

Are the Abnormal Eye Movements Binocular and Symmetric, Binocular and Asymmetric, or Monocular?

In assessing a patient with abnormal eye oscillations, it is first useful to note whether the oscillations are confined to one eye (monocular), involve mainly one eye (binocular asymmetric or dissociated), or both eyes symmetrically (binocular symmetric) (Burde, 1991).

What Causes Monocular Eye Oscillations and Asymmetric Binocular Eye Oscillations?

Monocular eye oscillations and asymmetric binocular eye oscillations may be due to spasmus nutans and its mimickers, monocular visual deprivation or loss, monocular pendular nystagmus, internuclear ophthalmoplegia and its mimickers, partial paresis of extraocular muscles, restrictive syndromes of extraocular muscles, or superior oblique myokymia.

Spasmus nutans is a benign syndrome characterized by a triad of head nodding, nystagmus, and abnormal head posture (Gottlob, 1995b; Gresty, 1976; Norton, 1954; Weissman, 1987; Young, 1997). This condition usually has its onset in the first year of life and remits spontaneously within one month to several years after onset. The syndrome is occasionally familial and has been reported in monozygotic twins (Hoyt, 1979; Katzman, 1981). The sinusoidal nystagmus is often intermittent, asymmetric or unilateral, and of high frequency and small amplitude with a "shimmering" quality. The nystagmus is usually horizontal, but may have a vertical or torsional component. It may be accentuated by near effort and usually is greater in an abducting eye. Rarely, convergence nystagmus may occur (Massry, 1996). The irregular head nodding with spasmus nutans has horizontal, vertical, or mixed components. Patients often also demonstrate a head turn or tilt.

In all children with spasmus nutans, monocular nystagmus, or asymmetric pendular nystagmus, one must consider that the nystagmus may be due to a tumor of the optic nerve, chiasm, third ventricle, or thalamus (Antony, 1980; Arnoldi, 1995; Baram, 1986; Donin, 1967; Farmer, 1984; Gottlob, 1990; Halpern, 1980; Kelly, 1970; King, 1986; Lavery, 1984; Newman, 1990; Schulman, 1979; Skkorin, 1986). These latter patients may also have visual loss, optic atrophy, or other signs of tumor. Other spasmus nutans mimickers include arachnoid cyst (Spaide, 1985–1986), Leigh's subacute necrotizing encephalomyelopathy (Sedwick, 1984), and congenital stationary night blindness (Gottlob, 1995a; Lambert, 1993).

All children with monocular nystagmus or spasmus nutans should undergo a complete ophthalmologic examination. Neuroimaging studies (preferably MR imaging) should be performed in all patients who develop monocular or predominantly monocular oscillations or a spasmus nutans-like clinical picture, especially with an older age of onset, atypical features, or associated visual loss (Farmer, 1984; Gottlob, 1990; Newman, 1990; Schulman, 1979; Skkorin, 1986). Some authors, however, have stated that the estimated prevalence of tumor in spasmus nutans is less than 1.4% and have suggested that without other evidence of an intracranial mass lesion, neuroimaging of infants initially diagnosed with spasmus nutans may not be immediately warranted (Arnoldi, 1995). A myopic child suspected of having spasmus nutans should also undergo electroretinographic testing to exclude the diagnosis of congenital stationary night blindness (Lambert, 1993).

Monocular nystagmus may occur in adults or children with acquired monocular visual loss and consists of small, slow vertical pendular oscillations in primary position of gaze.

It may develop years after uniocular visual loss (Heimann-Bielschowsky phenomenon) and may improve if vision is corrected (Pritchard, 1988; Smith, 1982; Yee, 1979). Monocular, small-amplitude, fast frequency, and predominantly horizontal nystagmus in children may be caused by unilateral anterior visual pathway disease (Good, 1993).

Acquired monocular pendular nystagmus may also occur with multiple sclerosis, neurosyphilis, and brainstem infarct (thalamus and upper midbrain) and may be vertical, horizontal, or multivectorial (Nathanson, 1955, 1956; Pritchard, 1988). Vertical pendular nystagmus, with greater amplitude in the involved eye, has been described in a patient with chronic monocular myositis of the medial and lateral rectus muscles (Goldberg, 1978). Monocular downbeat nystagmus may occur with acute infarction of the medial thalamus and upper midbrain and with pontocerebellar degeneration; this abnormality is likely the result of dysfunction of the ipsilateral brachium conjunctivum (Bogousslavsky, 1985; Jacome, 1986). Monocular rotatory nystagmus may occur with brainstem lesions (Kattah, 1983). Congenital nystagmus may rarely be uniocular (Kamel, 1974). All these rare monocular nystagmus entities require MR imaging for evaluation. One patient has been described who developed ictal monocular horizontal nystagmus during a generalized seizure triggered by photic stimulation (Jacome, 1982).

Nystagmus is seen only in the abducting eye in internuclear ophthalmoplegia (INO) and in pseudo-INO syndromes. These entities and their evaluation are discussed in Chapter 14. In patients with partial paresis of one of the extraocular muscles, a monocular oscillation may occur in the involved eye or its yoke during an ocular movement into the field of action of the involved muscle (Burde, 1991). Monocular oscillations may also occur in restrictive syndromes (e.g., thyroid ophthalmopathy) in the field of action in which the tethering is occurring (Burde, 1991).

Superior oblique myokymia (SOM) is a disorder of unknown etiology characterized symptomatically by oscillopsia, vertical or torsional diplopia, or both (Hoyt, 1970; Rosenberg, 1983). Affected patients show bursts of rotary oscillations of the eye of small amplitude and high frequency, slow-frequency large-amplitude intorsional movements, or a combination of these paroxysms. Most patients with SOM complain of brief episodes of rapid vertical or torsional movements of the environment or shimmering sensations, usually lasting only a few seconds.

Neuro-ophthalmologic examination of SOM patients often reveals brief episodes of rapid, fine, torsional movements of one eye that are best seen using either the slit lamp biomicroscope or the direct ophthalmoscope. The abnormal movements can be induced in some patients by having the patient move the affected eye downward and outward, tilting the patient's head toward the side of the affected eye, having the patient converge, or having the patient move the affected eye downward and then moving it back to primary position (Keltner, 1983; Kommerell, 1980).

Patients with SOM are usually young adults who are otherwise healthy (Keltner, 1983). Most patients report no precipitating event for the onset of their symptoms, but several cases have followed ipsilateral trochlear nerve palsies, leading some authors to suggest that SOM might be associated with the recovery stage of injury to this nerve (Herzau, 1978; Komai, 1992; Lee, 1984). SOM has occurred several months after removal of a cerebellar tumor (Inagki, 1983). In addition, two cases of SOM have occurred in patients with posterior fossa tumors (one an astrocytoma of the rostral cerebellar vermis with midbrain tectal compression and the other a pilocytic astrocytoma expanding within the fourth ventricle and compressing the midbrain tectum) (Haene, 1993; Morrow, 1990). The rare association of SOM with brainstem tectal disease has caused some authors to recommend neuroimaging examination of the course of the trochlear nerve in all patients with this diagnosis (Morrow, 1990); however, the association of SOM with a posterior fossa tumor is extremely uncommon (Brazis, 1994). Finally, Neetens and Martin described two cases of SOM, one associated with lead intoxication and the other with adrenoleukodytrophy (Neetens, 1983). These associations may well have been coincidental.

Rosenberg and Glaser obtained from 1 to 19 years (average 8 years) follow-up for nine patients with SOM (Rosenberg, 1983). These authors noted that the natural history of the disorder is one of spontaneous remissions and exacerbations with untreated patients frequently enjoying months or even years of remission before subsequent relapses. Indeed, seven of their nine patients continued to have some symptoms after prolonged follow-up.

The treatment for a majority of patients with SOM is reassurance, since most are not significantly disabled by their visual symptoms. If the condition disrupts the patient's work and lifestyle, medications such as carbamazepine (Susac, 1973) or propranolol (Tyler, 1990) may be considered. In Rosenberg and Glaser's series, 7 of 11 patients were tried on carbamazepine and 6 noted a prompt decrease or cessation of ocular symptoms (Rosenberg, 1983). All experienced at least one subsequent relapse days to months after the initial improvement, however, and only three chose to continue the medication. We have tried gabapentin in one patient with SOM without subjective or objective improvement.

Brazis et al. investigated the clinical presentations and long-term course of 16 patients with superior oblique myokymia (Brazis, 1994). Follow-up information was obtained for 14 of the 16 patients with time from onset of symptoms to most recent contact 3 to 29 years (mean, 12 years). The SOM gradually improved or resolved, at least temporarily, without treatment in a significant number of patients. Three of the patients had complete spontaneous resolution of symptoms for periods of 6 to 12 months without recurrence. Six of 7 patients treated with carbamazepine reported no significant response. One patient remained on the medication for 3 years with only rare symptoms that worsen when attempts were made to taper the drug. Two of the patients treated with propranolol reported no significant benefit, and a third noted dramatic but transient improvement in symptoms. Four of the patients were cured by superior oblique tenectomy combined with inferior oblique myectomy. All four surgical patients experienced disappearance of oscillopsia, although one patient developed postoperative vertical diplopia that gradually resolved. Brazis et al. concluded that because SOM is a much more chronic disease than formerly realized and because of the poor long-term effects and potential side effects of the medications used for treatment, medical treatment of SOM, at least with currently available medications, may not be the optimum way to manage the disease. They believe that surgery is the treatment of choice when symptoms of SOM are intolerable to the patient. Other authors have also reported successful treatment of SOM with surgery (de Sa, 1992; Hoyt, 1970; Keltner, 1983; Kommerell, 1980; Palmer, 1984; Staudenmaier, 1986; Susac, 1973). For example, Kosmorsky et al. performed a Harada-Ito procedure on a woman with SOM (Kosmorsky, 1995). This procedure involves nasally transposing the anterior portion of the superior oblique tendon, which is responsible for the cyclorotation, to create an effective weakening of the anterior portion of the tendon instead of temporal displacement utilized for superior oblique paresis. The SOM was abolished and vertical eye movements, including saccades, were unaffected.

The treatment of SOM may, thus, simply be reassurance and the condition may be self-limiting. When symptoms are intolerable, medical or surgical therapy may be considered. A weakening procedure of the affected superior oblique muscle combined with a weakening procedure of the ipsilateral inferior oblique muscle or the Harada-Ito procedure is an effective treatment for SOM after failure of medical treatment or as an alternative to such treatment and should be considered in patients with unacceptable visual symptoms.

The evaluation of monocular or asymmetric binocular oscillations is outlined in Figure 17–2.

What are the Causes of Disconjugate Bilateral Symmetric Eye Oscillations?

If the ocular oscillations involve both eyes to a relatively equal degree, the next step in evaluation involves determining whether the eye movements are disconjugate (the eyes

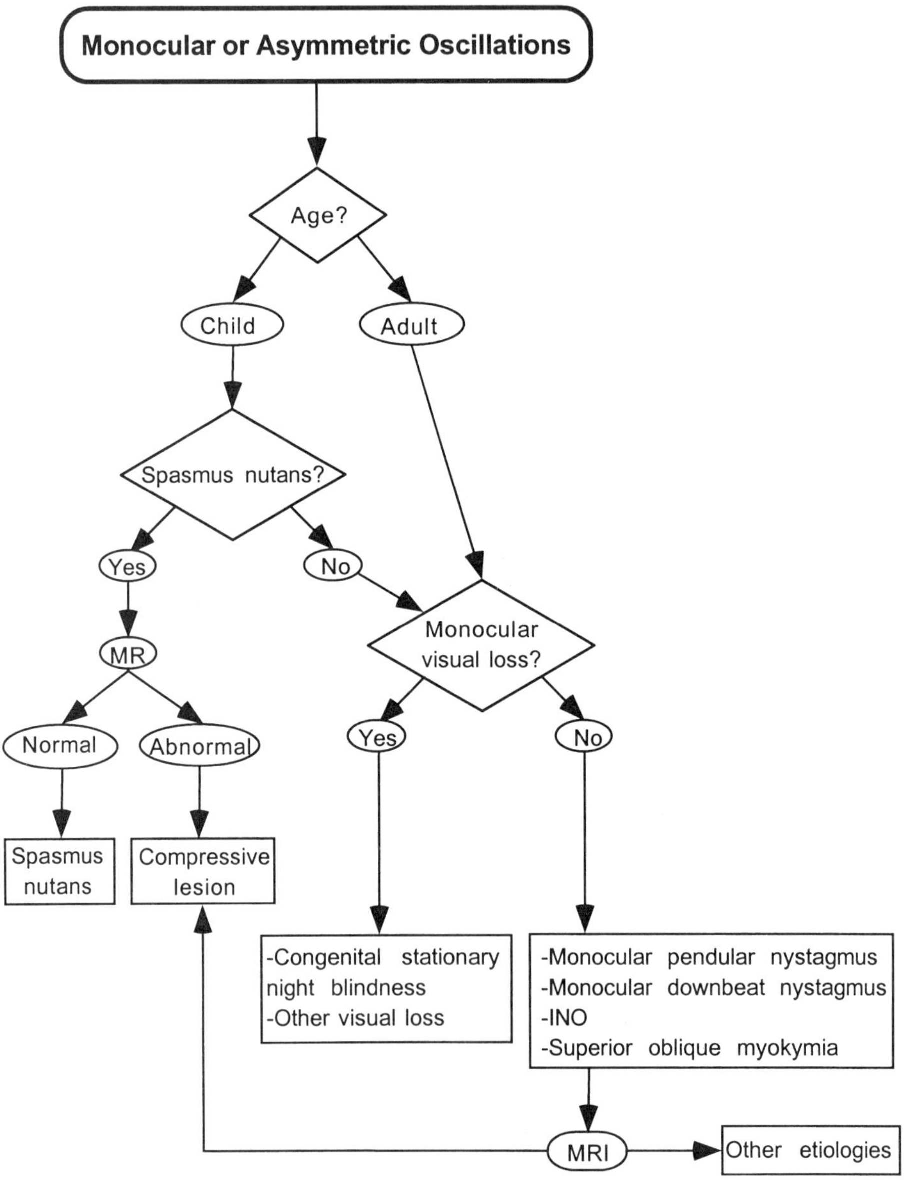

Figure 17–2. Monocular or asymmetric oscillations.

moving in opposite directions) or conjugate (both eyes moving in the same direction) (Burde, 1991). When the oscillations are disconjugate, the examiner should determine whether the oscillations are vertical or horizontal. Vertical disconjugate eye oscillations are usually due to see-saw nystagmus. Horizontal disconjugate eye oscillations include convergence-retraction nystagmus (nystagmus retractorius), divergence nystagmus, repetitive divergence, and oculomasticatory myorhythmia.

See-saw nystagmus is a cyclic movement of the eyes with a conjugate torsional component and a dysjunctive vertical component. While one eye rises and intorts, the other falls and extorts; the vertical and torsional movements are then reversed, completing the cycle (Daroff, 1965a; Nakada, 1988; Slatt, 1964; Williams, 1982). This nystagmus is usually pendular and due to a large suprasellar lesion compressing or invading the brainstem bilaterally at the mesodiencephalic junction. The nystagmus may also have an underlying jerk waveform caused by an intrinsic focal brainstem lesion, either in the lateral medulla (usually on the side opposite the torsional quick phases) or in the mesodiencephalon on the same side as the quick phases (Dehaene, 1984; Halmagyi, 1987, 1991, 1994). See-saw nystagmus likely represents oscillations involving central otolithic connections, especially the interstitial nucleus of Cajal (Halmagyi, 1987, 1991; Kanter, 1987). See-saw nystagmus may also be in part due to an unstable visuovestibular interaction control system. Lesions in the optic pathways may prevent retinal error signals, essential for vestibulocular reflex adaptation, from reaching the cerebellar flocculus and inferior olivary nucleus, thereby making the system less stable (Nakada, 1988). Etiologies responsible for see-saw nystagmus are outlined in Table 17–1.

The evaluation of a patient with see-saw nystagmus includes a complete ophthalmologic and neurologic examination. Patients with parasellar lesions often have bitemporal field defects and "bow-tie" optic atrophy associated with pendular seesaw nystagmus; those with jerk seesaw nystagmus usually demonstrate other neurologic signs of brainstem injury. Neuroimaging (preferably MR imaging attending to parasellar and posterior fossa regions) is warranted in all patients.

The treatment of see-saw nystagmus is directed at the responsible lesion. One patient with intermittent see-saw nystagmus responded to clonazepam, and the nystagmus did

Table 17–1. Etiologies of See-saw Nystagmus

Etiology	References
Parasellar masses	Barton, 1995; Daroff, 1965a; Drachman, 1966; Druckman, 1966; Rossazza, 1974; Safran, 1980
Brainstem and thalamic stroke	Daroff, 1965; Eber, 1982; Halmagyi, 1991, 1994; Kanter, 1987; Mastaglia, 1974; Williams, 1982
Multiple sclerosis	Samkoff, 1994
Trauma	Frisen, 1986; Keane, 1978; Sano, 1972; Schmidt, 1969
Arnold-Chiari malformation	Zimmerman, 1986
Hydrocephalus	Williams, 1982
Syringobulbia	Fein, 1969
Septo-optic dysplasia, retinitis pigmentosa, and cone degeneration	Bergin, 1986; Davis, 1975; Rych, 1974
Congenital see-saw nystagmus*	Daroff, 1965; Hoyt, 1984; Schmidt, 1974; Zauberman, 1969; Zelt, 1985

*Congenital see-saw nystagmus may lack the torsional component or even present with an opposite pattern (i.e., extorsion with eye elevation and intorsion with eye depression).

not recur after withdrawal of the medication (Cochin, 1995). Also, baclofen, with and without clonazepam, improved both nystagmus and associated oscillopsia in another patient, suggesting a possible GABA-ergic mechanism influencing the interstitial nucleus of Cajal (Carlow, 1986).

Convergence may evoke various forms of nystagmus (i.e., convergence-evoked nystagmus—see below). Convergence-retraction nystagmus is a disorder of ocular motility in which repetitive adducting saccades, which are often accompanied by retraction of the eyes into the orbit, occur spontaneously or on attempted up-gaze (Cogan, 1959; Gay, 1963; Ochs, 1979; Oohira, 1986). Sliding an optokinetic tape downward in front of the patient's eyes may also elicit convergence-retraction nystagmus. Convergence-retraction nystagmus is primarily a saccadic disorder as the convergence movements are not normal vergence movements but asynchronous, adducting saccades. Mesencephalic lesions affecting the pretectal region are most likely to cause this type of nystagmus that is often associated with abnormalities of vertical gaze. The localization and evaluation of these vertical gaze abnormalities and convergence-retraction nystagmus are discussed in Chapter 14. Convergence nystagmus has been described without vertical gaze abnormalities in patients with dorsal midbrain stroke and in patients with Arnold-Chiari malformation (Mossman, 1990; Schnyder, 1996). Whipple's disease may also cause convergence nystagmus at approximately one Hz (pendular vergence oscillations) (Selhorst, 1987). Convergence nystagmus has been described in a patient with spasmus nutans (Massry, 1996).

Divergence nystagmus (with divergent quick phases) may occur with hindbrain abnormalities (e.g., Arnold-Chiari malformation) and is associated with downbeat nystagmus (Cogan, 1959; Yee, 1979). These patients have slow phases directed upward and inward. Repetitive divergence consists of a slow divergent movement followed by a rapid return to the primary position at regular intervals (Noda, 1987). This rare disorder has been described with coma from hepatic encephalopathy. A similar disorder, probably related to seizures, was reported in a neonate in association with burst-suppression patterns of the electroencephalogram (Nelson, 1986).

Oculomasticatory myorhythmia refers to acquired pendular vergence oscillations of the eyes associated with concurrent contraction of the masticatory muscles (Adler, 1990; Grotta, 1987; Hausser-Hauw, 1988; Louis, 1996; Schwartz, 1986). When the myorhythmia also involves nonfacial skeletal muscles, it is called oculo-facial-skeletal myorhythmia. There is a smooth, rhythmic eye convergence, which cycles at a frequency of approximately 1 Hz, followed by divergence back to the primary position. Rhythmic elevation and depression of the mandible is synchronous with the ocular oscillations that persist in sleep and are unaltered by stimuli. The masticatory involvement may occasionally consist of a permanent bruxism leading to severe tooth abrasions (Tison, 1992). Patients with oculomasticatory myorhythmia may also have paralysis of vertical gaze, progressive somnolence, and intellectual deterioration. This distinct movement disorder has been recognized only in Whipple's disease. Therefore, if this condition is diagnosed, empiric antibiotic treatment of Whipple's disease must be instituted and attempts made to confirm the diagnosis of Whipple's by endoscopicically guided biopsy of multiple jejunal sites (Adler, 1990; Louis, 1996). Electron microscopy and PCR-based testing on tissue samples are often required to identify the Whipple's bacillus and confirm the diagnosis (Louis, 1996; Tison, 1992). If two small-bowel biopsies are not diagnostic, another tissue should be biopsied (lymph node, brain lesion, or vitreous fluid, where appropriate) (Louis, 1996).

The evaluation of disconjugate bilateral symmetric eye oscillations is outlined in Figure 17–3.

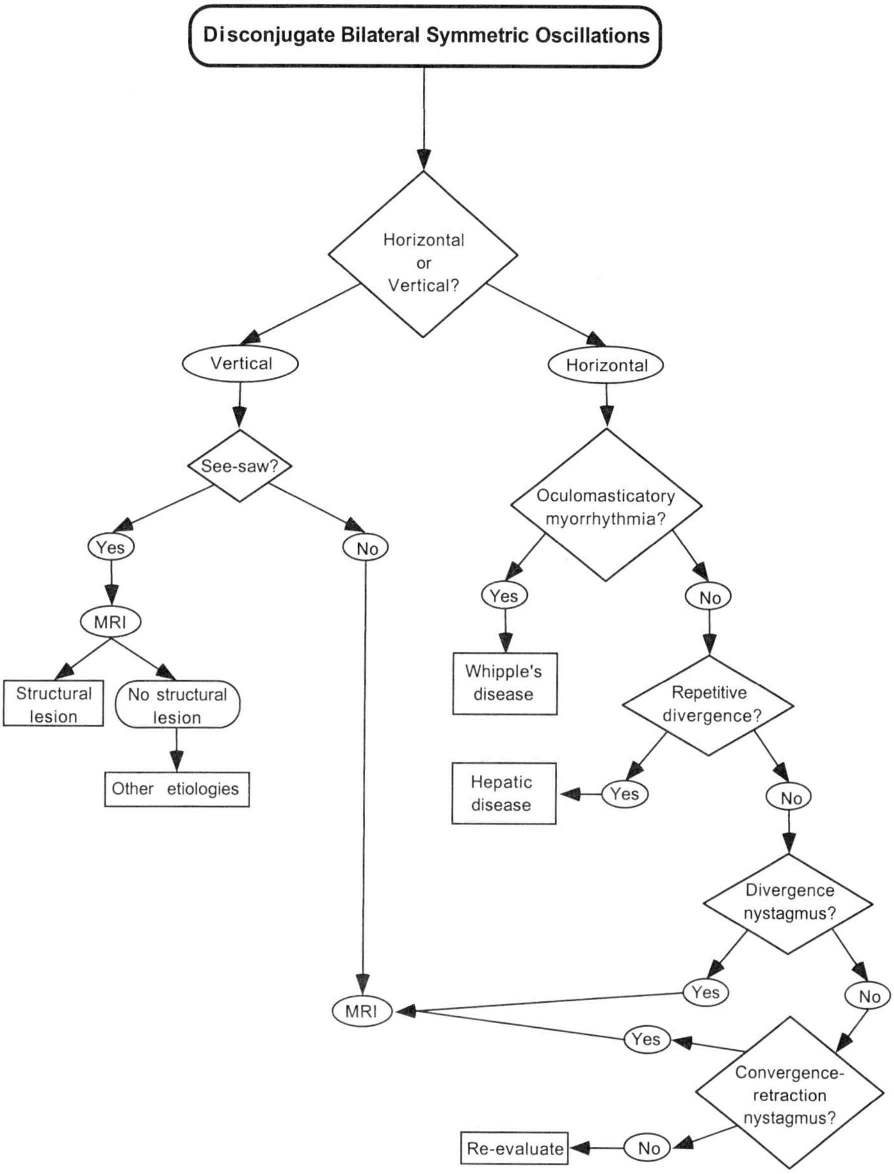

Figure 17–3. Disconjugate bilateral symmetric oscillations.

What Are the Causes of Binocular Symmetric Conjugate Eye Oscillations?

Binocular symmetric conjugate eye oscillations may be divided into pendular nystagmus, jerk nystagmus, and saccadic intrusions (Burde, 1991). Binocular symmetric pendular conjugate eye oscillations can be caused by congenital nystagmus, pendular nystagmus, oculopalatal myoclonus, spasmus nutans (discussed above), and visual deprivation nystagmus.

What Are the Causes of Binocular Symmetric Pendular Conjugate Eye Oscillations?

Congenital nystagmus may be noted at birth or in early infancy, or may emerge or enhance in teenage or adult life, often without apparent provocation (Dell'Osso, 1975, 1993; Gelbart, 1988; Gresty, 1984, 1991). It is seldom familial and most often idiopathic. Metabolic derangements and structural anomalies of the brain, including abnormalities of the eye or anterior visual pathways, have been occasionally responsible. More important, when it is found later in life it must be distinguished from other forms of nystagmus that have a potentially treatable cause. Congenital nystagmus may be wholly pendular or have both pendular and jerk components. Congenital jerk nystagmus has a slow phase with a velocity that increases exponentially as the eyes move in the direction of the slow phase. Occasionally congenital nystagmus may be purely vertical or torsional (Bixenman, 1983; Forsythe, 1955; Funahashi, 1988; Lambert, 1989; Marmor, 1973; Sogg, 1962). Although irregular, congenital nystagmus is generally conjugate and horizontal, even on up-gaze or down-gaze (uniplanar); visual fixation accentuates it and active eyelid closure or convergence attenuates it (Gresty, 1991). The nystagmus decreases in an eye position ("null region") that is specific for each patient. Despite the constant eye motion, these patients do not experience oscillopsia. When they are tested with a hand-held optokinetic tape or drum, the quick phase of the elicited nystagmus generally follows the direction of the tape (reversed optokinetic nystagmus) (Halmagyi, 1980).

The cause of congenital nystagmus is unknown, but it has been associated with many disease processes affecting the visual afferent system including ocular and oculocutaneous albinism, achromatopsia, optic nerve hypoplasia, Leber's amaurosis, coloboma, aniridia, cone dystrophies, corectopia, congenital stationary night blindness, Chédiak-Higashi syndrome, Joubert syndrome, and peroxisomal disorders (Abadi, 1989; Collewijn, 1985; Gelbart, 1988; Lambert, 1989; Simon, 1984; St. John, 1984). It has also been associated with hypothyroidism (Radhakrishnan, 1982; Schulman, 1969). The evaluation of children with congenital nystagmus should include a complete ophthalmologic examination, especially attending to symptoms of photophobia and paradoxical pupillary constriction in darkness as well as thyroid functions. An electroretinogram is indicated in all patients, even those with apparently normal afferent eye exams (Cibis, 1993; Good, 1989; Lambert, 1989; Price, 1988). For example, 56% of 105 consecutive patients with congenital nystagmus were found to have retinal disease when tested with ERG (Cibis, 1993).

Congenital nystagmus decreases in an eye position ("null region") that is specific for each patient and convergence often attenuates the nystagmus. Prisms can be used to take advantage of the dampening effect of convergence and the null region-lens combinations can be adjusted so that an asymmetric arrangement of base-out prisms both converge the eyes and turns them toward the null angle (Dell'Osso, 1979; Dickenson, 1986). Leigh et al. suggest 7.00-diopter base-out prisms with −1.00-diopter spheres added to compensate for accommodation (Leigh, 1994). Contact lenses may improve vision in patients with congenital nystagmus, possibly due to tactile feedback (Allen, 1983; Dell'Osso, 1988). Another approach for the treatment of severe nystagmus in general involves employing an optical system to stabilize images on the retina (Leigh, 1988, 1994; Rushton, 1987; Yaniglos, 1992). The combination of high "plus" (i.e., converging) spectacle lenses with high "minus" (i.e., diverging) contact lenses is used with the converging system focusing the image at the center of the eye rotation (thus stabilizing the image) and the diverging system moving the image back to focus on the retina. The contact lens moves with the eye so it does not negate the effect of image stabilization produced by the spectacle lens. This imaging system is theoretically beneficial but difficult to maintain in practice, especially because the system disables the vestibuloocular reflex and is thus only useful when the patient is stationary.

Congenital nystagmus may also be treated with botulinum toxin injections into the extraocular muscles or surgery. Acuity was restored in four patients, to the extent that they were able to receive daytime drivers licenses, by multiple horizontal recti injections of botulinum toxin (Carruthers, 1995). Surgical procedures effectively control congenital nystagmus by attempting to move the attachments of the extraocular muscles so that the null angle corresponds to the eyes' new primary position (the null region is shifted and broadened), to decrease nystagmus outside the null region, and to prolong foveation time by changing the waveform and dampening the nystagmus (Anderson, 1953; Bilska, 1995; Dell'Osso, 1979; D'Esposito, 1989; Flynn, 1981; Helveston, 1991; Kestenbaum, 1953; Spielmann, 1981; Von Noorden, 1991; Zubkov, 1993). Procedures used include the Anderson-Kestenbaum procedure, which moves the eyes to the null region, divergence procedures, large recessions of the horizontal rectus muscles, and combined procedures (Leigh, 1994). Finally, biofeedback has been reported to help some patients with this disorder (Abadi, 1980; Ciuffreda, 1982).

Latent nystagmus is common and generally congenital (Dell'Osso, 1979, 1983, 1987; Gresty, 1992; Wagner, 1990; Zubcov, 1990). It appears when one eye is covered. Both eyes then develop conjugate jerk nystagmus, with the viewing eye having a slow phase directed toward the nose (i.e., the quick phase of both eyes beat toward the side of the fixating eye). Although present at birth, latent nystagmus is often not recognized until later in life, when an attempt is made to determine monocular visual acuity during vision screening at school. Latent nystagmus is usually associated with strabismus, especially esotropia; amblyopia may occur and binocular vision with normal stereopsis is rare. In addition to horizontal strabismus, upward deviation of the covered eye (dissociated vertical deviation or alternating sursumduction) and a torsional, occasionally pendular, component to the nystagmus may occur (Clarke, 1988). Latent nystagmus is a marker for congenital ocular motor disturbance and does not indicate progressive structural brain disease (Burde, 1991).

Manifest latent nystagmus is an oscillation that occurs in patients with strabismus or acquired visual loss who have a jerk nystagmus in the direction of the fixing eye (i.e., right-beating nystagmus when fixing with the right eye and left-beating nystagmus when fixing with the left eye) (Burde, 1991). Patients with infantile uniocular blindness may have a bilateral horizontal nystagmus that represents a manifest nystagmus of the latent type (Kushner, 1995). These patients often have a family history of strabismus; the monocular blindness (opacity of the media or suppression) acts as an occluder, making manifest what would have been latent nystagmus. Therapy for latent nystagmus consists of measures to improve vision, such as patching for amblyopia in children or surgical correction of strabismus (Von Noorden, 1987; Zubkov, 1993).

As noted above, pendular nystagmus is often congenital. Acquired pendular nystagmus may be wholly horizontal, wholly vertical, or have mixed components (circular, elliptical, or windmill pendular nystagmus). Pendular nystagmus may be symmetric, dissociated, or even monocular and often causes distressing oscillopsia and decreased visual acuity (Aschoff, 1974; Averbuch-Heller, 1995; Barton, 1993; Lopez, 1996). Damage to the dentatorubroolivary pathways (Guillain-Mollaret triangle) is found in some cases of acquired pendular nystagmus, which is most often caused by multiple sclerosis, stroke, or tumor of the brainstem or other posterior fossa structures (Aschoff, 1974; Averbuch-Heller, 1995; Barton, 1993; Bender, 1952; Currie, 1986; Gresty, 1982; Herrman, 1967;

Herrmann, 1957; Keane, 1986; Lawrence, 1975; Lopez, 1996; Revol, 1990; Talks, 1997). In multiple sclerosis, pendular nystagmus may be a sign of cerebellar nuclear involvement (Aschoff, 1974), or result from optic neuropathy, but the most consistent finding on MR imaging is a lesion in the dorsal pontine tegmentum, perhaps affecting the central tegmental tract (Barton, 1993). In a study of 27 patients with acquired pendular nystagmus, MR images were characterized by multiple areas of abnormal signal with statistically significant ones occurring in areas containing the red nucleus, the central tegmental tract, the medial vestibular nucleus, and the inferior olive (Lopez, 1996). The abundance of abnormal MR imaging signals, predominantly in the pons but also in the midbrain and the medulla, suggests that large or multiple structural lesions may be required to elicit pendular nystagmus.

Other causes of acquired binocular pendular nystagmus include Pelizaeus-Merzbacher disease, mitochondrial cytopathy, Cockayne's syndrome, and toluene addiction (Coker, 1979; Mallinson, 1983; Maas, 1991; Rosenberg, 1988; Trobe, 1991). Congenital, familial, or acquired bilateral paralysis of horizontal gaze may be associated with pendular nystagmus; the familial type may also be associated with progressive scoliosis and facial contractures with myokymia (Sharpe, 1975; Yee, 1982). Pendular nystagmus may also appear with blindness or monocular loss of vision; in the latter case, it may be monocular (see above). Binocular visual loss may cause nystagmus that has both horizontal and vertical components that change direction over seconds or minutes (i.e., a wandering null point) (Good, 1990; Hoyt, 1984; Leigh, 1980). Blind patients may have windmill nystagmus, in which there are repeated oscillations in the vertical plane alternating with repeated oscillations in the horizontal plane.

Palatal myoclonus is a continuous rhythmic involuntary movement of the soft palate that may be accompanied by synchronous movements of other adjacent structures, such as the face, pharynx, larynx, or diaphragm. The association of pendular nystagmus with palatal myoclonus is not infrequent and the condition is then termed oculopalatal myoclonus (Bender, 1952; Gresty, 1982; Talks, 1997). Oculopalatal myoclonus may be of two types (Nakada, 1986):

1. A lateral form, consisting of jerky, nystagmoid movements with simultaneous oblique and rotatory components associated (and synchronous) with lateralized palatal myoclonus (in this form, the eye on the side of the myoclonus intorts as it rises and extorts as it falls while the opposite eye extorts as it rises and intorts as it falls).
2. A midline form in which vertical to and fro pendular eye movements occur synchronous with symmetric bilateral palatal myoclonus.

It has been postulated that the generation of oculopalatal myoclonus involves vestibuloocular reflex adaption mediated by the cerebellar flocculus as floccular integrity is preserved in most patients (Nakada, 1986). The lateral form implies unilateral disease while the midline form indicates bilateral disease. Damage to the dentatorubroolivary pathways (Guillain-Mollaret triangle) is found in cases of oculopalatal myoclonus, which is most often caused by multiple sclerosis or vascular lesions of the brainstem. MR imaging often shows enlargement of the inferior olivary nuclei (Talks, 1997).

The evaluation of the patient with pendular nystagmus depends on the clinical circumstances and associated neurologic findings. In patients with multiple sclerosis, the diagnosis is usually obvious by a history of remissions and exacerbations of neurologic signs and symptoms associated with abnormalities on neurologic examination, suggesting a disseminated process. Brainstem stroke or tumor is diagnosed by mode of onset of symptoms, associated neurologic signs and symptoms, and MR imaging. Ophthalmologic exam will reveal blindness as a cause for the nystagmus in some patients. MR imaging is warranted in all patients with palatal myoclonus.

The neurotransmitters involved in pendular nystagmus are unknown, but cholinergic and GABA-ergic pathways may be involved. Anticholinergic agents have been used for treatment with variable results (Barton, 1994; Jabbari, 1987; Leigh, 1991). In a randomized, double-blind study, trihexyphenidyl improved only one of five patients with pendular elliptical nystagmus; in another double-blind study, intravenous scopolamine reduced nystagmus and improved vision in all five patients treated (Barton, 1994; Jabbari, 1987). Isoniazid relieved nystagmus and oscillopsia in two of three patients with pendular elliptical nystagmus due to multiple sclerosis, but others have not found this drug to be helpful (Leigh, 1994; Traccis, 1990).

Although the mechanism of action of gabapentin is unknown, Stahl et al. have measured the effects of this agent on vision and eye movements in acquired pendular nystagmus in two patients with multiple sclerosis and one with brainstem stroke (Stahl, 1996). An oral dose of 600 mg produced improvement of vision due to changes in ocular oscillations in all three patients. The drug was well tolerated and was continued at 900 to 1500 mg daily in divided doses with long-term benefit. All the patients reported useful visual improvement that enabled them to read, watch television, and recognize faces.

Several reports have suggested that injection of botulinum toxin either into selected extraocular muscles or into the retrobulbar space might be effective in the treatment of acquired nystagmus (Carruthers, 1995; Helveston, 1988; Leigh, 1992; Repka, 1994; Ruben, 1994a, 1994b; Talks, 1997; Tomsak, 1995). Leigh et al. injected the horizontal rectus muscles of the right eye of two patients with acquired pendular nystagmus (Leigh, 1992). The treatment effectively abolished the horizontal component of the nystagmus in the injected eyes of both patients for two months. However, side effects including diplopia, ptosis, and worsening of the oscillopsia in the uninjected eye (attributed to plastic-adaptive changes in response to paresis caused by the botulinum toxin) limited the effectiveness of the treatment. In another study, botulinum toxin injection into the retrobulbar space of three patients with acquired pendular nystagmus abolished or reduced all components of the nystagmus (Tomsak, 1995). However, side effects of the treatment, including ptosis, diplopia, and keratitis, significantly limited the therapeutic value of the injections. Others have reported variable improvement in visual function and oscillopsia with retrobulbar or horizontal recti botulinum injection with transient ptosis the most common side effect (Ruben, 1994a, 1994b). Repka et al. injected 25 to 30 units of botulinum toxin into the retrobulbar space of six adults with acquired nystagmus (Repka, 1994). Each patient had subjective and objective improvement of distance visual acuity following injection with reduction of the amplitude but not the frequency of the nystagmus. Visual improvement lasted no more than eight weeks but persisted for six months in two patients with oculopalatal myoclonus. The authors concluded that retrobulbar botulinum toxin injection may improve visual function for patients with acquired nystagmus and that improvement seemed to be longer for patients with oculopalatal myoclonus. Further studies on the safety and efficacy of botulinum toxin injection for acquired nystagmus are warranted.

Lesions of the Guillain-Mollaret triangle are thought to induce cholinergic denervation supersensitivity of the inferior olive which results in the oculopalatal myoclonus (Matsuo, 1979). Anticholinergic agents (trihexyphenidyl) have thus been tried effectively in four patients with palatal myoclonus without ocular involvement (Jabbari, 1987) and in one patient with vertical pendular nystagmus identical to that seen with oculopalatal myoclonus but without palatal involvement (Herishanu, 1986). Valproate and carbamazepine have each been reported to reduce the nystagmus of palatal myoclonus

(Leftowitz, 1985; Sakai, 1981). Finally, as noted above, the nystagmus in patients with oculopalatal myoclonus may be especially sensitive to retrobulbar botulinum toxin injection (Repka, 1994).

The evaluation and treatment of pendular nystagmus is outlined in Figure 17–4.

What Are the Causes of Binocular Symmetric Jerk Nystagmus?

Binocular symmetric conjugate jerk nystagmus may be divided into that which is present spontaneously and that which is induced (Burde, 1991). Spontaneous jerk nystagmus may be further divided into forms present in primary position and forms present predominantly on eccentric gaze.

Spontaneous symmetric conjugate jerk nystagmus that occurs in primary position may be predominantly horizontal, predominantly torsional, or predominantly vertical. Spontaneous symmetric conjugate jerk nystagmus in primary gaze that is predominantly horizontal includes congenital nystagmus (above), latent nystagmus (above), vestibular nystagmus, periodic alternating nystagmus, drug-induced nystagmus, and epileptic nystagmus. Spontaneous symmetric conjugate jerk nystagmus in primary gaze that is purely

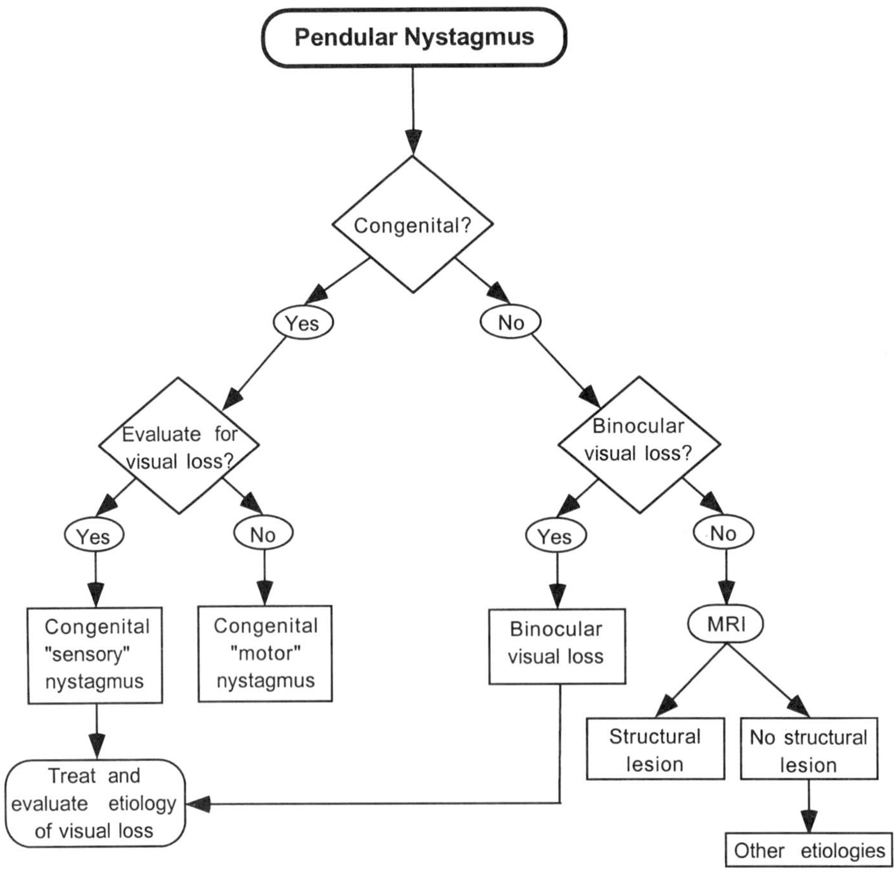

Figure 17–4. Pendular nystagmus.

torsional is a form of central vestibular nystagmus. Spontaneous symmetric conjugate jerk nystagmus in primary gaze that is predominantly vertical includes upbeat nystagmus and downbeat nystagmus.

Horizontal nystagmus in the primary position is often the result of peripheral vestibular disease. Peripheral vestibular lesions induce a tendency for the eyes to drift in a direction parallel to the plane in which the diseased canal lies. Horizontal nystagmus with the slow component toward the lesion (the opposite vestibular nuclei drive the eyes toward the diseased side) results from unilateral horizontal canal or total labyrinthine destruction. In the latter case there is a torsional slow component causing the upper part of the globe to rotate toward the lesioned side. Although constant for a particular position of gaze, the slow-phase velocity is greater when the eyes are turned in the direction of the quick component (Alexander's law). Nystagmus due to peripheral vestibular disease is most prominent, or only becomes apparent, when fixation is prevented. Both peripheral and central vestibular nystagmus may vary with head position and movement, but peripheral nystagmus changes after a latency period following the postural change and tends to fatigue.

Peripheral vestibular disease is suspected when the nystagmus is associated with subjective vertigo. Central vestibular disease (e.g., brainstem infarction) is suspected when associated neurological signs and symptoms of brainstem dysfunction are present. With the latter, MR imaging is warranted.

With periodic alternating nystagmus (PAN), the eyes exhibit primary position nystagmus, which, after 60 to 120 seconds, stops for a few seconds and then starts beating in the opposite direction (Baloh, 1976; DeBartolomeo, 1988). Horizontal jerk nystagmus in the primary position not associated with vertigo is usually periodic alternating nystagmus (Burde, 1991). This disorder may be associated with periodic alternating oscillopsia, periodic alternating gaze, or periodic alternating skew deviation (Kennard, 1981; Lewis, 1983; Troost, 1990). PAN may be congenital, but it is often acquired and caused by disease processes at the craniocervical junction. The nodulus and uvula of the cerebellum maintain inhibitory control over vestibular rotational responses by using GABA. Following ablation of these structures, the postrotational response is excessively prolonged, so that normal vestibular repair mechanisms act to reverse the direction of the nystagmus, which results in PAN (Leigh, 1991). PAN is thus thought to be produced by dysfunction of the GABA-ergic velocity-storage mechanism and may be controlled in most, but not all patients, by the GABA-B agonist baclofen (Furman, 1990; Halmmagyi, 1980; Troost, 1990; Uemura, 1988). Patients with congenital PAN may also respond to baclofen (Carlow, 1986; Isago, 1985). Etiologies for periodic alternating nystagmus are listed in Table 17–2.

Table 17–2. Etiologies of Periodic Alternating Nystagmus

Etiology	References
Congenital (may be associated with albinism)	Abadi, 1994; Baloh, 1976; Daroff, 1974; Guyer, 1986; Huygen, 1995; Isago, 1985
Arnold-Chiari malformation and other malformations of the craniocervical junction	Baloh, 1976; Furman, 1990; Leigh, 1981; Meienberg, 1980
Cerebellar degenerations	Baloh, 1976; DiBartolomeo, 1988; Furman, 1990; Gorman, 1950; Lewis, 1983; Plant, 1982; Sakakibara, 1993
Ataxia-telangiectasia	Stell, 1989
Cerebellar masses, including tumors, abscesses, and cysts	Kennard, 1981; Leigh, 1981; Towle, 1970

(continued)

Table 17–2. *(continued)*

Etiology	References
Brainstem infarction	Furman, 1990
Cerebellar infections, including syphilis and Creutzfeldt-Jacob disease	Grant, 1993; Leigh, 1981, 1991; Lewis, 1983; Reis, 1989; Yokota, 1991
Trauma	Leigh, 1991
Multiple sclerosis	Keane, 1974; Leigh, 1991
Anticonvulsant medications	Campbell, 1980; Schwankhaus, 1989
Following visual loss (e.g., due to cataract or vitreous hemorrhage)	Cross, 1982; Jay, 1985

The evaluation of a patient with PAN includes a complete neurological and ophthalmological exam. In many patients, the etiology of the nystagmus is evident by history (e.g., congenital onset, associated albinism, family history of cerebellar degeneration, anticonvulsant use, history of remissions and exacerbations of neurological signs and symptoms, acute onset of brainstem signs and symptoms, severe visual impairment, etc.). Otherwise, the evaluation should include MR imaging with attention to the cranio-cervical junction. If MR imaging is normal and the patient has a history of the subacute onset of progressive cerebellar signs and symptoms, Creutzfelt-Jacob disease should be suspected and an electroencephalogram looking for characteristic periodic complexes should be performed. Serology for syphilis is also warranted in these cases. If the patient develops progressive neurologic deterioration, then brain biopsy may be considered if Creutzfeldt-Jacob disease is a likely possibility.

Drug-induced nystagmus may be predominantly horizontal, predominantly vertical, predominantly rotatory, or, most commonly, mixed. It is most often seen with tranquilizing medications and anticonvulsants. Although drug-induced nystagmus is more often evident with eccentric gaze (see below), it may also be evident in primary gaze (Burde, 1991; Remler, 1990).

Nystagmus may occur as an epileptic phenomena. Epileptic nystagmus is usually horizontal, may be seen with epileptiform activity ipsilateral or contralateral to the direction of the slow component of the nystagmus, and often is associated with altered states of consciousness, although consciousness may be preserved during the attacks (Barry, 1986; Beun, 1984; Furman, 1990; Jacome, 1986; Kaplan, 1989, 1993; Stolz, 1991; Thurston, 1985; Tusa, 1990; Watanabe, 1984; White, 1971). There are two postulated mechanisms for the eye deviation in epileptic nystagmus (Furman, 1990; Kaplan, 1989, 1993; Tusa, 1990). Ipsiversive eye deviation, with eye movement recordings and EEG showing seizure-induced ipsilateral linear slow phases, is postulated to result from stimulation of the smooth pursuit region in the temporo-occipital cortex. If eye velocity is high or the eye reaches a far eccentric portion in the orbit, a normal resetting quick phase eye movement occurs after each slow phase, resulting in nystagmus. Contraversive eye deviations, with eye movement recordings and EEG showing seizure-induced contralateral quick phases, is thought due to stimulation of the saccade-controlling regions of the temporo-occipital or frontal cortex. If gaze-holding is defective (e.g., the neural integration is "leaky"), then velocity-decreasing slow phases bring the eyes back to the midline after each quick phase, resulting in nystagmus.

Epileptic nystagmus is rare and usually seen in patients with a history of epilepsy and in those with the nystagmus associated with altered levels of consciousness. Electroencephalography should be considered in patients with episodic nystagmus and oscillopsia, especially if other findings suggest a seizure disorder as a diagnostic possibility.

Spontaneous jerk nystagmus that is purely torsional is a rare form of central vestibular nystagmus. Purely torsional nystagmus may be present in primary gaze or elicited by head positioning or gaze deviation (Lopez, 1992). Purely torsional nystagmus may be seen with brainstem and posterior fossa lesions, such as tumors, syringobulbia, syringomyelia with Arnold-Chiari malformation, lateral medullary syndrome, multiple sclerosis, trauma, vascular anomalies, post-encephalitis, and sarcoidosis, and as part of the stiff-person syndrome (Bosley, 1985; Bronstein, 1987; Lepore, 1980; Lopez, 1992; Morrow, 1988; Noseworthy, 1988; Sabin, 1969; Stearns, 1993).

Contralesionally beating torsional nystagmus may be due to a midbrain lesion involving the rostral interstitial nucleus of the MLF, while lesions of the interstitial nucleus of Cajal in the midbrain cause ipsilesional torsional nystagmus (Helmchen, 1996). Torsional nystagmus occurring only during vertical pursuit has been described with cavernous angiomas of the middle cerebellar peduncle (FitzGibbon, 1996). MR imaging is thus warranted in all patients with purely torsional nystagmus. Nonrhythmic but continuous torsional eye movements have been reported as a paraneoplastic process (Rosenthal, 1987).

What Are the Causes of Predominantly Vertical Jerk Nystagmus?

Spontaneous jerk nystagmus in primary gaze that is predominantly vertical includes upbeat nystagmus and downbeat nystagmus (Baloh, 1989; Buttner, 1995).

Downbeat nystagmus is usually present in primary position, but is greatest when the patient looks down (Alexander's law) and to one side. On upward gaze, the nystagmus is less pronounced or disappears completely. Downbeat nystagmus may occur with cervicomedullary junction disease, midline medullary lesions, posterior midline cerebellar lesions, or diffuse cerebellar disease (Buttner, 1995; Wertenbaker, 1981; Yee, 1989). Deficient drive by the posterior semicircular canals, whose central projections cross in the floor of the fourth ventricle, has been postulated as an explanation for downbeat nystagmus. Interruption of downward vestibuloocular reflex pathways would result in upward smooth eye drift and a downward corrective saccade. Cerebellar, especially floccular and uvulonodular, lesions may cause this nystagmus by disinhibition of the cerebellar effect on the vestibular nuclei. The cerebellar flocculus contains Purkinje cells that send inhibitory projections to anterior canal but not posterior canal central pathways; therefore, disinhibition would lead to downbeat nystagmus. Damage to the nuclei propositus hypoglossi and the medial vestibular nuclei (the neural integrator) in the medulla has also been suggested as the cause of the nystagmus (Corbett, 1989). Etiologies of downbeat nystagmus are listed in Table 17–3.

Table 17–3. Etiologies of Downbeat Nystagmus

Etiology	References
Craniocervical anomalies, including cerebellar ectopia, Arnold-Chiari malformation, platybasia, basilar invagination, and Paget's disease	Abel, 1983; Baloh, 1981; Bogousslavsky, 1980, 1981; Bronstein, 1987; Chait, 1979; Cogan, 1968; Corkill, 1976; Faria, 1980; Halmagyi, 1983; Hortovsky, 1982; Pedersen, 1980; Russell, 1992; Senelick, 1981; Spooner, 1981; Yee, 1984, 1989; Yeow, 1989

(continued)

Table 17–3. *(continued)*

Etiology	References
Familial cerebellar degenerations	Baloh, 1981, 1989; Bronstein, 1987; Chambers, 1983; Donat, 1979; Farris, 1986; Halmagyi, 1983; Schott, 1980; Yee, 1989
Posterior fossa tumors	Bronstein, 1987; Chan, 1991; Halmagyi, 1983; Schmidt, 1981; Wolf, 1973; Yeow, 1989
Increased intracranial pressure (e.g., due to supra-tentorial mass) and hydrocephalus	Chan, 1991; Lavin, 1983; Phadke, 1981; Slavin, 1985
Brainstem or cerebellar infarction, anoxia, or hemorrhage	Baloh, 1981, 1989; Benjamin, 1986; Bronstein, 1987; Halmagyi, 1983; Rousseaux, 1991; Slavin, 1985; Yee, 1989
Dolichoectasia of the vertebrobasilar artery	Gans, 1990; Himi, 1995; Jacobson, 1989; Krespi, 1995
Intermittent vertebral artery compression by an osteophyte	Rosengart, 1993
Encephalitis, including herpes simplex encephalitis and HTLV-1 infection	Hirst, 1983; Shimizu, 1975; Waragai, 1995; Yoshimoto, 1991
Multiple sclerosis and other leukodystrophies	Baloh, 1981, 1989; Bronstein, 1987; Masucci, 1988; Tsuzuku, 1986; Yee, 1989
Syringomyelia/syringobulbia	Pinel, 1987
Trauma	Baloh, 1989
Alcohol, including alcohol-induced cerebellar degeneration	Costin, 1980; Halmagyi, 1983; Rosenberg, 1987; Zasorin, 1984
Wernicke's encephalopathy	Cox, 1981; Lavin, 1983
Paraneoplastic cerebellar degeneration	Anderson, 1988; Guy, 1988; Halmagyi, 1983; Hammack, 1992; Peterson, 1992
Congenital	Bixenman, 1983
Vitamin B12 deficiency	Mayfrank, 1986
Magnesium deficiency	Saul, 1981
Drugs, including lithium, toluene, and anticonvulsants (e.g., phenytoin, carbamazepine, felbamate)	Alpert, 1978; Berger, 1982; Chrousos, 1987; Coppeto, 1983; Corbett, 1989; Engelhardt, 1988; Gracia, 1985; Halmagyi, 1983, 1989; Hwang, 1995; Kitamura, 1984; Malm, 1980; Monteiro, 1993; Rosenberg, 1989; Wheeler, 1982; Williams, 1988; Yoshimoto, 1987
Transient finding in otherwise normal infants	Hoyt, 1987; Weissman, 1988
Idiopathic	Baloh, 1981; Yeow, 1989

The evaluation of downbeat nystagmus depends on the clinical circumstances and associated neurologic findings. Because downbeat nystagmus reflects abnormalities of posterior fossa structures, MR imaging is warranted in most cases to investigate the presence of a structural lesion (Bronstein, 1987; Himi, 1995; Pinel, 1987; Yeow, 1989). MR imaging will be normal or show diffuse cerebellar atrophy in patients with familial cerebellar degenerations. In patients taking anticonvulsants or lithium, drug levels should be measured and adjusted. If MR imaging is normal, B12 and magnesium levels should be measured, thiamine therapy should be considered and the possibility of alcohol or toluene abuse investigated. If there are signs suggestive of central nervous system infection, a spinal tap is warranted. In a patient with downbeat nystagmus with the acute or subacute onset of cerebellar signs and symptoms, a paraneoplastic process must be considered, especially due to small cell lung cancer, gynecological cancers (especially ovarian and breast cancer), and Hodgkin's disease. The work-up of these patients includes serum anti-Yo (anti-Purkinje cell) antibodies, serum anti-Hu antibodies (anti-neuronal nuclear antibodies type 1 or ANNA type 1), chest X ray and chest CT imaging, gynecological examination, CT or MR imaging of the abdomen and pelvis, mammography, and possibly hematologic consultation for bone marrow biopsy. Finally, in a significant number of individuals, no etiology for the downbeat nystagmus will be discovered.

Damage to the central projections of the anterior semicircular canals, which tend to deviate the eyes superiorly, has been suggested to explain upbeat nystagmus. Upbeat nystagmus is usually worse in upgaze (Alexander's law) and, unlike downbeat nystagmus, it usually does not increase on lateral gaze (Baloh, 1989). Convergence may increase or decrease the nystagmus, or convert downbeat nystagmus to upbeat nystagmus (Halmagyi, 1983; Hirose, 1991). Damage to the ventral tegmental pathways, which may link the superior vestibular nuclei to the superior rectus and inferior oblique subnuclei of the oculomotor nuclei, may cause the eyes to glide down, resulting in upbeat nystagmus (Ranalli, 1988). Medullary disease may cause upbeat nystagmus as may lesions of the anterior cerebellar vermis, perihypoglossal and inferior olivary nuclei of the medulla, pontine tegmentum, brachium conjunctivum, midbrain, and brainstem diffusely (Baloh, 1989; Buttner, 1995; Fisher, 1983; Hankey, 1987; Kanaya, 1994; Kato, 1985; Keane, 1987; Munro, 1993; Nakada, 1981). Bow-tie nystagmus, in which quick phases are directed obliquely upward with horizontal components alternating to the right and left, is probably a variant of upbeat nystagmus. Etiologies of upbeat nystagmus are outlined in Table 17–4.

Table 17–4. Etiologies of Upbeat Nystagmus

Etiology	References
Primary cerebellar degenerations and atrophies	Fujikane, 1992; Furman, 1985, 1986; Kattah, 1983; Mizuno, 1990
Arnold-Chiari malformation	Hatashita, 1980
Posterior fossa tumors	Elliott, 1989; Fisher, 1983; Gilman, 1977; Nakada, 1981; Troost, 1980; Traccis, 1989
Brainstem or cerebellum infarction or hemorrhage	Benjamin, 1986; Daroff, 1973; Hirose, 1990; Kato, 1985; Keane, 1987; Munro, 1993; Rousseaux, 1991; Yura, 1988
Multiple sclerosis	Fisher, 1983; Hirose, 1990, 1991
Meningitis and brainstem encephalitis	Furman, 1985; Holmes, 1981
Thalamic arteriovenous malformation	Nowack, 1986
Wernicke's encephalopathy	Cox, 1981; Fisher, 1983; Zumstein, 1982
Behçet's syndrome	Ishikawa, 1986
Congenital, including cases associated with Leber's congenital amaurosis and other congenital anterior visual pathway disorders	Good, 1990, 1993; Hoyt, 1984; Sogg, 1962
Pelizaeus-Merzbacher disease	Trobe, 1991
Fisher's syndrome (ataxia, areflexia, and ophthalmoplegia)	Yamazaki, 1994
Middle ear disease	Gresty, 1988
Organophosphate poisoning	Jay, 1982
Tobacco-induced	Sibony, 1987
Anticonvulsant intoxication	Isago, 1982
Transient finding in otherwise healthy neonates	Goldblum, 1994; Hoyt, 1987

The evaluation of upbeat nystagmus includes a complete neurological and ophthalmological examination. MR imaging is warranted in most cases to investigate the presence of a structural lesion. In children, MR imaging is indicated not only to investigate posterior fossa lesions, but also lesions of the anterior visual pathways. If imaging is normal in children, then ERG is warranted. Spinal tap is indicated in patients with signs or symptoms suggestive of meningeal irritation or central nervous system infection. In adults with negative neuroimaging studies, organophosphate or anticonvulsant intoxication should be investigated.

The treatment of vertical nystagmus is directed at the etiology (e.g., surgical correction of Arnold-Chiari malformation). Clinical evidence suggests involvement of gamma-aminobutyric acid (GABA-ergic) pathways and cholinergic transmission in vertical vestibuloocular reflexes (Leigh, 1994). GABA agonists and cholinergic drugs have thus been tried to relieve the visual impairment with vertical nystagmus. Clonazapam, a GABA-A agonist, and baclofen, a GABA-B agonist, have been shown to reduce nystagmus velocity and oscillopsia in some patients with downbeat or upbeat nystagmus (Currie, 1986; Dieterich, 1991). Intravenous physostigmine, an acetylcholinesterase inhibitor, worsened vertical nystagmus in five patients (Dieterich, 1991) while intravenous scopolamine, an anticholinergic drug, reduced nystagmus and oscillopsia in two patients with downbeat nystagmus (Barton, 1994). Anticholinergic drugs may thus be considered for patients with upbeat or downbeat nystagmus. Finally, downbeat nystagmus usually is present in primary position but is greatest when the patient looks down (Alexander's law) and subsides in upgaze. Patients may therefore benefit from symmetric base-down prisms that turn the eyes up.

What Are the Causes of Binocular Symmetric Jerk Nystagmus Present in Eccentric Gaze or Induced by Various Maneuvers?

Spontaneous binocular conjugate symmetric jerk nystagmus that is induced by eccentric gaze (gaze-evoked nystagmus) include nystagmus due to brainstem/cerebellar disease, Bruns' nystagmus, drug-induced nystagmus, physiologic nystagmus, rebound nystagmus, and convergence-induced nystagmus. Downbeat nystagmus and upbeat nystagmus may only occur on downward or upward gaze, respectively (see above).

With gaze-evoked nystagmus, the eyes fail to remain in an eccentric position of gaze but drift to midposition. The velocity of the slow component decreases exponentially as the eyes approach midposition. A "leaky" neural integrator or cerebellar (especially vestibulocerebellar) lesion may result in this type of nystagmus, which is more pronounced when the patient looks toward the lesion. Cerebellopontine angle tumors may cause Bruns' nystagmus, a combination of ipsilateral large-amplitude, low-frequency nystagmus that is due to impaired gaze holding, and contralateral small-amplitude, high-frequency nystagmus that is due to vestibular impairment (Baloh, 1976; Leigh, 1991). Gaze-evoked nystagmus may be a side effect of medications, including anticonvulsants, sedatives, and alcohol. Physiologic or endpoint nystagmus is a benign low-amplitude jerk nystagmus with the fast component directed toward the field of gaze. It usually ceases when the eyes are brought to a position somewhat less than the extremes of gaze. Rebound nystagmus is seen in some patients with cerebellar disease (e.g., olivocerebellar atrophy, cerebellar tumor, Marinesco-Sjogren syndrome, Dandy-Walker cyst, Gerstmann-Straussler-Scheinker disease, etc.) (Bondar, 1984; Cox, 1979; Hood, 1973; Morales-Garcia, 1978; Sharpe, 1974; Toupet, 1979; Yamazaki, 1979; Yee, 1992; Yoshimoto, 1987; Zee, 1976). After keeping the eyes eccentric for some time, the original gaze-evoked nystagmus may wane and actually reverse direction so that the slow component is directed centrifugally; it becomes obvious if the eyes are returned to midposition. Rebound nystagmus probably reflects an attempt by brainstem or cerebellar mechanisms to correct for the centripetal drift of gaze-evoked nystagmus (Leigh, 1991).

Patients with gaze-evoked nystagmus who are taking anticonvulsant or sedative medications and those with physiologic nystagmus require no further evaluation. Otherwise, patients with gaze-evoked or rebound nystagmus, especially if associated symptoms or signs of brainstem or cerebellar dysfunction or auditory impairment exist, require MR imaging, with special attention to the cerebellum and cerebello-pontine angle.

Convergence may change nystagmus by converting downbeat to upbeat, upbeat to downbeat, or pendular to upbeat. Convergence-evoked nystagmus is usually vertical (upbeat is more common than downbeat) and seen most commonly with multiple sclerosis or brainstem infarction (Oliva, 1990; Sharpe, 1975; Zak, 1983). MR imaging is thus warranted in patients with convergence-induced nystagmus. Convergence may also increase or decrease the amplitude of nystagmus and may evoke horizontal (congenital or acquired pendular and jerk) or vertical (upbeat or downbeat) nystagmus (Sharpe, 1975). Convergence-induced pendular nystagmus has been described as a congenital phenomenon (conjugate) and as an acquired phenomenon (disjunctive) with multiple sclerosis (Oliva, 1990; Sharpe, 1975; Zak, 1983). The effects of convergence on nystagmus are not to be confused with convergence nystagmus in which a slow abduction of the eyes is followed by quick adduction (see above).

Binocular symmetric conjugate jerk nystagmus that is induced includes optokinetic nystagmus, rotational/caloric vestibular nystagmus, positional nystagmus, Valsalva-induced nystagmus, and hyperventilation-induced nystagmus (Burde, 1991; Leigh, 1991). The first two types of induced nystagmus are physiological and, although abnormalities of these responses may aid in clinical diagnosis, they will not be further discussed.

Positional vertigo of the benign paroxysmal type, also known as benign paroxysmal positioning vertigo or positional nystagmus, is usually "idiopathic" and possibly related to degeneration of the macula of the otolith organ or to lesions of the posterior semicircular canal (Baloh, 1987, 1995; Brandt, 1990, 1991; Lawden, 1995; Lin, 1986; Weider, 1994). It has been proposed that otoconia detached from the otoconial layer (by degeneration or trauma) gravitate and settle on the cupula of the posterior canal causing it to become heavier than the surrounding endolymph and thus sensitive to changes in the direction of gravity (with positional change). After rapid head tilt toward the affected ear or following head extension, when the posterior semicircular canal is moved in the specific plane of stimulation, an ampullofugal deflection of the cupula occurs, with a rotational vertigo and concomitant nystagmus. Some patients show a strong horizontal nystagmus induced by lateral head positioning suggesting lateral (rather than posterior) semicircular canal irritation (lateral canal or horizontal canal variant of benign paroxysmal positional vertigo) (Baloh, 1993; De la Meilleure, 1996; Pagnini, 1989). Other causes of positional vertigo include trauma, infection, labyrinthine fistula, ischemia, demyelinating disease, Arnold-Chiari malformation, and, rarely, posterior fossa tumors or vascular malformations (Lawden, 1995; Sakata, 1987, 1991; Sweeney, 1980; Watson, 1982).

Besides paroxysmal positional nystagmus, patients often also exhibit static (persistent) positional nystagmus while lying in a lateral position. This static nystagmus is predominantly horizontal with minimal vertical component (Baloh, 1987). Paroxysmal vertigo induced by certain head positions is the most common complaint; the patient is asymptomatic between bouts. The Nylén-Bárány maneuver (briskly tilting the patient's head backward and turning it 45 degrees to one side) allows a differentiation between a peripheral and a central origin for positional vertigo.

With peripheral lesions, severe rotational vertigo associated with nausea (occasionally vomiting) and nystagmus appear several seconds (2–15 seconds) after the head position is changed. In benign paroxysmal positional (positioning) vertigo, it is unusual for the vertigo to have a duration of more than one minute. Cochlear or neurological symptoms are typically absent. The nystagmus is usually torsional, with the upper pole of the eye beating toward the ground. The vertigo and nystagmus then fatigue and abate within 10 seconds after appearance, and when the patient is rapidly brought back to a sitting position, vertigo recurs and nystagmus develops in the opposite direction (rebound). With repetition of the maneuver, the symptoms and nystagmus become progressively less severe (habituation), and the reproducibility of the abnormalities is inconstant. Mild transient nystagmus in one head position may occasionally be elicited in normal subjects. Patients with benign paroxysmal positional vertigo are often treated successfully with canalith repositioning procedures (Weider, 1994).

A central lesion should be suspected when: (1) the maneuver is positive with the head turned to either side; (2) the nystagmus is direction changing rather than fixed, appearing immediately after the shift in position and remaining for as long as the head is down; (3) the nystagmus is unaccompanied by nausea or a sense of discomfort; if present, vertigo is mild and lasts no longer than 60 seconds; and (4) repetition does not cause blunting of the effects. Typically, there are other associated central nervous system findings. Patients with the central form of positional nystagmus require MR imaging to investigate structural posterior fossa lesions. Occasionally, patients with benign paroxysmal positional vertigo will demonstrate findings during the Nylén-Bárány maneuver similar to those documented in patients with central lesions (Baloh, 1995).

Nystagmus induced by the Valsalva maneuver may occur with Arnold-Chiari malformation or perilymph fistulas (Leigh, 1991). Hyperventilation may induce nystagmus in patients with tumors of the eighth cranial nerve (e.g., acoustic neuroma or epidermoid tumors), after vestibular neuritis, or central demyelinating lesions (Leigh, 1991). Hyperventilation-induced nystagmus has the slow phase away from the side of the lesion (an excitatory or recovery nystagmus) and is likely due to the effect of hyperventilation upon serum pH and calcium concentration, which improve nerve conduction in a marginally functional, demyelinated nerve (Leigh, 1991).

The evaluation of patients with jerk nystagmus are outlined in Figure 17–5.

What Are the Characteristics of Saccadic Intrusions?

Inappropriate saccades, or saccadic intrusions, interfere with macular fixation of an object of interest. There are several types of saccadic intrusions.

Square-wave jerks take the eyes off the target and are followed after about 200 msec by a corrective saccade (Elidan, 1984; Feldon, 1977; Herishanu, 1981; Ohtsyka, 1986; Shallo-Hoffmann, 1989, 1990). They may appear normally in the young and the elderly, but when larger than 1 or 2 degrees they are pathologic, resulting from disorders including a variety of cerebral or cerebellar lesions, progressive supranuclear palsy, Huntington's chorea, Parkinson's disease, Wernicke-Korsakoff's syndrome, Friedreich's ataxia, AIDS-dementia complex, Gerstmann-Straussler-Scheinker disease, and schizophrenia (Friedman, 1992; Rascol, 1991; Yee, 1992). They may also occur with lithium or tobacco use. Very frequent square-wave jerks (square-wave oscillations) may be mistaken for nystagmus and may occur with cerebellar disease, progressive supranuclear palsy, and cerebral hemispheral

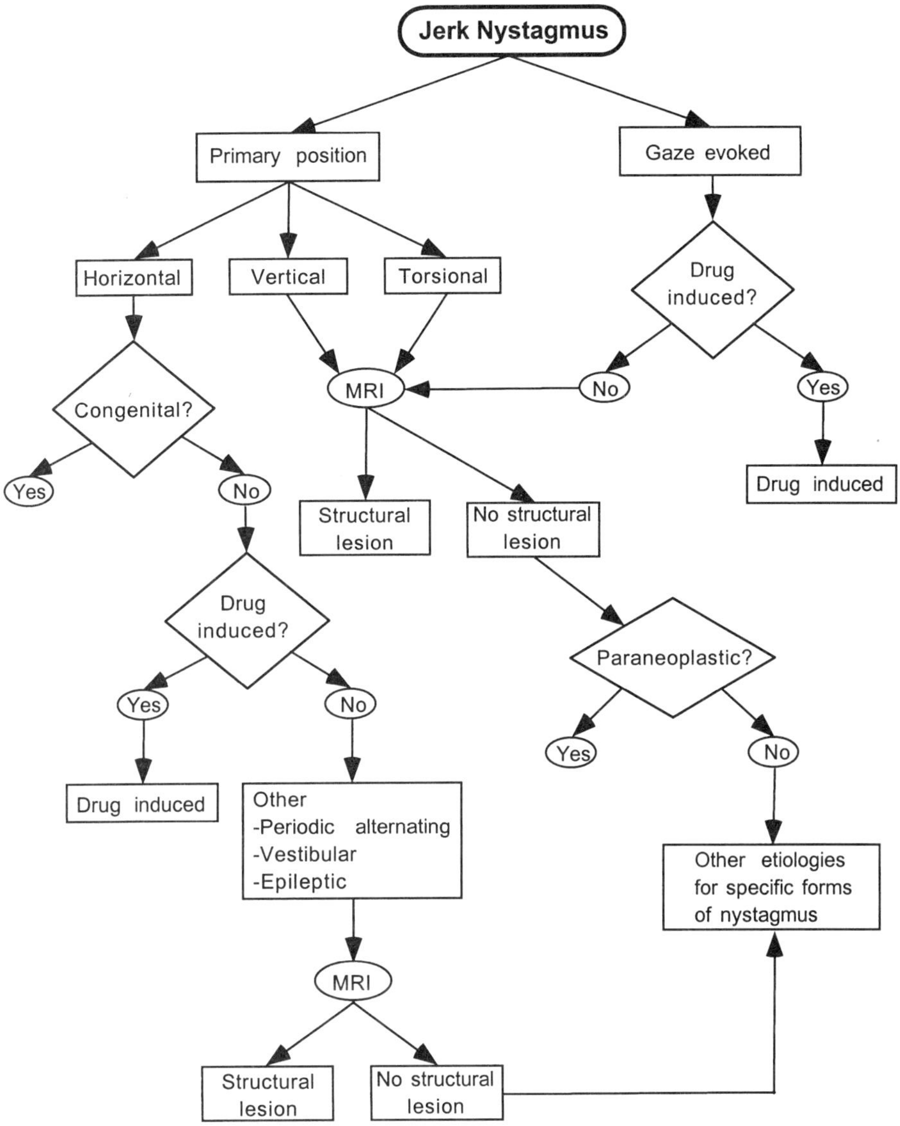

Figure 17–5. Jerk nystagmus.

disease (Abel, 1984; Friedman, 1992; Leigh, 1991; Sharpe, 1982; Troost, 1977). Macrosquare-wave jerks are similar to square-wave jerks but are of larger amplitude (20–40 degrees) (Dell'Osso, 1975, 1977; Fukazawa, 1986; Traccis, 1988). They are occasionally present in the vertical plane and have been noted in multiple sclerosis, cerebellar hemorrhage, olivopontocerebellar atrophy, multiple systems atrophy, and Arnold-Chiari malformation (Fukuda, 1984; Leigh, 1991; Neshige, 1984; Yamamoto, 1992).

Macrosaccadic oscillations are different from square wave jerks and consist of eye oscillations around the fixation angle with intersaccadic intervals approximately 200 msec (Leigh, 1991). They occur in patients with cerebellar disease, especially affecting the cerebellar midline and underlying nuclei (e.g., cerebellar hemorrhage or spinocerebellar degenerations) (Kase, 1985; Masson, 1986; Selhorst, 1976).

Square-wave jerks, square-wave oscillations, macrosquare-wave jerks, and macrosaccadic oscillations usually occur in the context of otherwise evident neurological diseases. If the nature of the causal degenerative process accounting for these intrusions is not evident on clinical history and neurological exam, MR imaging is warranted. Macrosaccadic oscillations and high-amplitude square-wave jerks may be treated with GABA-A agonists, benzodiazepines, and barbiturates (Fukazawa, 1986).

Voluntary nystagmus (psychogenic flutter) occurs in normal subjects, sometimes as a familial trait, and consists of bursts of high frequency horizontal oscillations composed of back-to-back saccades (Ciuffreda, 1980; Condon, 1970; Coren, 1972; Hotson, 1984; Jarrett, 1977; Keyes, 1973; Kondo, 1980; Lee, 1993; Lipman, 1972; Shults, 1977; Zahn, 1978). The movements may be vertical or torsional as well. This movement will completely disappear if patients are forced to keep their eyes open, since it requires tremendous volitional effort and cannot be sustained for prolonged periods of time (Burde, 1991). Voluntary nystagmus is often accompanied by a "fixed look" required to produce the symptoms, eyelid flutter, and convergence.

Occasionally, otherwise normal individuals show intermittent, 15 to 30 Hz frequency, low amplitude (0.1 to 0.5 degrees) horizontal oscillations (not detected on visual inspection but seen with the ophthalmoscope) termed microsaccadic flutter (Ashe, 1991). Patients with microsaccadic flutter often complain of "shimmering," "jiggling," "wavy," or "laser beams" with paroxysms of visual disturbances lasting seconds to hours. Dizziness or dysequilibrium often accompanies the visual symptoms. Most patients are otherwise normal, although one patient had multiple sclerosis. Clonazepam, propranolol, and verapamil may reduce visual symptoms in some patients (Ashe, 1991).

Ocular flutter is a burst of to-and-fro horizontal saccades without an intersaccadic interval. Opsoclonus (saccadomania) is similar to ocular flutter, except that in opsoclonus there are conjugate, involuntary, large amplitude saccades in all directions. Like ocular flutter, opsoclonus indicates brainstem, especially mesencephalic or pontine, or cerebellar disease (Digre, 1986; Hattori, 1988, 1993). Opsoclonus evident only during eye closure has been described with hereditary cerebellar ataxia (Hattori, 1993). Etiologies for ocular flutter and opsoclonus are outlined in Table 17–5.

Table 17–5. Etiologies of Ocular Flutter and Opsoclonus

Etiology	References
Viral encephalitis, meningitis, and other infections	Baringer, 1968; Blue, 1971; Bolthauser, 1979; Christoff, 1969; Cogan, 1968; Digre, 1986; Ellenberger, 1972; Estrin, 1977; Kalyanaranan, 1971; Kinsbourne, 1962; Lücking, 1975; McLean, 1970; Smith, 1960; Swanson, 1962; Tamura, 1971; Vejjajiva, 1977; Vignaendra, 1977; Zangemeister, 1979
Kinsbourne's myoclonic encephalopathy or dancing eyes and dancing feet or infantile polymyoclonia	Corrias, 1985; Digre, 1986; Dyken, 1968; Kaulfersch, 1984; Kinsbourne, 1962; Popescu, 1970
Neuroblastoma	Altman, 1976; Baker, 1985; Bolthauser, 1979; Brissaud, 1969; Digre, 1986; Farrelly, 1984; Fisher, 1994; Harel, 1987; Kinast, 1980; Larbrisseau, 1973; Mitchell, 1990; Moe, 1970; Sandok, 1971; Savino, 1975; Senelick, 1971; Soloman, 1968; Telander, 1989; Williams, 1972

Etiology	References
Paraneoplastic effect of other tumors, especially small-cell lung cancer and breast cancer	Alessi, 1940; Anderson, 1988; Bellur, 1975; Caviness, 1995; Corcia, 1997; Digre, 1986; Dropcho, 1986; Ellenberger, 1968; Furman, 1988; Graus, 1984; Herishanu, 1985; Herman, 1981; Hunter, 1986; Kilgo, 1984; Lechi, 1983; Luque, 1991; Nausieda, 1981; Ridley, 1987; Ross, 1967; Schwartz, 1990; Sheinman, 1982; Toupet, 1982; Tzuzaka, 1993; Wolprow, 1988
Intracranial tumors or cysts	Corcia, 1997; Digre, 1986; Tzuzaka, 1993
Trauma	Borodic, 1988; Robin, 1976; Turazzi, 1977
Hydrocephalus	Shetty, 1972
Hereditary cerebellar degeneration	Hattori, 1993
Thalamic hemorrhage, pontine hemorrhage, or vertebrobasilar vascular insufficiency	Boddie, 1972; Brichet, 1970; Keane, 1980
Multiple sclerosis	Francis, 1985; Gresty, 1980
Hyperosmolar stupor and coma	Matsamura, 1985; Noda, 1985; Weissman, 1989
Side effects of drugs, including: lithium; amitriptyline; cocaine; phenytoin and diazepam; phenelzine and imipramine	Au, 1979; Cohen, 1974; Dehaene, 1987; Fisher, 1990; Scharf, 1989
Toxic exposures, including thallium, toluene, chlordecone, strychnine, DDT, and organophosphates	Blain, 1982; Garcin, 1965; Lazar, 1983; Maccario, 1975; Pullicino, 1989; Taylor, 1978
Associated with other miscellaneous diseases, including acute polyradiculoneuritis, viral hepatitis, cherry-red spot-myoclonus syndrome, sarcoidosis, and AIDS	Gizzi, 1990; Jabs, 1989; Pepin, 1981; Rosa, 1988; Salonen, 1988; Sogg, 1979; Toupet, 1982
In neonates, as either a transient benign phenomenon or related to brain injury due to anoxia, intracranial hemorrhage, or Leber's congenital amaurosis	Bienfang, 1974; Hoyt, 1977, 1980

In patients with viral encephalitis, meningitis, and other infections, the opsoclonus may occur after a prodromal illness, including gastrointestinal tract symptoms, upper respiratory symptoms, malaise, and fever (Aikawa, 1984; Baringer, 1968; Blue, 1971; Bolthauser, 1979; Christoff, 1969; Cogan, 1954, 1968; Dalrymple, 1980; Delreaux, 1988; Digre, 1986; Ellenberger, 1972; Estrin, 1977; Evans, 1982; Hankey, 1987; Hashiba, 1984; Herve, 1988; Jabbari, 1981; Kalyanaraman, 1971; Kinsbourne, 1962; Kuban, 1983; Lucking, 1975; McLean, 1970; Nichelli, 1984; Rivner, 1982; Rosa, 1980; Sachdeva, 1984; Smith, 1960; Swanson, 1962; Tamura, 1971; Terao, 1986; Toupet, 1982; Vejjavjiva, 1977; Vignaendra, 1977; Wertenbaker, 1981; Zangemeister, 1979). The opsoclonus in these patients is often associated with truncal ataxia and other cerebellar signs, long tract signs, tremulousness, and myoclonus of the trunk and limbs. Spinal fluid studies often show increased protein and a mononuclear pleocytosis. The illness usually resolves in a few weeks or months, although the course may be protracted and recovery incomplete, especially in children (Kinsbourne's myoclonic encephalopathy or dancing eyes and dancing feet or infantile polymyoclonia) (Corrias, 1985; Digre, 1986; Dyken, 1968; Kaulfersch, 1984; Kinsbourne, 1962; Popescu, 1970). Opsoclonus occurs in 2% of children with neuroblastoma and, conversely, 50% of children with opsoclonus/myoclonus have neuroblastoma (Altman, 1976;

Baker, 1985; Bolthauser, 1979; Brissaud, 1969; Digre, 1986; Farrelly, 1984; Fisher, 1994; Harel, 1987; Kinast, 1980; Larbrisseau, 1973; Mitchell, 1990; Moe, 1970; Sandok, 1971; Savino, 1975; Senelick, 1971; Soloman, 1968; Telander, 1989; Warrier, 1985; Williams, 1972). Opsoclonus appears before the discovery of a neuroblastoma in over 50% of the cases and neuroblastomas associated with opsoclonus have a tendency to be located within the thorax. Opsoclonus may also develop as a paraneoplastic effect of other tumors, especially small-cell lung cancer and breast cancer (Alessi, 1940; Anderson, 1988; Bellur, 1975; Caviness, 1995; Corcia, 1997; Digre, 1986; Dropcho, 1986; Ellenberger, 1968; Furman, 1988; Graus, 1984; Herishanu, 1985; Herman, 1981; Hunter, 1986; Kilgo, 1983; Lechi, 1983; Luque, 1991; Nausieda, 1981; Ridley, 1987; Ross, 1967; Schwartz, 1990; Sheinman, 1982; Toupet, 1982; Tzuzaka, 1993; Wolprow, 1988). Approximately 20% of patients with opsoclonus-myoclonus in adults have an underlying tumor. In patients with small-cell lung cancer, opsoclonus usually antedates the diagnosis of the neoplasm, while in patients with breast cancer, opsoclonus develops before the diagnosis of the tumor in only half the patients. Although opsoclonus in these patients may occur as an isolated sign, it is more often associated with myoclonus, ataxia, and encephalopathy. The cerebrospinal fluid may show an elevated protein and a mild pleocytosis. Patients with breast cancer and opsoclonus/myoclonus may demonstrate an anti-Ri antibody (anti-neuronal nuclear antibody 2 or ANNA-2) in their serum.

The evaluation of ocular flutter and opsoclonus depends on the age of the patient and the clinical circumstances. In children or adults with prodromal symptoms and signs of systemic or central nervous system infection, neuroimaging (preferably MR imaging) followed by spinal tap are warranted. In children without apparent infection, a search for occult neuroblastoma is indicated with studies variably including chest X ray, CT or MR imaging of chest and abdomen, skeletal survey, intravenous pyelogram, bone marrow biopsy, and determination of urinary catecholamines. In adults, without signs of infection, an occult malignancy should be sought with work-up including: gynecological examination; chest X ray; CT or MR imaging of the chest, abdomen, and pelvis; mammogram; possible bone marrow biopsy; and serum anti-Ri antibody (anti-neuronal nuclear antibody 2 or ANNA-2). MR imaging of the brain is warranted for most patients. A history of drug or toxic exposures should be sought in all patients. In some circumstances, other blood studies to be considered include serum osmolality, HIV titers, and ACE levels for sarcoidosis.

The treatment of ocular flutter and opsoclonus is initially directed at the underlying etiology (e.g., underlying neoplasm). Symptomatic reduction of the eye movements has been reported with ACTH, corticosteroids, clonazepam, baclofen, propranolol, thiamine, reserpine, and valproic acid (Digre, 1986; Fowler, 1976; Harada, 1986; Leigh, 1991; Nausieda, 1981; Sheinman, 1982; Spalton, 1980). High-dose intravenous immunoglobulin has been successful in several cases (Fisher, 1994; Pless, 1996).

The evaluation and treatment of opsoclonus are outlined in Figure 17–6.

What Are the Characteristics of Spontaneous Eye Oscillations in Stuporous and Comatose Patients?

In comatose patients, if the brainstem is intact, the eyelids are closed, and the eyes, slightly divergent, drift slowly from side to side (roving eye movements). The roving eye movements of light coma cannot be voluntarily executed and are therefore incompatible

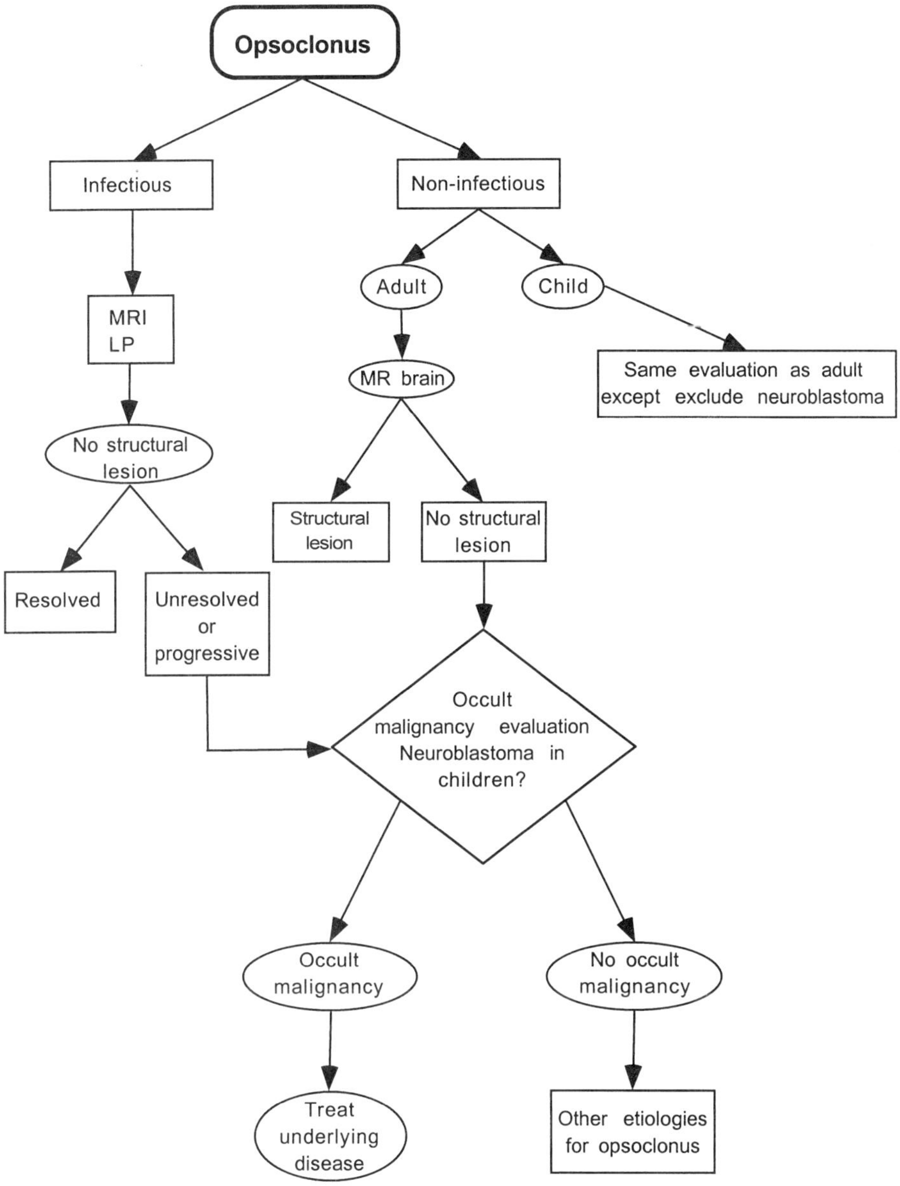

Figure 17–6. Opsoclonus.

with the diagnosis of feigned unresponsiveness. As coma deepens, roving eye movements disappear.

Other spontaneous eye movements seen in comatose patients include the following (see Table 17–6):

1. Short-cycle periodic alternating gaze (Ping-Pong gaze), which consists of roving of the eyes from one extreme of horizontal gaze to the other and back with each oscillating cycle taking 2.5 to 8 seconds (Ishikawa, 1993; Masucci, 1981; Stewart, 1979). This finding usually indicates bilateral cerebral damage (e.g., bilateral cerebral infarcts)

Table 17–6. Spontaneous Eye Movements in Comatose Patients

Movement	Description	Localization
Periodic alternating gaze (Ping-Pong gaze)	Cyclic horizontal roving	Bilateral cerebral damage, rarely posterior fossa lesion, hepatic, hypoxic, carbon monoxide, drug intoxication
Repetitive divergence	Slow deviation out, rapid return to primary	Metabolic encephalopathy
Nystagmoid jerk of a single eye	Vertical, horizontal, or rotatory movements	Middle or low pontine lesion
Status epilepticus	Small-amplitude vertical (occasionally horizontal) movements	Diffuse encephalopathy (hypoxia)
Ocular bobbing	Fast down, slow up	Pontine lesion, extra-axial posterior fossa mass, diffuse encephalopathy
Inverse ocular bobbing (ocular dipping)	Slow down, fast up	Anoxia, post status epilepticus (diffuse encephalopathy)
Reverse ocular bobbing	Fast up, slow down	Diffuse encephalopathy, rarely pontine lesion
Slow-upward ocular bobbing (converse ocular bobbing, reverse ocular dipping)	Slow up, fast down	Diffuse encephalopathy, rarely pontine lesion
Pretectal pseudobobbing	"V-pattern" down and in	Pretectal (hydrocephalus)
Vertical ocular myoclonus	Pendular, vertical isolated eye movements	Pontine lesion

Source: Adapted from Brazis PW, Masdeu JC, Biller J. *Localization in Clinical Neurology.* Third Edition. Little, Brown, Boston, 1996. With permission from the authors.

with an intact brainstem, but has also been described with posterior fossa hemorrhage, basal ganglia infarcts, bilateral cerebral peduncle lesions, hydrocephalus, hepatic encephalopathy, diffuse cerebral hypoxia, carbon monoxide intoxication, and overdose of the monoamine oxidase inhibitor trancypromine (Crevits, 1992; Ishikawa, 1993; Larmande, 1982, 1987a, 1987b; Masucci, 1981; Reynard, 1979; Senelick, 1976; Stewart, 1979; Watkins, 1989). The disorder may occasionally occur in coma with no structural hemispheric lesion (Larmande, 1987; Zegers, 1983).

Ping-Pong gaze must be differentiated from periodic alternating gaze deviation, which is an alternating horizontal conjugate gaze deviation lasting one to two minutes in each direction. Periodic alternating gaze deviation usually occurs in alert patients with structural lesions involving the cerebellum and brainstem, such as the Arnold-Chiari malformation or medulloblastoma, but has been described in obtunded or comatose patients with hepatic encephalopathy (Averbuch-Heller, 1995).

2. Repetitive divergence is rarely seen in patients with coma from metabolic encephalopathy (e.g., hepatic encephalopathy) (Noda, 1987). With this disorder, the eyes are midposition or slightly divergent at rest. They then slowly deviate out, become fully deviated for a brief period, and then rapidly return to primary position before repeating the cycle. These motions are synchronous in the two eyes.
3. Nystagmoid jerking of a single eye, in a vertical, horizontal, or rotatory fashion, may occur with mid- to lower pontine damage (Plum, 1980). Pontine lesions occasionally

give rise to disconjugate rotatory and vertical movements of the eyes, in which one eye may rise and intort as the other falls and extorts (Plum, 1980). This type of movement should not be confused with see-saw nystagmus, which is very seldom seen in comatose patients (Keane, 1978).

4. Electrographic status epilepticus without appendicular motor manifestations, due to anoxia, may result in brisk, small-amplitude, mainly vertical (occasionally horizontal) eye movements detectable by passive lid elevation (Simon, 1986).
5. Ocular bobbing refers to intermittent, often conjugate, brisk, bilateral downward movement of the eyes with slow return to midposition (Daroff, 1965; Fisher, 1964; Rosa, 1987). Ocular bobbing has been associated with intrinsic pontine lesions (e.g., hemorrhage, tumor, infarction, central pontine myelinolysis, etc.) (DeBeyl, 1983; Katz, 1982; Larmande, 1983; Mehler, 1988; Rosa, 1987; Tijssen, 1986), extra-axial posterior fossa masses (e.g., aneurysm rupture or cerebellar hemorrhage or infarction) (Bosch, 1975; Hameroff, 1969; Osenbach, 1986), diffuse encephalitis (Rudick, 1981), Jakob-Creutzfeldt disease (Rosa, 1987), and toxic-metabolic encephalopathies (e.g., acute organophosphate poisoning) (Drake, 1982; Hata, 1986; Susac, 1970). "Typical" ocular bobbing, which is associated with preserved horizontal eye movements, is thought to be specific but not pathognomonic of acute pontine injury, while "atypical" ocular bobbing, which is associated with absent horizontal eye movements, is thought to be less helpful in predicting the site of abnormality (Susac, 1970). Monocular bobbing (paretic bobbing), which consists of a quick downward movement of one eye and intorsion or no movement in the other eye, may occur if there is a coexistent unilateral fascicular oculomotor nerve palsy (Dehaene, 1993; Susac, 1970). Disconjugate ocular bobbing, with movements involving sometimes one eye and sometimes the other, may also occur without oculomotor nerve palsy (Gaymard, 1993).
6. Inverse ocular bobbing (ocular dipping or fast-upward ocular bobbing) (Goldschmidt, 1987; Knobler, 1981; Luda, 1982; Mehler, 1988; Ropper, 1981; Safran, 1983; Stark, 1984; Van Weerden, 1985) consists of a slow-downward eye movement with fast return to midposition, which may occur in anoxic coma or after prolonged status epilepticus (Knobler, 1981; Ropper, 1981; Stark, 1984). Ocular dipping has also been described associated with deafness in a patient with pinealblastoma (Toshniwal, 1986). Inverse/reverse ocular bobbing consists of inverse ocular bobbing in which the eyes do not stop on rapidly returning to primary position but shoot into upgaze and slowly return to midposition (Rosenberg, 1986; Titer, 1988).
7. Reverse ocular bobbing (fast-upward ocular bobbing) consists of fast-upward eye movement with a slow return to midposition, which may occur in patients with metabolic encephalopathy, viral encephalitis, or pontine hemorrhage (Brusa, 1984; Goldschmidt, 1986; Mehler, 1988). It has been described with coma due to combined phenothiazine and benzodiazepine poisoning (Lennox, 1993). Occasionally ocular bobbing, ocular dipping, and reverse bobbing may occur at different times in the same patient (Rosenberg, 1986).
8. Slow-upward ocular bobbing (converse ocular bobbing or reverse ocular dipping) is characterized by slow-upward eye movements followed by fast return to midposition (Goldschmidt, 1987; Mehler, 1988). This eye movement disorder has been described with pontine infarction (Brusa, 1984) and with metabolic or viral encephalopathy (i.e., diffuse cerebral dysfunction (Mehler, 1988).
9. Pretectal pseudobobbing has been described with acute hydrocephalus (Keane, 1985) and consists of arrhythmic, repetitive downward and inward ("V-pattern") eye movements at a rate ranging from 1 per 3 seconds to 2 per second and an amplitude of 1/5

to 1/2 of the full voluntary range. These movements may be mistaken for ocular bobbing, but their "V" pattern, their faster rate, and their pretectal rather than pontine-associated signs distinguish them from true pontine bobbing. Thus, patients with pretectal pseudobobbing may have abnormal pupillary light reactions, intact horizontal eye movements, open and often retracted eyelids, a blink frequently preceding each eye movement, and a mute or stuporous rather than a comatose state. Pretectal pseudobobbing probably represents a variety of convergence nystagmus and its presence usually indicates the need for prompt surgical attention (e.g., hydrocephalus decompression) (Keane, 1985). It is possible that some cases of "ocular bobbing" associated with thalamic hemorrhage or tentorial herniation may actually be cases of pretectal pseudobobbing.

10. Vertical ocular myoclonus consists of pendular, vertical isolated movements of the eyes noted in patients either locked-in or comatose after severe pontine strokes (Keane, 1986). Their frequency is 2 Hz, and other rhythmic body movements at a similar frequency occur after a 6-week to 9-month delay. These movements are generally associated with palatal myoclonus (palatal tremor), with which they share a common mechanism (Keane, 1986).

References

Abadi R, Pascal E. (1989). The recognition and management of albinism. *Ophthalmic Physiol Opt 9:*3–15.

Abadi RV, Pascal E. (1994). Periodic alternating nystagmus in humans with albinism. *Invest Ophthalmol Vis Sci 35:*4080–4086.

Abadi RV, Carden D, Simpson J. (1980). A new treatment for congenital nystagmus. *Br J Ophthalmol 64:*2–6.

Abel LA, Traccis S, Dell'Osso LF, Ansevin CF. (1983). Variable waveforms in downbeat nystagmus imply short-term gain changes. *Ann Neurol 13:*616–620.

Abel LA, Traccis S, Dell'Osso LF, et al. (1984). Square wave oscillation. The relationship of saccadic intrusions and oscillations. *Neuro-ophthalmology 4:*21–25.

Adler CH, Galetta SL. (1990). Oculo-facial-skeletal myorhythmia in Whipple disease: Treatment with ceftriaxone. *Ann Intern Med 112:*467–469.

Aikawa T, Takemiya T, Kobayoshi I, et al. (1984). An acute syndrome of opsoclonus and body tremulousness: A case of benign encephalitis. *No To Shinkei 36:*11–126.

Alessi D. (1940). Lesioni parenchimatose del cervelleto da carcinoma uterino (gliosi carcinotossica?). *Riv Pathol Nerv Ment 55:*1091–1094.

Allen ED, Davies PD. (1983). Role of contact lenses in the management of congenital nystagmus. *Br J Ophthalmol 67:*834–836.

Alpert JN. (1978). Downbeat nystagmus due to anticonvulsant toxicity. *Ann Neurol 4:*471–473.

Altman AJ, Baehner RL. (1976). (1986). Favorable prognosis for survival in children with coincident opsomyoclonus and neuroblastoma. *Cancer 37:*846–852. *Am Optom Assoc 57:*893–894.

Anderson JR. (1953). Causes and treatment of congenital eccentric nystagmus. *Br J Ophthalmol 37:*267–281.

Anderson NE, Budde-Steffen C, Rosenblum MK, et al. (1988). Opsoclonus, myoclonus, ataxia, and encephalopathy in adults with cancer: A distinct paraneoplastic syndrome. *Medicine 67:*100–109.

Anderson NE, Rosenblum MK, Posner JB. (1988). Paraneoplastic cerebellar degeneration: Clinical-immunological correlations. *Ann Neurol 24:*559–567.

Antony JH, Ouvier RA, Wise G. (1980). Spasmus nutans: A mistaken identity. *Arch Neurol 37:*373–375.

Arnoldi KA, Tychsen L. (1995). Prevalence of intracranial lesions in children initially diagnosed with disconjugate nystagmus (spasmus nutans). *J Pediatr Ophthalmol Strabismus 32:*296–301.

Aschoff JC, Conrad B, Kornhuber HH. (1974). Acquired pendular nystagmus with oscillopsia in multiple sclerosis: A sign of cerebellar nuclear disease. *J Neurol Neurosurg Psych 37:*570–577.

Ashe J, Hain TC, Zee DS, Schatz NJ. (1991). Microsaccadic flutter. *Brain 114:*461–472.

Au WJ, Keltner JL. (1979). Opsoclonus with amitriptyline overdose. *Ann Neurol 6:*87.

Averbuch-Heller L, Meiner Z. (1995). Reversible periodic alternating gaze deviation in hepatic encephalopathy. *Neurology 45:*191–192.

Averbuch-Heller L, Zivotofsky AZ, Das VE, et al. (1995). Investigations of the pathogenesis of acquired pendular nystagmus. *Brain 118:*369–378.

Baker ME, Kirks DR, Korobkin M, et al. (1985). The association of neuroblastoma and myoclonic encephalopathy: An imaging approach. *Pediatr Radiol 15:*185–189.

Baloh RW, Spooner JW. (1981). Downbeat nystagmus: A type of central vestibular nystagmus. *Neurology 31:*304–310.

Baloh RW, Yee RD. (1989). Spontaneous vertical nystagmus. *Rev Neurol 145:*527–532.

Baloh RW, Honrubia V, Jacobson K. (1987). Benign positional vertigo: Clinical and oculographic features in 240 cases. *Neurology 37:*371–378.

Baloh RW, Honrubia V, Konrad HR. (1976). Periodic alternating nystagmus. *Brain 99:*11–26.

Baloh RW, Jacobson K, Honrubia V. (1993). Horizontal semicircular canal variant of benign positional vertigo. *Neurology 43:*2542–2549.

Baloh RW, Konrad HR, Dirks D, Honrubia V. (1976). Cerebellar-pontine angle tumors: Results of quantitative vestibulo-ocular testing. *Arch Neurol 33:*507–512.

Baloh RW, Yue Q, Jacobson KM, Honrubia V. (1995). Persistent direction-changing positional nystagmus: Another variant of benign positional nystagmus? *Neurology 45:*1297–1301.

Baram TZ, Tang R. (1986). Atypical spasmus nutans as an initial sign of thalamic neoplasm. *Pediatr Neurol 2:*375–376.

Baringer JR, Sweeney VP, Winkler GF. (1968). An acute syndrome of ocular oscillations and truncal myoclonus. *Brain 91:*473–480.

Barry E. (1986). Epileptic gaze deviation and nystagmus. *Neurology 36:*875–876.

Barton JJS, Cox TA. (1993). Acquired pendular nystagmus in multiple sclerosis: Clinical observations and role of optic neuropathy. *J Neurol Neurosurg Psych 56:*262–267.

Barton JJS, Huaman AG, Sharpe JA. (1994). Muscarinic antagonists in the treatment of acquired pendular nystagmus: a double-blind, randomized trial of three intravenous drugs. *Ann Neurol 35:*319–325.

Barton JJS. (1995). Blink- and saccade-induced seesaw nystagmus. *Neurology 45:*831.

Bellur SN. (1975). Opsoclonus: Its clinical value. *Neurology 25:*502–507.

Bender MB, Nathanson M, Gordon GG. (1952). Myoclonus of muscles of the eye, face, and throat. *Arch Neurol Psych 67:*44–58.

Benjamin EE, Zimmerman CF, Troost BT. (1986). Lateropulsion and upbeat nystagmus are manifestations of central vestibular dysfunction. *Arch Neurol 43:*962–964.

Berger JR, Kovacs AG. (1982). Downbeat nystagmus with phenytoin. *J Clin Neuro-ophthalmol 2:*209–211.

Bergin DJ, Halpern J. (1986). Congenital see-saw nystagmus associated with retinitis pigmentosa. *Ann Ophthalmol 18:*346–349.

Beun AM, Beintema DJ, Binnie CD, et al. (1984). Epileptic nystagmus. *Epilepsia 25:*609–614.

Bienfang DC. (1974). Opsoclonus in infancy. *Arch Ophthalmol 91:*203–205.

Bilska C, Pociej-Zero M, Krzystkowa KM. (1995). Surgical treatment of congenital nystagmus in 463 children (Polish). *Klin Oczna 97:*140–141.

Bixenman WW. (1983). Congenital hereditary downbeat nystagmus. *Can J Ophthalmol 18:*344–348.

Blain PG, Nightingale S, Stodart JC. (1982). Strychnine poisoning: Abnormal eye movements. *J Toxicol 19:*215–217.

Blue SK, Janeway R, Stanley JA. (1971). Opsoclonus and body tremulousness: A case report with suggested cause. *Trans Am Neurol Assoc 96:*208–210.

Boddie HG. (1972). Ocular bobbing and opsoclonus. *J Neurol Neurosurg Psych 35:*739–742.

Bogousslavsky J, Regli F. (1985). Monocular downbeat nystagmus. *J Neurol 232:*99–101.

Bogousslavsky J, Regli F, Hungerbuhler JP. (1980). Downbeat nystagmus. *Neuro-ophthalmology 1:*137–143.

Bogousslavsky J. (1981). Downbeat nystagmus. Specificity in malformations of the cervico-occipital sulcus (French). *Rev Med Suisse Romande 101:*201–204.

Bolthauser E, Deonna T, Hirt HR. (1979). Myoclonic encephalopathy of infants or 'dancing eyes syndrome.' *Helv Paediatr Acta 34:*119–133.

Bondar RL, Sharpe JA, Lewis AJ. (1984). Rebound nystagmus in olivocerebellar atrophy: A clinico-pathologic correlation. *Ann Neurol 15:*474–477.

Borodic GE, Miller DC, Blenfang DC. (1988). Opsoclonus: Three cases and literature review. In Smith LJ (ed). *Neuro-ophthalmology Enters the Nineties*. Hialeah, Florida, Dutton Press, pp. 213–232.

Bosch EP, Kennedy SS, Aschenbrener CA. (1975). Ocular bobbing: The myth of its localizing value. *Neurology 25:*949–953.

Bosley TM, Cohen DA, Schatz NJ, et al. (1985). Comparison of metrizamide computed tomography and magnetic resonance imaging in the evaluation of lesions of the cervicomedullary junction. *Neurology 35:*485–492.

Brandt T. (1990). Positional and positioning vertigo and nystagmus. *J Neurol Sci 95:*3–28.

Brandt T. (1991). Man in motion. Historical and clinical aspects of vestibular function. *Brain 114:*2159–2174.

Brazis PW, Miller NR, Henderer JD, Lee AG. (1994). The natural history and results of treatment of superior oblique myokymia. *Arch Ophthalmol 112:*1063–1067.

Brichet B, André JM, Reny A, et al. (1970). Étude électromyographique d'opsoclonies survenues au cours d'un syndrome d'insuffisance vertebrobasilaire. *Rev Neurol 122:*439–443.

Brissaud HE, Beavais P. (1969). Opsoclonus and neuroblastoma. *New Eng J Med 280:*1242.

Bronstein AM, Miller DH, Rudge P, Kendall BE. (1987). Down beating nystagmus: Magnetic resonance imaging and neuro-otological findings. *J Neurol Sci 81:*173–184.

Brusa A, Firpo MP, Massa S, et al. (1984). Typical and reverse bobbing: A case with localizing value. *Eur Neurol 23:*151–155.

Burde RM, Savino PJ, Trobe JD. (1991). *Clinical decisions in Neuro-ophthalmology*. 2nd edition. St Louis, Mosby Yearbook, pp. 289–320.
Büttner U, Helmchen C, Büttner-Ennever JA. (1995). The localizing value of nystagmus in brainstem disorders. *Neuro-ophthalmology 15*:283–290.
Campbell WW Jr. (1980). Periodic alternating nystagmus in phenytoin intoxication. *Arch Neurol 37*:178–180.
Carlow TJ. (1986). Medical treatment of nystagmus and ocular motor disorders. In Beck RW, Smith CH, (eds). *Neuro-ophthalmology*. Boston, Little Brown, pp. 251–264.
Carruthers J. (1995). The treatment of congenital nystagmus with Botox. *J Pediatr Ophthalmol Strabismus 32*:306–308.
Caviness JN, Forsyth PA, Layton DD, McPhee TJ. (1995). The movement disorder of adult opsoclonus. *Movement Dis 10*:22–27.
Chait GE, Barber HO. (1979). Arnold-Chiari malformation—Some otoneurological features. *J Otolaryngol 8*:65–70.
Chambers BR, Ell JJ, Gresty MA. (1983). Case of downbeat nystagmus influenced by otolith stimulation. *Ann Neurol 13*:204–207.
Chan T, Logan P, Eustace P. (1991). Intermittent downbeat nystagmus secondary to veremian aracnoid cyst with associated obstructive hydrocephalus. *J Clin Neuro-ophthalmol 11*:293–296.
Christoff N. (1969). Myoclonic encephalopathy of infants. *Arch Neurol 21*:229–234.
Chrousos GA, Cowdry R, Schuelein M, et al. (1987). Two cases of downbeat nystagmus and oscillopsia associated with carbamazepine. *Am J Ophthalmol 103*:221–224.
Cibis GW, Fitzgerald KM. (1993). Electroretinography in congenital idiopathic nystagmus. *Pediatr Neurol 9*:369–371.
Ciuffreda KJ. (1980). Voluntary nystagmus: A new finding and clinical implications. *Am J Opyom Physiol Opt 57*:795–800.
Ciuffreda KJ, Goldrich SG, Neary C. (1982). Use of eye movement auditory biofeedback in the control of nystagmus. *Am J Optom Physiol Optics 59*:396–409.
Clarke WN, Noel L-P, Baylock JF. (1988). Rotatory nystagmus in infantile esotropia. *Can J Ophthalmol 23*:270–272.
Cochin JP, Hannequin D, Do Marcolino C, et al. (1995). Intermittent see-saw nystagmus successfully treated with clonazepam (French). *Rev Neurol (Paris) 151*:60–62.
Cogan DG. (1954). Ocular dysmetria: Flutter-like oscillation of eyes and opsoclonus. *Arch Ophthalmol 51*:318–335.
Cogan DG. (1959). Convergence nystagmus with notes on a single case of divergence nystagmus. *Arch Ophthalmol 62*:295–299.
Cogan DG. (1968). Down-beat nystagmus. *Arch Ophthalmol 80*:757–768.
Cogan DG. (1968). Opsoclonus, body tremulousness, and benign encephalitis. *Arch Ophthalmol 79*:545–551.
Cohen WJ, Cohen NH. (1974). Lithium carbonate, haloperidol, and irreversible brain damage. *JAMA 230*:1283–1287.
Coker S, Susac J, Sharpe J, Smallridge R. (1979). Cockayne's syndrome. Neuro-ophthalmic, CAT scan and endocrine observations. In Smith JL (ed). *Neuro-ophthalmology Focus 1980*. New York, Masson, pp. 379–385.
Collewijn H, Apkarian P, Spekrejjse H. (1985). The oculomotor behavior of human albinos. *Brain 108*:1–28.
Condon RM. (1970). Voluntary nystagmus. *Am J Arch Am Acad Optom 47*:415–417.
Coppeto JR, Monteiro ML, Lessell S, et al. (1983). Downbeat nystagmus. Long-term therapy with moderate-dose lithium carbonate. *Arch Neurol 40*:754–755.
Corbett JJ, Jacobson DM, Thompson HS, et al. (1989). Downbeating nystagmus and other ocular motor defects caused by lithium toxicity. *Neurology 39*:481–487.
Corcia P, De Toffol B, Hommet C, et al. (1997). Paraneoplastic opsoclonus associated with cancer of the gall bladder. *J Neurol Neurosurg Psych 60*:293.
Coren S, Komada MK. (1972). Eye movement control in voluntary nystagmus. *Am J Ophthalmol 74*:1161–1165.
Corkill G, Vijayan N. (1976). Saccadic visual suppression and down-beat nystagmus: A case of Arnold-Chiari malformation. *Surg Neurol 5*:95–96.
Corrias A, Nurchi AM, Rossi G, et al. (1985). Opsoclonic encephalopathy in childhood (Kinsbourne syndrome) (Italian). *Pediatr Med Chir 7*:437–441.
Costin JA, Smith JL, Emery S, Tomsak RL. (1980). Alcoholic downbeat nystagmus. *Ann Ophthalmol 12*:1127–1131.
Cox TA. (1979). Rebound nystagmus. An adult with Dandy-Walker syndrome. *J Kans Med Soc 80*:414–416.
Cox TA, Corbett JJ, Thompson HS, Lennarson L. (1981). Upbeat nystagmus changing to downbeat nystagmus with convergence. *Neurology 31*:891–892.
Crevits L, Decruyenaere J. (1992). 'Ping-pong' gaze. *Neuro-ophthalmology 12*:121–123.
Cross SA, Smith JL, Norton EWD. (1982). Periodic alternating nystagmus clearing after vitrectomy. *J Clin Neuro-ophthalmol 2*:5–11.
Currie JN, Matsuo V. (1986). The use of clonazepam in the treatment of nystagmus-induced oscillopsia. *Ophthalmology 93*:924–932.
D'Esposito M, Reccia R, Roberti G, Russo P. (1989). Amount of surgery in congenital nystagmus. *Ophthalmologica 198*:145–151.
Dalrymple JM. (1980). Opsoclonus and generalized tremulousness. *Clini-Pearls 3*:6–7.
Daroff RB. (1965a). See-saw nystagmus. *Neurology 15*:874–877.
Daroff RB, Dell'Osso LF. (1974). Periodic alternating nystagmus and the shifting null. *Can J Otolaryngol 3*:367–371.
Daroff RB, Troost BT. (1973). Upbeat nystagmus. *JAMA 225*:312.
Daroff RB, Waldman AL. (1965b). Ocular bobbing. *J Neurol Neurosurg Psych 28*:375–377.

Davis GV, Shock JP. (1975). Septo-optic dysplasia associated with see-saw nystagmus. *Arch Ophthalmol 93:*137–139.
De la Meilleure G, Dehaene I, Depondt M, et al. (1996). Benign paroxysmal positional vertigo of the horizontal canal. *J Neurol Neurosurg Psych 60:*68–71.
de Sa LC, Good WV, Hoyt CS. (1992). Surgical management of myokymia of the superior oblique muscle. *Am J Ophthalmol 114:*693–696.
DeBeyl DZ, Flament-Durand J, Borenstein S, Brunko E. (1983). Ocular bobbing and myoclonus in central pontine myelinolysis. *J Neurol Neurosurg Psych 46:*564–565.
Dehaene I, Van Vleymen B. (1987). Opsoclonus induced by phenytoin and diazepam. *Ann Neurol 21:*216.
Dehaene I, Van Zanddijcke M. (1984). See-saw jerk nystagmus. *Neuro-ophthalmol 4:*261–263.
Dehaene I, Lammens M, Marchau M. (1993). Paretic ocular bobbing. A clinicopathological study of two cases. *Neuro-ophthalmol 13:*143–146.
Dell'Osso LF, Daroff RB. (1975). Congenital nystagmus waveforms and foveation strategy. *Doc Ophthalmol 39:*155–182.
Dell'Osso LF, Flynn JT. (1979). Congenital nystagmus surgery. A quantitative evaluation of the effects. *Arch Ophthalmol 97:*462–469.
Dell'Osso LF, Abel LA, Daroff RB. (1977). "Inverse latent" macro square-wave jerks and macro saccadic oscillations. *Ann Neurol 2:*57–60.
Dell'Osso LF, Abel LA, Daroff RB. (1987). Latent/manifest latent nystagmus reversal using an ocular prosthesis: Implications for vision and ocular dominance. *Invest Ophthalmol Vis Sci 28:*1873–1876.
Dell'Osso LF, Schmidt D, Daroff RB. (1979). Latent, manifest latent, and congenital nystagmus. *Arch Ophthalmol 97:*1877–1885.
Dell'Osso LF, Traccis S, Abel LA, Erzurum SI. (1988). Contact lenses and congenital nystagmus. *Clin Vision Sci 3:*229–232.
Dell'Osso LF, Traccis S, Abel LA. (1983). Strabismus—A necessary condition for latent and manifest latent nystagmus. *Neuro-ophthalmology 3:*247–257.
Dell'Osso LF, Troost BT, Daroff RB. (1975). Macro square wave jerks. *Neurology 25:*975–979.
Dell'Osso LF, Weissman BM, Leigh RJ, et al. (1993). Hereditary congenital nystagmus and gaze-holding failure: The role of the neural integrator. *Neurology 43:*1741–1749.
Delreux V, Kever L, Sindic CJM, Callewaert A. (1988). Opsoclonus secondary to an Epstein-Barr virus infection. *Neuro-ophthalmology 8:*179–189.
DiBartolomeo JR, Yee RD. (1988). Periodic alternating nystagmus. *Otolaryngol Head Neck Surg 99:*552–557.
Dickenson CM. (1986). The elucidation and use of the effect of near fixation in congenital nystagmus. *Ophthalmic Physiol Opt 6:*303–311.
Dieterich M, Straube A, Brandt T, et al. (1991). The effects of baclofen and cholinergic drugs on upbeat and downbeat nystagmus. *J Neurol Neurosurg Psych 54:*627–632.
Digre KB. (1986). Opsoclonus in adults. Report of three cases and review of the literature. *Arch Neurol 43:*1165–1175.
Donat JR, Auger R. (1979). Familial periodic ataxia. *Arch Neurol 36:*568–569.
Donin JF. (1967). Acquired monocular nystagmus in children. *Can J Ophthalmol 2:*212–215.
Drachman DA. (1966). See-saw nystagmus. *J Neurol Neurosurg Psych 29:*356–361.
Drake ME Jr, Erwin CW, Massey EW. (1982). Ocular bobbing in metabolic encephalopathy: Clinical, pathologic, and electrophysiologic study. *Neurology 32:*1029–1031.
Dropcho E, Payne R. (1986). Paraneoplastic opsoclonus myoclonus. Association with medullary thyroid carcinoma and review of the literature. *Arch Neurol 43:*410–415.
Druckman R, Ellis P, Kleinfeld J, Waldman M. (1966). See-saw nystagmus. *Arch Ophthalmol 76:*668–675.
Dyken P, Kolar O. (1968). Dancing eyes, dancing feet: Infantile polymyoclonia. *Brain 91:*305–320.
Eber AM, Rumbach L, Bataillard M, et al. (1982). See-saw nystagmus and oculomotor disorders in unilateral thalmopeduncular softening (French). *Rev Otoneuro-ophthalmol 54:*173–178.
Elidan J, Gay I, Lev S. (1984). Square wave jerks—Incidence, characteristics, and significance. *J Otolaryngol 13:*375–381.
Ellenberger C, Campa JF, Netsky MG. (1968). Opsoclonus and parenchymatous degeneration of the cerebellum. *Neurology 18:*1041–1046.
Ellenberger C, Keltner JL, Stroud MH. (1972). Ocular dyskinesia in cerebellar disease. *Brain 95:*685–692.
Elliott AJ, Simpson EM, Oakhill A, Decock R. (1989). Nystagmus after medulloblastoma. *Dev Med Child Neurol 31:*43–46.
Engelhardt A, Neurndorfer B. (1988). Downbeat nystagmus in lithium medication (German). *Nervenarzt 59:*624–627.
Estrin WJ. (1977). The serological diagnosis of St Louis encephalitis in a patient with the syndrome of opsoclonia, body tremulousness, and benign encephalitis. *Ann Neurol 1:*596–598.
Evans RW, Welch KWA. (1982). Opsoclonus in a confirmed case of St Louis encephalitis. *J Neurol Neurosurg Psych 45:* 660–661.
Faria MA Jr, Spector RH, Tindall GT. (1980). Downbeat nystagmus as the salient manifestation of the Arnold-Chiari malformation. *Surg Neurol 13:*333–336.
Farmer J, Hoyt CS. (1984). Monocular nystagmus in infancy and early childhood. *Am J Ophthalmol 98:*504–509.
Farrelly C, Daneman A, Chan HSL, et al. (1984). Occult neuroblastoma presenting with opsomyoclonus. *Am J Rad 142:*807–810.

Farris BK, Smith JL, Ayyar DR. (1986). Neuro-ophthalmologic findings in vestibulocerebellar ataxia. *Arch Neurol 43:*1050–1053.

Fein JM, Williams RDB. (1969). See-saw nystagmus. *J Neurol Neurosurg Psych 32:*202–207.

Feldon SE, Langston JW. (1977). Square-wave jerks: A disorder of microsaccades? *Neurology 27:*278–281.

Fisher A, Gresty M, Chambers B, Rudge P. (1983). Primary position upbeating nystagmus. A variety of central positional nystagmus. *Brain 106:*949–964.

Fisher CM. (1964). Ocular bobbing. *Arch Neurol 11:*543–546.

Fisher CM. (1990). Ocular flutter. *J Clin Neuro-ophthalmol 10:*155–156.

Fisher PG, Wechsler DS, Singer HS. (1994). Anti-Hu antibody in a neuroblastoma-associated paraneoplastic syndrome. *Pediatr Neurol 10:*309–312.

FitzGibbon EJ, Calvert PC, Dieterich M, et al. (1996). Torsional nystagmus during vertical pursuit. *J Neuro-ophthamol 16:*79–90.

Flynn J, Dell'Osso LF. (1981). Surgery of congenital nystagmus. *Trans Ophthalmol Soc UK 101:*431–433.

Forsythe WI. (1955). Congenital hereditary vertical nystagmus. *J Neurol Neurosurg Psych 18:*196–198.

Fowler GW. (1976). Propranolol treatment of infantile polymyoclonia. *Neuropediatrics 7:*443–449.

Francis DA, Heron JR. (1985). Ocular flutter in suspected multiple sclerosis: A presenting paroxysmal manifestation. *Postgrad Med J 61:*333–371.

Friedman DI, Jankovic J, McCrary JA 3rd. (1992). Neuro-ophthalmic findings in progressive supranuclear palsy. *J Clin Neuro-ophthalmol 12:*104–109.

Frisen I, Wikkelso C. (1986). Posttraumatic seesaw nystagmus abolished by ethanol injestion. *Neurology 36:*841–844.

Fujikane M, Katayama S, Hirata K, Sunami S. (1992). Central diabetes insipidus complicated with upbeat nystagmus and cerebellar ataxia (Japanese). *Rinsho Shinkeigaku 32:*68–72.

Fukazawa T, Tashino K, Hamada T, Kase M. (1986). Multisystem degeneration: Drugs and square wave jerks. *Neurology 36:*1230–1233.

Fukuda Y, Shinoda K, Konishi S, et al. (1984). A case of Arnold-Chiari malformation with macrosquare wave jerks (Japanese). *Rinsho Shinkeigaku 24:*1035–1038.

Funahashi K, Kuwata T, Yabumoto M, et al. (1988). Congenital vertical pendular nystagmus in sisters. *Ophthalmologica 196:*137–142.

Furman JM, Baloh RW, Chugani JH, et al. (1985). Infantile cerebellar atrophy. *Ann Neurol 17:*399–402.

Furman JMR, Baloh RW, Yee RD. (1986). Eye movement abnormalities in a family with cerebellar vermian atrophy. *Acta Otolaryngol 101:*371–377.

Furman JM, Brownstone PK, Baloh RW. (1985). Atypical brainstem encephalitis: Magnetic resonance imaging and oculographic features. *Neurology 35:*438–440.

Furman JM, Crumrine PK, Reinmuth OM. (1990). Epileptic nystagmus. *Ann Neurol 27:*686–688.

Furman JMR, Eidelman BH, Fromm GH. (1988). Spontaneous remission of paraneoplastic ocular flutter and saccadic intrusions. *Neurology 38:*499–501.

Furman JMR, Wall C III, Pang D. (1990). Vestibular function in periodic alternating nystagmus. *Brain 113:*1425–1439.

Gans MS, Melmed CA. (1990). Downbeat nystagmus associated with dolichoectasia of the vertebrobasilar artery. *Arch Neurol 47:*843.

Garcin MR, Ginsbourg M, Godlewski ST, Emile J. (1965). Intoxication par le DDT: Syndrome méningo-encéphalique aigu régressif avec décharges cloniques diffuses et movements désordonnés "en salves" des globes oculaires. *Rev Neurol 113:*559–564.

Gay AJ, Brodkey J, Miller JE. (1963). Convergence retraction nystagmus. An electromyographic study. *Arch Ophthalmol 70:*456–461.

Gaymard B. (1993). Disconjugate ocular bobbing. *Neurology 43:*2151.

Gelbart SS, Hoyt CS. (1988). Congenital nystagmus: A clinical perspective in infancy. *Graefe's Arch Clin Exp Ophthalmol 226:*178–180.

Gilman N, Baloh RW, Tomiyasu U. (1977). Primary position upbeat nystagmus. A clinicopathologic study. *Neurology 27:*294–298.

Gizzi M, Randolph S, Perakis A. (1990). Ocular flutter in vidarabine toxicity. *Am J Ophthalmol 109:*105.

Goldberg RT. (1978). Vertical pendular nystagmus in chronic myositis of medial and lateral rectus. *Ann Ophthalmol 10:*1697–1702.

Goldblum TA, Effron LA. (1994). Upbeat nystagmus associated with tonic downward deviation in healthy neonates. *J Pediatr Ophthalmol Strabismus 31:*334–335.

Goldschmidt TJ, Wall M. (1987). Slow-upward ocular bobbing. *J Clin Neuro-ophthalmol 7:*241–243.

Good PA, Searle AET, Campbell S, Crews SJ. (1989). Value of the ERG in congenital nystagmus. *Br J Ophthalmol 73:*512–515.

Good WV, Brodsky MC, Hoyt CS, Ahn JC. (1990). Upbeating nystagmus in infants: A sign of anterior visual pathway disease. *Binocular Vision Quarterly 5:*13–18.

Good WV, Koch TS, Jan JE. (1993). Monocular nystagmus caused by unilateral anterior visual-pathway lesions. *Dev Med Child Neurol 35:*1106–1110.

Gorman WF, Brock S. (1950). Periodic alternating nystagmus in Friedreich's ataxia. *Am J Ophthalmol 33:*860–864.

Gottlob I, Wizov SS, Reincke RD. (1995a). Quantitative eye and head movement recordings of retinal disease mimicking spasmus nutans. *Am J Ophthalmol 119:*374–376.

Gottlob I, Wizov SS, Reincke RD. (1995b). Spasmus nutans. A long-term follow-up. *Invest Ophthalmol Vis Sci 36:*2768–2771.

Gottlob I, Zubcov A, Catalan RA, et al. (1990). Signs distinguishing spasmus nutans (with and without central nervous system lesions) from infantile nystagmus. *Ophthalmology 97:*1166–1175.

Gracia F, Koch J, Aziz N. (1985). Downbeat nystagmus as a side effect of lithium carbonate: Case report. *J Clin Psych 46:*292–293.

Grant MP, Cohen M, Petersen RB, et al. (1993). Abnormal eye movements in Creutzfeldt-Jacob disease. *Ann Neurol 34:*192–197.

Graus F, Cordon-Cardo C, Cho E, et al. (1984). Opsoclonus and oat cell carcinoma of the lung: Lack of evidence for anti-CNS antibodies. *Lancet 1:*1479.

Gresty M, Leech J, Sanders M, Eggars H. (1976). A study of head and eye movements in spasmus nutans. *Br J Ophthalmol 60:*652–654.

Gresty MA, Metcalfe T, Timms C, et al. (1992). Neurology of latent nystagmus. *Brain 115:*1303–1321.

Gresty M, Page N, Barratt H. (1984). The differential diagnosis of congenital nystagmus. *J Neurol Neurosurg Psych 47:*936–942.

Gresty MA, Bronstein AM, Brookes GB, Rudge P. (1988). Primary position upbeating nystagmus associated with middle ear disease. *Neuro-ophthalmology 8:*321–328.

Gresty MA, Bronstein AM, Page NG, Rudge P. (1991). Congenital-type nystagmus emerging in later life. *Neurology 41:*653–656.

Gresty MA, Ell JJ, Findley LJ. (1982). Acquired pendular nystagmus: its characteristics, localizing value and pathophysiology. *J Neurol Neurosurg Psych 45:*431–439.

Gresty MA, Findley LJ, Wade P. (1980). Mechanism of rotatory eye movements in opsoclonus. *Br J Ophthalmol 64:*923–925.

Grotta JC, Pettigrew LC, Schmidt WA, et al. (1987). Oculomasticatory myorhythmia. *Ann Neurol 22:*395–396.

Guy JR, Schatze NJ. (1988). Paraneoplastic downbeating nystagmus: A sign of occult malignancy. *J Clin Neuro-ophthalmol 8:*269–272.

Guyer DR, Lessell S. (1986). Periodic alternating nystagmus associated with albinism. *J Clin Neuroophthamol 6:*82–85.

Haene I, Casselman J. (1993). Left superior oblique myokymia and right superior oblique paralysis due to a posterior fossa tumor. *Neuro-ophthalmol 13:*13–16.

Halmagyi CM, Rudge P, Gresty MA, Sanders MD. (1983). Downbeating nystagmus. A review of 62 cases. *Arch Neurol 40:*777–784.

Halmagyi GM, Hoyt WF. (1991). See-saw nystagmus due to unilateral mesodiencephalic lesion. *J Clin Neuro-Ophthalmol 11:*79–84.

Halmagyi GM, Aw ST, Dehaene I, et al. (1994). Jerk-waveform see-saw nystagmus due to unilateral mesodiencephalic lesion. *Brain 117:*789–803.

Halmagyi GM, Curthoys IS, Gresty MA, et al. (1987). Hemi-see-saw nystagmus due to unilateral diencephalic lesion: A novel eye movement disorder. *Ann Neurol 22:*147.

Halmagyi GM, Gresty MA, Leech J. (1980). Reversed optokinetic nystagmus (OKN): Mechanism and clinical significance. *Ann Neurol 7:*429–435.

Halmagyi GM, Lessell I, Curthoys IS, et al. (1989). Lithium-induced downbeat nystagmus. *Am J Ophthalmol 107:*664–670.

Halmagyi GM, Rudge P, Gresty MA, et al. (1980). Treatment of periodic alternating nystagmus. *Ann Neurol 8:*609–611.

Halpern J. (1980). Spasmus nutans. *Arch Neurol 37:*737–738.

Hameroff SB, Garcia-Mullin R, Eckholdt J. (1969). Ocular bobbing. *Arch Ophthalmol 82:*774–780.

Hammack JE, Kotanides H, Rosenblum MK, Posner JB. (1992). Paraneoplastic cerebellar degeneration. II. Clinical and immunologic findings in 21 patients with Hodgkin's disease. *Neurology 42:*1938–1943.

Hankey GJ, Sadka M. (1987). Ocular flutter, postural body tremulousness and CSF pleocytosis: A rare postinfection syndrome. *J Neurol Neurosurg Psych 50:*1235–1236.

Hankey GJ, Silbert PL, Edis RH. (1987). Localising value of primary position upbeating nystagmus. *Aust NZ J Med 17:*333–335.

Harada Y, Ishimitsu H, Nishimoto K, et al. (1986). Opsoclonus-polymyoclonus syndrome suppressed with reserpine. *No To Shinkei 38:*359–362.

Harel S, Yurgenson U, Rechavi G, et al. (1987). Cerebellar ataxia and opsoclonus as the initial manifestations of myoclonic encephalopathy associated with neuroblastoma. *Childs Nerv Syst 3:*245–247.

Hashiba Y, Kuroda Y, Neshige R, et al. (1984). A case of opsoclonus-polymyoclonia syndrome: Suppression by TRH and 5-hydroxytryptophan. *Rinsho Shinkeigaku 11:*1091–1094.

Hata S, Bernstein F, Davis LE. (1986). Atypical ocular bobbing in a case of organophosphate poisoning. *Arch Neurol 43:*185–186.

Hatashita S, Shimoji T, Shimizu A, et al. (1980). A case of up-beat nystagmus associated with Chiari malformation type I (Japanese). *No Shinkei Geka 8:*989–994.

Hattori T, Hirayama K, Imai T, et al. (1988). Pontine lesions in opsoclonus-myoclonus syndrome shown by MRI. *J Neurol Neurosurg Psych 51:*1572–1575.

Hattori T, Takaya Y, Tsuboi Y, Hirayama K. (1993). Opsoclonus showing only during eye closure in hereditary cerebellar ataxia. *J Neurol Neurosurg Psych 56:*1037–1038.

Hausser-Hauw C, Roullet E, Robert R, Marteau R. (1988). Oculo-facio-skeletal myorhythmia as a cerebral complication of systemic Whipple's disease. *Movement Disorders 3:*179–184.
Helmchen C, Glasauer S, Bartl K, et al. (1996). Contralesionally beating torsional nystagmus in a unilateral rostral midbrain lesion. *Neurology 47:*482–486.
Helveston EM, Pogrebniak AE. (1988). Treatment of acquired nystagmus with botulinum A toxin. *Am J Ophthalmol 106:*584–586.
Helveston EM, Ellis FD, Plager DA. (1991). Large recession of the horizontal recti for treatment of nystagmus. *Ophthalmology 98:*1302–1305.
Herishanu Y, Louzoun Z. (1986). Trihexyphenidyl treatment of vertical pendular nystagmus. *Neurology 36:*82–84.
Herishanu Y, Apte R, Kuperman O. (1985). Immunologic abnormalities in opsoclonus cerebellopathy. *Neuro-ophthalmology 5:*271–275.
Herishanu YO, Sharpe JA. (1981). Normal square wave jerks. *Invest Ophthalmol Vis Sci 20:*268–270.
Herman P. (1981). Opsoclonus and oscillopsia. *Mt Sinai J Med 48:*412–417.
Herrman C Jr, Brown JW. (1967). Palatal myoclonus: A reappraisal. *J Neurol Sci 5:*473–492.
Herrmann C, Crandall PH, Fan HCH. (1957). Palatal myoclonus. A new approach to the understanding of its production. *Neurology 7:*37–51.
Herve F, Soulier J, Berger JP. (1988). Opso-myoclonic syndrome and Coxsackie B3 (French). *Arch Fr Pediatr 45:*597–598.
Herzau V, Körner F, Kommerell G, Friedel B. (1978). Superior oblique myokymia: A clinical and electromyographical study. In Kommerell G (ed). *Disorders of Ocular Motility, Neuro-physiological and Clinical Aspects.* Munich, JF Bergmann Verlag, pp. 81–90.
Himi T, Katura A, Tokuda S, et al. (1995). Downbeat nystagmus with compression of the medulla oblongata by the dolicoectatic vertebral arteries. *Am J Otol 16:*377–381.
Hirose G, Kawada J, Yoshioka A. (1990). Primary position upbeat nystagmus: Clinicopathologic study in three patients. *Neurology 40 Suppl:*312.
Hirose G, Kawada J, Tsukada K, et al. (1991). Upbeat nystagmus: Clinicopathological and pathophysiological considerations. *J Neurol Sci 105:*159–167.
Hirst LW, Clark AW, Wolinsky JS, et al. (1983). Downbeat nystagmus. A case report of herpetic brain stem encephalitis. *J Clin Neuro-ophthalmol 3:*245–249.
Holmes GL, Hafford J, Zimmerman AW. (1981). Primary position upbeat nystagmus following meningitis. *Ann Ophthalmol 13:*935–936.
Hood JD, Kayan A, Leech J. (1973). Rebound nystagmus. *Brain 96:*507–526.
Hostovsky M, Tubman DE, Wirtschafter JD. (1982). Intrathecal metrizamide computed tomography: Diagnosis of downbeat nystagmus in Arnold-Chiari I malformation. *Survey Ophthalmol 27:*123–125.
Hotson JR. (1984). Convergence-initiated voluntary flutter: A normal intrinsic capability in man. *Brain 294:*299–304.
Hoyt CS. (1977). Neonatal opsoclonus. *J Pediatr Ophthalmol 14:*274–277.
Hoyt CS. (1987). Nystagmus and other abnormal ocular movements in children. *Pediatr Clin North Am 34:*1415–1492.
Hoyt CS, Aicardi E. (1979). Acquired monocular nystagmus in monozygous twins. *J Pediatr Ophthalmol Strabismus 16:*115–118.
Hoyt CS, Gelbart SS. (1984). Vertical nystagmus in infants with congenital ocular motor abnormalities. *Ophthalmic Pediatr Genet 4:*155–162.
Hoyt CS, Mousel DK, Weber AA. (1980). Transient supranuclear disturbances of gaze in healthy neonates. *Am J Ophthalmol 89:*708–713.
Hoyt WF, Keane JR. (1970). Superior oblique myokymia. Report and discussion on five cases of benign intermittent uniocular microtremor. *Arch Ophthalmol 84:*461–467.
Hunter S, Kooistra C. (1986). Neuropathologic findings in idiopathic opsoclonus and myoclonus. Their similarities to those in paraneoplastic cerebellar cortical degeneration. *J Clin Neuro-ophthalmol 6:*236–241.
Huygen PLM, Verhagen WIM, Cruysberg JRM, Koch PAM. (1995). Familial congenital periodic alternating nystagmus with presumably X-linked dominant inheritance. *Neuro-ophthalmol 15:*149–155.
Hwang TL, Still CN, Jones JE. (1995). Reversible downbeat nystagmus and ataxia in felbamate intoxication. *Neurology 45:*846.
Inagki M, Suzuki T, Nakano N, et al. (1983). A case of superior oblique myokymia caused by cerebellar tumor. *Folia Ophthalmol Jpn 42:*59–61 (in Japanese).
Isago H, Asano K, Himi T, Kataura A. (1982). Upbeating nystagmus resulting from anticonvulsant intoxication. Report of a case. *Auris Nasus Larynx 9:*15–24.
Isago H, Tsuboya R, Kataura A. (1985). A case of periodic alternating nystagmus: with a special reference to the efficacy of baclofen treatment. *Auris Nasus Larynx 12:*15–21.
Ishikawa H, Ishikawa S, Mukuno K. (1993). Short-cycle periodic alternating (ping-pong) gaze. *Neurology 43:*1067–1070.
Ishikawa S, Nozaki S, Mukuno K. (1986). Upbeat and downbeat nystagmus in a single case. *Neuro-ophthalmology 6:*95–99.
Jabbari B, Urban E. (1981). Abnormal visual evoked responses and opsoclonus. *J Clin Neuro-ophthalmol 1:*269–271.

Jabbari B, Rosenberg M, Scherokman B, et al. (1987). Effectiveness of trihexiphenidyl against pendular nystagmus and palatal myoclonus: evidence of cholinergic dysfunction. *Mov Disord 2:*93–98.

Jabs DA, Green WR, Fox R, et al. (1989). Ocular manifestations of acquired immune deficiency syndrome. *Ophthalmology 96:*1092–1099.

Jacobson DM, Corbett JJ. (1989). Downbeat nystagmus associated with dolichoectasia of the vertebrobasilar artery. *Arch Neurol 46:*1005–1008.

Jacome DE, FitzGerald R. (1982). Monocular ictal nystagmus. *Arch Neurol 39:*653–656.

Jacome DE. (1986). Epileptic nystagmus and eye movements. *J Clin Neuro-ophthalmol 6:*269–270.

Jacome DE. (1986). Monocular downbeat nystagmus. *Ann Ophthalmol 18:*293–296.

Jarrett A, Emery JM, Coats AC, Justice J Jr. (1977). Voluntary nystagmus. *Ann Ophthalmol 9:*853–859.

Jay WM, Marcus RW, Jay MS. (1982). Primary position upbeat nystagmus with organophosphate poisoning. *J Pediatr Ophthalmol Strabismus 19:*318–319.

Jay WM, Williams BB, De Chicchis A. (1985). Periodic alternating nystagmus clearing after cataract surgery. *J Clin Neuro-ophthalmol 5:*149–152.

Kalyanaraman K, Jagannathan K. (1971). Opsoclonus with acute cerebellar ataxia (cerebellitis of pontine encephalitis) of childhood. *Neurology India 19:*87–91.

Kamel KS. (1974). Congenital nystagmus. Report of a rare case of uniocular congenital nystagmus. *Bull Ophthalmol Soc Egypt 67:*349–352.

Kanaya T, Nonaka S, Kamito M, et al. (1994). Primary position upbeat nystagmus—localizing value. ORL *J Otorhinolaryngol Relat Spec 56:*236–238.

Kanter DS, Ruff RL, Leigh RJ, et al. (1987). See-saw nystagmus and brainstem infarction: MRI findings. *J Neuro-ophthalmol 7:*279–283.

Kaplan PW, Lesser RP. (1989). Vertical and horizontal epileptic gaze deviation and nystagmus. *Neurology 39:*1391–1393.

Kaplan PW, Tusa RJ. (1993). Neurophysiologic and clinical correlations of epileptic nystagmus. *Neurology 43:*2508–2514.

Kase M, Nagata R, Arikado T. (1985). Macrosaccadic oscillation, saccadic dysmetria and motor error in spinocerebellar degeneration. *Jpn J Ophthalmol 29:*369–377.

Kato I, Nakamura T, Watanabe J, et al. (1985). Primary position upbeat nystagmus. Localizing value. *Arch Neurol 42:*819–821.

Kattah JC, Cohan SL, Cahill W, Buas M. (1983). Monocular rotatory nystagmus. *J Clin Neuro-ophthalmol 3:*49–51.

Kattah JC, Kolsky MP, Guy J, O'Doherty D. (1983). Primary position vertical nystagmus and cerebellar ataxia. *Arch Neurol 40:*310–314.

Katz B, Hoyt WF, Townsend J. (1982). Ocular bobbing and unilateral pontine hemorrhage. *J Clin Neuro-ophthalmol 2:*193–195.

Katzman B, Lu LW, Tiwari RP. (1981). Spasmus nutans in identical twins. *Ann Ophthalmol 13:*1193–1195.

Kaulfersch W, Urban C, Fritsch G, Maurer G. (1984). Myoclonic encephalopathy (Kinsbourne syndrome) (German). *Padiatr Padol 19:*279–285.

Keane JR. (1978). Intermittent see-saw nystagmus. Report of a patient in coma after hyperextension head injury. *Arch Neurol 34:*173–174.

Keane JR. (1986). Acute vertical ocular myoclonus. *Neurology 36:*86–89.

Keane JR. (1974). Periodic alternating nystagmus with downward beating nystagmus. A clinicoanatomical study of multiple sclerosis. *Arch Neurol 30:*399–402.

Keane JR. (1985). Pretectal pseudobobbing—Five patients with 'V'-pattern convergence nystagmus. *Arch Neurol 42:*592–594.

Keane JR. (1980). Transient opsoclonus with thalamic hemorrhage. *Arch Neurol 37:*423–424.

Keane JR, Devereaux MW. (1974). Opsoclonus associated with an intracranial tumor. *Arch Ophthalmol 92:*443–445.

Keane JR, Itabashi HH. (1987). Upbeat nystagmus: Clinicopathologic study of two patients. *Neurology 37:*491–494.

Kelly TW. (1970). Optic glioma presenting as spasmus nutans. *Pediatrics 45:*295–296.

Keltner JL, Miller NR, Gittinger JW, Burde RM. (1983). The monocular shimmers—Your patient isn't deluded! *Surv Ophthalmol 27:*313–316.

Kennard C, Barger G, Hoyt WF. (1981). The association of periodic alternating nystagmus with periodic alternating gaze. A case report. *J Clin Neuro-ophthalmol 1:*191–193.

Kestenbaum A. (1953). Nouvelle operation de nystagmus. *Bull Soc Ophthalmol Fr 6:*599–602.

Keyes MJ. (1973). Voluntary nystagmus in two generations. *Arch Neurol 29:*63–64.

Kilgo GR, Schwartze GM. (1984). Opsoclonus. *J Clin Neuro-ophthalmol 4:*109–119.

Kinast M, Levin HS, Rothner AD, et al. (1980). Cerebellar ataxia, opsoclonus, and occult neural crest tumor. *AJDC 134:*1057–1059.

King RA, Nelson LB, Wagner RS. (1986). Spasmus nutans—A benign clinical entity? *Arch Ophthalmol 104:*1501–1504.

Kinsbourne M. (1962). Myoclonic encephalopathy of infants. *J Neurol Neurosurg Psych 25:*271–276.

Kitamura K, Toriyama M. (1984). Downbeat nystagmus due to anticonvulsant intoxication (Japanese). *Rinsho Shinkeigaku 24:*137–144.

Knobler RL, Somasundaram M, Schutta HS. (1981). Inverse ocular bobbing. *Ann Neurol 9:*194–197.
Komai K, Mimura O, Uyama J, et al. (1992). Neuro-ophthalmological evaluation of superior oblique myokymia. *Neuro-ophthalmol 12:*135–140.
Kommerell G, Schaubele G. (1980). Superior oblique myokymia. An electromyographical analysis. *Trans Ophthalmol Soc UK 100:*504–506.
Kondo C, Miyanaga K, Kamei T. (1980). A case of voluntary nystagmus (Japanese). *Rinsho Shinkeigaku 20:*940–944.
Kosmorsky GS, Ellis BD, Fogt N, Leigh RJ. (1995). The treatment of superior oblique myokymia utilizing the Harada-Ito procedure. *J Neuro-ophthalmol 15:*142–146.
Krespi Y, Vertichel P, Masson C, Cambier J. (1995). Downbeat nystagmus and vertebrobasilar arterial dolichoectasia (French). *Rev Neurol 151:*196–197.
Kuban KC, Ephros MA, Freeman RL, et al. (1983). Syndrome of opsoclonus-myoclonus caused by Coxsackie B3 infection. *Ann Neurol 13:*69–71.
Kushner BJ. (1995). Infantile uniocular blindness with bilateral nystagmus. A syndrome. *Arch Ophthalmol 113:*1298–1300.
Lambert SR, Newman NJ. (1993). Retinal disease masquerading as spasmus nutans. *Neurology 43:*1607–1609.
Lambert SR, Kriss A, Gresty M, et al. (1989). Joubert syndrome. *Arch Ophthalmol 107:*709–713.
Lambert SR, Taylor D, Kriss A. (1989). The infant with nystagmus, normal appearing fundi, but an abnormal ERG. *Surv Ophthalmol 34:*173–186.
Larbrisseau A, Geoffroy G, Lasalle R. (1973). Neuroblastoma associated with polymyoclonia-opsoclonia syndrome (French). *Union Med Can 103:*1691–1694.
Larmande P, Dongmo L, Limodin J, Ruchoux M. (1987a). Periodic alternating gaze: A case without any hemispheric lesion. *Neurosurgery 20:*481–483.
Larmande P, Henin D, Jan M, Gouaze A. (1982). Periodic alternating gaze: Electro-oculographic and anatomical observation of a new case. *Neurosurgery 10:*263–265.
Larmande P, Limodin J, Dongmo L, Belin C. (1987b). Periodic alternating gaze. *Neurosurgery 20:*666–667.
Larmande P, Limodin J, Henin D, Lapierre F. (1983). Ocular bobbing: Abnormal eye movement or eye movement abnormality? *Ophthalmologica 187:*161–165.
Lavery MA, O'Neill JF, Chu FC, Martyn LJ. (1984). Acquired nystagmus in early childhood: A presenting sign of intracranial tumor. *Ophthalmology 91:*425–435.
Lavin PJM, Bahntge MF. (1983). Downbeat nystagmus with supra-tentorial disease. *Neuro-ophthalmol 3:*235–237.
Lavin PJM, Traccis S, Dell'Osso LF, et al. (1983). Downbeat nystagmus with a pseudocycloid waveform: Improvement with base-out prisms. *Ann Neurol 13:*621–624.
Lawden MC, Bronstein AM, Kennard C. (1995). Repetitive paroxysmal nystagmus and vertigo. *Neurology 45:*276–280.
Lawrence WH, Lightfoote WE. (1975). Continuous vertical pendular eye movements after brain-stem hemorrhage. *Neurology 225:*896–898.
Lazar RB, Ho SU, Melen O, Daghestani AN. (1983). Multifocal central nervous system damage caused by toluene abuse. *Neurology 33:*1337–1340.
Lechi A, Tedeschi F, Terzano MG, Trabattoni G. (1983). Opsoclonus and myoclonus in malignant disease: A case report. *Acta Neurol 5:*205–209.
Lee J, Gresty M. (1993). A case of "voluntary nystagmus" and head tremor. *J Neurol Neurosurg Psych 56:*1321–1322.
Lee JP. (1984). Superior oblique myokymia. A possible etiologic factor. *Arch Ophthalmol 102:*1178–1179.
Lefkowitz D, Harpold G. (1985). Treatment of ocular myoclonus with valproic acid. *Ann Neurol 17:*103–104.
Leigh RJ, Zee DS. (1980). Eye movements of the blind. *Invest Ophthalmol Vis Sci 19:*328–331.
Leigh RJ, Zee DS. (1991a). *The Neurology of Eye Movements*. 2nd edition. Philadelphia, FA Davis, pp. 378–421.
Leigh RJ, Averbuch-Heller L, Tomsak RL, et al. (1994). Treatment of abnormal eye movements that impair vision: Strategies based on current concepts of physiology and pharmacology. *Ann Neurol 36:*129–141.
Leigh RJ, Burnstine TH, Ruff RL, Kasmer RJ. (1991b). The effect of anticholinergic agents upon acquired pendular nystagmus. A double-blind study of trihexyphenidyl and tridihexethyl chloride. *Neurology 41:*1737–1741.
Leigh RJ, Robinson DA, Zee DS. (1981). A hypothetical explanation for periodic alternating nystagmus: Instability in the optokinetic-vestibular system. *Ann NY Acad Sci 374:*619–635.
Leigh RJ, Rushton DN, Thurston SE, et al. (1988). Effects of retinal image stabilization on acquired nystagmus due to neurological diseases. *Neurology 38:*122–127.
Leigh RJ, Tomsak RL, Grant MP, et al. (1992). Effectiveness of botulinum toxin administration to abolish acquired nystagmus. *Ann Neurol 32:*633–642.
Lennox G. (1993). Reverse ocular bobbing due to combined phenothiazine and benzodiazepine poisoning. *J Neurol Neurosurg Psych 56:*1137–1137.
Lepore FE, McKiernan JE Jr, Slevin JT. (1980). Bilateral nystagmus in syringobulbia. *Ann Ophthalmol 12:*304–306.
Lewis JM, Kline LB. (1983). Periodic alternating nystagmus associated with periodic alternating skew deviation. *J Clin Neuro-ophthalmol 3:*115–117.
Lin J, Elidan J, Baloh RW, Honrubia V. (1986). Direction-changing positional nystagmus: Incidence and meaning. *Am J Otolaryngol 7:*306–310.
Lipman IJ. (1972). "Voluntary nystagmus"—ocular shuddering. *Dis Nerv Syst 33:*200–201.

Lopez L, Bronstein AM, Gresty MA, et al. (1992). Torsional nystagmus. A neuro-otological and MRI study of thirty-five cases. *Brain 115:*1107–1124.

Lopez LI, Bronstein AM, Gresty MA, et al. (1996). Clinical and MRI correlates in 27 patients with acquired pendular nystagmus. *Brain 119:*465–472.

Louis ED, Lynch T, Kaufmann P, et al. (1996). Diagnostic guidelines in central nervous system Whipple's disease. *Ann Neurol 40:*561–568.

Lücking CH, Birnberger KL, Straschill M. (1975). Opsoclonus, truncal ataxia and myoclonus as signs of benign brain stem encephalitis. *Electroenceph Clin Neurophysiol 39:*212.

Luda E. (1982). Ocular dipping. *Arch Neurol 39:67.*

Luque FA, Furneaux HM, Ferziger R, et al. (1991). Anti-Ri: An antibody associated with paraneoplastic opsoclonus and breast cancer. *Ann Neurol 29:*241–251.

Maas EF, Ashe J, Spiegel P, et al. (1991). Acquired pendular nystagmus in toluene addiction. *Neurology 41:*282–285.

McLean DR. (1970). Polymyoclonia with opsoclonus. *Neurology 20:*508–512.

Maccario M, Seelinger D, Snyder R. (1975). Thallotoxicosis with coma and abnormal eye movements (opsoclonus). Clinical and EEG correlations. *Electroencephalogr Clin Neurophysiol 38:*98–99.

Mallinson AI, Longridge NS, Dunn HG, McCormick AQ. (1983). Vestibular studies in Pelizaeus-Merzbacher disease. *J Otolaryngol 12:*361–364.

Malm G, Lying-Tunell U. (1980). Cerebellar dysfunction related to toluene sniffing. *Acta Neurol Scand 62:*188–190.

Marmor MF. (1973). Hereditary vertical nystagmus. *Arch Ophthalmol 90:*107–111.

Masson C, Prier S, Masson M, Cambier J. (1986). Macrosaccadic oscillations as a symptom of cerebellar hemorrhage (French). *Rev Neurol 142:*98–930.

Massry GG, Bloom JN, Cruz OA. (1996). Convergence nystagmus associated with spasmus nutans. *J Neuro-ophthalmol 16:*196–198.

Mastaglia FL. (1974). See-saw nystagmus: An unusual sign of brain-stem infarction. *J Neurol Sci 22:*439–443.

Masucci EF, Kurtzke JF. (1988). Downbeat nystagmus secondary to multiple sclerosis. *Ann Ophthalmol 20:*347–348.

Masucci EF, Fabara JA, Saini N, Kurtzke JF. (1981). Periodic alternating ping-pong gaze. *Ann Ophthalmol 13:*1123–1127.

Matsamura K, Sonoh M, Tamaoka A, Sakuta M. (1985). Syndrome of opsoclonus-myoclonus in hyperosmolar nonketotic coma. *Ann Neurol 18:*623–624.

Matsuo F, Ajax ET. (1979). Palatal myoclonus, denervation supersensitivity in the central nervous system. *Ann Neurol 5:*72–78.

Mayfrank L, Thoden U. (1986). Downbeat nystagmus indicates cerebellar or brain-stem lesions in vitamin B12 deficiency. *J Neurol 233:*145–148.

Mehler MF. (1988). The clinical spectrum of ocular bobbing and ocular dipping. *J Neurol Neurosurg Psych 51:725–727.*

Meienberg O, Hoyt WF. (1980). Ocular motor control during the neutral phase of periodic alternating nystagmus. *J Neurol 223:*309–312.

Mitchell WG, Snodgrass SR. (1990). Opsoclonus-ataxia due to childhood neural crest tumors: A chronic neurologic syndrome. *J Child Neurol 5:*153–158.

Mizuno M, Kudo Y, Yamane M. (1990). Upbeat nystagmus influenced by postire: Report of two cases. *Auri Nasus Larynx 16:*215–221.

Moe PG, Nellhaus G. (1970). Infantile polymyoclonia-opsoclonus syndrome and neural crest tumors. *Neurology 20:*756–764.

Monteiro ML, Sampaio CM. (1993). Lithium-induced downbeat nystagmus in a patient with Arnold-Chiari malformation. *Am J Ophthalmol 116:*648–649.

Morales-Garcia C, Cardenas JL, Arrigada C, Otte J. (1978). Clinical significance of rebound nystagmus in neuro-otological diagnosis. *Ann Otol Rhinol Laryngol 87:*238–242.

Morrow MJ, Sharpe JA. (1988). Torsional nystagmus in the lateral medullary syndrome. *Ann Neurol 24:*390–398.

Morrow MJ, Sharpe JA, Ranalli PJ. (1990). Superior oblique myokymia associated with a posterior fossa tumor: Oculographic correlation with an idiopathic case. *Neurology 40:*367–370.

Mossman SS, Bronstein AM, Gresty MA, et al. (1990). Convergence nystagmus associated with Arnold-Chiari malformation. *Arch Neurol 47:*357–359.

Munro NAR, Gaymard B, Rivaud S, et al. (1993). Upbeat nystagmus in a patient with a small medullary infarct. *J Neurol Neurosurg Psych 56:*1126–1128.

Nakada T, Kwee IL. (1986). Oculopalatal myoclonus. *Brain 109:*431–441.

Nakada T, Kwee IL. (1988). Seesaw nystagmus. Role of visuovestibular interaction in its pathogenesis. *J Clin Neuro-ophthalmol 8:*171–177.

Nakada T, Remler MP. (1981). Primary position upbeat nystagmus. Another central vestibular nystagmus? *J Clin Neuro-ophthalmol 1:*185–189.

Nathanson M. (1956). Palatal myoclonus. Further clinical and pathophysiological observations. *Arch Neurol Psych 75:*285–296.

Nathanson M, Bergman PS, Bender MB. (1955). Monocular nystagmus. *Am J Ophthalmol 40:*685–692.

Nausieda PA, Tanner CM, Weiner WJ. (1981). Opsoclonus cerebellopathy: A paraneoplastic syndrome responsive to thiamine. *Arch Neurol 38:*780–781.

Neetens A, Martin JJ. (1983). Superior oblique myokymia in a case of adrenoleukodystrophy and in a case of lead intoxication. *Neuro-ophthalmol 3:*103–107.

Nelson KR, Brenner RP, Carlow T. (1986). Divergent-convergence eye movements and transient eyelid opening associated with an EEG burst-suppression pattern. *J Clin Neuro-ophthalmol 6:*43–46.

Neshige R, Kuroda Y, Oda K, Shibasaki H. (1984). A case of macro square wave jerks due to cerebellar hemorrhage (Japanese). *Rinsho Shinkeigaku 24:*912–915.

Newman SA, Hedges TR, Wall M, Sedwick LA. (1990). Spasmus nutans—or is it? *Surv Ophthalmol 34:*453–456.

Nichelli P, Bahmanian-Behbahani G, Di Pellegrino G. (1984). Opsoclonus-ataxia syndrome. Description of a case (Italian). *Riv Patol Nerv Ment 105:*239–248.

Noda S, Ide K, Umezaki H, et al. (1987). Repetitive divergence. *Ann Neurol 21:*109–110.

Noda S, Takao A, Itoh H, et al. (1985). Opsoclonus in hyperosmolar nonketotic coma. *J Neurol Neurosurg Psych 48:*1186–1187.

Norton EWD, Cogan DG. (1954). Spasmus nutans: A clinical study of twenty cases followed two years or more since onset. *Arch Ophthalmol 52:*442–446.

Noseworthy JH, Ebers GC, Leigh RJ, Dell'Osso LF. (1988). Torsional nystagmus: Quantitative features and possible pathogenesis. *Neurology 38:*992–994.

Nowack WJ, Clark GF. (1986). Vertical nystagmus and thalamic arteriovenous malformation. Report of a case. *Neuro-ophthalmology 6:*169–172.

Ochs AL, Stark L, Hoyt WF, D'Amico D. (1979). Opposed adducting saccades in convergence-retraction nystagmus. A patient with sylvian aqueduct syndrome. *Brain 102:*497–508.

Ohtsyka K, Mukuno K, Ukai K, Ishikawa S. (1986). The origin of square wave jerks: Conditions of fixation and microsaccades. *Jpn J Ophthalmol 30:*209–215.

Oliva A, Rosenberg ML. (1990). Convergence-evoked nystagmus. *Neurology 40:*161–162.

Oohira A, Goto K, Ozawa T. (1986). Convergence nystagmus. An observation of horizontal and vertical components. *Neuro-ophthalmol 6:*313–330.

Osenbach RK, Blumenkopf B, McComb B, Huggins MJ. (1986). Ocular bobbing with ruptured giant distal posterior inferior cerebellar artery aneurysm. *Surg Neurol 25:*149–152.

Pagnini P, Nuti D, Vannuchi P. (1989). Benign paroxysmal vertigo of the horizontal canal. *Otorhinolaryngology 51:*161–170.

Palmer EA, Shults WT. (1984). Superior oblique myokymia: Preliminary results of surgical treatment. *J Ped Ophthalmol Strabismus 21:*96–101.

Pedersen RA, Troost BT, Abel LA, Zorub D. (1980). Intermittent downbeat nystagmus and oscillopsia reversed by suboccipital craniectomy. *Neurology 30:*1239–1242.

Pepin B, Toupet M, de Gramont A, Lidy C. (1981). Ocular flutter in acute polyradiculoneuritis (French). *Nouv Presse Med 10:*1419.

Peterson K, Rosenblum MK, Kotanides H, Posner JB. (1992). Paraneoplastic cerebellar degeneration. I. A clinical analysis of 55 anti-Yo antibody-positive patients. *Neurology 42:*1931–1938.

Phadke JG, Hern JE, Blaiklock CT. (1981). Downbeat nystagmus—A false localizing sign due to communicating hydrocephalus. *J Neurol Neurosurg Psych 44:*459.

Pinel JF, Larmande P, Guegan Y, Iba-Zizen MT. (1987). Down-beat nystagmus: Case report with magnetic resonance imaging and surgical treatment. *Neurosurgery 21:*736–739.

Plant GT. (1982). Periodic alternating nystagmus in a case of hereditary ataxia and its treatment with baclofen. *J Neurol Neurosurg Psych 45:*937–938.

Pless M, Ronthal M. (1996). Treatment of opsoclonus-myoclonus with high-dose intravenous immunoglobulin. *Neurology 46:*583–584.

Plum F, Posner JB. (1980). *The Diagnosis of Stupor and Coma.* 3rd edition. Contemporary Neurology Series, Vol. 19, Philadelphia, Davis.

Popescu F. (1970). The dancing eye syndrome: Infantile polymyoclonus (Rumanian). *Neurol Psych Neurochir 15:*559–564.

Price MJ, Judisch GF, Thompson HS. (1988). X-linked congenital stationary night blindness with myopia and nystagmus without clinical complaints of nyctylopia. *J Pediatr Ophthalmol Strabismus 25:*33–36.

Pritchard C, Flynn JT, Smith JL. (1988). Wave form characteristics of vertical oscillations in longstanding visual loss. *J Pediatr Ophthalmol Strabismus 25:*233–236.

Pullicino P, Aquilina J. (1989). Opsoclonus in organophosphate poisoning. *Arch Neurol 46:*704–705.

Radhakrishnan K, Venkateswarlu K, Walia BN, Mann SB. (1982). Kocher-Debre-Semelaigne syndrome and congenital nystagmus. *Postgrad Med J 58:*307–310.

Ranalli PJ, Sharpe JA. (1988). Upbeat nystagmus and the ventral tegmental pathway of the upward vestibulo-ocular reflex. *Neurology 38:*1329–1330.

Rascol O, Sabatini U, Sinonetta-Moreau M, et al. (1991). Square-wave jerks in Parkinsonian syndromes. *J Neurol Neurosurg Psych 54:*599–602.

Reis J, Eber AM, Warter JM, et al. (1989). Alternating nystagmus and infectious mononucleosis. *Neuro-ophthalmol 9:*289–292.

Remler BF, Leigh RJ, Osoria I, et al. (1990). The characteristics and mechanisms of visual disturbance associated with anticonvulsant therapy. *Neurology 40:*791–796.

Repka MX, Savino PJ, Reincke RD. (1994). Treatment of acquired nystagmus with botulinum neurotoxin A. *Arch Ophthalmol 112:*1320–1324.

Revol A, Vighetto A, Confavreux C, et al. (1990). Oculo-palatal myoclonus and multiple sclerosis (French). *Rev Neurol 146:*518–521.

Reynard M, Wertenbaker C, Behrens M, et al. (1979). "Ping-pong gaze" amplified. *Neurology 29:*757–758.

Ridley A, Kennard C, Scholtz CL, et al. (1987). Omnipause neurons in two cases of opsoclonus associated with oat cell carcinoma of the lung. *Brain 110:*1699–1709.

Rivner MH, Jay WM, Green JB, Dyken PR. (1982). Opsoclonus in Hemophilus influenza meningitis. *Neurology 32:*661–663.

Robin A, Vallat M, Tapie P, et al. (1976). Opsoclonus et troubles neurologiques associes. *Arch Ophthalmol 36:*645–656.

Ropper AH. (1981a). Atypical ocular bobbing. *Ann Neurol 10:*400.

Ropper AH. (1981b). Ocular dipping in anoxic coma. *Arch Neurol 38:*297–299.

Rosa A, Mizon JP. (1980). Opsoclonus. *Rev Otoneuro-ophthalmol 52:*459–461.

Rosa A, Masmoudi K, Mizon JP. (1987). Typical and atypical ocular bobbing: Pathology through five case reports. *Neuro Ophthalmol 7:*285–290.

Rosa A, Masmoudi K, Barvieux D, et al. (1988). Opsoclonus and virus A hepatitis. *Neuro-Ophthalmol 8:*275–279.

Rosenberg ML. (1986). Spontaneous vertical eye movements in coma. *Ann Neurol 20:*635–637.

Rosenberg ML. (1987). Reversible downbeat nystagmus secondary to excessive alcohol intake. *J Clin Neuro-ophthalmol 7:*23–25.

Rosenberg ML. (1989). Permanent lithium-induced downbeating nystagmus. *Arch Neurol 46:*839.

Rosenberg ML, Glaser JS. (1983). Superior oblique myokymia. *Ann Neurol 13:*667–669.

Rosenberg NL, Kleinschmidt-DeMasters BJ, Davis KA, et al. (1988). Toluene abuse causes diffuse central nervous system white matter changes. *Ann Neurol 23:*611–614.

Rosengart A, Hedges TR 3rd, Teal PA, et al. (1993). Intermittent downbeat nystagmus due to vertebral artery compression. *Neurology 43:*216–218.

Rosenthal JG, Selhorst JB. (1987). Continuous non-rhythmic cycloversion. A possible paraneoplastic disorder. *Neuro-ophthalmology 7:*291–295.

Ross AT, Zeman W. (1967). Opsoclonus, occult carcinoma, and chemical pathology in dentate nuclei. *Arch Neurol 17:*546–551.

Rossazza C, Delplace MP, Larmande A. (1974). The see-saw nystagmus in hypophyseal adenomas (French). *Rev Otoneuro-ophthalmol 46:*367–368.

Rousseaux M, Dupard T, Lesoin F, et al. (1991). Upbeat and downbeat nystagmus occurring successively in a patient with posterior medullary haemorrhage. *J Neurol Neurosurg Psych 54:*367–369.

Ruben S, Dunlop IS, Elston J. (1994a). Retrobulbar botulinum toxin for treatment of oscillopsia. *Aust NZ J Ophthalmol 22:*65–67.

Ruben S, Lee JP, O'Neill D, et al. (1994b). The use of botulinum toxin for treatment of acquired nystagmus and oscillopsia. *Ophthalmology 101:*783–787.

Rudick R, Satran R, Eskin TA. (1981). Ocular bobbing in encephalitis. *J Neurol Neurosurg Psych 44:*441–443.

Rushton D, Cox N. (1987). A new optical treatment for oscillopsia. *J Neurol Neurosurg Psych 50:*411–415.

Russell GE, Wick B, Tang RA. (1992). Arnold-Chiari malformation. *Optom Vis Sci 69:*242–247.

Rych K. (1974). See-saw nystagmus and cone degeneration (German). *Klin Monatsbl Augenheilkd 165:*930–935.

Sabin TD, Poche JA. (1969). Pure torsional nystagmus as a consequence of head trauma. *J Neurol Neurosurg Psych 32:*265–267.

Sachdeva JR, Singh N, Mann GS. (1984). Acute cerebellar ataxia with myoclonus. *J Assoc Physicians India 32:*460.

Safran AB, Berney J. (1983). Synchronism of reverse ocular bobbing and blinking. *Am J Ophthalmol 95:*863–864.

Safran AB, Berney J, Panchaud A. (1980). See-saw nystagmus in a case of giant adenoma of the hypophysis (French). *Rev Med Suisse Romande 100:*343–347.

Sakai T, Shiraishi S, Murakami S. (1981). Palatal myoclonus responding to carbamazepine. *Ann Neurol 9:*199–200.

Sakakibara R, Hirayama K, Takaya Y, et al. (1993). Periodic alternating nystagmus in familial congenital cerebellar ataxia (Japanese). *Rinsho Shinkeigaku 33:*1–7.

Sakata E, Ohtsu K, Itoh Y. (1991). Positional nystagmus of benign paroxysmal type (BPPN) due to cerebellar vernmis lesions. Pseudo-BPPN. *Acta Otolaryngol Suppl 481:*254–257.

Sakata E, Ohtsu K, Shimura H, Sakai S. (1987). Positional nystagmus of benign type (BPPN) due to cerebellar vermis lesions. *Auris Nasus Larynx 14:*17–21.

Salonen R, Nikoskelainen E, Aantaa E, Marttila R. (1988). Ocular flutter associated with sarcoidosis. *Neuro-ophthalmology 8:77–79.*

Samkoff LM, Smith CR. (1994). See-saw nystagmus in a patient with clinically definite MS. *Eur Neurol 34:*228–229.

Sandok BA, Kranz H. (1971). Opsoclonus as the initial manifestation of occult neuroblastoma. *Arch Ophthalmol 86:*235–236.

Sano K, Sekino H, Tsukamoio Y, et al. (1972). Stimulation and destruction of the region of the interstitial nucleus in cases of torticollis and see-saw nystagmus. *Confinia Neurologica 34:*331–338.

Saul RF, Selhorst JB. (1981). Downbeat nystagmus with magnesium depletion. *Arch Neurol 38:*650–652.

Savino PJ, Glaser JS. (1975). Opsoclonus. Pattern of regression in a child with neuroblastoma. *Br J Ophthalmol 59:*696–698.

Scharf D. (1989). Opsoclonus-myoclonus following the intranasal usage of cocaine. *J Neurol Neurosurg Psych 52:*1447–1448.
Schmidt D, Kommerell G. (1974). Congenital seesaw nystagmus. *Albrecht Von Graefes Arch Klin Exp Ophthalmol 191:*265–272.
Schmidt D, Kommerell G. (1969). Seesaw nystagmus with bitemporal hemianopia following head traumas (German). *Albrecht Von Graefes Arch Klin Exp Ophthalmol 178:*349–366.
Schmidt D, Neumann HP, Eggert HR, Friedburg H. (1988). Neuro-ophthalmologic findings in hemangioblastoma of the cerebellum and brain stem—downbeat nystagmus as the first symptom of hemangioblastoma in Hippel-Lindau disease (German). *Fortschr Ophthalmol 85:*427–433.
Schnyder H, Bassetti C. (1996). Bilateral convergence nystagmus in unilateral dorsal midbrain stroke due to occlusion of the superior cerebellar artery. *Neuro-ophthalmology 16:*59–63.
Schott GD. (1980). Familial cerebellar ataxia presenting with down beat nystagmus. *J Med Genet 17:*115–118.
Schulman JD, Crawford JD. (1969). Congenital nystagmus and hypothyroidism. *N Eng J Med 280:*708–710.
Schulman JA, Shults WT, Jones JM Jr. (1979). Monocular vertical nystagmus as an initial sign of chiasmal glioma. *Am J Ophthalmol 87:*87–90.
Schwankhaus JD, Kattah JC, Lux WE, et al. (1989). Primidone/phenobarbital-induced periodic alternating nystagmus. *Ann Ophthalmol 21:*230–232.
Schwart M, Sharf B, Zidan J. (1990). Opsoclonus as a presenting symptom in thymic cancer. *J Neurol Neurosurg Psych 53:*534.
Schwartz MA, Selhorst JB, Ochs AL, et al. (1986). Oculomasticatory myorhythmia: A unique movement disorder occurring in Whipple's disease. *Ann Neurol 20:*677–683.
Sedwick LA, Burde RM, Hodges FJ 3rd. (1984). Leigh's subacute necrotizing encephalomyelopathy manifesting as spasmus nutans. *Arch Ophthalmol 102:*1046–1048.
Selhorst JB. (1987). Pendular vergence oscillations. In Ishikawa H (ed). *Highlights in Neuro-Ophthalmology.* Proceedings of the Sixth Meeting of the International Neuro-Ophthalmology Society. Aeolus, Amsterdam, pp. 153–162.
Selhorst JB, Stark L, Ochs AL, Hoyt WF. (1976). Disorders in cerebellar ocular motor control. II. Macrosaccadic oscillation. An oculographic, control system and clinico-anatomical analysis. *Brain 99:*509–522.
Senelick RC. (1976). "Ping-pong" gaze: Periodic alternating gaze deviation. *Neurology 26:*532–535.
Senelick RC. (1981). Total alleviation of downbeat nystagmus in basilar impression by transoral removal of the odontoid process. *J Clin Neuro-ophthalmol 1:*265–267.
Senelick RC, Bray PF, Lahey ME, et al. (1971). Neuroblastoma and myoclonic encephalopathy: Two cases and a review of the literature. *J Pediatr Surg 86:*235–236.
Shallo-Hoffmann J, Petersen J, Mühlendyck H. (1989). How normal are "normal" square wave jerks? *Invest Ophthalmol Vis Sci 30:*225–227.
Shallo-Hoffmann J, Sendler B, Mühlendyck H. (1990). Normal square wave jerks in differing age groups. *Invest Ophthalmol Vis Sci 31:*1649–1652.
Sharpe JA. (1974). Rebound nystagmus—A cerebellar sign? *JAMA 227:*648–649.
Sharpe JA, Hershanu YO, White OB. (1982). Cerebral square wave jerks. *Neurology 32:*57–62.
Sharpe JA, Hoyt WF, Rosenberg MA. (1975). Convergence-evoked nystagmus. Congenital and acquired forms. *Arch Neurol 32:*191–194.
Sharpe JA, Silversides JL, Blair RD. (1975). Familial paralysis of horizontal gaze. Associated with pendular nystagmus, progressive scoliosis, and facial contraction with myokymia. *Neurology 25:*1035–1040.
Sheinman BD, Gawler J. (1982). Opsoclonus and polymyoclonia complicating oat-cell carcinoma of the bronchus. *Postgrad Med J 58:*704–705.
Shetty T, Rosman NP. (1972). Opsoclonus in hydrocephalus. *Arch Ophthalmol 88:*585–589.
Shimizu N, Weinberger J, Yahr MD. (1975). Downbeat nystagmus as a sign of brainstem involvement in acute meningoencephalitis. *Neurology 25:*267–270.
Shults WT, Stark L, Hoyt WF, Ochs AL. (1977). Normal saccadic structure of voluntary nystagmus. *Arch Ophthalmol 95:*1399–1404.
Sibony PA, Evinger C, Manning KA. (1987). Tobacco-induced primary-position upbeat nystagmus. *Ann Neurol 21:*53–58.
Simon JW, Kandel GL, Krohel GB, Nelsen PT. (1984). Albinotic characteristics in congenital nystagmus. *Am J Ophthalmol 97:*320–327.
Simon RP, Aminoff MJ. (1986). Electrographic status epilepticus in fatal anoxic coma. *Ann Neurol 20:*351–355.
Skkorin L Jr, Briggs KS, Multack RF. Spasmus nutans: A pediatric enigma. *J Am Optom Assoc 57:*893–894.
Slatt B, Nykiel F. (1964). See-saw nystagmus. *Am J Ophthalmol 58:*1016–1021.
Slavin ML, Rosenberg ML. (1985). Unusual associations of downbeat nystagmus. *Neuro-ophthalmology 5:*265–270.
Smith JL, Flynn JT, Spiro HJ. (1982). Monocular visual oscillations of amblyopia. *J Clin Neuro-ophthalmol 2:*85–91.
Smith JL, Walsh FB. (1960). Opsoclonus-ataxic conjugate movements of the eyes. *Arch Ophthalmol 64:*244–250.
Sogg RL, Hoyt WF. (1962). Intermittent vertical nystagmus in a father and son. *Arch Ophthalmol 68:*515–517.
Sogg RL, Steinman L, Rathjen B, et al. (1979). Cherry-red spot-myoclonus syndrome. *Ophthalmology 86:*1861–1874.
Soloman GE, Chutrian AM. (1968). Opsoclonus and occult neuroblastoma. *New Eng J Med 279:*475–477.
Spaide RF, Klara PM, Restuccia RD. (1985–1986). Spasmus nutans as a presenting sign of an arachnoid cyst. *Pediatr Neurosci 12:*311–314.

Spalton DJ, Sanders MD, Gresty M, et al. (1980). Ocular myoclonus and oscillopsia. *Trans Ophthalmol Soc UK 100*:507–508.

Spielmann A. (1981). Congenital nystagmus: Clinical types and their surgical treatment. *Ophthalmologica 182*:65–72.

Spooner JW, Baloh RW. (1981). Arnold-Chiari malformation: Improvement in eye movements after surgical treatment. *Brain 104*:51–60.

St. John R, Fisk JD, Timney B, Goodale MA. (1984). Eye movements of human albinos. *Am J Optom Physiol Opt 61*:377–385.

Stahl JS, Rottach KG, Averbuch-Heller L, et al. (1996). A pilot study of gabapentin as treatment for acquired nystagmus. *Neuro-ophthalmology 16*:107–113.

Stark SR, Masucci EF, Kurtzke JF. (1984). Ocular dipping. *Neurology 34*:391–393.

Staudenmaier C. (1986). Superior oblique myokymia: When treatment is necessary. *Can J Ophthalmol 21*:236–241.

Stearns MQ, Sinoff SE, Rosenberg ML. (1993). Purely torsional nystagmus in a patient with stiff-man syndrome: A case report. *Neurology 43*:220.

Stell R, Bronstein AM, Plant GT, Harding AE. (1989). Ataxia telangiectasia: A reappraisal of the ocular motor features and their value in the diagnosis of atypical cases. *Mov Disord 4*:320–329.

Stewart JD, Kirkham TH, Mathieson G. (1979). Periodic alternating gaze. *Neurology 29*:222–224.

Stolz SE, Chatrian GE, Spence AM. (1991). Epileptic nystagmus. *Epilepsia 32*:910–918.

Susac JO, Hoyt WF, Daroff RB, Lawrence W. (1970). Clinical spectrum of ocular bobbing. *J Neurol Neurosurg Psych 33*:771–775.

Susac JO, Smith JLS, Schatz NJ. (1973). Superior oblique myokymia. *Arch Neurol 29*:4342–4434.

Swanson PD, Luttrell CN, Magladery JW. (1962). Myoclonus: A report of 67 cases and review of the literature. *Medicine 41*:339–356.

Sweeney PJ, Hahn JF, McHenry MC, Mitsumoto H. (1980). Mucormycosis presenting as positional nystagmus and hydrocephalus. *J Neurosurg 52*:270–272.

Talks SJ, Elston JS. (1997). Oculopalatal myoclonus: Eye movement studies, MRI findings, and the difficulty of treatment. *Eye 11*:19–24.

Tamura K, Kuroiwa Y. (1971). Opsoclonus-myoclonus syndrome in acute cerebellar ataxia—Clinical and electrophysiological observations of an adult case. *Folia Psychiatr Neurol Jpn 25*:129–135.

Taylor JR, Selhorst JB, Houff SA, Martinez AJ. (1978). Chlordecone intoxication in man. I. Clinical observations. *Neurology 28*:626–630.

Telander RL, Smithson WA, Groover RV. (1989). Clinical outcome in children with acute cerebellar encephalopathy and neuroblastoma. *J Pediatr Surg 24*:11–14.

Terao S, Sahashi K, Tsuchiya I, et al. (1986). Benign encephalopathy with flutter-like oscillations, truncal ataxia and shivering of the head: Report of two cases (Japanese). *Rinsho Shinkeigaku 26*:910–914.

Thurston SE, Leigh RJ, Osorio I. (1985). Epileptic gaze deviation and nystagmus. *Neurology 35*:1518–1521.

Tijssen CC, Ter Bruggen JP. (1986). Locked-in syndrome associated with ocular bobbing. *Acta Neurol Scand 73*:444–446.

Tison F, Louvet-Giendaj C, Henry P, et al. (1992). Permanent bruxism as a manifestation of the oculo-facial syndrome related to systemic Whipple's disease. *Mov Dis 7*:82–85.

Titer EM, Laureno R. (1988). Inverse/reverse ocular bobbing. *Ann Neurol 23*:103–104.

Tomsak RL, Remler BF, Averbuch-Heller L, et al. (1995). Unsatisfactory treatment of acquired nystagmus with retrobulbar injection of botulinum toxin. *Am J Ophthalmol 119*:489–496.

Toshniwal P, Yadava R, Goldbarg H. (1986). Presentation of pinealoblastoma with ocular dipping and deafness. *J Clin NeuroOphthalmol 6*:128–136.

Toupet M, Pialoux P. (1979). Rebound nystagmus: A new cerebellar sign (French). *Ann Otolaryngol Chir Cervicofac 96*:813–819.

Toupet M, de Gramont A, Bacri D, et al. (1982). Flutter-myoclonus: Report on three cases (French). *Rev Neurol 138*:219–239.

Towle PA, Romanul F. (1970). Periodic alternating nystagmus: First pathologically studied case. *Neurology 20*:408.

Traccis S. Rosati G, Aiello I, et al. (1989). Upbeat nystagmus as an early sign of cerebellar astrocytoma. *J Neurol 236*:359–360.

Traccis S, Rosati G, Monaco MF, et al. (1988). Alternating esotropia, monocular and binocular macro square wave jerks. *Neuro-ophthalmology 8*:43–49.

Traccis S, Rosati G, Monaco MF, et al. (1990). Successful treatment of acquired pendular elliptical nystagmus in multiple sclerosis with isoniazid and base-out prisms. *Neurology 40*:492–494.

Trobe JD, Sharpe JA, Hirsh DK, Gebarski SS. (1991). Nystagmus in Pelizaeus-Merzbacher disease. A magnetic search-coil study. *Arch Neurol 48*:87–91.

Troost BT, Daroff RB. (1977). The ocular motor defects in progressive supranuclear palsy. *Ann Neurol 2*:397–403.

Troost BT, Janton F, Weaver R. (1990). Periodic alternating oscillopsia: A symptom of periodic alternating nystagmus abolished by baclofen. *J Clin Neuro-ophthalmol 10*:273–277.

Troost BT, Martinez J, Abel LA, Heros RC. (1980). Upbeat nystagmus and internuclear ophthalmoplegia with brainstem glioma. *Arch Neurol 37*:453–456.

Tsuzuku T, Kaga K. (1986). Spontaneous downbeat nystagmus in two sisters with suanophilic leukodystrophy. *Auris Nasus Larynx 13 Suppl 2*:S131–S138.

Turazzi S, Alexandre A, Bricole A, et al. (1977). Opsoclonus and palatal myoclonus during prolonged post-traumatic coma. *Eur Neurol 15:*257–263.

Tusa RJ, Kaplan PW, Hain TC, Naidu S. (1990). Ipsiversive eye deviation and epileptic nystagmus. *Neurology 40:*662–665.

Tyler TD, Ruiz RS. (1990). Propranolol in the treatment of superior oblique myokymia. *Arch Ophth 108:*175–176.

Tzuzaka K, et al. (1993). A case of primary intracranial malignant lymphoma presenting as opsoclonus-myoclonus syndrome. *Rinsho Shinkeigaku 33:*194–196.

Uemura T, Inoue H, Hirano T. (1988). The effect of baclofen on periodic alternating nystagmus and experimentally induced nystagmus. *Adv Otorhinolaryngol 42:*254–259.

Van Weerden TW, van Woerkom TCAM. (1985). Ocular dipping. *Neurology 35:*135.

Vejjajiva A, Lerdverasirikul P. (1977). Opsoclonus in Salmonella infection. *Br Med J 2:*1260.

Vignaendra V, Lim CL. (1977). Electro-oculographic analysis of opsoclonus: Its relationship to saccadic and non-saccadic eye movements. *Neurology 27:*1129–1133.

Von Noorden GK, Sprunger DT. (1991). Large rectus muscle recession for the treatment of congenital nystagmus. *Arch Ophthalmol 109:*221–224.

Von Noorden GK, Avilla C, Sidokaro Y, LaRoche R. (1987). Latent nystagmus and strabismic amblyopia. *Am J Ophthalmol 103:*87–89.

Wagner RS, Caputo AR, Reynolds RD. (1990). Nystagmus in Down's syndrome. *Ophthalmology 97:*1439–1444.

Waragai M, Takaya Y, Hayashi M. (1995). HTLV–1 associated myelopathy (HAM) with cerebellar atrophy presenting as down-beat nystagmus (Japanese). *Rinsho Shinkeigaku 35:*549–552.

Warrier RP, Kini R, Besser A, et al. (1985). Opsomyoclonus and neuroblastoma. *Clin Pediatr 24:*32–34.

Watanabe K, Negoro T, Matsumoto A, et al. (1984). Epileptic nystagmus associated with typical absence seizures. *Epilepsia 25:*22–24.

Watkins HC, Ellis CJK. (1989). Ping pong gaze in reversible coma due to overdose of monoamine oxidase inhibitor. *J Neurol Neurosurg Psych 52:*539.

Watson CP, Terbrugge K. (1982). Positional nystagmus of the benign paroxysmal type with posterior fossa medulloblastoma. *Arch Neurol 39:*601–602.

Weider DJ, Ryder CJ, Stram JR. (1994). Benign paroxysmal positional vertigo: Analysis of 44 cases treated by the canalith repositioning procedure of Epley. *Am J Otol 15:*321–326.

Weissman B, Devereaux M, Krishan C. (1989). Opsoclonus and hyperosmolar stupor. *Neurology 39:*1401–1402.

Weissman BM, Dell'Osso LF, Abel LA, et al. (1987). Spasmus nutans: A quantitative prospective study. *Arch Ophthalmol 105:*525–528.

Weissman BM, Dell'Osso LF, DiScenna A. (1988). Downbeat nystagmus in an infant. Spontaneous resolution during infancy. *Neuro-ophthalmology 8:*317–319.

Wertenbaker C, Behrens MM, Hunter SB, et al. (1981). Opsoclonus: A cerebellar disorder? *Neuro-ophthalmol 2:*73–83.

Wertenbaker C, Henkind P, Keltner JL, et al. (1981). Downbeat nystagmus. *Survey Oph 25:*263–269.

Wheeler SD, Ramsay RE, Weiss J. (1982). Drug-induced downbeat nystagmus. *Ann Neurol 12:*227–228.

White JC. (1971). Epileptic nystagmus. *Epilepsia 12:*157–164.

Williams IM, Dickinson P, Ramsay RJ, et al. (1982). See-saw nystagmus. *Aust J Ophthalmol 10:*19–25.

Williams TH, House RF Jr, Burgert EO Jr, Lynn HB. (1972). Unusual manifestations of neuroblastoma: Chronic diarrhea, polymyoclonia-opsoclonus, and erythrocyte abnormalities. *Cancer 29:*475–480.

Williams DP, Troost BT, Rogers J. (1988). Lithium-induced downbeat nystagmus. *Arch Neurol 45:*1022–1023.

Wolf SM. (1973). An unusual case of brain stem glioma with prolonged spontaneous remission and downbeat nystagmus. *Bull Los Angeles Neurol Soc 38:*202–208.

Wolprow ER, Richardson EP Jr. (1988). Case records of the Massachusetts General Hospital. Case 9–1988. *New Eng J Med 318:*563–570.

Yamamoto K, Fukusako T, Nogaki H, Morimatsu M. (1992). Multiple system atrophy with macro square wave jerks and pendular nystagmus (Japanese). *Rinsho Shinkeigaku 32:*1261–1265.

Yamazaki A, Zee DS. (1979). Rebound nystagmus: EOG analysis of a case with a floccular tumor. *Br J Ophthalmol 63:*782–786.

Yamazaki K, Katayama S, Ishihara T, Hirata K. (1994). A case of Fisher's syndrome with upbeat nystagmus (Japanese). *Rinsho Shinkeigaku 34:*489–492.

Yaniglos SS, Leigh RJ. (1992). Refinement of an optical device that stabilizes vision in patients with nystagmus. *Optom Vis Sci 69:*447–450.

Yee RD, Baloh RW, Honrubia V. (1984). Episodic vertical oscillopsia and downbeating nystagmus in a Chiari malformation. *Arch Ophthalmol 102:*723–725.

Yee RD, Baloh RW, Honrubia V, et al. (1979). Slow build-up of optokinetic nystagmus associated with downbeat nystagmus. *Invest Ophthalmol Vis Sci 18:*622–629.

Yee RD, Duffin RM, Baloh RW, Isenberg SJ. (1982). Familial congenital paralysis of horizontal gaze. *Arch Ophthalmol 100:*1449–1452.

Yee RD, Farlow MR, Suzuki DA, et al. (1992). Abnormal eye movements in Gerstmann-Straussler-Scheinker disease. *Arch Ophthalmol 110:*68–74, 178.

Yee RD, Jelks GW, Baloh RW, Honrubia V. (1979). Uniocular nystagmus in monocular visual loss. *Ophthalmology 86:*511–522.

Yee RD. (1989). Downbeat nystagmus: Characteristics and localization of lesions. *Trans Am Ophthalmol Soc 87:*984–1032.
Yeow YK, Tjia TL. (1989). The localizing value of downbeat nystagmus. *Singapore Med J 30:*273–276.
Yokota T, Tsuchiya K, Yamane M, et al. (1991). Geotrophic ocular deviation with skew and absence of saccades in Creutzfeldt-Jacob disease. *J Neurol Sci 106:*175–178.
Yoshimoto Y. (1987a). A case of lithium intoxication with downbeat vertical nystagmus. *Auris Nasus Larynx 14:*71–75.
Yoshimoto Y. (1987b). Neuro-otological findings in a case of Marinesco-Sjogren syndrome with nystagmus. *Auris Nasus Larynx 14:*171–176.
Yoshimoto Y, Koyama S. (1991). A case of acquired nystagmus alternans associated with acute cerebellitis. *Acta Otolaryngol Suppl 481:*371–373.
Young TL, Weis JR, Summers G, Egbert JE. (1997). The association of strabismus, amblyopia, and refractive errors in spasmus nutans. *Ophthalmology 104:*112–117.
Yura S, Sako K, Yonemasu Y. (1988). Primary midbrain hemorrhage with upbeat nystagmus. *Acta Neurol 10:*239–245.
Zahn JR. (1978). Incidence and characteristics of voluntary nystagmus. *J Neurol Neurosurg Psych 41:*617–623.
Zak TA. (1983). Infantile convergence-evoked nystagmus. *Ann Ophthalmol 15:*368–369.
Zangemeister WH, Mueller-Jensen A, Zschocke S. (1979). Benign encephalitis: Electro-oculographic analysis of opsoclonus. *J Neurol 222:*95–108.
Zasorin NL, Baloh RW. (1984). Downbeat nystagmus with alcoholic cerebellar degeneration. *Arch Neurol 41:*1301–1302.
Zauberman H, Magora A. (1969). Congenital "see-saw" movement. *Br J Ophthalmol 53:*418–421.
Zee DS, Yee RD, Cogan DG, et al. (1976). Ocular motor abnormalities in hereditary cerebellar ataxia. *Brain 99:*207–234.
Zegers Beyl DZ, Flament-Durand J, Borenstein S, Brunko E. (1983). Ocular bobbing and myoclonus in central pontine myelinolysis. *J Neurol Neurosurg Psych 46:*564–565.
Zelt RP, Biglan AW. (1985). Congenital seesaw nystagmus. *J Pediatr Ophthalmol Strabismus 22:*13–16.
Zimmerman CF, Roach ES, Troost BT. (1986). See-saw nystagmus associated with Chiari malformation. *Arch Neurol 43:*299–300.
Zubcov AA, Reinencke RD, Gottlob I, et al. (1990). Treatment of manifest latent nystagmus. *Am J Ophthalmol 110:*160–167.
Zubkov AA, Staark N, Weber A, et al. (1993). Improvement of visual acuity after surgery for nystagmus. *Ophthalmology 100:*1488–1497.
Zumstein H, Meienberg O. (1982). Upbeat nystagmus and visual system disorders in Wernicke's encephalopathy due to starvation. *Neuro-ophthalmology 2:*157–162.

18

Ptosis

Ptosis is present when the upper eyelid is less than 2 mm from the center of the pupil (Small, 1989). Ptosis may be classified into mechanical, neurogenic, myogenic, and neuromuscular junction causes (Anderson, 1979b; Beard, 1971, 1978; Caplan, 1974; Collin, 1988; Fox, 1972; Frueh, 1980; Katz, 1968; Kersten, 1995; Leone, 1985a, 1985b; McCord, 1988; Oosterhuis, 1996; Werb, 1976).

What Distinguishes Ptosis from Pseudoptosis?

A number of conditions may cause downward displacement of the eyelid without true ptosis (pseudoptosis) (Hornblass, 1981). These are listed in Table 18–1.

What Is Blepharospasm or Hemifacial Spasm?

Blepharospasm or hemifacial spasm may produce a pseudoptosis due to the intermittent (voluntary or involuntary) closure (spasm) of the upper and lower eyelid(s) resulting from contraction of the orbicularis oculi muscles. The lid position during the periods

Table 18–1. Causes of Pseudoptosis

Aberrant regeneration of the facial nerve
Anophthalmic socket (Vistner, 1976)
Apraxia of lid opening (Goldstein, 1965; Johnston, 1989)
Downgaze paralysis and pseudoblepharoptosis (Cogan, 1974; LoBue, 1983)
Blepharospasm or hemifacial spasm (Krueger, 1978)
Hypertropia or hyperglobus (Gay, 1967; Gonnering, 1988; Kratky, 1992; Lepore, 1988; Lohman, 1984; Lyon, 1993; Meyer, 1991; Schecter, 1978; Sevel, 1984)
Lid retraction in the contralateral eye (Lohman, 1984)
Microphthalmia or phthisis bulbi

without contraction of the orbicularis muscles is normal. Voluntary lid closure may create pseudoptosis and occur as a conversion reaction (Krueger, 1978).

What Is Apraxia of Eyelid Opening?

Apraxia of eyelid opening is a supranuclear inability to open the eyelids voluntarily. Spontaneous and reflex eyelid opening are normal and patients may manually open the lids or employ a head thrust as a compensatory movement. Unilateral or bilateral hemispheric disease and extrapyramidal disease may produce apraxia of lid opening (Goldstein, 1965; Johnston, 1989).

What Is Hypertropia or Hyperglobus?

Hypertropia or hyperglobus may result in an abnormal position of the eye under a normal eyelid. Fixation with the hypertropic eye may eliminate the pseudoptosis. Likewise, contralateral eyelid retraction (e.g., thyroid eye disease) may produce an apparent ptosis in the fellow (normal) eye (Gay, 1967; Gonnering, 1988; Kratky, 1992; Lepore, 1988; Lohman, 1984; Lyon, 1993; Meyer, 1991; Schecter, 1978).

Is the Ptosis Acquired or Congenital?

Ptosis may occur on a congenital or acquired basis (Wobig, 1982). Long-standing isolated and static congenital ptosis with no other signs of systemic neurogenic (e.g., third nerve palsy), myogenic (e.g., chronic progressive external ophthalmoplegia), or neuromuscular disease (e.g., myasthenia gravis) does not require additional evaluation. Other forms of congenital non-isolated ptosis necessitate the same evaluation as the patients with acquired non-isolated ptosis. Table 18–2 lists the various forms of congenital ptosis. Congenital ptosis may be associated with other ocular and non-ocular defects.

Although children with congenital ptosis in isolation do not usually require any further evaluation, they may need surgical therapy to avoid amblyopia (Anderson, 1980a, 1980b; Beneish, 1983; Beyer-Machule, 1988; Cibis, 1995; Cohen, 1972; Crawford, 1986; Harrad,

Table 18–2. Congenital Ptosis

- Isolated
- Nonisolated
  - Associated other ocular defects
    - Congenital cataracts
    - Epicanthus
    - Punctal abnormalities
    - Refractive error/anisometropia
    - Strabismus and amblyopia
  - Associated non-ocular defects (e.g., skeletal, CNS)
  - Blepharophimosis syndrome (Kohn, 1971)
  - Synkinetic ptosis (e.g., Marcus-Gunn jaw winking ptosis)
  - Myogenic (e.g., congenital fibrosis)
  - Neurogenic (e.g., third nerve palsy)
  - Neuromuscular junction (e.g., myasthenia gravis)

1988; Hornblass, 1995; Larned, 1986; Merriam, 1980; McCulloch, 1993; Steel, 1996; Wobig, 1982). Intermittent lid retraction of a ptotic eyelid may occur during chewing, jaw movement, or sucking in a child due to aberrant innervation of the oculomotor (levator) and trigeminal nerves (the Marcus-Gunn jaw winking phenomenon). No evaluation is required in children with the jaw winking phenomenon.

Patients with acquired forms of ptosis should undergo further diagnostic evaluation (Pearl, 1985; Tye, 1971; Waller, 1975; Wilkins, 1982a, 1982b).

Is the Ptosis Isolated or Non-isolated?

A non-isolated acquired ptosis is defined as ptosis associated with other findings that may suggest a specific etiology as listed in Table 18–3 (Wilkins, 1982a, 1982b).

Is the Ptosis due to Mechanical Causes?

Any mechanical disturbance of the upper eyelid may result in ptosis. Mechanical causes of ptosis are listed in Table 18–4.

Table 18–3. Etiologies of Non-isolated Ptosis

Mechanical (e.g., lid mass, infection, or inflammation)
Myogenic (e.g., external ophthalmoplegia)
Neurogenic (e.g., ocular motor deficit and/or diplopia, other neurologic findings)
Horner's syndrome (e.g., miosis, upside down ptosis)
Neuromuscular junction disease (e.g., signs of myasthenia gravis such as fatigue, enhancement, variability, Cogan's lid twitch sign)

Table 18–4. Mechanical Causes of Ptosis

Redundant skin or fat on the upper eyelid (dermatochalasis)
Tumors or cysts of the conjunctiva (Limbert, 1978; Sameshima, 1988) or eyelid (Avisar, 1991)
Infection (e.g., preseptal or orbital cellulitis)
Cicatricial scarring (e.g., post-traumatic, post-surgical, or post-inflammatory)
Inflammation and edema
Graves' disease (Leonard, 1984)
Blepharochalasis (Stiegler, 1974)
Dermatomyositis
Infiltration
Amyloid (Cohen, 1979; Liesegang, 1983; Richlin, 1962; Savino, 1976)
Sarcoid
Neoplastic (e.g., breast cancer) (Po, 1996)
Primary or metastatic tumors or orbital pseudotumor (Cahill, 1986; Dunnaway, 1985; Gonnering, 1987; Liesgang, 1983; Po, 1996)
Neurofibroma
Hemangioma
Dermoid

(continued)

Table 18–4. *(continued)*

Contact lenses (Epstein, 1981; Fonn, 1986; Kersten, 1995; Levy, 1992; Sheldon, 1979; Shenkin, 1969; Uchinuma, 1983; van der Bosch, 1992; Yassin, 1971)
Foreign body reaction
Giant papillary conjunctivitis (Molinari, 1983)
Contact lens migration (Yassin, 1971)
Disinsertion of the levator from excessive eyelid manipulation (Epstein, 1981)

Is the Ptosis due to Myogenic Causes?

Chronic progressive external ophthalmoplegia (CPEO) includes a spectrum of disorders that may result in a syndrome of painless, pupil-sparing, slowly progressive, and generally symmetric ophthalmoplegia. One subset of CPEO, the Kearns-Sayre syndrome, is characterized by the clinical triad of early onset (usually less than 20 years old), CPEO, pigmentary degeneration of the retina, and cardiac abnormalities (e.g., intraventricular conduction defects, bundle branch block, and complete heart block). Other features of Kearns-Sayre syndrome include elevation of cerebrospinal fluid protein, other neurologic dysfunction (e.g., cerebellar, auditory, and vestibular dysfunction), cognitive dysfunction, short stature, or developmental delay. Muscle biopsy may show "ragged red fibers" or other changes in mitochondria (Gross-Jendroska, 1992; Simonsz, 1992). Pathologic examination of the brain may demonstrate spongiform degeneration (Shorr, 1987).

Other systemic and ocular myopathies may cause ptosis but are usually associated with myopathic signs and symptoms due to involvement of extraocular and other muscles (Olenius, 1987; Parmeggiani, 1992). Detailed discussion of these myogenic forms of ptosis is beyond the scope of this text. Myopathies that may cause ptosis are listed in Table 18–5.

Table 18–5. Myopathies Associated with Ptosis

Chronic progressive external ophthalmoplegia (Koerner, 1972; Shorr, 1987)
Congenital fibrosis (Engle, 1995; Gillies, 1995; Leone, 1972; Tandon, 1993; von Noorden, 1970)
Congenital myopathy
- Central core myopathy
- Centronuclear myopathy (Jadro-Santel, 1980)
- Multicore myopathy (Engel, 1971)
- Nemaline myopathy
- Fiber type disproportion (Ohtaki, 1990; Owen, 1981)

Congenital muscular dystrophy (Tsutsumi, 1989)
Diabetes (? hypoxia to levator)
Familial periodic paralysis
Myotonia congenita and myotonic dystrophy (Ashizawa, 1992)
Oculopharyngeal dystrophy (Blumen, 1993; Johnson, 1974; Lacomis, 1991; Murphy, 1968)
Inflammatory and infiltrative myopathies
Hypothyroid myopathy (Green, 1977)

Table 18–6. Neurogenic Conditions Associated with Ptosis

Third nerve palsy
Aberrant regeneration
Alternating ptosis in abetaliproteinemia (Yee, 1976)
Horner's syndrome
Fisher syndrome
Cerebral ptosis (Afifi, 1990; Averbuch-Heller, 1996; Barton, 1995; Caplan, 1975; Krohel, 1978; Nutt, 1977; Lepore, 1987; Lowenstein, 1987; Walsh, 1969; Zachariah, 1994)
Paradoxic supranuclear inhibition of levator tonus (Hepler, 1968)
Seizure-induced (Afifi, 1987)
Chronic inflammatory polyradiculoneuropathy (CIDP) (Chalmers, 1986)
Thiamine deficiency (Varavithya, 1975)
Wernicke's disease (Vogel, 1967)

Is the Ptosis due to a Neurogenic Cause?

The neurogenic causes of ptosis are listed in Table 18–6.

Denervation of the levator muscle due to a third nerve palsy may result in partial or complete ptosis. Levator excursion will be decreased in all of these patients (Frueh, 1980). As noted in Chapter 11, nuclear third nerve palsies result in bilateral ptosis or no ptosis because both levator muscles are innervated by a single central caudal nucleus (Bogousslavsky, 1983; Conway, 1983; Growdon, 1974; Meienberg, 1979). This type of ptosis is usually associated with other features of a third nerve palsy (e.g., pupil involvement, extraocular muscle dysfunction), but may rarely occur with minimal other third nerve signs (Bartleson, 1986; Good, 1990; Wand, 1972). Midbrain lesions may result in ptosis with or without downgaze paralysis, fatiguable ptosis (Ragge, 1992), or pseudoptosis (Buttner-Ennever, 1989; Conway, 1983; Dehaene, 1985; Fleet, 1988; Galetta, 1993; Johnson, 1992; Lagreze, 1996; LoBue, 1989; Meienberg, 1979; Tomecek, 1994).

Ptosis and ipsilateral miosis may be due to a Horner's syndrome. The associated features of the Horner's syndrome are discussed in more detail in Chapter 20.

The Fisher variant of Guillain-Barré syndrome may present with supranuclear ptosis, ophthalmoplegia, ataxia, and areflexia (Becker, 1981; Ishikawa, 1990; Meinenberg, 1983; Yip, 1991).

Unilateral or bilateral hemispheric dysfunction (e.g., stroke, arteriovenous malformation, seizure) may produce ptosis (Afifi, 1990; Averbuch-Heller, 1996; Barton, 1995; Caplan, 1975; Krohel, 1978; Nutt, 1977; Lepore, 1987; Lowenstein, 1987; Walsh, 1969; Zachariah, 1994).

Is Neuromuscular Junction Disease Responsible for the Ptosis?

Myasthenia gravis may result in a ptosis that is often variable and may worsen after sustained effort or fatigue. As noted in Chapter 15, myasthenia gravis may result in ptosis with or without other extraocular muscle dysfunction (Castronuovo, 1983; Kapetansky, 1972; Norman, 1984). Other rare causes of neuromuscular junction ptosis includes wound botulism (Miller, 1977); Eaton-Lambert syndrome (Cruciger, 1983), and topical neuromuscular blockade (e.g., topical timolol) (Berstein, 1981).

What Are the Causes of Isolated Ptosis?

The causes of isolated ptosis include congenital ptosis, trauma (including surgery), steroid-induced ptosis, and aponeurotic ptosis.

Is the Ptosis Secondary to Trauma?

Trauma may damage the skin, soft tissues, muscles, levator complex, or nerve supply of the eyelid (Berke, 1971; Crawford, 1974; Keane, 1993; Marion, 1983; Silkiss, 1987; Smith, 1967). Surgical trauma and/or myotoxicity from the local anesthetic agents during orbital or ocular (including strabismus, retinal, corneal, cataract, glaucoma, and refractive) surgery may also damage the eyelid structures and cause ptosis (Alpar, 1982; Bonham, 1987; Bullock, 1986; Deady, 1989; Feibel, 1993; Kaplan, 1985; Liu, 1992; Linberg, 1986; Loeffler, 1990; Paris, 1973, 1976; Rainin, 1985; Ropo, 1992). Kaplan et al. performed a prospective analysis of ptosis and cataract surgery and felt that trauma to the superior rectus complex was the most critical factor (Kaplan, 1985).

Is the Ptosis Steroid Induced?

Topical steroids have been implicated in some cases of ptosis (Burde, 1992; Dortzbach, 1980; Newsome, 1971). Discontinuation of the steroids may reverse the ptosis in these cases.

Is Aponeurotic Ptosis Present?

Levator aponeurosis thinning and/or dehiscence may occur as a result of trauma, surgery (Paris, 1976), lid swelling, patching, or, most commonly, as an age-related phenomenon (Anderson, 1979; Berlin, 1989; Collin, 1985; Dortzbach, 1980; Frueh, 1980, 1996; Liu, 1993; Martin, 1985; Mehta, 1985; Older, 1978, 1995; Patipa, 1984; Ring, 1982; Sanke, 1984; Shore, 1984; Smith, 1969; Tyers, 1985; Werb, 1985). The characteristic features of aponeurotic ptosis are listed in Table 18–7.

Patients with aponeurotic ptosis may have significant ptosis in downgaze more than primary position (Dryden, 1992; Wojno, 1993). In the absence of findings to suggest mechanical, neurogenic, myogenic, or neuromuscular etiologies for ptosis, no further evaluation is necessary (Collin, 1986). Superior visual field loss may occur due to ptosis and may be an indication for surgical correction (Cahill, 1987). The surgical treatment of aponeurotic ptosis is well described in the literature and is not reviewed here (Anderson, 1979; Berlin, 1989; Collin, 1985; Dortzbach, 1980; Frueh, 1996; Jones, 1975; Jordan, 1987; Liu, 1993; Martin, 1985; Mehta, 1985; Older, 1978, 1983, 1995; Patipa, 1984; Ring, 1982; Sanke, 1984; Shore, 1984; Smith, 1969; Tyers, 1985; Werb, 1985).

Table 18–7. Clinical Features of Aponeurotic Ptosis

Clinical Features
Acquired
Good to excellent levator function (> 12 mm)
Elevated or absent lid crease
Thinning of the eyelid above the tarsus
Bilateral
Elderly population

An approach to the evaluation of ptosis is outlined in Figure 18–1.

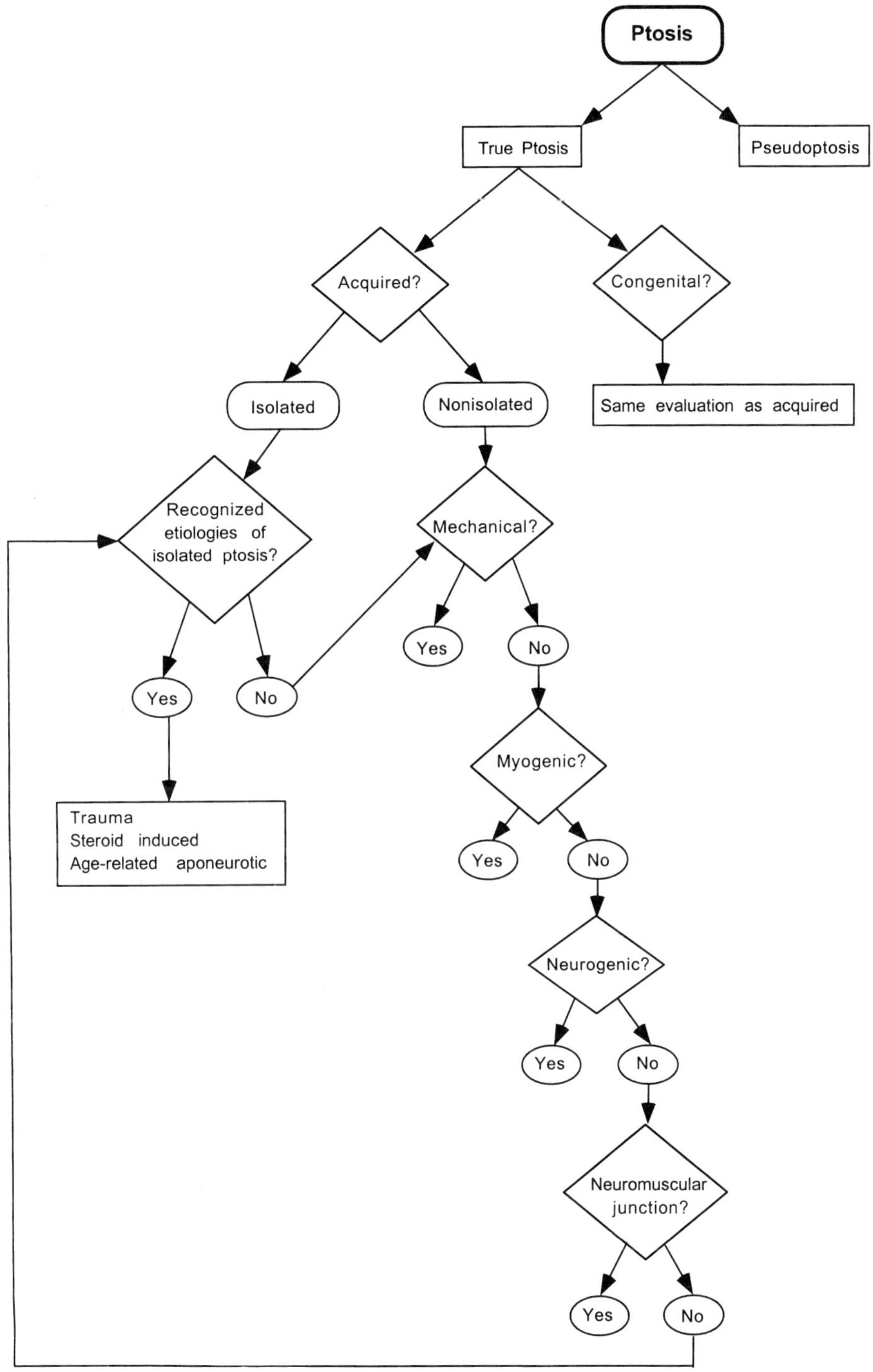

Figure 18–1. Ptosis.

References

Afifi AK, Corbett JJ, Thompson HS, Wells KK. (1990). Seizure-induced miosis and ptosis: Association with temporal lobe magnetic resonance imaging abnormalities. *J Child Neurol 5:*142–146.

Alpar JJ. (1982). Acquired ptosis following cataract and glaucoma surgery. *Glaucoma 4:*66–68.

Anderson RL, Baumgartner SA. (1980a). Amblyopia in ptosis. *Arch Ophthalmol 98:*1068–1069.

Anderson RL, Baumgartner SA. (1980b). Strabismus in ptosis. *Arch Ophthalmol 98:*1062–1067.

Anderson RL, Dixon RS. (1979a). Aponeurotic ptosis surgery. *Arch Ophthalmol 97:*1123–1128.

Anderson RL, Dixon RS. (1979b). Neuromyopathic ptosis: A new surgical approach. *Arch Ophthalmol 97:*1129–1131.

Arden RL, Moore GK. (1989). Complete post-traumatic ptosis: A mechanism for recovery? *Laryngoscope 99:*1175–1179.

Ashizawa T, Hejtmancki JF, Liu J, Perryman MB, Epstein MF, Koch DD. (1992). Diagnostic value of ophthalmologic findings in myotonic dystrophy: Comparison with risks calculated by haplotype analysis of closely linked restriction fragment length polymorphisms. *Am J Med Genet 42:*55–60.

Averbuch-Heller L, Stahl JS, Remler BR, Leigh RJ. (1996). Bilateral ptosis and upgaze palsy with right hemispheric lesions. *Ann Neurol 40:*465–468.

Avisar R, Leshem Y, Savir H. (1991). Unilateral congenital ptosis due to plexiform neurofibroma, causing refraction error and secondary amblyopia. *Met Pediatr System Ophthalmol 14:*62–63.

Bartleson JD, Trautmann JC, Sundt TM Jr. (1986). Minimal oculomotor nerve paresis secondary to unruptured intracranial aneurysm. *Arch Neurol 43:*1015–1020.

Barton JJ, Kardon RH, Slagel D, Thompson HS. (1995). Bilateral central ptosis in acquired immunodeficiency syndrome (review). *Can J Neurol Sci 22:*52–55.

Beard C. (1971). Ptosis: Some newer concepts. *Ann Ophthalmol 3:*1047–1048.

Beard C, Sullivan JH. (1978). Ptosis—current concepts. *Int Ophthalmol Clin 18:*53–73.

Becker WJ, Watters GV, Humphreys P. (1981). Fischer syndrome in childhood. *Neurology 31:*555–560.

Beneish R, Williams F, Polomeno RC, Little JM, Ramsey B. (1983). Unilateral congenital ptosis and amblyopia. *Can J Ophthalmol 18:*127–130.

Berke RN. (1971). Surgical treatment of traumatic blepharoptosis. *Am J Ophthalmol 72:*691.

Berlin AJ, Vestal KP. (1989). Levator aponeurosis surgery. A retrospective review. *Ophthalmology 96:*1033–1037.

Berstein LP, Henkind P. (1981). Additional information on adverse reactions to timolol. *Am J Ophthalmol 92:*295–296.

Beyer-Machule CK. (1988). Congenital ptosis and complications of ptosis surgery. *Plast Reconstr Surg 81:*789–799.

Blumen SC, Nisipeanu P, Sadeh M, Asherov A, Tome F, Korczyn AD. (1993). Clinical features of oculopharyngeal muscular dystrophy among Bukhara Jews. *Neuromusc Dis 3:*575–577.

Bonham RD, Iliff WF, Stark WF, Smith PW, Whitney CE. (1987). Ptosis following refractive corneal surgery. Case report. *Arch Ophthalmol 105:*25.

Bogousslavsky J, Regli F, Ghika J, Hunderbuhler JP. (1983). Internuclear ophthalmoplegia, prenuclear paresis of contralateral superior rectus, and bilateral ptosis. *J Neurol 230:*197–203.

Bullock JD. (1986). Prevention of post-cataract extraction ptosis (letter). *Arch Ophthalmol 104:*972.

Buttner-Ennever JA, Acheson JF, Buttner U, et al. (1989). Ptosis and supranuclear downgaze paralysis. *Neurology 39:*385–389.

Cahill KV, Buerger GF, Jr, Johnson BL. (1986). Ptosis associated with fatty infiltration of Muller's muscle and levator muscle. *Ophthalm Plast Reconstr Surg 2:*213–217.

Cahill KV, Burns JA, Weber PA. (1987). The effect of blepharoptosis on the field of vision. *Ophthalm Plast Reconstr Surg 3:*121–125.

Caplan LR. (1974). Ptosis. *J Neurol Neurosurg Psychiatr 37:*1–7.

Castonuovo S, Krohel GB, Kristan RW. (1983). Blepharoptosis in myasthenia gravis. *Ann Ophthalmol 15:*751–754.

Chalmers AC, Miller RG. (1986). Chronic inflammatory polyradiculoneuropathy with ophthalmoplegia. *J Clin Neuro-ophthalmol 6:*166–168.

Cibis GW, Fitzgerald KM. (1995). Amblyopia in unilateral congenital ptosis: Early detection by sweep visual evoked potential. *Graefes Arch Clin Exp Ophthalmol 233:*605–609.

Cogan DG. (1974). Paralysis of down-gaze. *Arch Ophthalmol 91:*192–199.

Cohen HB. (1972). Congenital ptosis: A new pedigree and classification. *Arch Ophthalmol 87:*161–163.

Cohen MM, Lessell S. (1979). Amyloid tumor of the orbit. *Neuroradiology 18:*157–159.

Collin JR. (1986). Involutional ptosis. *Austral N Z J Ophthalmol 14:*109–112.

Collin JR. (1988). New concepts in the management of ptosis. *Eye 2:*185–188.

Collin JR, Tyers AG. (1985). Senile ptosis II: posterior approach and complications. *Trans Ophthalmol Soc UK 104:*(pt 1):17–21.

Conway VH, Rozdilsky B, Schneider RJ, Sundaram M. (1983). Isolated bilateral complete ptosis. *Can J Ophthalmol 18:*37–40.

Crawford JS. (1974). Ptosis as a result of trauma. *Can J Ophthalmol 9:*244–248.

Crawford JS. (1986). Congenital ptosis: Examination and treatment. *Trans New Orleans Acad Ophthalmol 34:*173–191.

Cruciger MP, Brown B, Denys EH, et al. (1983). Clinical and subclinical oculomotor findings in the Eaton-Lambert syndrome. *J Clin Neuro-ophthalmol 3:*19–21.

Deady JP, Price NJ, Sutton GA. (1989). Ptosis following cataract and trabeculectomy surgery. *Br J Ophthalmol 73:*283–285.

D'Esposito M, Bonavolonta G, Magli A, Aurilia P. (1989). Ptosis correction in the context of the treatment of external congenital ophthalmoplegia. *Ophthalm Plast Reconstr Surg 5:*176–181.

Dehaene I, Dom R, Marchau M, Geens K. (1985). Locked-in syndrome with bilateral ptosis: Combination of bilateral horizontal pontine paralysis and nuclear oculomotor nerve paralysis. *J Neurol 232:*366–367.

Dortzbach RK, Sutula FC. (1980). Involutional blepharoptosis: a histopathological study. *Arch Ophthalmol 98:*2045–2049.

Dryden RM, Kahanic DA. (1992). Worsening of blepharoptosis in downgaze. *Ophthalm Plast Reconstr Surg 8:*126–129.

Dunnaway RL. (1985). Ptosis as the presenting sign of orbital involvement from metastatic bronchogenic carcinoma. *Am J Optom Physiol Optics 62:*908–912.

Engel AG, Gomez MR, Groover RV. (1971). Multicore disease: A recently recognized congenital myopathy associated with multifocal degeneration of muscle fibers. *Mayo Clin Proc 46:*666–681.

Engle EC, Marondel I, Houtman WA, et al. (1995). Congenital fibrosis of the extraocular muscles (autosomal dominant congenital external ophthalmoplegia): Genetic homogeneity, linkage refinement, and physical mapping on chromosome 12. *Am J Hum Genet 57:*1086–1094.

Epstein FA, Putterman AM. (1984). Super-maximum levator resection for severe unilateral congenital blepharoptosis. *Ophthalmic Surg 15:*971.

Epstein G, Putterman AM. (1981). Acquired blepharoptosis secondary to contact-lens wear. *Am J Ophthalmol 91:*634–639.

Etzihe S. (1966). Congenital ptosis with paradoxic eyelid movements. *Am J Ophthalmol 61:*793–795.

Feibel RM, Custer PL, Gordon MO. (1993). Postcataract ptosis: A randomized, double-masked comparison of peribulbar and retrobulbar anesthesia. *Ophthalmol 100:*660–665.

Fleet WS, Rapcsak SZ, Huntley WW, Watson RT. (1988). Pupil-sparing oculomotor palsy from midbrain hemorrhage. *Ann Ophthalmol 20:*345–346.

Fonn D, Holden BA. (1986). Extended wear of hard gas permeable contact lenses can induce ptosis. *CLAO Journal 12:*93–94.

Fox SA. (1971). Surgery for progressive familial myopathic ptosis. *Ann Ophthalmol* 1033–1039.

Fox SA. (1972). A new ptosis classification. Late spontaneous ptosis. *Arch Ophthalmol 88:*590–593.

Frueh BR. (1980). The mechanistic classification of ptosis. *Ophthalmology 87:*1019–1021.

Frueh BR, Musch DC. (1996). Evaluation of levator muscle integrity in ptosis with levator force measurement. *Ophthalmology 103:*244–250.

Galetta SL, Gray LG, Raps EC, Grossman RI, Schatz NJ. (1993). Unilateral ptosis and contralateral eyelid retraction from a thalamic-midbrain infarction. Magnetic resonance imaging correlation. *J Clin Neuro-ophthalmol 13:*221–224.

Gay AJ, Salmon ML, Windsor CE. (1967). Hering's law, the levators and their relationship in disease states. *Arch Ophthalmol 77:*157–160.

Gillies WE, Harris AJ, Brooks AM, Rivers MR, Wolfe RJ. (1995). Congenital fibrosis of the vertically acting extraocular muscles. A new group of dominantly inherited ocular fibrosis with radiologic findings. *Ophthalmology 102:*607–612.

Goldstein JE, Cogan DG. (1965). Apraxia of lid opening. *Arch Ophthalmol 73:*155–159.

Gonnering RS. (1988). Pseudoretraction of the eyelid in thyroid associated orbitopathy. *Arch Ophthalmol 106:*1078–1080.

Gonnering RS, Sonneland PR. (1987). Ptosis and dermatochalasis as presenting signs in a case of occult primary systemic amyloidosis (AL). *Ophthalmic Surg 18:*495–497.

Good EF. (1990). Ptosis as the sole manifestation of compression of the oculomotor nerve by an aneurysm of the posterior communicating artery. *J Clin Neuro-ophthalmol 10:*59–61.

Green HP. (1977). Bilateral ptosis and proximal myopathy—muscular manifestations of hypothyroidism. *Aust N Z J Med 7:*418–419.

Gross-Jendroska M, Schatz H, McDonald HR, Johnson RN. (1992). Kearns-Sayre syndrome: A case report and review (review). *Eur J Ophthalmol 2:*15–20.

Growdon JH, Winkler GF, Wray SH. (1974). Midbrain ptosis: A case with clinico-pathologic correlation. *Arch Neurol 30:*179–181.

Harrad RA, Graham CM, Collin JRO. (1988). Amblyopia and strabismus in congenital ptosis. *Eye 2:*625–627.

Hepler RS, Hoyt WF, Loeffler JD. (1968). Paradoxical synkinetic levator inhibition and excitation: An electromyographic study of unilateral oculopalpebral and bilateral mandibulopalpebral (Marcus Gunn) synkinesis in a 74-year-old man. *Arch Neurol 18:*416–424.

Hornblass A. (1981). Ptosis and pseudoptosis and blepharoplasty. *Clin Plast Surg 8:*811–830.

Hornblass A, Kass LG, Ziffer AJ. (1995). Amblyopia in congenital ptosis. *Ophthalm Surg 26:*334–337.

Ishikawa H, Wakakura M, Ishikawa S. (1990). Enhanced ptosis in Fisher's syndrome after Epstein Barr virus infection. *J Clin Neuro-ophthalmol 10:*197–200.

Jadro-Santel D, Grcevvic N, Dogan S, et al. (1980). Centronuclear myopathy with type I fibre hypotrophy and "fingerprint" inclusions associated with Marfan's syndrome. *J Neurol Sci 45:*43–56.

Johnson CC, Kuwabara T. (1974). Oculopharyngeal muscular dystrophy. *Am J Ophthalmol 77:*872–879.

Johnson LN, Castro D. (1992). Monocular elevation paresis and incomplete ptosis due to midbrain infarction involving the fascicular segment of the oculomotor nerve (letter). *J Clin Neuro-ophthalmol 12:*73.

Johnston JC, Rosenbaum DM, Picone CM, et al. (1989). Apraxia of eyelid opening secondary to right hemisphere infarction. *Ann Neurol 25:*622–624.

Jones LT, Quickert MH, Wobig JL. (1975). The cure of ptosis by aponeurotic repair. *Arch Ophthalmol 93:*629–634.

Jordan DR, Anderson RL. (1987). A simple procedure for adjusting eyelid position after aponeurotic ptosis surgery. *Arch Ophthalmol 105:*1288–1291.

Kapetansky DI. (1972). Surgical correction of blepharoptosis in myasthenia gravis. *Am J Ophthalmol 74:*818–820.

Kaplan LJ, Jaffe NS, Clayman HM. (1985). Ptosis and cataract surgery. A multivariant computer analysis of a prospective study. *Ophthalmology 92:*237–242.

Katz AH, Kuder GG. (1968). Ptosis: A ten year review. *Can J Ophthalmol 3:*353–357.

Keane JR. (1993). Ptosis and levator paralysis caused by orbital roof fractures. Three cases with subfrontal epidural hematomas. *J Clin Neuro-ophthalmol 13:*225–228.

Kersten RC, De Concillis C, Kulwin DR. (1995). Acquired ptosis in the young and middle-aged adult population. *Ophthalmology 102:*924–928.

Koerner F, Schlote W. (1972). Chronic progressive external ophthalmoplegia. *Arch Ophthalmol 88:*155.

Kohn R, Romano PE. (1971). Blepharoptosis, blepharophimosis, epicanthus inversus and telecanthus—a syndrome with no name. *Am J Ophthalmol 72:*625.

Kratky V, Harvey JT. (1992). Tests for contralateral pseudoretraction in blepharoptosis. *Ophthalm Plast Reconstr Surg 8:*22–25.

Krohel GB, Griffin JF. (1978). Cortical blepharoptosis. *Am J Ophthalmol 85:*632–634.

Krueger DW. (1978). Unilateral ptosis as a conversion reaction. *J Clin Psychiatr 39:*351, 355–356.

Lacomis D, Kupsky WJ, Kuban KK, Specht LA. (1991). Childhood onset oculopharyngeal muscular dystrophy. *Pediatr Neurol 7:*382–384.

Lagreze WD, Warner JE, Zamani AA, Gouras GK, Koralnik IJ, Bienfang DC. (1996). Mesencephalic clefts with associated eye movement disorders. *Arch Ophthalmol 114:*429–432.

Larned DC, Flanagan JC, Nelson LE, Harley RD, Wilson TW. (1986). The association of congenital ptosis and congenital heart disease. *Ophthalmol 93:*492–494.

Leonard TJ, Graham EM, Stanford MR, Sanders MD. (1984). Graves' disease presenting with bilateral acute painful proptosis, ptosis, ophthalmoplegia, and visual loss. *Lancet 2:*431–433.

Leone CR Jr, Shore JW. (1985a). The management of the ptosis patient: Part I. *Ophthalm Surg 16:*666–670.

Leone CR Jr, Shore JW. (1985b). The management of the ptosis patient: Part II. *Ophthalm Surg 16:*720–727.

Leone CR Jr, Weinstein GW. (1972). Orbital fibrosis and enophthalmos. *Ophthalm Surg 3:*71.

Lepore FE. (1988). Unilateral ptosis and Hering's law. *Neurology 38:*319–322.

Lepore FE. (1987). Bilateral cerebral ptosis. *Neurology 37:*1043–1046.

Levy B, Stamper RL. (1992). Acute ptosis secondary to contact lens wear. *Optom Vis Sci 69:*565–566.

Liesgang TJ. (1983). Amyloid infiltration of the levator palpebrae superioris muscle: Case report. *Ann Ophthalmol 15:*610–613.

Limbert JG, Levine MR, Rutti PJ, Kohn HD. (1978). Acquired ptosis secondary to conjunctival cysts. *Ophthalm Surg 9:*86–91.

Linberg JV, McDonald MB, Safir A, Googe JM. (1986). Ptosis following radial keratotomy. Performed using a rigid eyelid speculum. *Ophthalmology 93:*1509–1512.

Liu D. (1993). Ptosis repair by single suture aponeurotic tuck. Surgical technique and long-term results. *Ophthalmology 100:*251–259.

Liu D, Bachynski BN. (1992). Complete ptosis as a result of removal of epibulbar lipodermoid. *Ophthalm Plast Reconstr Surg 8:*134–136.

LoBue TD, Feldon SE. (1983). Reverse Collier's sign: Pseudoblepharoptosis associated with downgaze paralysis (letter). *Am J Ophthalmol 95:*120–121.

Loeffler M, Solomon LD, Renaud M. (1990). Postcataract extraction ptosis: Effect of the bridle suture. *J Cat Refract Surg 16:*501–504.

Lohman L, Burns JA, Penland WR, Cahill KV. (1984). Unilateral eyelid retraction secondary to contralateral ptosis in dysthyroid ophthalmopathy. *J Clin Neuro-ophthalmol 4:*163–166.

Lowenstein DH, Koch TK, Edwards MS. (1987). Cerebral ptosis with contralateral arteriovenous malformation: a report of two cases. *Ann Neurol 21:*404–407.

Lyon DB, Gonnering RS, Dorztbach RK, Lemke BN. (1993). Unilateral ptosis and eye dominance. *Ophthalm Plast Reconstr Surg 9:*237–240.

McCord CD Jr. (1988). The evaluation and management of the patient with ptosis. *Clin Plast Surg 15:*169–184.

McCulloch DL, Wright KW. (1993). Unilateral congenital ptosis: Compensatory head posturing and amblyopia. *Ophthalm Plast Reconstr Surg 9:*196–200.

Marion JR. (1983). Dehiscence or tear of the levator aponeurosis as a cause of ptosis in children. *No Carolina Med J 44:*635–636.

Martin JJ Jr, Tenzel RR. (1992). Acquired ptosis: Dehiscences and disinsertions. Are they real or iatrogenic? *Ophthalm Plast Reconstr Surg 8:*130–132.

Martin PA, Rogers PA. (1985). Involutional ptosis: Recognition and management. *Austr N Z J Ophthalmol 13:*185–187.

Martin PA, Rogers PA. (1988). Congenital aponeurotic ptosis. *Austr N Z J Ophthalmol 16:*291–294.

Mehta HK. (1985). Day surgery management of senile ptosis. *Trans Ophthalmol Soc UK 104:*(pt 2):171–175.
Mehta HK. (1979). The contralateral upper eyelid in ptosis: Some observations pertinent to ptosis corrective surgery. *Br J Ophthalmol 63:*120–124.
Meienberg O, Mumenthaler M, Karbowski K. (1979). Quadriparesis and nuclear oculomotor palsy with total bilateral ptosis mimicking coma: A mesencephalic "locked-in syndrome"? *Arch Neurol 38:*708–710.
Meienberg O, Ryffel E. (1983). Supranuclear eye movement disorders in Fisher's syndrome of ophthalmoplegia, ataxia, and areflexia. Report of a case and literature review. *Arch Neurol 40:*402–405.
Merriam WW, Ellis FD, Helveston EM. (1980). Congenital blepharoptosis, anisometropia, and amblyopia. *Am J Ophthalmol 89:*401–407.
Meyer DR, Wobig JL. (1991). Detection of contralateral eyelid retraction associated with blepharoptosis. *Ophthalmology 98:*366–375.
Miller NR, Moses H. (1977). Ocular involvement in wound botulism. *Arch Ophthalmol 95:*1788–1789.
Molinari JF. (1983). Transient ptosis secondary to giant papillary conjunctivitis in a hydrogel lens patient. *J Amer Optom Assoc 54:*1007–1009.
Murphy SF, Drachman DB. (1968). The oculopharyngeal syndrome. *JAMA 203:*1003.
Newsome DA, Wong VG, Cameron TP, Anderson RR. (1971). "Steroid-induced" mydriasis and ptosis. *Invest Ophthalmol 10:*424–429.
Norman RA. (1984). Differential diagnosis of ptosis: Report of a case of myasthenia gravis in a patient with diabetes and thyroid disease. *J Amer Osteopath Assoc 83:*523–526.
Nutt JG. (1977). Lid abnormalities secondary to cerebral hemispheric lesions. *Ann Neurol 1:*149–151.
Ohtaki E, Yamaguch Y, Yamashita Y, et al. (1990). Complete external ophthalmoplegia in a patient with congenital myopathy without specific features (minimal change myopathy). *Brain Dev 12:*427–430.
Older JJ. (1978). Levator aponeurosis disinsertion in the young adult. *Arch Ophthalmol 96:*1857–1858.
Older JJ. (1983). Levator aponeurosis surgery for the correction of acquired ptosis: Analysis of 113 procedures. *Ophthalmology 90:*1056–1059.
Older JJ. (1995). Ptosis repair and blepharoplasty in the adult (Review). *Ophthalm Surg 26:*304–308.
Olenius M, Nylen B. (1987). Ocular myopathy with palpebral ptosis. *Ann Plast Surg 19:*146–153.
Oosterhuis HJ. (1996). Acquired blepharoptosis. *Clin Neurol Neurosurg 98:*1–7.
Owen JS, Kline LB, Oh SJ, Miles NE, Benton JW. (1981). Ophthalmoplegia and ptosis in congenital fiber type disproportion. *J Ped Ophthalmol Strab 18:*55–60.
Paris GL, Beard C. (1973). Blepharoptosis following dermolipoma surgery. *Ann Ophthalmol 5:*697–699.
Paris GL, Quickert MH. (1976). Disinsertion of the aponeurosis of the levator palpebral superioris muscle after cataract extraction. *Am J Ophthalmol 81:*337–340.
Parmeggiani A, Posar A, Leonardi M, Rossi PG. (1992). Neurological impairment in congenital bilateral ptosis with ophthalmoplegia. *Brain Dev 14:*107–109.
Patipa M, Wilkins RB. (1984). Acquired ptosis in patients undergoing upper eyelid blepharoplasty. *Ann Ophthalmol 16:*266–270.
Pearl RM. (1985). Acquired ptosis: A reexamination of etiology and treatment. *Plast Reconstr Surg 76:*56–64.
Po SM, Custer PL, Smith ME. (1996). Bilateral lagophthalmos. An unusual presentation of metastatic breast carcinoma. *Arch Ophthalmol 114:*1139–1141.
Ragge NK, Hoyt WF. (1992). Midbrain myasthenia: Fatiguable ptosis, lid twitch sign, and ophthalmoparesis from a dorsal midbrain glioma. *Neurol 42:*917–919.
Rainin EA, Carlson BM. (1985). Postoperative diplopia and ptosis. A clinical hypothesis based on myotoxicity of local anesthesia. *Arch Ophthalmol 103:*1337–1339.
Richlin JJ, Kuwubara T. (1962) Amyloid disease of the eyelid and conjunctiva. *Arch Ophthalmol 67:*138–142.
Ring CP. (1982). Management of ptosis due to defects of the levator aponeurosis. *Trans Ophthalmol Soc NZ 34:*64–69.
Ropo A, Ruusuvaara P, Nikki P. (1992). Ptosis following periocular or general anesthesia in cataract surgery. *Acta Ophthalmol 70:*262–265.
Sameshima SS, Beyer-Machule CK. (1988). Acquired ptosis associated with a conjunctival cyst. *Ophthalm Plast Reconstr Surg 4:*159–162.
Sanke RF. (1984). Relationship of senile ptosis to age. *Ann Ophthalmol 16:*928–931.
Savino PJ, Schatz NJ, Rodrigues MM. (1976). Orbital amyloidosis. *Can J Ophthalmol 11:*252–255.
Schecter RJ. (1978). Ptosis with contralateral lid retraction due to excessive innervation of the levator palpebral superioris. *Ann Ophthalmol 10:*1324–1328.
Sevel D. (1984). Ptosis and underaction of the superior rectus muscle. *Ophthalmology 91:*1080–1085.
Sheldon L, Biedner B, Geltman C, Sachs U. (1979). Giant papillary conjunctivitis and ptosis in contact lens wearer. *J Ped Ophthalmol Strab 16:*136–137.
Shenkin E. (1969). Traumatic dislocation of a contact lens into the eyelid. *Can Med Assoc J 101:*295–296.
Shore JW, McCord CD. (1984). Anatomic changes in involutional blepharoptosis. *Am J Ophthalmol 98:*21–27.
Shorr N, Christenbury JD, Goldberg RA. (1987). Management of ptosis in chronic progressive external ophthalmoplegia. *Ophthalmic Plast Reconstr Surg 3:*141–145.
Silkiss RZ, Baylis H. (1987). Management of traumatic ptosis. *Adv Ophthalm Plast Reconstr Surg 7:*149–155.
Simonsz HJ, Barlocher K, Rotig A. (1992). Kearns-Sayre syndrome developing in a boy who survived Pearson's syndrome caused by mitochondrial DNA deletion. *Doc Ophthalmol 82:*73–79.
Small RG, Sabates NR, Burrows D. (1989). The measurement and definition of ptosis. *Ophthal Plast Reconstr Surg 5:*171–175.

Smith B, McCord CD, Baylis H. (1969). Surgical treatment of blepharoptosis. *Am J Ophthalmol 68:*92–99.
Smith B, Obear MF. (1967). Traumatic blepharoptosis. *Surg Clin No Amer 47:*515.
Steel DH, Harrad RA. (1996). Unilateral congenital ptosis with ipsilateral superior rectus muscle overaction. *Am J Ophthalmol 122:*550–556.
Stiegler LN, Crawford JS. (1974). Blepharochalasis. *Am J Ophthalmol 77:*100.
Tandon RK, Burke JP, Strachan IM. (1993). Unilateral congenital fibrosis syndrome presenting with hypertropia. *Acta Ophthalmol 71:*860–862.
Tomecek FJ, Morgan JK. (1994). Ophthalmoplegia with bilateral ptosis secondary to midbrain hemorrhage. A case with clinical and radiologic correlation. *Surg Neurol 41:*131–136.
Tsutsumi A, Uchida Y, Osawa M, Fukuyama Y. (1989). Ocular findings in Fukuyama type congenital muscular dystrophy. *Brain Dev 11:*413–419.
Tye AA. (1971). Neurological aspects of ptosis. *Trans Austr Coll Ophthalmol 3:*76–79.
Tyers AG, Collin JR. (1985). Senile ptosis—introduction and anterior approach. *Trans Ophthalmol Soc UK 104:*(pt 1):11–16.
Uchinuma E, Torkia K, Shioya N, Mukuno K. (1983). Repair of ptosis possibly attributable to the long-term wearing of contact lenses. *Ann Plast Surg 11:*252–254.
van der Bosch WA, Lemij HG. (1992). Blepharoptosis induced by prolonged hard contact lens wear. *Ophthalmology 99:*1759–1765.
Varavithya W, Dhanamitta S, Valyasevi A. (1975). Bilateral ptosis as a sign of thiamine deficiency in childhood. Response to corrective therapy is rapid. *Clin Pediatr 14:*1063–1065.
Vistner LM. (1976). Mechanism of upper lid ptosis in the anophthalmic orbit. *Plast Reconstr Surg 58:*539–545.
Vogel RM, Lee RV. (1967). Bilateral ptosis in Wernicke's disease. *Neurology 17:*85–86.
von Noorden GK. (1970). Congenital hereditary ptosis with inferior rectus fibrosis. Report of two cases. *Arch Ophthalmol 83:*378–380.
Waller RR. (1975). Management of myogenic (myopathic) ptosis. *Trans Am Acad Ophthalm Otolaryngol 79:*697–702.
Walsh FB, Hoyt WF. (1969). *Clinical Neuro-ophthalmology.* 3rd edition. Williams & Wilkins, Baltimore, Maryland, vol. 1, p. 298.
Wand O. (1972). Ptosis associated with aseptic meningitis. *Arch Ophthalmol 88:*334–335.
Werb A. (1985). Senile ptosis. *Trans Ophthalmol Soc UK 104:*(pt 1):22–25.
Werb A. (1976). Ptosis. *Trans Ophthalmol Soc NZ 28:*29–32.
Wilkins RB, Patipa M. (1982a). Acquired ptosis and current treatment. *Trans New Orleans Acad Ophthalm 30:*93–104.
Wilkins RB, Patipa M. (1982b). The recognition of acquired ptosis in patients considered for upper-eyelid blepharoplasty. *Plast Reconstruc Surg 70:*431–434.
Wobig JL. (1982). Congenital ptosis and levator resection. *Trans New Orleans Acad Ophthalmol 30:*86–92.
Wojno TH. (1993). Downgaze ptosis. *Ophthalm Plast Reconstr Surg 9:*83–89.
Yassin JG, White RH, Shannon GM. (1971). Blepharoptosis as a complication of contact lens migration. *Am J Ophthalmol 72:*536.
Yee RD, Cogan DG, Zee DS. (1976). Ophthalmoplegia and dissociated nystagmus in abetalipoproteinemia. *Arch Ophthalmol 94:*571–575.
Yip PK. (1991). Bilateral ptosis, ataxia and areflexia—a variant of Fisher's syndrome (letter). *J Neurol Neurosurg Psychiatr 54:*1121.
Zachariah SB, Wilson MC, Zachariah B. (1994). Bilateral lid ptosis on a supranuclear basis in the elderly. *J Am Geriatr Soc 42:*215–217.

♦ 19 ♦

Lid Retraction and Lid Lag

In normal adults, the upper lid just covers the superior cornea (1–2 mm) and the lower lid lies slightly below the inferior corneal margin. Eyelid elevation occurs with contraction of the levator palpebrae superioris (LPS) muscle innervated by the oculomotor nerve. Accessory muscles include Müller's muscle (sympathetic innervation), which is embedded in the LPS and inserts mainly on the tarsal plate, and the frontalis muscle (innervated by the temporal branch of the facial nerve), which helps to retract the lid in extreme upgaze (Schmidtke, 1992). Tone in the LPS normally parallels that to the superior rectus muscle and in extreme downgaze both muscles are completely inhibited. However, there is an inverse relationship between the LPS and the superior rectus during forced lid closure where the eye elevates (Bell's phenomenon). The motor neurons for both levator muscles are in the unpaired central caudal nucleus (CCN), located at the dorsal caudal pole of the oculomotor complex adjacent to the medial rectus and superior rectus subdivisions. Within the CCN, motor neurons of both LPS muscles are intermixed. The region of the nuclear complex of the posterior commissure is involved in lid–eye movement coordination (Schmidtke, 1992).

The upper lid position is abnormal if it exposes a white band of sclera between the lid margin and the upper corneal limbus. This may be due to lid retraction (related to overactivity of the LPS, contracture of the LPS, or hyperactivity of Müller's muscle), or lid lag, which is noted on attempted downgaze. Bartley has reviewed the differential diagnosis and classification of eyelid retraction and divided etiologies into four categories: neurogenic, myogenic (including disease processes affecting the neuromuscular junction), mechanical, and miscellaneous (Bartley, 1996). We will adopt his classification in this chapter, discuss the etiologies of lid lag and lid retraction, and suggest a diagnostic approach.

What Are the Neurogenic Causes of Lid Retraction and Lid Lag?

Neurogenic eyelid retraction and lid lag may be due to supranuclear, nuclear, or infranuclear lesions affecting the LPS or conditions that produce hyperactivity of the sympathetically innervated Müller's muscle (Miller, 1985).

Preterm infants may have a benign transient conjugate downward gaze deviation with eyelid retraction thought to be due to immature myelination of vertical eye movement control pathways (Kleinman, 1994; Miller, 1985). Approximately 80% of normal infants of 14 to 18 weeks of age may demonstrate bilateral transient lid retraction ("eye popping reflex") when ambient light levels are suddenly reduced (Perez, 1972). Both of these phenomena are benign and require no evaluation.

Dorsal mesencephalic supranuclear lesions may result in eyelid retraction, which is noted when the eyes are in the primary position of gaze or on looking upward (Collier's sign or "posterior fossa stare"). Unlike the retraction from thyroid orbitopathy (see below), with midbrain lid retraction, there is no retraction in downgaze. Patients with dorsal mesencephalic lesions often have associated vertical gaze palsies; the etiologies of the dorsal midbrain syndrome and the work-up of these patients are discussed in Chapter 14. Spells of lid retraction lasting 20 to 30 seconds that may be seen with impending tentorial brain herniation may well be due to a dorsal mesencephalic mechanism (Miller, 1985).

Lesions of the medial and/or principal portion of the nuclear complex of the posterior commissure (NPC) are essential for the production of lid retraction because these structures are assumed to be involved in lid–eye coordination by providing inhibitory modulation of levator motor neuronal activity (Schmidtke, 1992). Clinical and experimental evidence suggests that there is an inhibitory premotor network in the periaqueductal gray (the supraoculomotor area or supra III), dorsal to the third cranial nerve nucleus, that projects from the NPC to the central caudal subnucleus (Schmidtke, 1992; Galetta, 1993a, 1993b,1996). Lesions in the region of NPC may produce excessive innervation to the lids and consequently lid retraction in primary position; thus, bilateral eyelid retraction and eyelid lag with minimal impairment of vertical gaze has been described with a circumscribed unilateral lesion immediately rostral and dorsal to the red nucleus involving the lateral periaqueductal gray area in the region of the NPC (Galetta, 1993a, 1993b, 1996). Eyelid lag without retraction has also been described in pretectal disease, implying that these lid signs may have separate neural mechanisms (Galetta, 1996). Conversely, vertical gaze paralysis without eyelid retraction may occur; in these cases the fibers and nucleus of the posterior commissure are spared and the lesions are more rostral, involving the rostral interstitial nucleus of the medial longitudinal fasciculus (MLF), the interstitial nucleus of Cajal, and the periaqueductal gray area (Schmidtke, 1992). Ipsilateral ptosis and contralateral superior eyelid retraction may be due to a nuclear oculomotor nerve syndrome (plus-minus lid syndrome) (Galetta, 1993b; Gaymard, 1992). The plus-minus syndrome results from a unilateral lesion of the third nerve fascicle with extension rostrally and dorsally to involve the nucleus of the posterior commissure or its connections.

Paroxysmal superior rectus and levator palpabrae spasm is a rare and unique disorder described in a single patient with multiple sclerosis (Ezra, 1996). Paroxysms of vertical diplopia and lid retraction in this patient lasted 3 to 4 seconds and examination revealed intermittent right hypertropia, lid retraction, and restriction of downgaze. MR imaging revealed multiple lesions consistent with multiple sclerosis, including a lesion in the midbrain in the region of the third nerve fascicle. Carbamazepine stopped all the symptoms that were thought due to spontaneous spasm of the superior rectus/levator complex.

Bilateral episodic retraction of the eyelids may occur as a manifestation of epileptic discharges associated with petit mal or myoclonic seizures or due to "levator spasms" during an oculogyric crisis (Miller, 1985). Lid lag may occur on a supranuclear basis in progressive supranuclear palsy, likely due to defective inhibition of the levator nuclei during downward gaze (Friedman, 1992; Miller, 1985). Lid lag may occur in the acute phases of Guillain-Barré syndrome (Keane, 1975; Tan, 1990) and lid retraction may also occur with parkinsonism (Miller, 1985; Tan, 1990).

Rhythmic upward jerking of the lids (eyelid nystagmus) refers to eyelid twitches that are synchronous with the fast phase of horizontal nystagmus on lateral gaze. It has been ascribed to lateral medullary disease where it may be inhibited by near effort (Daroff, 1968; Safran, 1982; Sanders, 1968). Lid nystagmus may also be provoked by convergence (Pick's sign) in patients with cerebellar or medullary pathology (Daroff, 1968; Safran, 1982; Sanders, 1968). In this situation, it consists of a slow down drift of the lid corrected by an upward flick. Rhythmic upward jerking of the eyelids may also be associated with vertical nystagmus, palatal myoclonus, or convergence-retraction nystagmus (Askenasy, 1953; Cooper, 1958; Miller, 1985) (see Chapters 14 and 17).

Eyelid retraction may also occur from paradoxic levator excitation that may be congenital or acquired and from lesions of the supranuclear, nuclear, or infranuclear pathways (Miller, 1985). Paradoxic lid retraction may occur with jaw movement or swallowing (the Marcus Gunn jaw-winking phenomenon) (Kirkham, 1971; Pratt, 1984; Sano, 1959). This trigemino-oculomotor synkinesis occurs on a congenital basis. Levator contraction with contraction of the external pterygoid muscle is the most common form of trigemino-oculomotor synkinesis (Miller, 1985). The involved eyelid is usually ptotic, but may be normal or even retracted while the jaw muscles are inactive. Elevation of the lid occurs when the mandible is moved to the opposite side, when the mandible is projected forward or the tongue protruded, or on wide opening of the mouth. These patients commonly have other associated ocular abnormalities including strabismus (e.g., double elevator palsy or superior rectus palsy), amblyopia, and anisometropia (Doucet, 1981; Miller, 1985; Pratt, 1984). Another rare form of trigemino-oculomotor synkinesis is levator contraction with contraction of the internal pterygoid muscle (i.e., eyelid elevation with closure of the mouth or clenching of the teeth) (Sano, 1959). Treatment of cases of Marcus Gunn jaw-winking phenomenon includes occlusion therapy for amblyopia, strabismus surgery, and surgery to correct the ptosis or retraction (Miller, 1985). Paradoxical eyelid retraction may also occur ipsilaterally in patients with congenital or acquired horizontal gaze or abducens palsies (Miller, 1985; Ticho, 1971).

Eyelid retraction may also occur with aberrant regeneration of the third nerve when the eye adducts, elevates, or depresses (Stout, 1993) (see Chapter 11), with partial paresis of the superior rectus muscle (Mauriello, 1993), or with orbital floor "blowout" fractures with globe hypotropia and increased innervation to the superior rectus and levator or Müllers muscle (Putterman, 1976). Eyelid retraction (pseudoretraction) may also occur if there is ptosis of the opposite eyelid (especially when the ptosis is due to disease at or distal to the neuromuscular junction) when fixating with the eye with the unilateral ptosis (due to Hering's law) (Gay, 1967; Lepore, 1988; Schecheter, 1978). Compensatory unilateral orbicularis oculi contraction may mask lid retraction; therefore, if the orbicularis oculi muscle is also weakened as in myasthenia gravis, contralateral lid retraction becomes more evident. Occlusion of the eye on the side of the ptosis will restore the retracted eyelid to a normal position.

Sympathetic overactivity may also cause lid retraction by contraction of Müller's muscle. Intermittent oculosympathetic irritation may cause cyclic sympathetic spasm, in which the pupil dilates for 40 to 60 seconds, which may be associated with lid retraction, facial hyperhidrosis, and headache (Claude-Bernard syndrome) (Burde, 1992). Sympathetic overactivity may also play a role in the lid retraction rarely noted in patients with ipsilateral orbital blowout fractures (Putterman, 1976). Sympathomimetic drops used in routine dilation of the pupils for ophthalmoscopy (e.g., phenylephrine) may also cause lid retraction. Finally, volitional bilateral lid retraction may occur in anxious or psychotic patients (Burde, 1992).

What Are the Neuromuscular and Myopathic Causes of Lid Retraction and Lid Lag?

Congenital maldevelopment or fibrosis of the LPS muscle or tendon may cause eyelid retraction or entropion at birth (Ballen, 1987; Collin, 1990; Gillies, 1995; Hiles, 1969; Leone, 1976; Stout, 1993; Zak, 1984). This eyelid retraction may be unilateral or bilateral and may be associated with congenital abnormalities (Miller, 1985). Other causes of congenital eyelid retraction include maternal hyperthyroidism (transient), congenital myotonia, and myotonic dystrophy (Lewis, 1957).

Dysthyroid disease (Graves' ophthalmopathy) with involvement of the LPS is the most common cause of acquired unilateral or bilateral sustained eyelid retraction (Burde, 1992; Miller, 1985). Patients may show retraction of the upper eyelid associated with infrequent or incomplete blinking (Stellwag's sign) and abnormal widening of the palpebral fissure (Dalrymple's sign). When the patient looks downward, there is often lid lag; the upper eyelid pauses and then incompletely follows the eye down (Graefe's sign). The retracted upper eyelid remains elevated in downgaze in dysthyroid disease; this differentiates dysthyroid eyelid retraction from dorsal midbrain eyelid retraction (Collier's sign), where the eyelids are also retracted in primary position but are normal in downgaze (Burde, 1992).

Eyelid retraction in patients with thyroid ophthalmopathy may result from excessive sympathetic activity, LPS fibrosis, local adhesions of the LPS to fixed orbital tissues, or contracture of the inferior rectus muscle (Feldon, 1990). The lid retraction may be controlled by botulinum toxin injection into the LPS (Biglan, 1994; Ebner, 1993). Surgical procedures are available to improve eyelid retraction with options including lateral tarsorrhaphy, Müller's muscle and LPS muscle lengthening, lower eyelid elevation, and blepharoplasty with orbital fat excision (Ceisler, 1995). Orbital decompression may improve lid retraction that is due to distortion from the proptotic globe. Strabismus surgery may relieve the compensatory component of lid retraction related to restrictive extraocular muscles, but recessions of the inferior rectus muscle often worsen the eyelid retraction. Therefore, the order of surgery for patients with thyroid ophthalmopathy should in general be: orbital decompression followed by strabismus surgery followed by lid surgery.

Myasthenia gravis may also be associated with three types of eyelid retraction:

1. Patients with unilateral ptosis may develop contralateral eyelid retraction as they attempt to elevate the ptotic lid due to bilateral excessive innervation to the eyelids.
2. Patients with ptosis may develop brief eyelid retraction lasting only seconds following a saccade from downgaze to primary position (Cogan's lid twitch sign).
3. Patients may develop transient eyelid retraction lasting seconds or minutes after staring straight ahead or looking upward for several seconds (possibly due to post-tetanic facilitation of the levator muscle) (Johns, 1962; Kansu, 1987; Lepore, 1988; Miller, 1985; Pukin, 1976).

Other myopathic causes of lid retraction include hypokalemic or hyperkalemic periodic paralysis and myotonic muscular dystrophy (Cohen, 1979; Davidons, 1961; Layzer, 1967; Lepore, 1988; Resnick, 1967; Van't Hoff, 1962). Myogenic eyelid retraction may also occur after botulinum toxin injections of the eyelids and after eye surgery, including superior rectus recession, ptosis repair, and enucleation (Bartley, 1996; Leatherbarrow, 1994; Miller, 1985; Zolli, 1983).

What Are the Mechanical and Miscellaneous Etiologies of Lid Lag and Lid Retraction?

The eyelid retraction noted with mechanical causes often responds to correction of the underlying abnormality (Bartley, 1996). Prominence of the globe, such as may occur with severe myopia, buphthalmos, proptosis, cherubism, craniosynostosis, or Paget's disease may cause apparent lid retraction (Bartley, 1996; Leatherbarrow, 1994; Lepore, 1988; Mauriello, 1993; Stout, 1993). Cicatricial scarring of the eyelid and LPS fibrosis from eyelid tumors, hemangioma of the orbit, herpes zoster ophthalmicus, atopic dermatitis, scleroderma, or thermal or chemical burns may also mechanically retract or distort the eyelids (Bartley, 1996; Burde, 1992; Stout, 1993). Blowout fractures of the orbital floor may cause upper eyelid retraction on either a neurogenic or mechanistic basis: hypotropia of the globe can stimulate increased innervation of the superior rectus and LPS or traction on the connective sheath of the LPS can elevate the upper eyelid mechanically (Bartley, 1996; Conway, 1988; Putterman, 1976). Contact lens wear may also cause upper eyelid retraction, presumably by mechanical irritation of the palpebral conjunctiva (Bartley, 1996). Lid retraction due to a lost hard contact lens becoming embedded in the upper eyelid has also been described (Weinstein, 1993).

Eyelid retraction, often associated with enophthalmos and hypoglobus, may occur with chronic maxillary sinusitis, maxillary sinus hypoplasia, and orbital floor resorption (silent sinus syndrome) (Rubin, 1994; Sporarkar, 1994; Wilkins, 1981). Radiation or trauma to the orbit or sinus may also be associated with eyelid retraction (Smitt, 1993). A retracted eyelid may also be a complication of surgical procedures, including trabeculectomy for glaucoma, scleral buckle, frontal sinusotomy, blepharoplasty, orbicularis myectomy, and cataract extraction (Bartley, 1996; Mauriello, 1993; Miller, 1985; Putterman, 1975; Shore, 1987).

Other miscellaneous entities that have been reported to be associated with eyelid retraction include optic nerve hypoplasia, microphthalmos, Down syndrome, hypertension, meningitis, sphenoid wing meningioma, and superior cul-de-sac lymphoma (Bartley, 1996; Friedgood, 1930; Rovit, 1988; Stout, 1993). Also, bilateral upper and lower lid retraction may occur with hepatic cirrhosis (Summerskill's sign); the existence of this sign has been questioned, as many of the original patients described may well have had Graves' ophthalmopathy in addition to liver disease, but rare cases without thyroid disease have been documented (Bartley, 1991, 1996; Miller, 1985, 1991; Summerskill, 1962).

Etiologies of upper lid retraction and lid lag are listed in Table 19–1.

Table 19–1. Etiologies of Upper Lid Retraction and Lid Lag

Neurogenic
- Benign transient lid retraction in preterm infants
- "Eye popping reflex" in infants
- Dorsal midbrain syndrome

(continued)

Table 19–1. *(continued)*

- Paroxysmal superior rectus and levator spasm in multiple sclerosis
- Seizures
  - Petit mal
  - Myoclonic
- Oculogyric crisis
- Progressive supranuclear palsy
- Parkinson's disease
- Guillain-Barré syndrome
- Lid nystagmus
  - Cerebellar or medullary lesions
  - Associated with vertical nystagmus
  - Associated with palatal myoclonus
  - Associated with convergence-retraction nystagmus
- Paradoxic levator excitation
  - Marcus Gunn jaw-winking phenomenon
- Abducens nerve palsy
- Aberrent regeneration of the third nerve
- Partial superior rectus paresis
- Orbital floor fracture
- Pseudoretraction
- Sympathetic overactivity
  - Claude-Bernard syndrome
  - Sympathomimetic drops
- Volitional lid retraction

Neuromuscular and myopathic
- Congenital
  - Congenital maldevelopment or fibrosis of the levator
  - Maternal hyperthyroidism
  - Congenital myotonia
  - Myotonic dystrophy
- Graves' ophthalmopathy
- Hypokalemic or hyperkalemic periodic paralysis
- Myotonic muscular dystrophy
- After botulinum injection into lids
- After eye surgery
  - Superior rectus recession
  - Ptosis repair
  - Enucleation

Mechanical
- Prominence of the globe
  - Myopia
  - Buphthalmos
  - Proptosis
  - Cherubism
  - Craniosynostosis
  - Paget's disease
- Cicatricial scarring and fibrosis
  - Eyelid tumors

- Hemangioma of the orbit
- Herpes zoster ophthalmicus
- Atopic dermatitis
- Scleroderma
- Thermal or chemical burns
- Blowout fracture of the orbital floor
- Contact lens wear
- Contact lens embedded in upper lid
- Enophthalmos and hypoglobus
  - Silent sinus syndrome
- Radiation therapy
- Trauma
- Surgical procedures
  - Trabeculectomy
  - Scleral buckle
  - Frontal sinus surgery
  - Blepharoplasty
  - Orbicularis myectomy
  - Cataract extraction
- Miscellaneous
  - Optic nerve hypoplasia
  - Microphthalmos
  - Down's syndrome
  - Hypertension
  - Meningitis
  - Sphenoid wing meningioma
  - Superior cul-de-sac lymphoma
  - Hepatic cirrhosis

Source: Adapted from Bartley 1996.

An approach to the diagnosis of unilateral or bilateral upper eyelid retraction is outlined in Figure 19–1. Most of the etiologies can be delineated by history, ophthalmologic examination, and neurologic examination.

What Are the Etiologies of Lower Eyelid Retraction?

Retraction of the lower eyelid may also be due to neurogenic, myogenic and mechanical causes (Brazis, 1991; Cohen, 1979). Congenital paradoxical lower eyelid retraction on upgaze and unilateral congenital lower eyelid retraction, due to the lid being tethered to the orbital margin, have been described (Aggarwal, 1974; Yee, 1974). Lower eyelid retraction may be the earliest clinical lid sign of a lesion of the facial nerve and facial nerve lesions are the most common cause of lower lid retraction (Brazis, 1991; Cohen, 1979; Pochin, 1939). Flaccidity of the lower lid may be an early manifestation of facial muscle paresis in myasthenia and myopathies and lower lid retraction may occur with dysthyroid orbitopathy (with or without proptosis), with proptosis, with senile entropion or ectropion, with enophthalmos, after eye muscle (e.g., inferior rectus recession) or orbital

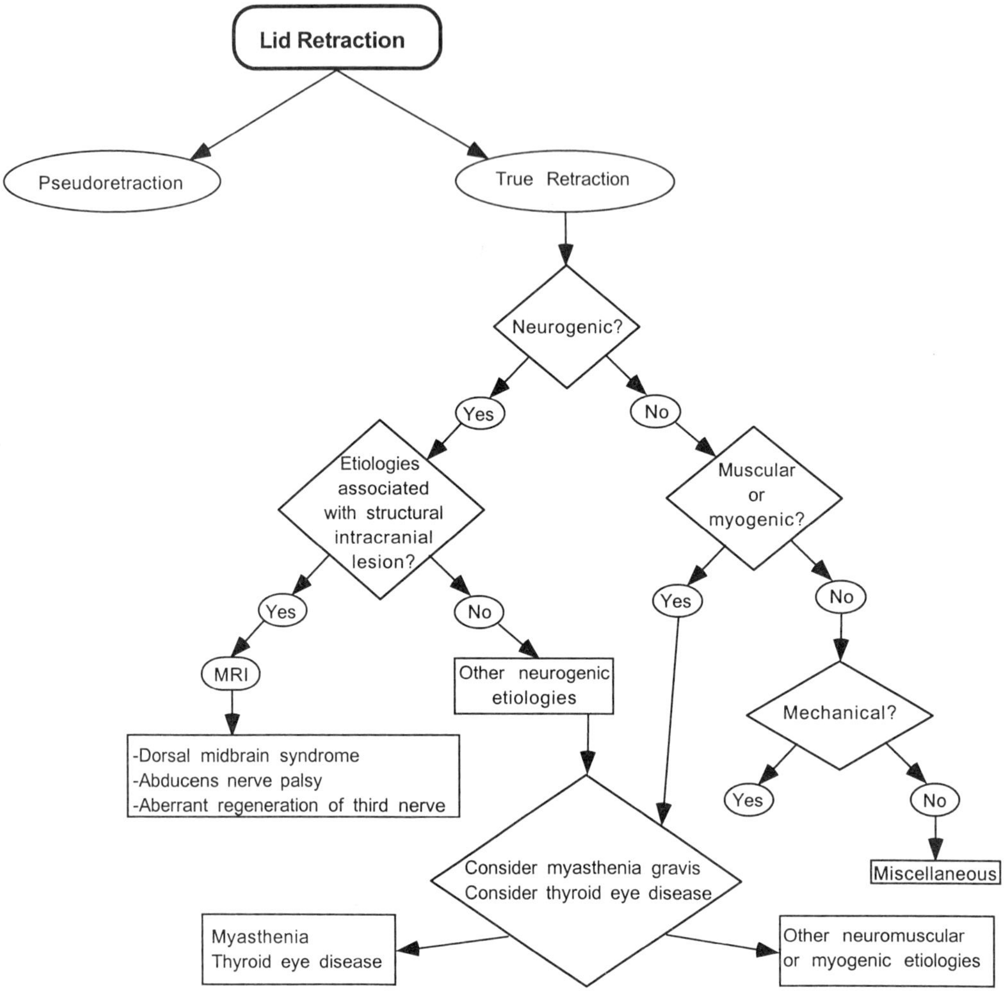

Figure 19–1. Lid retraction.

surgery (e.g., orbital floor "blowout" fracture repair, orbitotomy, or maxillectomy), or with scarring and contraction of lid tissue (e.g., from burns, tumors, trauma, granulomas of the orbital septum, dermatoses, or surgery) (Bartley, 1996; Cohen, 1979). With a hypertropia, the ipsilateral lid may appear to be retracted, while with a hypotropia there may be an illusion of contralateral lid retraction. Lid retraction may occur when there is elevation of the contralateral lower eyelid with facial contracture following Bell's palsy, spastic-paretic facial contracture with myokymia, hemifacial spasm, enophthalmus, or Horner's syndrome "upside-down" ptosis (Cohen 1979).

The etiologies of lower eyelid retraction are outlined in Table 19–2.

Table 19–2. Lower Eyelid Retraction

- Neurogenic causes
  - Congenital paradoxical lower eyelid retraction on upgaze
  - Unilateral congenital lower eyelid retraction due to the lid being tethered to the orbital margin
  - Lesion of the facial nerve
- Myogenic causes
  - Myasthenia
  - Myopathies
  - Dysthyroid orbitopathy
- Mechanical causes
  - Proptosis
  - Senile entropion or ectropion
  - Enophthalmos
  - After eye muscle or orbital surgery, including inferior rectus recession, orbital floor "blowout" fracture repair, orbitotomy, or maxillectomy
  - With scarring and contraction of lid tissue (e.g., burns, tumors, granulomas of the orbital septum, dermatoses, or surgery)
  - Apparent lid retraction
    - Ipsilateral with hypertropia
    - Contralateral with hypotropia
  - With elevation of the contralateral lower eyelid from:
    - Facial contracture following Bell's palsy
    - Spastic-paretic facial contracture with myokymia
    - Hemifacial spasm
    - Enophthalmus
    - Horner's syndrome ("upside-down" ptosis)

References

Aggarwal J. (1974). Congenital abnormality of the lower eyelid. *Br J Ophthalmol 58*:633.

Askenasy H, Wijsenbeek H, Herzberger E. (1953). Retraction nystagmus and retraction of the eyelids due to arteriovenous aneurysm of the midbrain. *Arch Neurol Psych 69*:236–241.

Ballen PH, Rochkopf L. (1987). Congenital retraction of the upper lid. *Ophthalmic Surg 18*:689–690.

Bartley GB. (1996). The differential diagnosis and classification of eyelid retraction. *Ophthalmology 103*:168–176.

Bartley GB, Gorman CA. (1991). Hepatic cirrhosis as a doubtful cause of eyelid retraction. *Am J Ophthalmol 111*:109–110.

Biglan AW. (1994). Control of eyelid retraction associated with Graves' disease with botulinum A toxin. *Ophthalmic Surg 25*:186–188.

Brazis PW, Vogler JB, Shaw KE. (1991). The "numb-cheek-limp lower lid" syndrome. *Neurology 41*:327–328.

Burde RM, Savino PJ, Trobe JD. (1992). *Clinical Decisions in Neuro-ophthalmology*. 2nd edition. St Louis, Mosby, pp. 362–364.

Ceisler EJ, Bilyk JA, Rubin PA, et al. (1995). Results of Mullerectomy and levator aponeurosis transposition for the correction of upper eyelid retraction in Graves' disease. *Ophthalmology 102*:483–492.

Cohen MM, Lessell S. (1979). Retraction of lower eyelids. *Neurology 29*:386–389.

Collin JR, Allen L, Castronuovo S. (1990). Congenital eyelid retraction. *Br J Ophthalmol 74*:542–544.

Conway ST. (1988). Lid retraction following blow-out fracture of the orbit. *Ophthalmic Surg 19*:279–281.

Cooper JC. (1958). Eye movements associated with myoclonus. *Am J Ophthalmol 46*:205–210.

Corin MS, Elizan TS, Bender MB. (1972). Oculomotor function in patients with Parkinson's disease. *J Neurol Sci 15*:251–265.

Daroff RB, Hoyt WF, Sanders MD, Nelson LR. (1968). Gaze-evoked eyelid and ocular nystagmus inhibited by the near reflex: Unusual ocular motor phenomena in a lateral medullary syndrome. *J Neurol Neurosurg Psych 31*:362–367.

Davidson SI. (1961). The eye in dystrophia myotonica: with a report on electromyography of the extra-ocular muscles. *Br J Ophthalmol 45*:183–196.

Doucet TW, Crawford JS. (1981). The quantification, natural course, and surgical results in 57 eyes with Marcus Gunn (jaw-winking) syndrome. *Am J Ophthalmol 92*:702–707.

Ebner A. (1993). Botulinum toxin type A in upper lid retraction of Graves' ophthalmopathy. *J Clin Neuro-ophthalmol 13*:258–261.

Ezra E, Plant GT. (1996). Paroxysmal superior rectus and levator palpabrae spasm: A unique presentation of multiple sclerosis. *Br J Ophthalmol 80*:187–188.

Feldon SE, Levin L. (1990). Graves' ophthalmopathy: V. Aetiology of upper eyelid retraction in Graves' ophthalmopathy. *Br J Ophthalmol 74*:484–485.

Friedgood HB. (1930). The ocular manifestations of sympathetic nervous system hyperactivity in conditions other than exophthalmic goiter and especially in essential hypertension: "Lidspasm:" A new eye sign. *Am J Med Sci 180*:836–848.

Friedman DI, Jankovic J, McCrary JA. (1992). Neuro-ophthalmic findings in progressive supranuclear palsy. *J Clin Neuro-ophthalmol 12*:104–109.

Galetta SL, Gray LG, Raps EC, Schatz NJ. (1993a). Pretectal eyelid retraction and lag. *Ann Neurol 33*:554–557.

Galetta SL, Gray LG, Raps EC, et al. (1993b). Unilateral ptosis and contralateral eyelid retraction from a thalamic-midbrain infarction. Magnetic resonance imaging correlation. *J Clin Neuro-ophthalmol 13*:221–224.

Galetta SL, Raps EC, Liu GT, et al. (1996). Eyelid lag without retraction in pretectal disease. *J Neuro-ophthalmol 16*:96–98.

Gay AJ, Salmon ML, Windsor CE. (1967). Hering's law, the levators, and their relationship in disease states. *Arch Ophthalmol 77*:157–160.

Gaymard B, Lafitte C, Gelot A, de Toffol BL. (1992). Plus-minus syndrome. *J Neurol Neurosurg Psych 55*:846–848.

Gillies WE, Harris AJ, Brooks AM, et al. (1995). Congenital fibrosis of the vertically acting extraocular muscles: A new group of dominantly inherited ocular fibrosis with radiologic findings. *Ophthalmology 102*:607–612.

Hawes MJ. (1989). Cherubism and its orbital manifestations. *Ophthal Plas Reconstruc Surg 5*:133–140.

Hiles DA, Wilder LW. (1969). Congenital entropion of the upper lids. *J Pediatr Ophthalmol 6*:157–161.

Johns RJ, Knox DL, Walsh FB, Renken HJ. (1962). Involuntary eye movements in a patient with myasthenia and hyperthyroidism. *Arch Ophthalmol 67*:455–472.

Kansu T, Subutay N. (1987). Lid retraction in myasthenia gravis. *J Clin Neuro-ophthalmol 7*:145–148.

Keane JR. (1975). Lid-lag in the Guillain-Barré syndrome. *Arch Neurol 32*:478–479.

Kirkham TH. (1971). Paradoxic elevation of eyelid on smiling. *Am J Ophthalmol 72*:207–208.

Kleinman MD, DiMario FJ Jr, Leconche DA, Zalneraitis EL. (1994). Benign transient downward gaze in preterm infants. *Pediatr Neurol 10*:313–316.

Layzer RB, Lovelace RE, Rowland LP. (1967). Hyperkalemic periodic paralysis. *Arch Neurol 16*:455–472.

Leatherbarrow B, Kwartz J, Sunderland S, et al. (1994). The 'baselball' orbital implant: A prospective study. *Eye 8*:569–576.

Leone CR Jr, Lewis R. (1976). Congenital upper eyelid retraction. *J Pediatr Ophthalmol 13*:350–352.

Lepore FE. (1988). Unilateral ptosis and Hering's law. *Neurology 38*:319–322.

Lewis IC, MacGregor AG. (1957). Congenital hyperthyroidism. *Lancet 1*:14–16.

Mauriello JA Jr, Palydowycz SB. (1993). Upper eyelid retraction after retinal detachment repair. *Ophthalmic Surg 24*:694–697.

Miller NR. (1985). Anatomy and physiology of normal and abnormal eyelid position and movement. In Miller NR: *Walsh and Hoyt's Clinical Neuro-ophthalmology*. 4th edition. Baltimore, Williams & Wilkins, pp 932–995.

Miller NR. (1991). Hepatic cirrhosis as a cause of eyelid retraction. *Am J Ophthalmol 112*:94–95.

Perez RB. (1972). The eye-popping reflex in infants. *J Pediatr 81*:87–89.

Pochin EE. (1939). The mechanism of lid retraction in Graves' disease. *Clin Sci 4*:91–101.

Pratt SG, Beyer CK, Johnson CC. (1984). The Marcus Gunn phenomenon. A review of 71 cases. *Ophthalmology 91*:27–30.

Puklin JE, Sacks JG, Boshes B. (1976). Transient eyelid retraction in myasthenia gravis. *J Neurol Neurosurg Psych 39*:44–47.

Putterman AM, Urist MJ. (1975). Upper eyelid retraction after glaucoma filtering procedures. *Ann Ophthalmol 7*:263–266.

Putterman AM, Usist MJ. (1976). Upper eyelid retraction after blowout fracture. *Arch Ophthalmol 94*:112–116.

Resnick JS, Engel WK. (1967). Myotonic lid lag in hypokalemic periodic paralysis. *J Neurol Neurosurg Psych 30*:47–51.

Rovit AJ, Deupree DM, Zang Y-F, Biglan AW. (1988). Treatment of congenital unilateral upper eyelid retraction with a marginal myotomy procedure. *Ophthalmic Surg 19*:872–875.

Rubin PAD, Bilyk JR, Shore JW. (1994). Orbital reconstruction using porous polyethylene sheets. *Ophthalmology 101*:1679–1708.

Safran AB, Berney J, Safran E. (1982). Convergence-evoked eyelid nystagmus. *Am J Ophthalmol 93:*48–51.
Sanders MD, Hoyt WF, Daroff RB. (1968). Lid nystagmus evoked by ocular convergence: An ocular electromyographic study. *J Neurol Neurosurg Psych 31:*368–371.
Sano K. (1959). Trigemino-oculomotor synkineses. *Neurologia 1:*29–51.
Schechter RJ. (1978). Ptosis with contralateral lid retraction due to excessive innervation of the levator palpebrae superioris. *Ann Ophthalmol 10:*1324–1328.
Schmidtke K, Buttner-Ennever JA. (1992). Nervous control of eyelid function. A review of clinical, experimental and pathologic data. *Brain 115:*227–247.
Shore JW, Westfall CT, Leone CR Jr, et al. (1987). Enophthalmos and upper eyelid retraction following osteoplastic frontal sinusotomy. *Ophthal Plas Reconstr Surg 3:*13–15.
Smitt MC, Donaldson SS. (1993). Radiotherapy is successful treatment of orbital lymphoma. *Int J Rad Oncol Biol Phys 26:*59–66.
Sporarkar CNS, Patrinely JR, Cuaycong MJ, et al. (1994). The silent sinus syndrome. A cause of spontaneous enophthalmos. *Ophthalmology 101:*772–778.
Stout AU, Borchert M. (1993). Etiology of eyelid retraction in children: A retrospective study. *J Pediatr Ophthalmol Strabismus 30:*96–99.
Summerskill WHJ, Molnar GD. (1962). Eye signs in hepatic cirrhosis. *New Eng J Med 266:*1244–1248.
Tan E, Kansu T, Kirkali P, Zileli T. (1990). Lid lag and the Guillain-Barré syndrome. *J Clin Neuro-ophthalmol 10:*121–123.
Ticho U. (1971). Synkinesis of upper lid elevation occurring in horizontal eye movements. *Acta Ophthalmol 49:*232–238.
Van't Hoff W. (1962). Familial myotonic periodic paralysis. *Q J Med 31:*385–402.
Weinstein GS, Myers BB. (1993). Eyelid retraction as a complication of an embedded hard contact lens. *Am J Ophthalmol 116:*102–103.
Wilkins RB, Kulwin DR. (1981). Spontaneous enophthalmos associated with chronic maxillary sinusitis. *Am J Ophthalmol 88:*981–985.
Yee RD, Odeh-Nasrala N. (1974). Congenital, paradoxical retraction of the lower eyelid. *Am J Ophthalmol 78:*1027–1029.
Zak TA. (1984). Congenital primary upper eyelid entropion. *J Pediatr Ophthalmol Strabismus 21:*69–73.
Zolli CI. (1983). Upper eyelid retraction in long-standing anophthalmic sockets. *Ann Ophthalmol 15:*621–626.

◆ 20 ◆

Anisocoria and Pupillary Abnormalities

Careful examination of pupillary reaction to light and near and attention to distinctive associated signs and symptoms allows differentiation of the abnormalities in pupil size and response to stimuli. Old photographs may be helpful in defining the duration of an anisocoria (Czarnecki, 1979; Safran, 1983; Zito, 1982). Generally the history and examination will distinguish the major entities causing an abnormal large pupil (e.g., third nerve palsy, tonic pupil, iris damage, pharmacological dilation, or sympathetic irritation) or small pupil (e.g., Horner's syndrome, simple anisocoria, pharmacologic miosis). Pharmacologic testing further confirms the diagnosis and allows topographical localization in many cases.

Is the Pupillary Light Reaction Abnormal?

If a large pupil is poorly reactive to light and the visual afferent system is normal, then a defect in the efferent parasympathetic innervation to this pupil is likely (Burde, 1977, 1992a,b; Carter, 1979; Multak, 1989; Selhorst, 1983; Thompson, 1977). If the light reaction is difficult to compare to the fellow eye, then a measurement of the anisocoria in light and dark may help to determine the pupillary abnormality. If the anisocoria is greater in dim light (stimulates dilation of the normal pupil), then the defect is in the sympathetic innervation to the pupil. If the anisocoria is less in dim light, then the lesion is in the parasympathetic innervation to the pupil (Thompson, 1976).

Is Light-Near Dissociation Present?

If the light reaction is poor in both eyes but the near reaction is intact, the patient has bilateral light-near dissociation of the pupils (Thompson, 1984). The reader is referred to the extensive critical survey of the pupillary literature by Loewenfeld (1969) for more details regarding the Argyll Robertson pupil and light-near dissociation. Table 20–1 lists the causes of light-near dissociation.

The Argyll Robertson pupils are classically described as small and irregular pupils with light-near dissociation and variable iris atrophy in a patient with relatively normal afferent visual function (Loewenfeld, 1969). The reader is referred to the review by Loewenfeld for further details on this entity (Loewenfeld, 1969). Patients with diabetes may also have small, poorly reactive pupils with light-near dissociation (Sigsbee, 1974).

Is There Other Evidence for a Third Nerve Palsy?

Patients with anisocoria and a poorly reactive pupil should be evaluated for an ipsilateral third nerve palsy. Although Sunderland and Hughes suggested that an extra-axial lesion compressing the third nerve (e.g., unruptured intracranial aneurysm) may cause a dilated pupil in isolation (or with minimal ocular motor nerve paresis) (Bartleson, 1986), in the absence of an extraocular motility deficit and/or ptosis, an isolated dilated pupil is usually not due to third nerve paresis (Sunderland, 1952). In addition, although intracranial aneurysms, especially those involving the posterior communicating artery-internal carotid artery junction, often produce a fixed and dilated pupil, this is almost always associated with other signs of a third nerve palsy (Miller, 1985). Walsh and Hoyt reported a patient with headache and a unilateral dilated pupil who was found to have an aneurysm at the junction of the superior cerebellar artery and basilar artery (Walsh, 1969). One week later, however, the patient developed other signs of a third nerve palsy. Payne and Adamkiewicz reported a case of unilateral internal ophthalmoplegia with a posterior communicating aneurysm, but this patient also had an intermittent exotropia and variable ptosis (Payne, 1969). Crompton and Moore reported 2 cases of isolated pupil dilation due to aneurysm but these patients developed severe headache and eventual signs of a third nerve palsy (Crompton, 1981). Fujiwara et al. reviewed 26 patients with an oculomotor

Table 20–1. Etiologies of Light-Near Dissociation

Bilateral afferent disease
Bilateral anterior visual pathway (optic nerve, chiasm, tract)
Bilateral retinopathy
Midbrain lesions (Seybold, 1971)
Dorsal midbrain syndrome (Parinaud's syndrome)
Encephalitis/meningitis
Wernicke's encephalopathy and alcoholism
Demyelination
Pineal tumors
Vascular disease
Argyll Robertson pupil
Diabetes
Tonic pupils (e.g., local, neuropathic, Adie's)
Aberrent third nerve regeneration
Syringomyelia (rare)

palsy due to cerebral aneurysm and reported three with only ptosis and anisocoria (Fujiwara, 1989). Gale and Crockard observed transient unilateral mydriasis in a patient with a basilar aneurysm (Gale, 1982). Miller reported an isolated internal ophthalmoplegia in a patient with a basilar aneurysm (Miller, 1985). Wilhelm et al. described an oculomotor nerve paresis that began as an isolated internal ophthalmoplegia in 1979 and then developed into a more typical third nerve palsy in 1993 due to a neurinoma of the third nerve (Wilhelm, 1995). Kaye-Wilson et al. also described a patient who initially had only minimal pupil signs due to a neurinoma of the third nerve (Kaye-Wilson, 1994).

Other rare cases of interpeduncular cyst, mesencephalic hemorrhage (Shuaib, 1989), presumed ocular motor nerve inflammation due to meningitis (e.g., bacterial, cryptococcal or tuberculous basal) (Fisher, 1967; Lesser, 1979; McGravey, 1989; Sandyk, 1982), and direct head trauma to the third nerve at the posterior petroclinoid ligament (Nageseki, 1989) have been described which presented with an isolated, unilateral, fixed and dilated pupil. Other neurologic signs of a third nerve palsy, however, were present or appeared over time in almost all these patients. In a patient with an isolated dilated pupil in the presence of normal extraocular motility, a third nerve palsy can be safely excluded in almost every circumstance simply with close follow-up.

In indeterminate cases, topical pilocarpine 1% can be used as a simple test for third nerve palsy versus pharmacologic blockade (see below) (Anastasi, 1968; Thompson, 1971). A pupil dilated from a third nerve palsy will constrict to pilocarpine 1%, but one with a parasympathetic pharmacological blockade will not.

Is There Evidence for Pharmacologic (or Toxic) Mydriasis or Miosis?

A careful history is usually all that is required in patients with inadvertent or intentional (e.g., glaucoma medication, treatment with topical cycloplegics for uveitis) exposure to agents that may affect pupil size. Table 20–2 lists some environmental agents that may result in mydriasis or miosis.

Nurses, physicians, and other health care workers are particularly prone to inadvertent or intentional exposure to pharmacological mydriatics. The pupil size of patients with pharmacologic blockade is often quite large, on the order of 10 to 12 mm in diameter, which is much greater than the mydriasis usually seen in a typical third nerve palsy or tonic pupil syndromes. As stated above, in poorly reactive pupils of uncertain origin, topical pilocarpine 1% can be used as a simple test for pharmacologic blockade (Anastasi, 1968; Thompson, 1971). A pupil dilated from a third nerve palsy will constrict to pilocarpine 1%, but a pupil with a parasympathetic pharmacological blockade will not. Adrenergic pharmacologic mydriasis (e.g., phenylephrine) may be clinically distinguished by blanched conjunctival vessels, residual light reaction, and a retracted upper lid due to sympathetic stimulation of the upper lid retractor muscle (Robin, 1988; Thompson, 1971).

Exposure to anticholinesterases can result in a miotic pupil (Apt, 1995; Ellenberg, 1992; Flach, 1995). In most cases the history and a simple confirmatory pharmacologic test are all that are required for the diagnosis. Simple reassurance with close follow-up as the effect wears off is sufficient. It is important to remember, however, that an acute tonic pupil may be unreactive to either light or near stimuli (Slamovits, 1987) and may be difficult to distinguish from a pharmacologically dilated pupil or acute traumatic iridoplegia.

Table 20–2. Environmental Agents Associated with Mydriasis or Miosis

- Medications
  - Topical
    - Ocular mydriatics
      - Topical parasympatholytics
        - Atropine
        - Cyclopentolate
        - Eucatropine
        - Homatropine
        - Oxyphenonium
        - Scopolamine
        - Tropicamide
      - Topical sympathomimetics
        - Epinephrine
        - Dipivalyl epinephrine (Propine)
        - Phenylephrine
      - Topical dexamethasone (Spaeth, 1980)
        - Vehicle in Decadron (Newsome, 1971)
      - Topical apraclonidine (Robin, 1988)
    - Ocular miotics
      - Parasympathomimetics
        - Aceclidine
        - Carbachol
        - Methacholine
        - Organophosphate esters
        - Physostigmine
        - Pilocarpine
      - Sympatholytics
        - Guanethidine (Riley, 1970)
        - Timolol with epinephrine
    - Anesthetic agents for the airway
      - Phenylephrine/lidocaine spray (Prielepp)
    - Nasal vasoconstrictor (phenylephrine) (Stirt, 1985)
  - Local and systemic mydriatics (Miller, 1985)
    - Atropine (IV) in general anesthesia (Schwartz, 1979)
    - Benztropine (Crawford, 1971)
    - Barracuda meat
    - Calcium
    - Diphenhydramine (Delaney, 1980)
    - Epinephrine (Perlman, 1991)
    - Fenfluramine/norfenfluramine
    - Glutethimide (Brown, 1971)
    - Levodopa (Weintraub, 1970)
    - Lidocaine local injection
    - Lysergica acid dethylamide
    - Magnesium
    - Nalorphine
    - Nutmeg (? may not have an effect on pupils) (Ahmad, 1975)
    - Pimozide (? patient also treated with benztropine) (Crawford, 1971)
    - Propantheline bromide (Pro-Banthine) (Gokhale, 1970; Nissen, 1977)
    - Thiopental (Larson, 1981)
    - Transdermal scopolamine patches (Bienia, 1983; Carlson, 1982; Chiaramonte, 1982; Lepore, 1982; Roper, 1982; Verdier, 1982)
    - Tricyclic antidepressants
  - Systemic miotics
    - Adrenergic blockers
    - Chlorpromazine
    - Heroin (Mitchell, 1976; Tress, 1979)
    - Lidocaine (extradural anesthesia)
    - Marijuana (Brown, 1977)
    - Methadone (Campbell, 1979)
    - Morphine and other narcotics
    - Phenothiazines (Mitchell, 1976)
  - Aerosolized agents
    - Atropine (Nakagawa, 1993)
    - Ipatropium bromide (Helprin, 1986)
- Plants
  - Alkaloids
    - Jimson weed (Datura stramonium) (Thompson, 1971)
    - Blue nightshade or European bittersweet (Solanum dulcamara) (Rubinfeld, 1987)
    - Deadly nightshade (Atropa belladona)
    - Henbane (Hyoscamus niger)
    - Moonflower (Datura wrightii or D. meteloides) (Reader, 1977)
    - Other Datura species (D. suaveolans, aurea, candida, sanguinea, stramonium, wrightii) (Reader, 1977; Wilhelm, 1994)
- Others
  - Hypromellose viscoelastic in cataract surgery (Tan, 1993)
  - Flea collar (miosis)
  - Pyrithns and piperonyl butoxide (insecticide) (Weintraub, 1971)
  - Siderosis bulbi/iron mydriasis
    - Occult intraocular iron foreign body (Monteiro, 1984, 1993; Scotcher, 1995; Talamo, 1985; Welch, 1975)

Are Intermittent or Transient Pupillary Phenomenon Present?

Transient mydriasis or miosis has been reported in patients with cluster (Salvesen, 1989) or migraine headaches (Drummond, 1991; Herman, 1970; Woods, 1984) and migraine aura without headache (Soriani, 1996); in a patient with an astrocytoma (Berreen, 1990); with Horner's syndrome (Kline, 1984; Smolin, 1969; Voorhies, 1981); after carotid puncture; during or after seizure activity (Gadoth, 1981; Pant, 1966; Zee, 1974) and even in normal individuals (Edelson, 1974; Zak, 1983). Tadpole-shaped pupils due to segmental spasm may also be related to migraine phenomenon (Thompson, 1983). Some of these phenomena represent true sympathetic irritation or excess (Cole, 1970), but the mechanism remains controversial. If the transient or intermittent nature of the mydriasis can be firmly established, then these patients should not undergo arteriography or other testing and should simply be followed for 24 to 48 hours at which point improvement would indicate the benign nature of the mydriasis. Transient anisocoria was reported by Stromberg following reduction of bilateral orbital floor fractures (Stromberg, 1988).

Is a Structural Iris Abnormality Present?

Careful slit lamp biomicroscopy of the iris should be performed in all patients with anisocoria to exclude structural iris abnormalities or damage. In many cases, the pupil is irregular and the structural abnormality can easily be identified. Table 20–3 lists some etiologies of structural damage to the iris.

Is a Tonic Pupil Present?

The clinical features of a tonic pupil are listed in Table 20–4 (Harriman, 1970; Levy, 1967; Thompson, 1977a, 1977b, 1978, 1979; Ulrich, 1980). The diagnosis of a tonic pupil can usually be made on clinical grounds alone.

Pharmacological testing with low dose pilocarpine (1/8% to 1/10%) may demonstrate cholinergic supersensitivity in the tonic pupil (a more miotic response than the fellow eye) (Bourgon, 1978; Cohen, 1975; Harriman, 1968; Laties, 1965; Loewenfeld, 1967; Pilley, 1975;

Table 20–3. Abnormalities of Iris Structure

Congenital aplasia of the iris sphincter and dilator muscles (Buys, 1993)
Increased intraocular pressure due to acute angle closure glaucoma (sphincter paresis due to iris ischemia)
Intraocular inflammation (e.g., iritis)
Ischemia (e.g., ocular ischemic syndrome)
Mechanical (e.g., iris tumor, intraocular lens)
Surgical (e.g., iridectomy, iridotomy, iris damage)
Trauma
Blunt trauma (traumatic iridoplegia)
Sphincter tears at the pupillary margin

Table 20–4. Clinical Features of a Tonic Pupil

Clinical Features
Poor pupillary light reaction
Segmental palsy of the sphincter
Tonic pupillary near response with light-near dissociation
Cholinergic supersensitivity of the denervated muscles
Accommodation paresis (that tends to recover)
Induced astigmatism at near
Tonicity of accommodation
Occasional ciliary cramp with near work

Ponsford, 1982; Ramsay, 1986; Younge, 1976). Unfortunately, cholinergic supersensitivity is not uniformly present in tonic pupils (80% with topical pilocarpine testing) and is not specific for postganglionic parasympathetic denervation. Supersensitivity has been reported after oculomotor nerve palsy (Coppetto, 1985; Cox, 1991; Jacobson, 1990, 1994; Mindel, 1981; Ponsford, 1982; Slamovits, 1987; Thompson, 1975). In addition, larger-sized pupils normally constrict more than smaller pupils to the same dose of topical cholinergics. Jacobson recommends evaluating cholinergic supersensitivity responses in darkness to minimize the mechanical resistance factors of large and small pupil size (Jacobson, 1990, 1994). A larger pupil that becomes the smaller pupil in darkness after topical cholinergics is more likely a supersensitive response (Jacobson, 1990, 1994).

Is the Tonic Pupil Isolated?

The history and examination should be able to differentiate the various associations of secondary pupils from idiopathic Adie's tonic pupil syndrome. Table 20–5 lists the causes of a tonic pupil.

Table 20–5. Etiologies of a Tonic Pupil

- Local (ocular or orbital) lesion affecting ciliary ganglion or nerve
  - Infection (Caputo, 1992)
    - Cellulitus
    - Chickenpox (Noel, 1976; Rogers, 1964)
    - Choroiditis
    - Diphtheria
    - Herpes simplex virus (Sammartino, 1981; Tokumaru, 1975)
    - Herpes zoster virus (Dubois, 1977; Sen, 1979)
    - Influenza
    - Measles
    - Parvovirus B19 (Corridan, 1991)
    - Pertussis
    - Scarlet fever
    - Sinusitis
    - Syphilis
    - Varicella virus (Goldsmith, 1968; Hodgkins, 1993; Rogers, 1964)
    - Viral hepatitis

- Inflammation
  - Iritis/uveitis damage to ciliary ganglion (Loewenfeld, 1967)
  - Rheumatoid arthritis (Victor, 1977)
  - Sarcoidosis (Henkind, 1973; Kupersmith, 1984; Rosenberg, 1989)
  - Vogt-Koyanagi-Harada syndrome (Levy, 1970)
- Ischemia
  - Orbital vasculitis
  - Lymphomatoid granulomatosis (Haider, 1993)
  - Migraine (Massey, 1981; Purvin, 1995)
  - Giant cell arteritis (Bronster, 1983; Currie, 1984; Davis, 1968; Dimant, 1980; Rabinowich, 1988)
- Orbital or chroidal tumor (Haider, 1993)
- Local anesthesia (Blaxter, 1967; Hales, 1970; Holmgren, 1979; Perlman, 1991)
  - Inferior dental block (O'Connor, 1983)
  - Injection of retrobulbar alcohol
- Surgery (Bodker, 1993; Golnik, 1995; Halpern, 1995; Salz, 1991)
- Cataract surgery (Lam, 1989; Monson, 1992; Olson, 1987; Percival, 1977; Saiz, 1991)
  - Cryotherapy (Pruett, 1979)
  - Diathermy
  - Penetrating keratoplasty (Bertelsen, 1974; Davies, 1975; Gassett, 1977; Uribe, 1967; Urrets-Zavilla, 1963)
  - Retinal surgery (Newsome, 1971)
  - Strabismus surgery (Bajart, 1979)
  - Orbital surgery (Bodker, 1993; Horblass, 1979; Stillwater, 1981; Stromberg, 1988)
- Laser therapy (Lobes, 1985; Rogell, 1979)
- Toxicity
  - Quinine (Gangitano, 1980)
  - Trichloroethylene (Feldman, 1968, 1984)
- Trauma (non-surgical)
  - Blunt trauma to ciliary plexus (Thompson, 1971)
  - Orbital floor fracture (Hornblass, 1979)
  - Retrobulbar hemorrhage
  - Damage to short ciliary nerves

Neuropathic (Loewenfeld, 1969; Spector, 1984; Thompson, 1977a, 1977b)

- Peripheral or autonomic neuropathy
  - Amyloidosis
  - Diabetes (Friedman, 1967; Gilmore, 1980; Sigsbee, 1974; Smith, 1978)
  - Alcohol-related (Thompson, 1977a)
  - Familial dysautonomia (Goldberg, 1968)
  - Hereditary neuropathy (Mateer, 1980; Miller, 1976)
    - Shy-Drager syndrome
    - Charcot-Marie-Tooth disease (Keltner, 1975; Kilimov, 1973)
    - Guillain-Barré syndrome (Keane, 1977; Okajima, 1977; Weintraub, 1971; Williams, 1979)
    - Fisher syndrome
  - Pandysautonomia (Anderson, 1972; Appenzeller, 1973; Hopkins, 1974; Low, 1983; Okada, 1975, 1988; Thomashefsky, 1972; Wichler, 1972; Yee, 1976; Young, 1969, 1975)
  - Progressive autonomic failure (Clark, 1988)
  - Ross' syndrome (tonic pupil, hyporeflexia segmental anhidrosis) (Hedges, 1975; Lucy, 1967; Ross, 1958; Weller, 1992; Wolfe, 1995)

(continued)

Table 20–5. *(continued)*

Sjogren's syndrome (Gemignani, 1988)
Systemic infectious
Syphilis (congenital or acquired) (Sundaram, 1985)
Paraneoplastic (Maitland, 1985)
Eaton-Lambert syndrome (Rubenstein, 1979)
Carcinomatous neuropathy (Bell, 1986)
Following oculomotor nerve palsy (Coppetto, 1985; Cox, 1991; Ponsford, 1982)
Adie's tonic pupil syndrome

Source: Loewenfeld, 1967; Thompson, 1977a, 1977b, 1978, 1979.

Is this Adie's Tonic Pupil Syndrome?

The clinical features of Adie's tonic pupil syndrome based on Thompson's extensive review of his patients (Thompson, 1977a, 1977b) and the literature is reported in Table 20–6.

What Causes the Adie's Tonic Pupil Syndrome?

The pathophysiology of Adie's tonic pupil is damage to the ciliary ganglion (Adie, 1932b; Adler, 1940; Harriman, 1968; Loewenfeld, 1967). More than 90% of the ciliary ganglion cells normally serve the ciliary body and only 3% serve the iris sphincter. After damage to the ciliary ganglion, aberrant regeneration of fibers originally destined for the ciliary body now innervate the iris sphincter. The initially mydriatic pupil may become smaller over time ("little old Adie's") and indeed Adie's tonic pupil may present as a miotic pupil (Rosenberg, 1989b; Thompson, 1979). Although most Adie's tonic pupils present unilaterally, bilateral involvement may develop at a rate of 4% per year (Thompson, 1977a). Thompson reviewed 220 cases from the literature and reported that 20% were bilateral (Thompson, 1977b).

Table 20–6. Clinical Features of Adie's Syndrome

Prevalence	2 cases per 1000 population
Mean age	32 years
Female to male ratio	2.6:1
Unilateral	80%
Reduced deep tendon reflexes	89%
Sector palsy	100%*
Accommodative paresis	66%
Bilateral	4% per year
Cholinergic supersensitivity	80%
Decreased regional corneal sensation	90%

*In patients with some degree of light reaction.

Should Neuroimaging Studies Be Performed in Adie's Syndrome?

Once the diagnosis of the Adie's tonic pupil is confirmed clinically and/or pharmacologically, no neuroimaging studies are required.

What Treatment Is Recommended for Adie's Syndrome?

Treatment of Adie's tonic pupil includes reassurance and unequal bifocal reading adds or a unilateral frosted bifocal segment in patients with permanent accommodative paresis (Press, 1981; Rouse, 1984). The use of topical low-dose pilocarpine or eserine has been suggested by some authors for Adie's syndrome (Flach, 1984, 1985; Hepler, 1976; Wirtschafter, 1980) but may precipitate ciliary spasm, induced myopia, cause browache, or worsen anisocoria due to miosis (Thompson, 1977a, 1977b).

When Does One Perform Syphilis Serology in Bilateral Tonic or Miotic, Irregular Pupils with Light-Near Dissociation?

Thompson recommends that all patients with bilateral tonic pupils should have serologic testing for syphilis (Thompson, 1977b). Fletcher and Sharpe reported that 5 of 60 consecutive patients with tonic pupils had positive serology for syphilis (Fletcher, 1986). Of these patients, all were bilateral tonic pupils and none presented with acute mydriasis or cycloplegia.

The Argyll Robertson pupil consists of bilateral miotic, irregular, pupils with light-near dissociation. Although classically described with neurosyphilis, other entities (Dacso, 1989; Sears, 1971) may produce a similar clinical syndrome (Loewenfeld, 1969). These etiologies include diabetes, chronic alcoholism, encephalitis, multiple sclerosis, degenerative diseases of the CNS (e.g., Charcot-Marie-Tooth) (Salichas, 1977), rare midbrain tumors, herpes zoster (Sammartino, 1981), neurosarcoidosis (Kirkham, 1976; Poole, 1984), and lymphocytic meningoradiculitis (Koudstaal, 1987).

Is the Pupillary Light Reaction Normal?

If the pupillary light reaction is normal in both eyes, then physiologic (simple) anisocoria (Lam, 1996; Loewenfeld, 1977), a Horner's syndrome, or sympathetic irritation should be considered.

Is the Anisocoria Isolated?

If the patient has an isolated anisocoria (e.g., no ptosis or dilation lag, no evidence of iris injury or drugs, and not related to Adie's tonic pupil or other innervational defects), then simple (physiologic or central) anisocoria is likely to be present (Lam, 1996; Thompson, 1976). Simple anisocoria may have a prevalence of up to 21% (range 1 to 90% in various studies), and most of these patients have an anisocoria of less than 0.4 mm that is usually only intermittently present (Lam, 1996; Loewenfeld, 1977). Topical cocaine will dilate both pupils equally (see pharmacologic testing for Horner's syndrome below).

Is a Horner's Syndrome Present?

Interruption of the ocular sympathetic pathway is known as a Horner's syndrome (HS). HS is characterized clinically by the signs listed in Table 20–7.

HS may result from a lesion anywhere along a three-neuron pathway that arises as a first order (central) neuron from the posterolateral hypothalamus, descends in the brainstem and lateral column of the spinal cord to exit at the cervical (C8) and thoracic (T1-T2) levels (ciliospinal center of Budge) of the spinal cord as a second order neuron. This second order (intermediate) preganglionic neuron exits the ventral root and arches over the apex of the lung to ascend in the cervical sympathetic chain. The second order neurons synapse in the superior cervical ganglion and exit as a third order neuron. The neural fibers for sweating of the face travel with the external carotid artery. The third order postganglionic neuron travels with the carotid artery into the cavernous sinus, on to the abducens nerve for a short course, and then travels with the ophthalmic division of the trigeminal nerve to join the nasociliary branch of the trigeminal nerve, pass through the ciliary ganglion, and reach the eye as long and short ciliary nerves (Burde, 1992a; Jaffe, 1950; Johnston, 1974; Maloney, 1980; Miller, 1985; Parkinson, 1978, 1979; Thompson, 1977a; Weisfeld, 1978).

The evaluation of HS includes two stages (Burde, 1992; Miller, 1985; Thompson, 1977; van der Wiel, 1982):

1. Recognition of the clinical syndrome
2. Confirmation and localization by pharmacological testing

Table 20–7. Clinical Findings in Horner's Syndrome

Ipsilateral mild ptosis (due to denervation of the Müller's muscle of the upper eyelid)
"Upside down ptosis" (from sympathetic denervation to the lower eyelid retractors) (Lepore, 1983; Nielsen, 1983)
Apparent enophthalmos (Lepore, 1983)
Anisocoria due to ipsilateral miosis
Dilation lag (slow dilation of the pupil after the lights are dimmed) (Pilley, 1976; Thompson, 1977a; van Der Wiel, 1982)
Increased accommodative amplitude or accommodative paresis (Giles, 1958; Miller, 1985; Weisfeld, 1978)
Transient (acute phase) ocular hypotony and conjunctival hyperemia
Variable ipsilateral facial anhidrosis
Ipsilateral straight hair in congenital cases (Shewmon, 1983)
Heterochromia of the iris (usually congenital but rarely acquired) (Dissenhouse, 1992; Makley, 1965; Miller, 1985; Simon, 1982)

Is the Horner's Syndrome Isolated?

Non-isolated HS should undergo imaging with attention to the topographical localization of the clinical findings.

Is a Central HS Present?

Patients with a central HS can usually be identified by the presence of associated hypothalamic or brainstem signs or symptoms (e.g., contralateral fourth nerve palsy, diabetes insipidus, disturbed temperature or sleep regulation, meningeal signs, vertigo, sensory deficits, anhidrosis of the body, etc.). The etiologies of central HS are listed in Table 20–8.

Is a Preganglionic (Intermediate) HS Present?

The preganglionic (intermediate) HS patient may have neck or arm pain, anhidrosis involving the face and neck, brachial plexopathy, vocal cord paralysis, or phrenic nerve palsy (Burde, 1992a; Ismail, 1988; Kori, 1981). The etiologies of preganglionic intermediate HS are listed in Table 20–9.

Is a Postganglionic HS Present?

The postganglionic HS patient may have ipsilateral pain and other symptoms suggestive of cluster or migraine headaches (e.g., tearing, facial flushing, rhinorrhea) (DeMarinis, 1994; Manzoni, 1991). Anhidrosis in postganglionic HS is often absent (Thompson, 1977a),

Table 20–8. Central Causes of Horner's Syndrome

Neoplasm
Pituitary
Third ventricle
Brainstem
Spinal cord
Infection
Syphilis
Poliomyelitis
Meningitis
Demyelination
Inflammation (e.g., sarcoid)
Trauma
Ischemia or infarction
Hypothalamic (Austin, 1991; Mustschler, 1994; Stone, 1986)
Wallenberg syndrome (Kim, 1994)

Source: Austin, 1991; Burde, 1992a; Coppeto, 1983; Crill, 1966; Custer, 1982; Guy, 1988; Jaffe, 1950; Kellen, 1988; Liu, 1981; Miller, 1985; Mutschler, 1994; Spencer, 1983; Stone, 1986.

Table 20–9. Etiologies of Preganglionic Intermediate Horner's Syndrome

Neoplasm (including neck, head, brachial plexus, lung)
Glomus tumors
Breast cancer
Sarcomas
Lung cancer
Lymphreticular neoplasms
Neurofibroma
Thyroid adenoma
Mediastinal or neck lymphadenopathy
Cervicothoracic abnormalities
Cervical rib
Pachymeningitis
Hypertrophic spinal arthritis
Foraminal osteophyte (Bernad, 1980)
Ruptured intervertebral disc
Thoracic aneurysm
Neck, brachial plexus or lung trauma or surgery
Birth trauma (Klumpke's paralysis)
Surgical or procedural trauma
Upper cervical sympathectomies
Anterior C3-C6 fusion
Radical thyroid surgery
Thoracic aneurysms
Infection or inflammation

Source: Bernad, 1980; Burde, 1992; Jaffe, 1950; Kori, 1981; Miller, 1985; Spector, 1976.

but because the sweat glands of the forehead are supplied by the terminal branches of the internal carotid nerve, involvement of these fibers after they have separated from the remaining facial sweat fibers may explain the occurrence of anhidrosis of the forehead with sparing of the rest of the face in these patients (Morris, 1984; Vijayan, 1978). Postganglionic HS due to cavernous sinus lesions (e.g., thrombosis, infection, neoplasm) usually are associated with other localizing signs such as ipsilateral third, fourth, or sixth nerve palsy or trigeminal nerve dysfunction (Abad, 1981; Boxley, 1983; Gelber, 1980; Gutman, 1986; Hartmann, 1987; Johnston, 1974; Miller, 1985; Parkinson, 1978, 1979; Striph, 1988).

Dissection of the internal carotid artery (e.g., traumatic, spontaneous) may result in a HS. Table 20–10 lists the associated signs and symptoms of a possible carotid artery dissection (Bogousslavsky, 1987; Burde, 1992a; Cullom, 1994; Fisher, 1982; Kline, 1987; Mokri, 1979; West, 1976). Patients with these signs should undergo imaging of the head and neck (e.g., MR imaging and MR angiography of the head and neck, carotid angiography).

Other etiologies of a postganglionic HS are listed in Table 20–11.

Although facial sweating abnormalities may be helpful in localizing a HS, the performance of clinical testing with starch and iodine (e.g., thermoregulatory sweat test) as described by some authors (Morris, 1984) is somewhat time consuming, messy, and may be difficult to perform in the outpatient setting. Other tests of facial sweating may not add to the clinical or pharmacological localization of HS (Rosenberg, 1989).

Table 20–10. Associated Signs and Symptoms of a Possible Carotid Artery Dissection

Ipsilateral orbital, facial or neck pain
Diplopia if cavernous carotid involvement
Transient carotid distribution ischemic attacks (e.g., amaurosis fugax)
Retinal artery occlusion
Neck bruit or swelling
Neurologic deficits
Dysgeusia
Tinnitus
Syncope
Cranial neuropathy (VI, IX, X, XI, XII)

Source: Bougouslavsky, 1987; Burde, 1992a; Cullom, 1994; Fisher, 1982; Kline, 1987; Mokri, 1979; West, 1976.

Table 20–11. Etiologies of a Postganglionic HS

Cavernous sinus lesions (Abad, 1981; Boxley, 1983; Gelber, 1980; Gutman, 1986; Hartmann, 1987; Johnston, 1974; Miller, 1985; Parkinson, 1978, 1979, 1988; Striph, 1988)
Infection (e.g., thrombosis, herpes zoster) (Smith, 1993; Wimlarantna, 1987)
Inflammatory (e.g., sarcoid, Tolosa-Hunt syndrome)
Intracavernous aneurysm
Neoplasm (e.g., meningioma, metastatic)
Headache syndromes (e.g., cluster or migraine) (DeMarinis, 1994; Herman, 1983; Manzoni, 1991; Sjaastad, 1985, 1988)
Inflammatory lesions of adjacent structures
Cervical lymphadenopathy
Otitis media (caroticotympanic plexus)
Petrositis
Sphenoid sinus mucocoele
Infectious
Severe purulent otitis media (caroticotympanic plexus)
Herpetic geniculate neuralgia (Jarrett, 1967)
Meningitis
Sinusitis
Neoplasm
Cavernous sinus
Cervical node metastasis
Metastatic
Orbital
Systemic peripheral or autonomic disorders
Diabetes
Fisher's syndrome
Shy-Drager syndrome
Trauma including surgery
Basilar skull fracture
Orbital fractures
Radical middle ear surgery

(continued)

Table 20–11. *(continued)*

Injection or surgery of the Gasserian ganglion
Intraoral trauma to internal carotid sympathetic plexus (Pruett, 1967)
Tonsillectomy
Vascular abnormalities of the internal carotid artery
Congenital anomalies
Fibromuscular dysplasia
Carotid artery aneurysms or dissection (Assaf, 1993; Cullom, 1995; Foster, 1991; Milandre, 1989; Mokri, 1992; Vighetto, 1990)
Arteriosclerosis or thrombosis of the internal carotid artery (Casto, 1989; Stern, 1989)

Source: Burde, 1992a; Giles, 1958; Grimson, 1979; Keane, 1979; Maloney, 1980; Miller, 1985.

What Is Alternating HS?

HS that alternates from one eye to the other (usually over days to weeks) is an uncommon finding but has been reported in multiple system atrophy (Shy-Drager syndrome) and in cervical spinal cord lesions (Ben Zur, 1975). Tan et al. reported a case and reviewed 25 cases from the literature (1 vertebral luxation, 14 cervical cord injuries, 8 Shy-Drager syndromes, 1 syringomyelia, 1 unknown, and 1 radiation myelopathy) (Ben Zur, 1975; Freeman, 1955; Fujita, 1973; Furukawa, 1974; Makibayashi, 1973; Nirankari, 1982; Ottomo, 1980; Shy, 1960; Tan, 1990).

Generalized peripheral or autonomic neuropathies (e.g., diabetes, Fisher's syndrome, Shy-Drager syndrome) may also result in a HS (Ben Zur, 1975; Freeman, 1955; Fujita, 1973; Makibayashi, 1973; Miller, 1985; Nirankari, 1982; Okajima, 1977; Ottomo, 1980; Shy, 1960).

Is the HS Related to Trauma?

Patients with a clear temporal association of the onset of HS with surgical or nonsurgical trauma to the sympathetic chain in the neck or chest do not require additional evaluation. The etiologies of traumatic HS are listed in Table 20–12.

What Is Congenital HS?

Weinstein et al. reported 11 patients with congenital HS and divided them into three groups based on clinical and pharmacological testing (Weinstein, 1980):

1. Obstetric perinatal forceps (high forceps and rotation for fetal malposition) trauma to the carotid sympathetic plexus
2. Presumed superior cervical ganglion lesions (postganglionic lesions with facial anhidrosis)
3. Surgical (thoracic) or obstetric trauma (brachial plexus) to the preganglionic pathway

Congenital HS may result in heterochromia of the irides as the sympathetic innervation of the iris determines iris pigmentation. Acquired HS, however, has also been rarely reported to cause iris heterochromia (Dissenhouse, 1992; Makley, 1965; Miller, 1985; Simon, 1982).

Table 20–12. Traumatic Horner's Syndrome

Direct or indirect trauma to the sympathetic chain
Medical procedures
Chest tube above the third posterior rib (Burde, 1992a; Bertino, 1987; Bourque, 1986; Campbell, 1989; Fleischman, 1983; Gasch, 1996; Miller, 1985; Resnick, 1993; Rossegger, 1980)
Extradural analgesia (Carrie, 1976; Mohan, 1973)
Lumbar epidural anesthesia (Schachner, 1982)
Percutaneous catheterization of the internal jugular vein (Briscoe, 1974; Davis, 1982; Gomez, 1993; Guccione, 1992; Lozano, 1983; Parikh, 1972; Peake, 1990; Vaswani, 1991; Vrints, 1989; Zelligowsky, 1991)
Swan-Ganz catheterization via the internal jugular vein (Birrer, 1981; Teich, 1985)
Carotid artery damage
Carotid angiography (Amundsen, 1963; Maloney, 1980)
Injection into the carotid artery of heroin by a drug addict (Hawkins, 1977)
Surgery (Burde, 1992a; Bertino, 1987; Bourque, 1986; Campbell, 1989; Fleischman, 1983; Gasch, 1996; Resnick, 1993; Romano, 1979; Rosner, 1970; Rossegger, 1980; Seltzer, 1977; Miller, 1985; Winnie, 1974)
Cardiac surgery (Lederman, 1982; Shaw, 1987)
Median sternotomy (Treasure, 1980)
Intentional surgical damage (e.g., sympathectomy)
Thoracic esophageal surgery (Szawlowski, 1991)
Other
After patient malpositioning (Jaffe, 1982)
Interscalene brachial plexus block (Al-Khafaji, 1986)
Stereotactic thalamotomy (Carmel, 1968)
Intrathecal bicillin injections in the neck (Keane, 1983)

What Is Pharmacological Localization of HS?

Patients with a HS that cannot be localized by clinical examination alone should undergo pharmacological studies to confirm the diagnosis of HS and localize it to the preganglionic or postganglionic levels. Although the clinical features of HS are classic, they are not pathognomonic. Ipsilateral ptosis and miosis may occur in patients without a HS (e.g., levator dehiscence and physiologic anisocoria). Pharmacological confirmation is relatively easy to perform (Skarf, 1982; Thompson, 1982) and is more specific and sensitive than clinical diagnosis alone (Van der Wiel, 1988).

Cocaine inhibits the reuptake of norepinephrine at the neuromuscular junction. Therefore, topical 5 to 10% cocaine will dilate a normal pupil (the mydriatic effect is small and usually about 1 mm) but will not dilate a pupil with a HS (regardless of the location of the affected sympathetic neuron) as well as the normal pupil. Therefore, there will be an increase in the degree of anisocoria after the cocaine test in a patient with a HS (Friedman, 1984). Minimal dilation of the pupil may occur in patients with partial disruption of the oculosympathetic pathway or first order neuron involvement (Burde, 1992a; Giles, 1958; Miller, 1985; Thompson, 1971). Minimal or no dilation of the pupil after topical cocaine confirms that a HS exists, but does not localize the responsible process to a preganglionic or postganglionic location. Friedman et al. reported the response to topical cocaine 10% in 24 normal volunteers and felt that 0.5 mm or more of anisocoria was necessary for the diagnosis of HS (Friedman, 1984). Van der Wiel and Van Gijn compared 12

Table 20–13. Post-Cocaine Test Anisocoria and the Mean Odds of Horner's Syndrome

Anisocoria (mm)	Mean Odds
0.0	1:1
0.1	2:1
0.2	6:1
0.3	14:1
0.4	32:1
0.5	77:1
0.6	185:1
0.7	441:1
0.8	1050:1
0.9	2510:1
1.0	5990:1

Source: Kardon, 1990.

patients with HS and 20 normals and found that an anisocoria of 1.0 mm after topical 5% cocaine was sufficient to diagnose a HS (Van der Wiel, 1986). Kardon et al. administered the cocaine test to 50 normals and 119 patients with HS (Kardon, 1990). A post-cocaine test anisocoria value of 1.0 mm gave a mean odds ratio using logistic regression analysis of about 5990:1 that a HS was present (lower 95% confidence limit 37:1). These authors felt that simply measuring the post-cocaine anisocoria (versus measuring the net change in anisocoria) was the best predictor of a HS (Kardon, 1990). The amount of post-cocaine anisocoria and the mean odds (that a patient has a HS) are listed in Table 20–13.

Hydroxyamphetamine releases stored norepinephrine from the postganglionic adrenergic nerve endings at the dilator muscle of the pupil (Heitman, 1986; Salvesen, 1989). Therefore, a preganglionic HS (with intact postganglionic third order neuron) will dilate after administration of topical hydroxyamphetamine 1% (Paredrine) while a postganglionic HS pupil will not dilate (no norepinephrine stores). The suggested procedure for pharmacologic testing for HS is outlined in Table 20–14.

A positive test result is noted if the anisocoria increases after the test versus a negative result if the anisocoria is diminished or unchanged (this measurement accounts for any preexisting anisocoria and psychosensory transient dilation effects) (Cremer, 1990a,b).

In intermediate and central preganglionic lesions, the affected pupil usually dilates more in response to hydroxyamphetamine possibly because of enhanced receptor sensitivity at the dilator muscle (Cremer, 1990a,b). There is no effective pharmacological test to differentiate central from intermediate preganglionic HS. The hydroxyamphetamine test should be deferred for 24 to 48 hours following the cocaine test because cocaine will block

Table 20–14. Pharmacological Testing for Horner's Syndrome

One drop of 1% hydroxyamphetamine or cocaine (4% or 10%) is instilled in the conjunctival sac of each eye
Both eyes are wiped with a tissue
20 to 40 seconds later a second drop is applied to each eye (to balance the dosage)
The amount of mydriasis (dilation) is measured and the difference in the amount of dilation between the eyes compared
The cocaine test and the hydroxyamphetamine test cannot be given on the same day

the effects of the hydroxyamphetamine (Cremer, 1990a,b; Thompson, 1971). Topical pharmacological testing should be performed in both eyes (the fellow eye serves as a control) and iatrogenic disruption of the corneal epithelium (e.g., applanation tonometry or corneal sensitivity testing) should be avoided prior to testing (Thompson, 1971). Patients with congenital HS may fail to dilate after topical hydroxyamphetamine due to orthograde transynaptic dysgenesis of the postganglionic neuron and may in reality have a preganglionic lesion (Grimson, 1979; Weinstein, 1980). Friedman et al. noted that the pupils of black patients (with heavily pigmented irides) dilated poorly with cocaine and, therefore, the test should be interpreted with more caution in black patients (Friedman, 1984; Kardon, 1990). Patients undergoing topical pharmacological testing should be informed that urine drug screening tests (for occupational hiring reasons) will remain positive for 24 to 48 hours following topical testing (Braillar, 1989).

Maloney et al. reviewed the clinical accuracy of the pharmacological localization of HS in 267 patients (Maloney, 1980). The hydroxyamphetamine test correctly localized in peripheral postganglionic HS in 75 (84%) of 89 patients. The reported sensitivity for identification of a postganglionic HS by hydroxyamphetamine was 96% (Maloney, 1980). Van der Wiel and Van Gijn reported a sensitivity of only 40% (Van der Wiel, 1983), but had a relatively smaller number of patients and excluded patients with cluster headache from their study. Cremer et al. described the results of hydroxyamphetamine testing in 54 patients with HS and reported a sensitivity of 93% and specificity of 83% (Cremer, 1990a,b). Patients with an isolated postganglionic HS usually have a benign HS whereas patients with a preganglionic HS are at risk for harboring an underlying malignancy (Maloney, 1980; Thompson, 1977). Grimson and Thompson described 67 patients with HS (Grimson, 1975). The incidence of malignant neoplasm in the preganglionic HS was almost 50% versus 2% in postganglionic HS. Some authors have recommended a screening chest radiograph for all cases of HS of undetermined etiology due to the small risk of misdiagnosis of a preganglionic HS by the hydroxyamphetamine test (Gasch, 1996). Wilhelm et al. reviewed 90 cases of HS and reported a specificity of 90% for postganglionic HS and 88% for preganglionic HS (Wilhelm, 1992).

Grimson and Thompson reported 120 patients with HS (Grimson, 1979). Of these 120 patients, 41% were preganglionic and one-half of these were due to underlying neoplasm (Grimson, 1979). Maloney et al. reported an etiology in 270 (60%) of 450 cases of HS (Maloney, 1980). Of the 180 cases without a defined etiology, 65 (35%) were reexamined (6 months to 28 years later) without a definite etiology and the authors thus felt this indicated a benign and stable origin of the HS. The etiology of the remaining 270 cases included: 60 (13%) tumors (23 benign lesions and 37 malignant lesions); 54 (12%) cluster headaches; 45 (10%) iatrogenic cases (e.g., neck surgery and carotid angiography); 18 (4%) Raeder's syndromes; 18 (4%) trauma; 13 (3%) cervical disc protrusions; 13 (3%) congenital cases; 13 (3%) vascular occlusions; 9 (2%) vascular anomalies, and 27 (6%) miscellaneous (e.g., pneumothorax, herpes zoster, cervical rib, and mediastinal lymphadenopathy) cases. Of these 270 cases, 34 (13%) were central preganglionic HS, 120 (44%) were intermediate preganglionic HS, and 116 (43%) were peripheral postganglionic HS. Of particular interest, 13 patients in this series had undetected malignancy, and 10 were due to primary or metastatic tumor involving the pulmonary apex. Nine of these 10 (90%) patients had arm pain (due to presumed involvement of the adjacent sympathetic chain and C8-T2 nerves).

Giles and Henderson reported a 35.6% incidence (77 cases) of HS due to underlying neoplasm (Giles, 1958). Of these 77 cases, 58 were malignant (mostly bronchogenic carcinoma and metastatic disease) and 19 were benign (e.g., neurofibroma and thyroid adenoma) (Giles, 1958).

Is the Evaluation of HS Different for Children?

Giles and Henderson reported birth trauma to be the most common etiology of HS in children (Giles, 1958). In children, cervical or thoracic tumors (e.g., neuroblastoma, neurilemmoma, and other congenital or acquired tumors) may cause a HS and, therefore, a complete evaluation including imaging (e.g., computed tomography scan) of the cervicothoracic region is indicated in all children with an unexplained HS (e.g., no history of birth trauma to the brachial plexus or other iatrogenic etiology) (Burde, 1992a; Beckerman, 1978; Garvin, 1993; Gibbs, 1992; Gilboa, 1976; Jaffe, 1975; Miller, 1985; Musarella, 1984; Sayed, 1983; Shewmon, 1983; Spigelblatt, 1976; Woodruff, 1988). Musarella et al. reviewed 405 children with neuroblastoma and 14 had HS; 9 of these 14 patients presented with HS (Murasella, 1984). Woodruff et al. reported that 2 out of 10 children with HS had neuroblastoma (Woodruff, 1988). Sauer and Levinsohn described seven patients (less than 11 years old) with HS due to spinal cord tumor, traumatic brachial plexus palsy, intrathoracic aneurysm, embryonal cell carcinoma, neuroblastoma, rhabdomyosarcoma, and thrombosis of the internal carotid artery (Sauer, 1976). Iris coloration is not established until several months of age and therefore iris heterochromia is not a helpful differential feature of HS in these patients after the perinatal period (Burde, 1992b). Patients with a substantial history of perinatal head trauma, such as forceps delivery or with evidence of brachial plexus injury (Klumpke's paralysis), and pharmacologic evidence of a postganglionic HS do not require additional evaluation (Leone, 1970). Childhood HS without a history of clear trauma (including surgical and birth trauma) to the sympathetic chain often have a preganglionic (intermediate) lesion and, therefore, should undergo evaluation for an underlying neoplasm such as neuroblastoma (Burde, 1992; Jaffe, 1975, 1976; Miller, 1985; Sauer, 1976; Shewmon, 1983; Woodruff, 1984). Other etiologies of congenital HS include viral infections (e.g., cytomegalovirus or varicella) (Bayatpour, 1982; Borzyskowski, 1981); fibromuscular dysplasia of the internal carotid artery (possibly posttraumatic) (Reader, 1980); and a HS in association with other congenital anomalies (e.g., facial hemiatrophy, enterogenous cyst and cervical vertebral anomaly) (Miller, 1985).

What Are the Indications for Imaging Based on Clinical and Pharmacological Localization?

Digre et al. prospectively performed magnetic resonance (MR) imaging studies in 33 patients with HS (Digre, 1992). Of these 33 patients, 13 were preganglionic HS and 20 were postganglionic HS. Patients with preganglionic HS without brainstem signs or symptoms underwent T1 weighted sagittal imaging of the entire neck, offset to the ipsilateral side; coronal imaging of the posterior spinal cord through anterior neck, and axial T1 and T2 weighted imaging from cervical level 2 (C2) to thoracic level 6 (T6). Preganglionic HS patients with brainstem signs or symptoms underwent sagittal imaging of the entire brain and axial T1 and T2 weighted sagittal brain and upper cervical spine imaging offset to the side of interest; coronal T2 weighted imaging of the carotid and cavernous sinuses and axial T1 and T2 weighted images from the optic chiasm to C4. These authors reported 4 patients with a lateral medullary infarct out of 6 central preganglionic HS; 2 patients with spinal cord/root compression secondary to disc disease, 1 apical Pancoast lung tumor, and 1 paravertebral metastatic mass out of 7 preganglionic HS; and 3 carotid dissections out of 20 postganglionic HS.

What Is the Evaluation for an Isolated Postganglionic HS?

Isolated postganglionic HS do not usually require further evaluation (Burde, 1992a; Havelius, 1985). A number of headache syndromes may be associated with a postganglionic HS, including cluster headache (Vijayan, 1981), migraine (Drummond, 1991), and Raeder's syndrome (Boniuk, 1962; Grimson, 1979; Kunkle, 1961; Pimental, 1993; Riley, 1971). Cluster headache is typically characterized by the following ipsilateral clinical manifestations in addition to headache: conjunctival injection, tearing, miosis or mydriasis, ptosis, bradycardia, nasal stuffiness, rhinorrhea, facial hyperhidrosis or flushing. These cluster accompaniments are thought to be related to a combination of sympathetic hypofunction and parasympathetic hyperfunction (e.g., tearing and rhinorrhea) (Vijayan, 1981). Cremer et al. reported that 19 of 39 (63%) postganglionic HS were due to cluster headache (Cremer, 1990a,b).

An approach to anisocoria is outlined in Figure 20–1. (See pp. 376–377.)

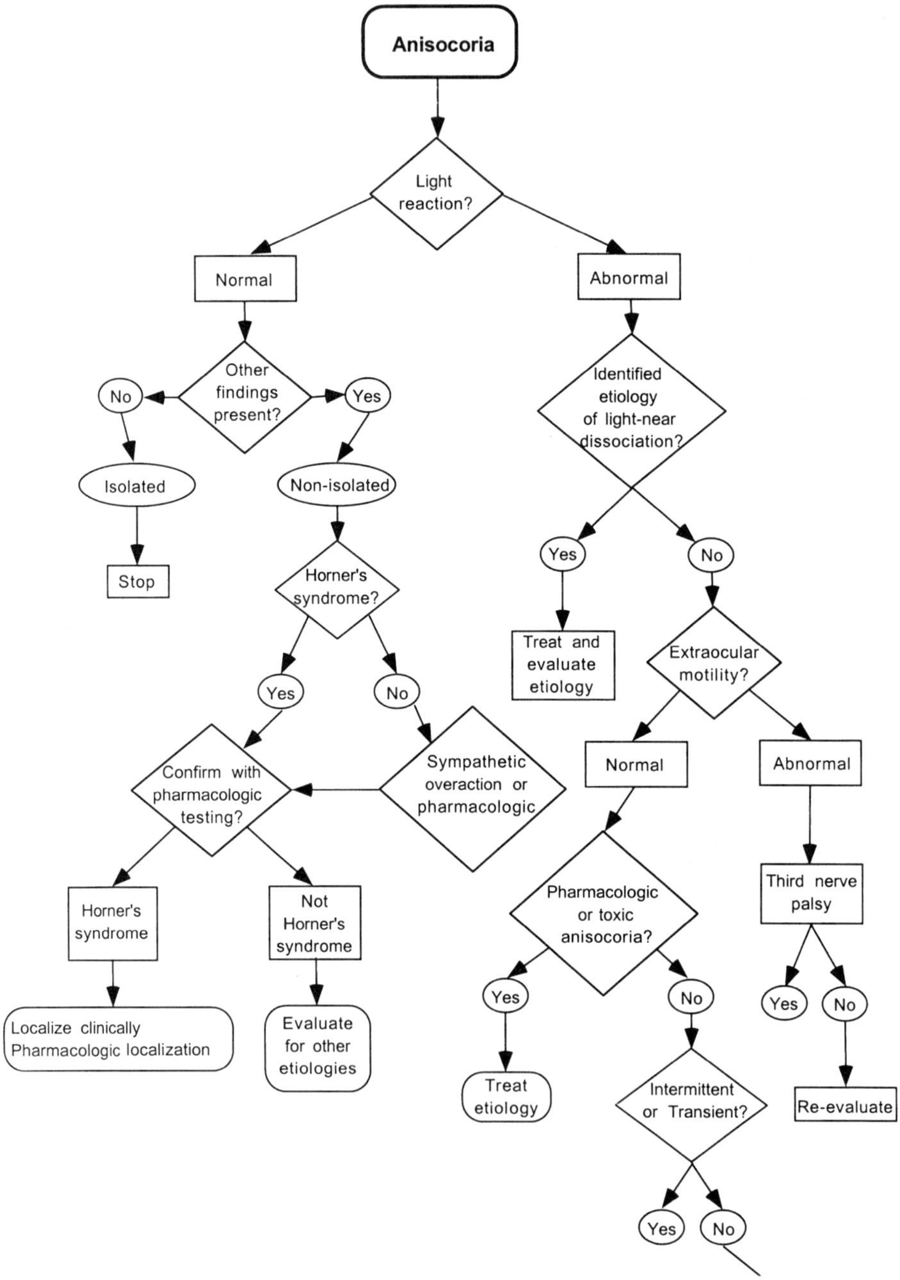

Figure 20–1. Anisocoria. *(continued)*

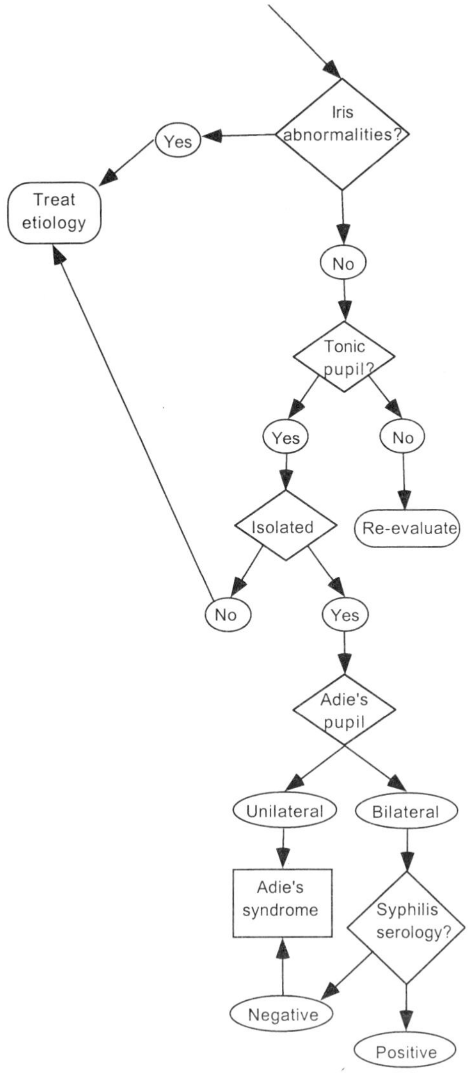
Iris abnormalities?
Yes
Treat etiology
No
Tonic pupil?
Yes
No
Isolated
Re-evaluate
No
Yes
Adie's pupil
Unilateral
Bilateral
Adie's syndrome
Syphilis serology?
Negative
Positive

Figure 20–1.

References

Abad J, Alvarez F, Blazquez M. (1981). An unrecognized neurological syndrome: Sixth nerve palsy and Horner's syndrome due to traumatic intracavernous carotid aneurysm. *Surg Neurol 16:*140–144.

Abramson SJ, Berdon WE, Ruzal-Shapiro C, Stolar C, Garvin J. (1993). Cervical neuroblastoma in eleven infants—a tumor with favorable prognosis. Clinical and radiologic (US, CT, MRI) findings. *Pediatr Radiol 23:*253–257.

Adie WG. (1932a). Complete and incomplete forms of the benign disorder characterized by tonic pupils and absent tendon reflexes. *Br J Ophthalmol 16:*449–461.

Adie WJ. (1932b). Tonic pupils and absent tendon reflexes: a benign disorder sui generis: Its complete and incomplete forms. *Brain 55:*98–113.

Adler FH, Scheie HG. (1940). Site of the disturbance in tonic pupils. *Trans Am Ophthalmol Soc 38:*183–189.

Ahmad A, Thompson HS. (1975). Nutmeg mydriasis. *JAMA 234:*274.

Al-Khafaji JM, Elias MA. (1986). Incidence of Horner syndrome with interscalene brachial plexus block and its importance in the management of head injury (letter). *Anesthesiology 64:*127.

Amundsen P, Dietrichson P, Enge I, Williams R. (1963). Cerebral angiography by catheterization: Complications and side effects. *Acta Radiol 1:*164–172.

Anastasi LM, Ogle KN, Kearnes TP. (1968). Effect of pilocarpine in counteracting mydriasis. *Arch Ophthalmol 79:*710–715.

Anderson O, Lindberg J, Modigh K, Reske-Nielsen E. (1972). Subacute dysautonomia with incomplete recovery. *Acta Neurol Scand 48:*510–519.

Appenzeller O, Kornfeld M. (1973). Acute pandysautonomia: Clinical and morphologic study. *Arch Neurol 29:*334–339.

Apt L. (1995). Flea collar anisocoria. *Arch Ophthalmol 113:*403–404.

Assaf M, Sweeney PJ, Kosmorsky G, Masaryk T. (1993). Horner's syndrome secondary to angiogram negative subadventitial carotid artery dissection. *Can J Neurol Sci 20:*62–64.

Austin CP, Lessel S. (1991). Horner's syndrome from hypothalamic infarction. *Arch Neurol 48:*332–334.

Bajart AM, Robb RM. (1979). Internal ophthalmoplegia following inferior oblique myectomy: A report of three cases. *Ophthalmology 86:*1401–1406.

Bartleson JT, Trautmann JC, Sundt TF. (1986). Minimal ocular motor nerve paresis secondary to unruptured intracranial aneurysm. *Arch Neurol 43:*1015–1029.

Bayatpour M, Logan J, Perry HP, Finley M. (1982). Horner's syndrome due to congenital cytomegalovirus infection. *South Med J 75:*220–221.

Beckerman BL, Seaver R. (1978). Congenital Horner's syndrome and thoracic neuroblastoma. *J Pediatr Ophthalmol Strab 15:*24–25.

Behrens M. (1977). Failure of the light reaction. *Trans Am Acad Ophthalmol Otolaryngol 83:*827–831.

Bell RA, Thompson HS. (1978). Ciliary muscle dysfunction in Adie's syndrome. *Arch Ophthalmol 96:*638–642.

Bell TA. (1986). Adie's tonic pupil in a patient with carcinomatous neuropathy (letter). *Arch Ophthalmol 104:*331–332.

Ben Zur PH. (1975). Intermittent Horner's syndrome: recurrent alternate Horner's syndrome in cervical cord injury. *Ann Ophthalmol 7:*955–962.

Bernad PG, Perlo VP. (1980). Horner syndrome with causalgia. *Neurology 30:*534–535.

Berreen JP, Vrabec MP, Penar PL. (1990). Intermittent pupillary dilatation associated with astrocytoma (letter). *Am J Ophthalmol 109:*237–239.

Bertelsen TI, Seim V. (1974). The cause of irreversible mydriasis following keratoplasty in keratoconus: A preliminary report. *Ophthalmic Surg 5:*56–58.

Bertino RE, Wesby GE, Johnson RJ. (1987). Horner syndrome occurring as a complication of chest tube placement. *Radiology 164:*745.

Bienia RA, Smith M, Pellegrino T. (1983). Scopolamine skin-disks and anisocoria (letter). *Ann Intern Med 99:*572–573.

Birrer RB, Plorz CM. (1981). Bernard-Horner syndrome associated with Swan-Ganz catheter. *NY State J Med 3:*362–364.

Blaxter PL, Britten MJA. (1967). Transient amaurosis after mandibular block. *Br Med J 1:*681.

Bodker FS, Cytryn AS, Putterman AM, Marschall MA. (1993). Postoperative mydriasis after repair of orbital floor fracture. *Am J Ophthalmol 115:*372–375.

Boghen D. (1975). Transient benign unilateral pupillary dilation [Letter]. *Arch Neurol 32:*68–69.

Bogousslavsky J, Despland PA, Regli F. (1987). Spontaneous carotid dissection with acute stroke. *Arch Neurol 44:*137.

Boniuk M, Schlezinger NS. (1962). Raeder's paratrigeminal syndrome. *Am J Ophthalmol 54:*1074–1078.

Borzyskowski M, Harris RF, Jones RWA. (1981). The congenital varicella syndrome. *Eur J Pediatr 137:*335–338.

Bourgon P, Pilley SFJ, Thompson HS. (1978). Cholinergic supersensitivity of the iris sphincter in Adie's tonic pupil. *Am J Ophthalmol 85:*373–377.

Bourque PR, Paulus EM. (1986). Chest-tube thoracostomy causing Horner's syndrome. *Can J Surg 29:*202–203.

Boxley TM, Schatz NJ. (1983). Clinical diagnosis of cavernous sinus syndromes. *Neurol Clin 1:*929–953.

Brailliar BB, Skarf B, Owens JB. (1989). Ophthalmic use of cocaine and the urine test for benzoylecgonine. *New Eng J Med 320:*1757.
Brazier DJ. (1983). Ocular sympathetic denervation associated with ocular hypertension. A case report. *Br J Ophthalmol 67:*297–301.
Briscoe CE, Bushman JA, McDonald WI. (1974). Extensive neurological damage after cannulation of the internal jugular vein. *Br Med J 1:*314.
Bronster DJ, Rudolph SH, Shanzer S. (1983). Pupillary light-near dissociation in cranial arteritis: a case report. *J Neuro-ophthalmol 3:*65–70.
Brown B, Adams AJ, Haegerstrom-Portnoy G, Jones RT, Flom MC. (1977). Pupil size after use of marijuana and alcohol. *Am J Ophthalmol 83:*350–354.
Brown DG, Hammill JF. (1971). Glutethimide poisoning: Unilateral pupillary abnormalities. *N Engl J Med 285:*806.
Burde RM, Savino PJ, Trobe JD. (1992a). *Clinical Decisions in Neuro-ophthalmology*. St. Louis, Mosby Year Book, pp. 330–332.
Burde RM, Savino PJ, Trobe JD. (1992b). *Clinical Decisions in Neuro-ophthalmology*. St. Louis, Mosby, pp. 326–327.
Burde RM, Thompson HS. (1991). Hydroxyamphetamine. A good drug lost? (editorial). *Am J Ophthalmol 111:*100–102.
Burde RM. (1977). Clinician's guide to the pupil. *Int Ophthalmol Clin 17:*139–156.
Buys Y, Buncic JR, Enzenauer RW, Mednick E, O'Keefe M. (1993). Congenital aplasia of the iris sphincter and dilator muscles. *Can J Ophthalmol 28:*72–75.
Campbell KB, Mandelzys N, Mills GK. (1979). Pupillary correlates of methadone treatment in heroin post-addicts. *Int J Addict 14:*627–638.
Campbell P, Neil T, Wake PN. (1989). Horner's syndrome caused by an intercostal chest drain. *Thorax 44:*305–306.
Capputo AR, Mickey KJ, Guo S. (1992). A varicella-induced pupil abnormality (letter). *Pediatrics 89:*685–686.
Carlston JA. (1982). Unilateral dilated pupil from scopolamine disk (letter). *JAMA 248:*31.
Carmel PW. (1968). Sympathetic deficits following thalamotomy. *Arch Neurol 18:*378–387.
Carrie LES, Mohan J. (1976). Horner's syndrome following obstetric extradural block. *Br J Anaesth 48:*611.
Carter JH. (1979). Diagnosis of pupillary anomalies. *J Am Optometr Assoc 50:*671–680.
Casto L, Ferraro B, Camerlingo M, Gazzaniga GC, Moschini L, Mamoli A. (1989). A case of "young stroke" with ICA intracranial occlusion; pathogenetic implication for dissection in migraine. *Rivista di Neurologia 59:*172–175.
Chiaramonte JS. (1982). Cycloplegia from transdermal scopolamine. *N Engl J Med 306:*174.
Clark CV, Ewing JD. (1988). Ocular autonomic function in progressive autonomic failure. *Doc Ophthalm 70:*309–321.
Cohen DN, Zakov ZN. (1975). The diagnosis of Adie's pupil using 0.0625% pilocarpine solution. *Am J Ophthalmol 79:*883–885.
Cole M, Berguis J. (1970). The reverse Horner syndrome. *J Thorac Cardiovasc Surg 59:*603–606.
Coppeto JR. (1983). Superior oblique paresis and contralateral Horner's syndrome. *Ann Ophthalmol 15:*681.
Coppetto R, Ribeiro Monteiro ML, Young D. (1985). Tonic pupils following oculomotor nerve palsies. *Ann Ophthalmol 17:*585–588.
Corridan PG, Laws DR, Morrell AJ, Murray PI. (1991). Tonic pupils and human parvovirus (B19) infection. *J Clin Neuro-ophthalmol 11:*109–110.
Cox TA, Goldberg RA, Rootman J. (1991). Tonic pupil and Czarnecki's sign following third nerve palsy. *J Clin Neuro-ophthalmol 11:*55.
Crawford R. (1971). Pupillary paralysis after tranquilizer. *Br Med J 3:*530–531.
Cremer SA, Thompson HS, Digre KB, Kardon RH. (1990b). Hydroxyamphetamine mydriasis in Horner's syndrome. *Am J Ophthalmol 110:*71–76.
Cremer SA, Thompson HS, Digre KB, Kardon RH. (1990a). Hydroxyamphetamine mydriasis in normal subjects. *Am J Ophthalmol 110:*66–70.
Crill WE. (1966). Horner's syndrome secondary to deep cerebral lesions. *Neurology 16:*325.
Crompton JL, Moore CF. (1981). Painful third nerve palsy; How not to miss an intracranial aneurysm. *Aust J Ophthalmol 9:*113–115.
Cullom RD, Cullom ME. (1995). Two Neuro-ophthalmic episodes separated in time and space. *Surv Ophthalmol 40:*217–224.
Currie J, Lessell S. (1984). Tonic pupil with giant cell arteritis. *Br J Ophthalmol 68:*135–138.
Custer P, Breen L, Burde RM. (1982). Cryptococcal meningitis: An atypical presentation. *J Clin Neuro-ophthalmol 2:*33–37.
Czarnecki JSC, Pilley SFJ, Thompson HS. (1979). The analysis of anisocoria: The use of photography in the clinical evaluation of unequal pupils. *Can J Ophthalmol 14:*297–302.
Dasco CC, Bortz DL. (1989). Significance of the Argyll-Robertson pupil in clinical medicine. *Am J Med 86:*199–202.
Davies PD, Ruben M. (1975). The paretic pupil: Its incidence and aetiology after keratoplasty for keratoconus. *Br J Ophthalmol 59:*223–228.
Davis P, Watson D. (1982). Horner's syndrome and vocal cord paralysis as a complication of percutaneous internal jugular vein catheterization in adults. *Anaesthesia 37:*587–588.

Davis RH, Daroff RB, Hoyt WF. (1968). Tonic pupil after temporal arteritis. *Lancet 1*:822.

DeMarinis M. (1994). Pupillary abnormalities due to sympathetic dysfunction in different forms of idiopathic headache. *Clin Autonomic Res 4*:331–338.

Digre KB, Smoker WRK, Johnston P, et al. (1992). Selective MR imaging approach for evaluation of patients with Horner's syndrome. *AJNR 13*:223–227.

Dimant J, Grob D, Brunner NG. (1980). Ophthalmoplegia, ptosis, and miosis in temporal arteritis. *Neurology 30*:1054–1058.

Dissenhouse MC, Palay DA, Newman NJ, To K, ALbert DM. (1992). Acquired heterochromia with Horner's syndrome in two adults. *Ophthalmology 99*:1815–1817.

Drummond PD. (1991). Cervical sympathetic deficit in unilateral migraine headache. *Headache 31*:669–672.

Dubois HF, van Bijsteveld OP. (1977). Internal ophthalmoparesis: An uncommon complication of varicella, a common disease. *Ophthalmologica 175*:263–268.

Edelson RN, Levy DE. (1974). Transient benign unilateral pupillary dilatation in young adults. *Arch Neurol 31*:12–14.

Ellenberg DJ, Spector LD, Lee A. (1992). Flea collar pupil (letter). *Ann Emerg Med 21*:1170.

Esterly NB, Cantolino SJ, Alter BP, et al. (1968). Pupillotonia, hyporeflexia, and segmental hypohidrosis: Autonomic dysfunction in a child. *J Pediatr 73*:852.

Feldman RG, Lessell S, Travers PH, White RF, Currie J. (1984). Neuro-ophthalmolog and neuropsychological effects of trichloroethylene intoxication. 18-year follow-up. *Neurology 34*:242.

Feldman RG, Mayer RF. (1968). Studies of trichloroethylene intoxication in man. *Neurology 18*:309.

Fisher CM. (1983). Observations concerning brain herniation. *Ann Neurol 14*:110.

Fisher CM. (1967). Some neuro-ophthalmological observations. *J Neurol Neurosurg Psychiatr 30*:383–392.

Fisher CM. (1982). The headache and pain of spontaneous carotid dissection. *Headache 22*:6065.

Flach AJ, Dolan BJ. (1984). Adie's syndrome: A medical treatment for symptomatic patients. *Ann Ophthalmol 16*:1151–1154.

Flach AJ, Dolan BJ. (1985). The therapy of Adie's syndrome with dilute pilocarpine hydrochloride solutions. *J Ocular Pharm 1*:353–362.

Fleishman JA, Bullock JD, Rossett JS, Beck RW. (1983). Iatrogenic Horner's syndrome secondary to chest tube thoracostomy. *J Clin Neuro-ophthalmol 3*:205–210.

Fletcher WA, Sharpe JA. (1986). Tonic pupils in neurosyphilis. *Neurol 36*:188–192.

Forestner JE. (1980). Ipsilateral mydriasis following carotid-artery puncture during attempted cannulation of the internal jugular vein. *Anesthesiology 52*:438–439.

Foster RE, Kosmorsky GS, Sweeney PJ, Masaryk TJ. (1991). Horner's syndrome secondary to spontaneous carotid artery dissection with normal angiographic findings (letter). *Arch Ophthalmol 109*:1499–1500.

Freeman LW, Russell FR. (1955). The significance of temporary and alternating ptosis, miosis and anhydrosis. *J Neurosurg 12*:584–590.

Frewin DB, Gilmore HR, Ho JQK, Scroop GC. (1968). Clinical, physiological and pathological observations in a case of progressive autonomic nervous system degeneration associated with Homes-Adie syndrome and peripheral neuropathy. *Aust Ann Med 17*:141–147.

Friedman JR, Whiting DW, Kosmorsky GS, Burde RM. (1984). The cocaine test in normal patients. *Am J Ophthalmol 98*:808–810.

Friedman SA, Feinberg R, Podolak E, Bedell RHS. (1967). Pupillary abnormalities in diabetic neuropathy: A preliminary study. *Ann Intern Med 67*:977–983.

Fujita M, Miyazaki M. (1973). A case of Shy-Drager syndrome. *Neurol Topics 3*:42–48.

Fujiwara S, Fujii K, Nishio S, Matsushima T, Fukui M. (1989). Oculomotor nerve palsy in patients with cerebral aneurysms. *Neurosurg Rev 12*:123–132.

Furukawa T, Toyokura Y. (1974). Alternating Horner syndrome. *Arch Neurol 30*:311–313.

Gadoth N, Margalith D, Bechar M. (1981). Unilateral pupillary dilatation during focal seizures. *J Neurol 225*:227–230.

Gale A, Crockard HA. (1982). Transient unilateral mydriasis with basilar aneurysm. *J Neurol Neurosurg Psych 45*:565–566.

Gangitano JL, Keltner JL. (1980). Abnormalities of the pupil and visual-evoked potentials in quinine amblyopia. *Am J Ophthalmol 89*:425–430.

Gasch AT. (1996). Horner's syndrome secondary to chest tube placement. *Ann Ophthalmol 28*:235–239.

Gassett A. (1977). Fixed dilated pupil following penetrating keratoplasty in keratoconus (Castroviejo syndrome). *Ann Ophthalmol 9*:623–628.

Gelber B, Sundt T. (1980). Treatment of intracavernous and giant carotid aneurysm by combined internal carotid ligation and extra to intracranial bypass. *J Neurosurg 52*:1–10.

Gemignani F, Manganelli P, Pavesi G, Marbini A. (1988). Polyneuropathy in Sjogren's syndrome. A case of prevalently autonomic neuropathy with tonic pupil and hypohidrosis. *Funct Neurol 3*:337–348.

Gibbs J, Appleton RE, Martin J, Findlay G. (1992). Congenital Horner syndrome associated with non-cervical neuroblastoma. *Dev Med Child Neurol 34*:642–644.

Gilboa N, Campbell JR. (1976). Neuroblastoma in a newborn with Horner syndrome and respiratory distress (letter). *Am J Dis Child 130*:218.

Giles CL, Henderson JW. (1958). Horner's syndrome: an analysis of 216 cases. *Am J Ophthalmol 46*:289–296.

Gilmore PC, Carlow TJ. (1980). Diabetic oculomotor paresis with pupil fixed to light. *Neurology 30*:1229–1230.

Glauser TA, Brennan PJ, Galetta SL. (1989). Reversible Horner's syndrome and Lyme disease. *J Clin Neuro-ophthalmology 9:*225.

Gokhale AM, Gokhale SA. (1970). Ocular effects of Pro-Banthine. *Br J Ophthalmol 54:*683–686.

Goldberg HI, Grossman RI, Gomori JM, Asbury AK, Bilaniak LT, Zimmerman RA. (1986). Cervical internal carotid artery dissecting hemorrhage: Diagnosis using MR. *Radiology 158:*157–161.

Goldberg MF, Payne JW, Brunt PW. (1968). Ophthalmologic studies of familial dysautonomia: The Riley-Day syndrome. *Arch Ophthalmol 80:*732.

Goldsmith MO. (1968). Tonic pupil following varicella. *Am J Ophthalmol 60:*551–554.

Golnik KC, Hund PW III, Apple DJ. (1995). Atonic pupil after cataract surgery. *J Cat Refract Surg 21:*170–175.

Gomez ME, Gonzales I, Loinaz C, et al. (1993). Neurologic complications in liver transplantation. *Acta Neurol Scand 87:*25–31.

Graveson GS. (1949). The tonic pupil. *J Neurol Neurosurg Psych 12:*219–230.

Grimson BS, Thompson HS. (1975). Drug testing in Horner's syndrome. In Glaser et al. *Neuro-ophthalmology Symposium of the University of Miami and the Bascom Palmer Eye Institute.* St Louis, Mosby Year Book, vol. 8, p. 265.

Grimson BS, Thompson HS. (1979). Horner's syndrome: Overall view of 120 cases. In. Thompson HS, (ed). *Topics in Neuro-ophthalmology.* Baltimore, Williams and Wilkins, pp. 151–156.

Grimson BS, Thompson HS. (1980). Raeder's syndrome. A clinical review. *Surv Ophthalmol 24:*199.

Guccione P, Gagliardi G, Bevilacqua M, Parisi F, Marino B. (1992). Cardiac catheterization through the internal jugular vein in pediatric patients. *Chest 101:*1512–1514.

Gutman I, Levartovski S, Goldhammer Y, Tadmor R, Findler G. (1986). Sixth nerve palsy and unilateral Horner's syndrome. *Ophthalmology 93:*913–916.

Guy J, Day AL, Mickle JP, et al. (1988). Contralateral trochlear nerve paresis and ipsilateral Horner syndrome. *Am J Ophthalmol 107:*73–76.

Haider S. (1993). Tonic pupil in lymphomatoid granulomatosis. *J Clin Neuro-ophthalmol 13:*38–39.

Hales RH. (1970). Ocular injuries sustained in the dental office. *Am J Ophthalmol 70:*221–223.

Hallett M, Cogan DG. (1970). Episodic unilateral mydriasis in otherwise normal patients. *Arch Ophthalmol 84:*130–136.

Halpern BL, Pavilack MA, Gallagher SP. (1995). The incidence of atonic pupil following cataract surgery. *Arch Ophthalmol 113:*448–450.

Harriman DG, Garland H. (1968). The pathology of Adie's syndrome. *Brain 91:*401–418.

Harriman DGF. (1970). Pathological aspects of Adie's syndrome. *Adv Ophthalmol 23:*55.

Hartmann B, Kremer I, Gutman I, Krakowski D, Kam J. (1987). Cavernous sinus infection manifested by Horner's syndrome and ipsilateral sixth nerve palsy. *J Clin Neuro-ophthalmol 7:*223–226.

Havelius U, Hindfelt B. (1985). Minor vessels leaving the extracranial internal carotid artery. Possible clinical implications. *Neuro-ophthalmol 5:*51–56.

Hawkins KA, Bruckstein HA, Guthrie TC. (1977). Percutaneous heroin injection causing Horner syndrome. *JAMA 237:*1963–1964.

Hedges TR, Gerner EW. (1975). Ross's syndrome (tonic pupil plus). *Br J Ophthalmol 59:*387–391.

Heitman K, Bode DD. (1986). The Paredrine test in normal eyes: A controlled study. *J Clin Neuro-ophthalmol 6:*228–231.

Helprin GA, Clarke GM. (1986). Unilateral fixed dilated pupil associated with nebulised ipratropium bromide (letter). *Lancet 2:*1469.

Henkind P, Gottlieb MB. (1973). Bilateral internal ophthalmoplegia in a patient with sarcoidosis. *Br J Ophthalmol 57:*792–796.

Hepler RS. (1977). Adie's tonic pupil. Symposium: pupil in clinical diagnosis. *Trans Am Acad Ophthalmol Otol 83:*843–846.

Herman P. (1970). Severe headaches, large pupils, and mitral valve prolapse in young women. *Neurol* 33 *(Suppl 2):*144.

Herman P. (1983). The pupil and headaches. *Headache 23:*102–105.

Hodgkins PR, Luff AJ, Absolon MJ. (1993). Internal ophthalmoplegia—a compilation of ocular varicella. *Aust NZ J Ophthalmol 21:*53–54.

Holmes G. (1931). Partial iridoplegia associated with symptoms of other diseases of the nervous system. *Trans Ophthalmol Soc UK 51:*209–228.

Holmgren WC, Badour HM, Tilson HB. (1979). Unilateral mydriasis during general anesthesia. *J Oral Surg 37:*740–742.

Hopkins A, Neville B, Bannister R. (1974). Autonomic neuropathy of acute onset. *Lancet 1:*769–771.

Hornblass A. (1979). Pupillary dilatation in fractures of the floor of the orbit. *Ophthalmic Surg 10:*44–46.

Ismail M, Hodkinson H, Tuling B. (1988). Horner's syndrome and tuberculosis. *S Afr Med J 74:*586.

Itzachaki M, Herishanu Y. (1977). Dislocation of the cervical spine with Horner's syndrome and a lesion of the spinal trigeminal tract. *J Neurol 217:*139–143.

Jacobson DM. (1994). A prospective evaluation of cholinergic supersensitivity of the iris sphincter in patients with oculomotor nerve palsies. *Am J Ophthalmol 118:*377–383.

Jacobson DM. (1995). Benign episodic unilateral mydriasis. *Ophthalmology 102:*1623–1627.

Jacobson DM. (1990). Pupillary responses to dilute pilocarpine in preganglionic third nerve disorders. *Neurology 40:*804–808.

Jaffe N, Cassady R, Filler R, Petersen R, Traggis D. (1975). Heterochromia and Horner syndrome associated with cervical and mediastinal neuroblastoma. *J Ped 87:*75–77.

Jaffe N. (1976). Neuroblastoma with heterochromia and Horner syndrome [letter]. *J Pediatr 88:*1067–1068.

Jaffe NS. (1950). Localization of lesions causing Horner's syndrome. *Arch Ophthalmol 44:*710–728.

Jaffe TB, McLeskey CH. (1982). Position induced Horner's syndrome. *Anesthesiology 56:*49–50.

Jammes JL. (1980). Fixed dilated pupils in petit mal attacks. *Neuro-ophthalmology 1:*155–159.

Jarrett WH. (1967). Horner's syndrome with geniculate zoster: Occurring in association with trigeminal herpes in which the ophthalmic division was spared. *Am J Ophthalmol 63:*326–330.

Johnston M, Parkinson D. (1974). Intracranial sympathetic pathways associated with the sixth cranial nerve. *J Neurosurg 40:*236–243.

Kardon RH, Denison CE, Brown CK, Thompson HS. (1990). Critical evaluation of the cocaine test in the diagnosis of Horner's syndrome. *Arch Ophthalmol 108:*384–387.

Kaye-Wilson LG, Gibson R, Bell JE, Steers AJW. (1994). Oculomotor nerve neurinoma, early detection by magnetic resonance imaging. *Neuro-ophthalmology 14:*37–41.

Keane JR. (1983). *J Neuro-ophthalmology 3:*223.

Keane JR. (1979). Oculosympathetic paresis. Analysis of 100 hospitalized patients. *Arch Neurol 36:*13–16.

Keane JR. (1977). Tonic pupils with acute ophthalmoplegic polyneuritis. *Ann Neurol 2:*393–396.

Kellen RI, Burde RM, Hodges TF III, et al. (1988). Central bilateral sixth nerve palsy associated with a unilateral preganglionic Horner's syndrome. *J Clin Neuro-ophthalmol 8:*179–184.

Keltner JL, Swisher CN, Gay AJ, Hepler RS. (1975). Myotonic pupils in Charcot-Marie-Tooth disease: Successful relief of symptoms with 0.025% pilocarpine. *Arch Ophthalmol 93:*1141–1148.

Kilimov N. (1973). Charcot-Marie-Tooth neural muscular atrophy with pupillary anomalies. *Eur Neurol 10:*292–300.

Kim JS, Lee JH, Suh DC, Lee MC. (1994). Spectrum of lateral medullary syndrome. Correlation between clinical findings and magnetic resonance imaging in 33 subjects. *Stroke 25:*1405–1410.

Kirkham TH, Kline LB. (1976). Monocular elevation paresis, Argyll-Robertson pupils and sarcoidosis. *Can J Ophthalmol 11:*330–335.

Kline LB, McCluer SM, Bonikowski FP. (1984). Oculosympathetic spasm with cervical spinal cord injury. *Arch Neurol 41:*61–64.

Kline LB, Vitek JJ, Raymon BC. (1987). Painful Horner's syndrome due to spontaneous carotid artery dissection. *Ophthalmol 94:*226–230.

Koehler MP, Sholiton DB, Solomon OD. (1983). A new iatrogenic cause of anisocoria. *J Fam Pract 16:*675–676.

Kori SH, Foley KM, Posner JB. (1981). Brachial plexus lesions in patients with cancer. 100 cases. *Neurology 31:*45–50.

Koudstaal PJ, Vermeulen M, Wokke JH. (1987). Argyll Robertson pupils in lymphocytic meningoradiculitis (letter). *J Neurol Neurosurg Psych 50:*363–365.

Kunkle EC, Anderson WB. (1961). Significance of minor eye signs in headache of migraine type. *Arch Ophthalmol 65:*504–508.

Kupersmith MJ, Aleksic SN. (1984). Bilateral pupillary cholinergic supersensitivity in a case of sarcoidosis. *Neuro-ophthalmology 4:*15–20.

Lam BL, Thompson HS, Walls RC. (1996). Effect of light on the prevalence of simple anisocoria. *Ophthalmology 103:*790–793.

Lam BL, Thompson HS, Walls RC. (1987). The prevalence of simple anisocoria. *Am J Ophthalmol 104:*69.

Lam S, Beck RW, Hall D, Creighton JB. (1989). Atonic pupil after cataract surgery. *Ophthalmol 96:*589–590.

Langham ME, Weinstein GW. (1967). Horner's syndrome. Ocular supersensitivity to adrenergic amines. *Arch Ophthalmol 78:*462–469.

Larson MD. (1981). Dilation of the pupil in human subjects after intravenous thiopental. *Anesthesiology 54:*246–249.

Laties AM, Scheie HG. (1965). Adie's syndrome. Duration of methacholine sensitivity. *Arch Ophthalmol 74:*458–459.

Lederman RJ, Breur AC, Hanson MR, et al. (1982). Peripheral nervous system complications of coronary artery bypass graft surgery. *Ann Neurol 12:*297–301.

Leone CR, Russell DA. (1970). Congenital Horner's syndrome. *J Pediatr Ophthalmol Strab 7:*152.

Lepore FE. (1993). Amaurotic mydriasis. *J Clin Neuro-ophthalmol 13:*200.

Lepore FE. (1983). Enophthalmos and Horner's syndrome. *Arch Neurol 40:*460.

Lepore FE. (1982). More on cycloplegia from transdermal scopolamine (letter). *N Engl J Med 307:*824.

Lesser RL, Simon RM, Leon H, Siegel N. (1979). Cryptococcal meningitis and internal ophthalmoplegia. *Am J Ophthalmol 87:*682–687.

Levy NS, Kramer SG, de Barros T. (1970). Pupillary and accommodative abnormalities in the Vogt-Koyanagi-Harada syndrome. *Am J Ophthalmol 69:*582–588.

Levy R. (1967). The tendon reflexes in the Holmes-Adie syndrome. *Neurology 17:*1213–1216.

Liu JP, Bender MB. (1981). Horner's syndrome, bilateral sensory motor trigeminal and other cranial neuropathies in a patient with sarcoidosis. *Neuro-ophthalmology 2:*117–122.

Lobes LA, Bourgon P. (1985). Pupillary abnormalities induced by argon laser photocoagulation. *Ophthalmology 92:*234–236.

Loewenfeld IE. (1969). The Argyll-Robertson pupil, 1869–1969. A critical survey of the literature. *Surv Ophthalmol 14:*199–299.

Loewenfeld IE. (1977). Simple central anisocoria: A common condition seldom recognized. *Trans Am Acad Ophthalmol Otolaryngol 83:*832–839.

Loewenfeld IE. (1979). Pupillary changes related to age. In Thompson et al. *Topics in Neuro-ophthalmology.* Baltimore, Williams & Wilkins, p. 129.

Loewenfeld IE, Newsome DA. (1971). Iris mechanics influence of pupillary size on dynamics of pupillary movement. *Am J Ophthalmol 71:*347–362.

Loewenfeld IE, Thompson HS. (1967). The tonic pupil: A re-evaluation. *Am J Ophthalmol 63:*46–87.

Lopez-Ibor B, Schwartz AD. (1985). Neuroblastoma. *Ped Clin of No Amer 32:*755–758.

Low PA, Dyck PJ, Lambert EH, et al. (1983). Acute panautonomic neuropathy. *Ann Neurol 13:*412–417.

Lowenstein O, Levine AS. (1944). Pupillographic studies: V. Periodic sympathetic spasm and relaxation and role of sympathetic nervous system in pupillary innervation. *Arch Ophthalmol 31:*74–94.

Lowenstein O, Loewenfeld IE. (1965). Pupillotonic pseudotabes (syndrome of Markus-Weill and Reys-Holmes-Adie). A critical review of the literature. *Surv Ophthalmol 10:*129–185.

Lozano AM. (1983). Horner's syndrome following internal jugular vein catheterization. *Can Med Assoc J 129:*540.

Lucy DD, Van Allen MW, Thompson HS. (1967). Holmes-Adie's syndrome with segmental hypohidrosis. *Neurology 17:*763–769.

Maitland CG, Scherokman BJ, Schiffman J, Harlan JW, Galdi AP. (1985). Paraneoplastic tonic pupils. *J Clin Neuro-ophthalmol 5:*99–104.

Makibayashi C, Kurata M, Ueda A. (1973). A probable case of Shy-Drager syndrome. *Neurol Topics 3:*27–35.

Makley TA, Abbott K. (1965). Neurogenic heterochromia: report of an interesting case. *Am J Ophthalmol 59:*927–928.

Maloney WF, Younge BR, Moyer NJ. (1980). Evaluation of the causes and accuracy of pharmacologic localization in Horner's syndrome. *Am J Ophthalmol 90:*394–402.

Manzoni GC, Micieli G, Zanferrari S, et al. (1991). Cluster headache. Recent developments in clinical characterization and pathogenesis. *Acta Neurologica 13:*506–513.

Massey EW. (1981). Pupillary dysautonomia and migraine: Is Adie's pupil caused by migraine? *Headache 21:*143–146.

Mateer JE, Louden MB, Crosby TW. (1980). Hereditary sensory neuropathy, tonic pupils, and cyclic vomiting in siblings. *Neurology 30:*441.

McGravey AR. (1989). A dilated unreactive pupil in acute bacterial meningitis: oculomotor nerve inflammation versus herniation. *Ped Emerg Care 5:*187–188.

Menken M. (1977). Horner syndrome of benign origin. *Postgrad Med 62:*225–226.

Milandre L, Perot S, Salamon G, Khahil R. (1989). Spontaneous dissection of both extracranial internal carotid arteries. *Neuroradiology 31:*435–439.

Miller NR. (1986). Intermittent pupillary dilation in a young woman. *Surv Ophthalmol 31:*65–68.

Miller NR. (1985). *Walsh and Hoyt's Clinical Neuro-ophthalmology.* 4th edition. Baltimore, Williams and Wilkins, pp. 425–428, 500–511, 703–705, 1012–1015.

Miller NR. (1982). *Walsh and Hoyt's Clinical Neuro-ophthalmology.* Baltimore, Williams and Wilkins, vol. 2, pp. 492–494.

Miller RG, Nielsen SL, Sumner AJ. (1976). Hereditary sensory neuropathy and tonic pupils. *Neurology 26:*931–935.

Mindel JS. (1981). Miosis from echothiophate in patients with total oculomotor nerve paralysis from intracranial abnormalities. *Am J Ophthalmol 91:*373.

Mindell JS. (1975). Hydroxyamphetamine test in Horner's syndrome. *Am J Ophthalmol 79:*523–525.

Mitchell AA, Lovejoy FH, Jr., Goldman P. (1976). Drug ingestions associated with miosis in comatose children. *J Pediatr 89:*303–305.

Mohan J, Lloyd JW, Potter JM. (1973). Pupillary constriction following extradural analgesia. *Injury 5:*151–152.

Mokri B, Schievink WI, Olsen KD, Piepgras DG. (1992). Spontaneous dissection of the cervical internal carotid artery. Presentation with lower cranial nerve palsies. *Arch Otolaryngol Head Neck Surg 118:*431–435.

Mokri B, Sundt TM, Houser OW. (1979). Spontaneous internal carotid dissection, hemicrania, and Horner's syndrome. *Arch Neurol 36:*677–680.

Monson MC, Mamalis N, Olson RJ. (1992). Toxic anterior segment inflammation following cataract surgery. *J Cat Refract Surg 18:*184–189.

Monteiro ML, Coppeto JR, Milani JA. (1993). Iron mydriasis. Pupillary paresis from occult intraocular foreign body. *J Clin Neuro-ophthalmol 13:*254–257.

Monteiro ML, Ulrich RF, Imes RK, Fung WE, Hoyt WF. (1984). Iron mydriasis. *Am J Ophthalmol 97:*794–796.

Morris JGL, Lee J, Lim CL. (1984). Facial sweating in Horner's syndrome. *Brain 107:*751–758.

Multack RF, Lannin WC, Olbum FR. (1989). Improving diagnostic acumen in pupillary evaluation. A review for the primary care physician. *J Am Osteopath Assoc 89:*917–924.

Murasella MA, Chan HS, DeBoer G, Gallie BL. (1984). Ocular involvement in neuroblastoma: Prognostic implications. *Ophthalmol 91:*936–940.

Mutschler V, Sellal F, Maillot C, Maton B, Collard M. (1994). Horner's syndrome and thalamic lesions. *Neuro-ophthalmology 14:*231–236.

Nageseki Y, Shimizu T, Kakizawa T, Fukamachi A, Nukui H. (1989). Primary internal ophthalmoplegia due to head injury. *Acta Neurochir 97:*117–122.

Nakagawa TA, Geurra L, Storgion SA. (1993). Aerosolized atropine as an unusual cause of anisocoria in a child with asthma. *Ped Emerg Care 9:*153–154.

Newsome DA, Einaugler RB. (1971). Tonic pupil following retinal detachment surgery. *Arch Ophthalmol 86:*233–234.

Newsome DA, Wong VG, Cameron P, Anderson RR. (1971). "Steroid-induced" mydriasis and ptosis. *Invest Ophthalmol 10:*424–429.

Nielsen PJ. (1983). Upside down ptosis in patients with Horner's syndrome. *Acta Ophthalmologica 61:*952–957.

Nirankari VS, Khurana RK, Lakhanpal V. (1982). Ocular manifestations of Shy-Drager syndrome. *Ann Ophthalmol 14:*635–638.

Nishino H, Rubino FA. (1993). Horner's syndrome in Wegener's granulomatosis. Report of four cases. *J Neurol Neurosurg Psych 56:*897.

Nissen SH, Nielsen PG. (1977). Unilateral mydriasis after use of propantheline bromide in an antiperspirant. *Lancet 2:*1134.

Noel L-P, Watson AG. (1976). Internal ophthalmoplegia following chickenpox. *Can J Ophthalmol 11:*267–269.

O'Connor M, Eustace P. (1983). Tonic pupil and lateral rectus palsy following dental anaesthesia. *Neuro-ophthalmology 3:*205–208.

Okada F, Shintomi Y, Kase M. (1988). Pupillary symptoms in three patients with pandysautonomia. *Neuro-ophthalmol 8:*87–93.

Okada K, Yamashita I, Suwa N. (1975). Two cases of acute pandysautonomia. *Arch Neurol 32:*146–151.

Okajima T, Imamura S, Kawasaki S, Ideta T, Tokuomi H. (1977). Fisher's syndrome: A pharmacological study of the pupils. *Ann Neurol 2:*63–65.

Olson RJ, Apple DJ. (1987). Unexplained intraocular toxicity after cataract-intraocular lens surgery (letter). *J Cat Refract Surg 13:*688–689.

Ottomo M, Heimburger RF. (1980). Alternating Horner syndrome and hyperhidrosis due to dural adhesions following cervical spinal cord injury. *J Neurosurg 53:*97–100.

Pant SS, Benton JW, Dodge PR. (1966). Unilateral pupillary dilatation during and immediately following seizures. *Neurology 16:*837–840.

Parikh RK. (1972). Horner's syndrome: A complication of percutaneous catheterization of internal jugular vein. *Anaesthesia 27:*327–329.

Parkinson D. (1988). Further observations on the sympathetic pathways to the pupil. *Anat Record 220:*108–109.

Parkinson D, Bernard, Mitchell. (1979). Horner syndrome and others? *Surg Neurol 11:*221.

Parkinson D, Johnston J, Chaudhari A. (1978). Sympathetic connections of the fifth and sixth cranial nerves. *Anat Res 191:*221–226.

Payne JW, Adamkiewicz J. (1969). Unilateral internal ophthalmoplegia with intracranial aneurysm. *Am J Ophthalmol 68:*349–352.

Peake ST, Bollen B. (1990). Unilateral fixed dilated pupil after aortic valve replacement: An unusual combination of causes. *J Cardiothor Anesthesia 4:*737–739.

Pearson J, Budzilovich G, Finegold MJ. (1971). Sensory, motor, and autonomic dysfunction. The nervous system in familial dysautonomia. *Neurology 21:*486–493.

Pearson R. (1971). Pupillary paralysis after tranquilizer. *Br Med J 3:*639.

Pelton JJ, Ratner IA. (1990). Neuroblastoma of the thoracic inlet. *J Ped Surg 25:*547–549.

Percival SPB. (1977). Results after intracapsular extraction: the atonic pupil. *Ophthalmic Surg 8:*138–143.

Perkin GD. (1994). The pupil. *J Neurol Neurosurg Psych 57:*1179.

Perlman JP, Conn H. (1991). Transient internal ophthalmoplegia during blepharoplasty. A report of three cases. *Adv Ophthalm Plast Reconstr Surg 7:*141–143.

Pilley SFJ, Thompson HS. (1975). Cholinergic supersensitivity in Adie's syndrome. Pilocarpine vs Mecholyl. *Am J Ophthalmol 80:*955.

Pilley SFJ, Thompson HS. (1975). Pupillary "dilation lag" in Horner's syndrome. *Br J Ophthalmol 59:*731–735.

Pimentel J, Martins IP. (1993). Raeder's syndrome. A case with an unusual localization. *Cephalgia 13:*135.

Ponsford JR, Bannister R, Paul EA. (1982). Methacholine pupillary responses in third nerve palsy and Adie's syndrome. *Brain 105:*583–597.

Poole CJ. (1984). Argyll Robertson pupils due to neurosarcoidosis: evidence for site of lesion. *Br Med J Clin Res 289:*356.

Press LJ. (1981). Management of Adie syndrome. *Am J Optometr Physiol Optics 58:*235–238.

Prielipp RC. (1994). Unilateral mydriasis after induction of anaesthesia. *Can J Anaesth 41:*140–143.

Pruett RC. (1967). Horner's syndrome following intra-oral trauma. *Arch Ophthalmol 78:*420–421.

Pruett RC. (1979). Internal ophthalmoplegia after panretinal therapy (letter). *Arch Ophthalmol 97:*2212.

Purcell JJ, Krachmer JH, Thompson HS. (1977). Corneal sensation in Adie's syndrome. *Am J Ophthalmol 84:*496–500.

Purvin VA. (1995). Adie's tonic pupil secondary to migraine. *J Neuro-ophthalmol 15:*43–44.

Rabinowich L, Mehler MF. (1988). Parasympathetic involvement in biopsy-proven temporal arteritis. *Ann Ophthalmol 20:*400–402.

Ramsay DA. (1986). Dilute solutions of phenylephrine and pilocarpine in the diagnosis of disordered autonomic innervation of the iris: observations in normal subjects and in the syndromes of Horner and Holmes-Adie. *J Neurol Sci 73:*125–134.
Reader AL III. (1977). Mydriasis from Datura wrightii. *Am J Ophthalmol 84:*263–264.
Reader AL, Massey EW. (1980). Fibromuscular dysplasia of the carotid artery: A cause of congenital Horner's syndrome? *Ann Ophthalmol 12:*326–330.
Reid WL, Cone WV. (1939). The mechanism of fixed dilation of the pupil resulting from ipsilateral cerebral compression. *JAMA 112:*2030–2034.
Resnick DK. (1993). Delayed pulmonary perforation. A rare complication of tube thoracostomy. *Chest 103:*311–313.
Rieke H, Benecke R, DeVivie ER, Turner E, Crozier T, Kettler D. (1989). Brachial plexus lesions following cardiac surgery with median sternotomy and cannulation of the internal jugular vein. *J Cardiothorac Anesth 3:*286–289.
Riley FC, Moyer NJ. (1970). Experimental Horner's syndrome: A pupillographic evaluation of guanethidine-induced adrenergic blockade in humans. *Am J Ophthalmol 69:*442–447.
Riley FC, Jr., Moyer NJ. (1971). Oculosympathetic paresis associated with cluster headaches. *Am J Ophthalmol 72:*763.
Roarty JD, Keltner JL. (1990). Normal pupil size and anisocoria in newborn infants. *Arch Ophthalmol 108:*94–95.
Robin AL. (1988). Short-term effects of unilateral 1% apraclonidine therapy. *Arch Ophthalmol 106:*912–915.
Rogell GD. (1979). Internal ophthalmoplegia after argon laser panretinal photocoagulation. *Arch Ophthalmol 97:*904–905.
Rogers JW. (1964). Internal ophthalmoplegia following chickenpox. *Arch Ophthalmol 71:*617–618.
Romano PE, Kurchin A, Rudich R, Adar R. (1979). Ocular manifestations after upper dorsal sympathectomy. *Ann Ophthalmol 11:*1083–1086.
Roper DL, Hale LL. (1982). A case report: Unilateral cycloplegia resulting from careless use of Transderm-V. *Aviation Space Environ Med 53:*1129–1130.
Rosenberg ML. (1989a). The friction test as a new method for detecting facial anhidrosis in patients with Horner's syndrome. *Am J Ophthalmol 108:*443–447.
Rosenberg ML. (1989b). Miotic Adie's pupils. *J Clin Neuro-ophthalmol 9:*43–45.
Rosner S. (1970). The physiology of bilateral cervical sympathectomy and Horner's syndrome. *Vasc Surg 4:*44–45.
Ross AT. (1958). Progressive selective sudomotor denervation: A case with coexisting Adie's syndrome. *Neurol 8:*809–817.
Rossegger H, Fritsch G. (1980). Horner's syndrome after treatment of tension pneumothorax with tube thoracostomy in a newborn infant. *Eur J Pediatr 113:*67–68.
Rouse MW, Polte L. (1984). Accommodative involvement with Adie's pupil. *Am J Optometr Physiol Optics 61:*54–55.
Rubenstein AE, Horowitz SH, Bender AN. (1979). Cholinergic dysautonomia and Eaton-Lambert syndrome. *Neurology 29:*720–723.
Rubinfeld RS, Currie JN. (1987). Accidental mydriasis from blue nightshade "lipstick." *J Clin Neuro-ophthalmol 7:*34–37.
Safran AB, Roth A. (1983). Using a slit lamp for the neuro-ophthalmologic evaluation of old photographs. *Am J Ophthalmol 95:*558.
Saiz A, Angulo S, Fernandez M. (1991). Atonic pupil: An unusual complication of cataract surgery. *Ophthalmic Surg 22:*20–22.
Salichas P, Lapresle J. (1977). Argyll-Robertson like pupils in the neural type of Charcot-Marie-Tooth disease. *Eur Neurol 16:*172–175.
Salvesen R, de Souza CD, Sjaastad O. (1989a). Horner's syndrome. Sweat gland and pupillary response in two cases with a probable 3rd neurone dysfunction. *Cephalgia 9:*63–70.
Salvesen R, Sand T, Zhao JM, Sjaastad O. (1989b). Cluster headache: Pupillometric patterns as a function of the degree of anisocoria. *Cephalgia 9:*131–138.
Sammartino A, Fusco R, de Crecchio G, Magli A. (1981). Unilateral inferior altitudinal hemianopsia, Argyll-Robertson pupil and dendritic keratitis in a young patient with herpes zoster. *Ophthalmologica 183:*143–147.
Sandyk R. (1982). Pupillary signs in tuberculous meningitis. *S Afr Med J 61:*69.
Sauer C, Levinsohn MW. (1976). Horner's syndrome in childhood. *Neurology 26:*216–220.
Sayed AK, Miller BA, Lacke II, Sallan SE, Levey RH. (1983). Heterochromia iridis and Horner's syndrome due to paravertebral neurilemmoma. *J Surg Oncol 22:*15.
Schachner SM, Reynolds AC. (1982). Horner syndrome during lumbar epidural analgesia for obstetrics. *Obstetr Gynecol 59:*31S–32S.
Scheie HG. (1940). Site of disturbance in Adie's syndrome. *Arch Ophthalmol 24:*225–237.
Schiffter R. (1987). Telodiencephalic ischemic syndrome [letter]. *Arch Neurol 44:*1218–1219.
Schwartz H, Apt L. (1979). Mydriatic effect of anticholinergic drugs used during reversal of nondepolarizing muscle relaxants. *Am J Ophthalmol 88:*609–612.
Scotcher SM, Canning CR, Dorrell D. (1995). Siderosis bulbi: An unusual cause of a unilaterally dilated pupil. *Br J Hosp Med 54:*110–111.

Sears ML, Kier EL, Chavis RM. (1974). Horner's syndrome caused by occlusion of the vascular supply to the sympathetic ganglia. *Am J Ophthalmol 77:*717.

Sears ML. (1971). The cause of Argyll-Robertson pupil. *Am J Ophthalmol 72:*488–489.

Selhorst JB, Hoyt WF, Feinsod M, Hosobuch Y. (1977). Midbrain corectopia. *Arch Neurol 33:*193–195.

Selhorst JB. (1983). The pupil and its disorders. *Neurol Clin 1:*859–881.

Selhorst JB, Madge G, Ghatak M. (1984). The neuropathology of the Holmes-Adies syndrome. *Ann Neurol 16:*138.

Seltzer JL. (1977). Hoarseness and Horner's syndrome after intrascalene brachila plexus block. *Anesth Analg 56:*585–586.

Sen DK. (1979). Isolated pupillary paralysis in a case of herpes zoster. *J Pediatr Ophthalmol Strab 16:*33–34.

Seybold ME, Yoss RE, Hollenhorst RW, Moyer NJ. (1971). Pupillary abnormalities associated with tumors of the pineal region. *Neurology 21:*232–237.

Shaw PJ, Bates NEF, Cartlidge D, et al. (1987). Neuroophthalmological complications of coronary artery bypass graft surgery. *Acta Neurol Scand 76:*1–7.

Shewmon DA. (1983). Unilateral straight hair in congenital Horner syndrome due to stellate ganglion tumor. *Ann Neurol 13:*345–346.

Shuaib A, Israelian G, Lee MA. (1989). Mesencephalic hemorrhage and unilateral pupillary deficit. *J Clin Neuro-ophthalmol 9:*47.

Shy GM, Drager GA. (1960). A neurological syndrome associated with orthostatic hypotension. A clinical-pathological study. *Arch Neurol 2:*511–527.

Sigsbee B, Torkelson R, Kadis G, et al. (1974). Parasympathetic denervation of the iris in diabetes mellitus: A clinical study. *J Neurol Neurosurg Psych 37:*1031–1035.

Simon D, Austin J, Forstot L. (1982). Heterochromia pardus: Implications of the spotted pale iris. *Neuro-ophthalmology 2:*279–291.

Sjaastad O. (1985). The so-called "partial Horner syndrome" in cluster headache. An editorial. *Cephalgia 5:*59–61.

Sjaastad O, Antonaci F, Fragoso YD. (1988). Cluster headache: further observations on the dissociation of pain and autonomic findings. *Cephalgia 8:*127–132.

Skarf B, Czarnecki JSC. (1982). Distinguishing postganglionic from preganglionic lesions. *Arch Ophthalmol 100:*1319–1322.

Slamovits TL. (1987). The pupil in neuro-ophthalmology: Abnormal pupillary reactions and anisocoria. *Semin Ophthalmol 2:*209–228.

Slamovits TL, Miller NR, Burde RM. (1987). Intracranial oculomotor nerve paresis with anisocoria and pupillary parasympathetic hypersensitivity. *Am J Ophthalmol 104:*401–406.

Smith AA, Dancis J, Breinin G. (1965). Ocular responses to autonomic drugs in familial dysautonomia. *Invest Ophthalmol 4:*358–361.

Smith EF, Santamarina L, Wolintz AH. (1993). Herpes zoster ophthalmicus as a cause of Horner syndrome. *J Clin Neuro-ophthalmol 13:*250–253.

Smith RB, Read S, Oczypok PM. (1976). Mydriatic effect of phenylephrine. *Eye Ear Nose Throat J 55:*36–37.

Smith SA, Smith SE. (1983). Evidence of a neuropathic aetiology in the small pupil of diabetes mellitus. *Br J Ophthalmol 67:*89–93.

Smith SE, Smith SA, Brown PM, Cox C, Sonksen PH. (1978). Pupillary signs in diabetic autonomic neuropathy. *Br Med J 2:*924–927.

Smolin G. (1969). Unilateral intermittent pupillary dilatation. *Arch Ophthalmol 81:*705–706.

Soriani S, Scarpa P, Arnaldi C, De Carlo L, Pausini L, Montagna P. (1996). Migraine aura without headache and ictal fast EEG activity in an 11-year-old boy. *Eur J Pediatr 155:*126–129.

Spaeth GL. (1980). The effect of autonomic agents on the pupil and the intraocular pressure of eyes treated with dexamethasone. *Br J Ophthalmol 64:*426–429.

Spector GJ, Druck NS, Gado M. (1976). Neurologic manifestations of glomus tumors in the head and neck. *Arch Neurol 33:*270–274.

Spector RH, Bachman DL. (1984). Bilateral Adie's tonic pupil with anhidrosis and hyperthermia. *Arch Neurol 41:*342–343.

Spencer JA, Czarnecki JS. (1983). The pupil in stroke. *Can J Ophthalmol 18:*226–227.

Spigelblatt L, Benoit P, Jacob JL. (1976). Neuroblastoma with heterochromia and Horner syndrome. *J Ped 88:*1067–1068.

Stern MJ, Patel M, Davis J, Friedwald J, Slavin M. (1989). Painful Horner syndrome associated with occlusion of the extracranial internal carotid artery: MR imaging. *J Comput Assist Tomogr 13:*918–920.

Stillwater LB, Levine PA. (1981). Anisocoria with orbital floor fractures. Worry and wait. *Otolaryngol Head Neck Surg 89:*882.

Stirt JA, Shuptrine JR, Sternick CS, Korbbon GA. (1985). Anisocoria after anesthesia. *Can Anaesth Soc J 32:*422–424.

Stone WM, de Toledo J, Romanul FCA. (1986). Horner's syndrome due to hypothalamic infarction, clinical radiologic and pathologic correlation. *Arch Neurol 43:*199–200.

Striph GG, Burde RM. (1988). Abducens nerve palsy and Horner's syndrome revisited. *J Clin Neuro-ophthalmol 8:*13–17.

Stromberg BC, Knibbe M. (1988). Anisocoria following reduction of bilateral orbital floor fractures. *Ann Plast Surg 21:*486–488.

Sundaram MB. (1985). Pupillary abnormalities in congenital neurosyphilis. *Can J Neurol Sci 12:*134–135.

Sunderland S. (1952). Mechanism responsible for changes in the pupil unaccompanied by disturbances of extraocular muscle function. *Br J Ophthalmol 36:*638–644.

Szawlowski AW, Falkowski S, Morysinski T, et al. (1991). Preoperative concurrent chemotherapy and radiotherapy for local-regional and advanced squamous cell carcinoma of the thoracic oesophagus: Preliminary results of a pilot study. *Eur J Surg Oncol 17:*575–580.

Talamo JH, Topping TM, Maumenee AE, Green WR. (1985). Ultrastructural studies of cornea, iris and lens in a case of siderosis bulbi. *Ophthalmology 92:*1675–1680.

Tan AK, Humphry RC. (1993). The fixed pupil after cataract surgery—is it related to intraocular use of hypromellose? *Br J Ophthalmol 77:*639–641.

Tan E, Kansu T, Saygi S, Zileli T. (1990). Alternating Horner's syndrome. A case report and review of the literature. *Neuro-ophthalmology 10:*19–22.

Teich SA, Halpin SL, Tay S. (1985). Horner's syndrome secondary to Swan Ganz catheterization. *Am J Med 78:*168–170.

Thomashefsky AJ, Horwitz SJ, Feingold MH. (1972). Acute autonomic neuropathy. *Neurology 22:*251–255.

Thompson HS, Bourgon P, Van Allen MW. (1979). The tendon reflexes in Adie's syndrome. In Thompson HS, Daroff R, Frisen L, et al., (eds). *Topics in Neuro-ophthalmology*. Baltimore, Williams and Wilkins, pp. 104–113.

Thompson HS, Corbett JJ, Kline LB, et al. (1982). Pseudo-Horner's syndrome. *Arch Neurol 39:*108–111.

Thompson HS, Mensher JH. (1971). Adrenergic mydriasis in Horner's syndrome. Hydroxyamphetamine test for diagnosis of postganglionic defects. *Am J Ophthalmol 72:*472–480.

Thompson HS, Mensher JH, Serrs ML. (1975). Hydroxyamphetamine test in Horner's syndrome. *Reply Am J Ophthalmol 79:*525.

Thompson HS, Newsome DA, Loewenfeld IE. (1971). The fixed dilated pupil: Sudden iridoplegia or mydriatic drops? A simple diagnostic test. *Arch Ophthalmol 86:*21–27.

Thompson HS, Pilley SFJ. (1976). Unequal pupils: A flow chart for sorting out the anisocorias. *Surv Ophthalmol 21:*45–48.

Thompson HS, Pilley SJ. (1976). Unequal pupils: A flow chart for sorting out the anisocorias. *Surv Ophthalmol 21:*45–48.

Thompson HS, Zackon DH, Czarnecki JSC. (1983). Tadpole-shaped pupils caused by segmental spasm of the iris dilator muscle. *Am J Ophthalmol 96:*467–477.

Thompson HS. (1979). A classification of "tonic pupils." In Thompson HS, Daroff R, Frisen L, et al., (eds). *Topics in Neuro-ophthalmology*. Baltimore, Williams and Wilkins, pp. 95–96.

Thompson HS. (1977b). Adie's syndrome: Some new observations. *Trans Am Ophthalmol Soc 75:*587–626.

Thompson HS. (1971). Cornpicker's pupil: Jimson weed mydriasis. *J Iowa Med Soc 61:*475–477.

Thompson HS. (1977a). Diagnosing Horner's syndrome. *Trans Am Acad Ophthalmol Otolaryngol 83:*840–842.

Thompson HS. (1975). Pupillary light-near dissociation. A classification. *Surv Ophthalmol 19:*290–293.

Thompson HS. (1984). Pupillary light-near dissociation. *Ophthalmologica 189:*21–23.

Thompson HS. (1978). Segmental palsy of the iris sphincter in Adie's syndrome. *Arch Ophthalmol 96:*1615–1620.

Thompson HS. (1977c). Symposium: Pupil in clinical diagnosis. *Trans Am Acad Ophthalmol Otol 83:*847–848.

Thompson HS. (1975). Tables of diagnostic pupillary drug tests. *Bristol Medico-Chiru J 90:*37–38.

Treasure R, Garnett R, O'Connor J, et al. (1980). Injury to the lower trunk of the brachial plexus as a complication of median sternotomy for cardiac surgery. *Ann R Coll Surg Engl 62:*378.

Tress KH, El-Sobky AA. (1979). Pupil responses to intravenous heroin (diamorphine) in dependent and non-dependent humans. *Br J Clin Pharmacol 7:*213–217.

Ulrich J. (1980). Morphologic basis of Adie's syndrome. *Eur Neurol 19:*390–395.

Uribe LE. (1967). Fixed pupil following keratoplasty: Evaluation of six cases. *Am J Ophthalmol 63:*1682–1686.

Urrets-Zavalia A Jr. (1963). Fixed dilated pupil, iris atrophy and secondary glaucoma: A distinct clinical entity following penetrating keratoplasty in keratoconus. *Am J Ophthalmol 56:*257–265.

Van Der Weil HL, Van Gijn J. (1982). Localization of Horner's syndrome. Criteria for oculosympathetic denervation. *J Neurol Sci 56:*293–298.

Van Der Weil HL, Van Gijn J. (1983). Localization of Horner's syndrome: Use and limitations of the hydroxyamphetamine test. *J Neurol Sci 59:*229–235.

Van Der Weil HL, Van Gijn J. (1988). The diagnosis of Horner's syndrome. *Clin Neurol Neurosurg 90:*103–108.

Van Der Weil HL, Van Gijn J. (1986). The diagnosis of Horner's syndrome: Use and limitations of the cocaine test. *J Neurol Sci 73:*311–316.

Vaswani S, Garvin L, Matuschak GM. (1991). Postganglionic Horner's syndrome after insertion of a pulmonary artery catheter through the internal jugular vein. *Cr Care Med 19:*1215–1216.

Verdier DD, Kennerdall JS. (1982). Fixed dilated pupil resulting from transdermal scopolamine (letter). *Am J Ophthalmol 93:*803–804.

Victor DI, Green WR, Stark WJ, Walsh FB. (1977). A non-permanent tonic pupil in rheumatoid arteritis. *Can J Neurol Sci 4:*209–212.

Vighetto A, Lisovoski F, Revol A, Trillet M, Almard G. (1990). Internal carotid artery dissection and ipsilateral hyoglossal nerve palsy (letter). *J Neurol Neurosurg Psych 53:*530–531.

Vijayan N. (1977). A new post-traumatic headache syndrome: Clinical and therapeutic observations. *Headache 17*:19–22.
Vijayan N, Watson C. (1978). Pericarotid syndrome. *Headache 18*:244–254.
Vijayan N, Watson C. (1982). Evaluation of oculosympathetic function in vascular headache syndrome. II. Oculocephalic sympathetic function in cluster headaches. *Headache 22*:200–202.
Voorhies RM, Fraser RA. (1981). Transient mydriasis: In Horner's syndrome following surgery. *Neuro-ophthalmology 1*:295–296.
Vrints J, Vanhemelrijck J, Vandermeersch E, Van Aken H. (1989). Perioperative anisocoria after extravasal loss of iv fluids in the neck. *Acta Anaesthesiol Belg 40*:85–86.
Watson C, Vijayan N. (1982). Evaluation of oculocephalic sympathetic function in vascular headache syndromes. Part I: Methods of evaluation. *Headache 22*:192–199.
Weinstein JM, Zweifel TJ, Thompson HS. (1980). Congenital Horner's syndrome. *Arch Ophthalmol 98*:1074–1078.
Weintraub MI, Gaasterland D, Van Woert MH. (1970). Pupillary effects of levodopa therapy: Development of anisocoria in latent Horner's syndrome. *N Engl J Med 283*:120–123.
Weintraub MI, Ribner JA, Gallagher BB. (1971). Transient internal ophthalmoplegia. *Arch Ophthalmol 86*:595–598.
Weisfeld L, Streeten BW. (1978). Horner's syndrome with ipsilateral accommodative paresis. *Am J Ophthalmol 86*:114–114.
Welch RB. (1975). Two remarkable events in the field of intraocular foreign body: 1) The reversal of siderosis bulbi. 2) The spontaneous extrusion of an intraocular foreign copper body. *Trans Am Ophthalmol Soc 73*:187–199.
Weller M, Wilhelm H, Sommer N, Dichgans J, Wietholter H. (1992). Tonic pupil, areflexia, and segmental anhidrosis: Two additional cases of Ross syndrome and review of the literature. *J Neurol 239*:231–234.
Wentworth WO, Brubaker RF. (1981). Aqueous humor dynamics in a series of patients with third order neuron Horner's syndrome. *Am J Ophthalmol 92*:407–415.
West TET, Davies RJ, Kelly RE. (1976). Horner's syndrome and headache due to carotid artery disease. *Br Med J 1*:818–820.
Wichler J, Vijayan N, Dreyfus PM. (1972). Dysautonomia: Its significance in neurologic disease. *Calif Med 117*:28–37.
Wilhelm H. (1994). Pupil examination and evaluation of pupillary disorders. *Neuro-ophthalmology 14*:283–295.
Wilhelm H, Klier R, Toth B, Wilhelm B. (1995). Oculomotor nerve paresis starting as isolated internal ophthalmoplegia. *Neuro-ophthalmology 15*:211–215.
Wilhelm H, Ochsner H, Kopycziok E, et al. (1992). Horner's syndrome: a retrospective analysis of 90 cases and recommendations for clinical handling. *German J Ophthalmol 1*:96–102.
Williams D, Brust JCM, Abrams G, Challenor Y, Devereaux M. (1979). Landry-Guillain-Barré syndrome with abnormal pupils and normal eye movements. *Neurology 29*:1033–1036.
Wimlararatna HSK, Capildeo R, Lee HY. (1987). Herpes zoster of second and third segments causing ipsilateral Horner's syndrome. *Br Med J 294*:1463.
Winnie AP, Ramamurthy S, Durrani Z, Radonjic R, Shaker MH. (1974). Pharmacologic reversal of Horner's syndrome following stellate ganglionic block. *Anesthesiology 41*:615–617.
Wirtschafter JD, Herman WK. (1980). Low concentration eserine therapy for tonic pupil (Adie) syndrome. *Ophthalmol 87*:1037–1043.
Wolfe GI, Galetta SL, Teener JW, Katz JS, Bird SJ. (1995). Site of autonomic dysfunction in a patient with Ross' syndrome and postganglionic Horner's syndrome. *Neurology 45*:2094–2096.
Woodruff G, Buncic JR, Morin JD. (1988). Horner's syndrome in children. *J Ped Ophthalmol Strab 25*:40–44.
Woods D, O'Connor PS, Fleming R. (1984). Episodic unilateral mydriasis and migraine. *Am J Ophthalmol 98*:229–234.
Yee RD, Trese M, Zee DS, Kollarits CR, Cogan DG. (1976). Ocular manifestations of acute pandysautonomia. *Am J Ophthalmol 81*:740–744.
Young RR, Asbury AK, Adams RD, Corbett JL. (1969). Pure dysautonomia with recovery. *Trans Am Neurol Assoc 94*:355–347.
Young RR, Asbury AK, Adams RD, Corbett JL. (1975). Pure dysautonomia with recovery. Description and diagnostic criteria. *Brain 98*:613–636.
Younge RB, Buski ZJ. (1976). Tonic pupil. A simple screening test. *Can J Ophthalmol 11*:295–299.
Zak TA. (1983). Benign episodic bilateral juvenile internal ophthalmoplegia. *J Pediatr Ophthalmol Strab 20*:8–10.
Zee DS, Griffin J, Price DL. (1974). Unilateral pupillary dilatation during adversive seizures. *Arch Neurol 30*:403–405.
Zelligowsky A, Szold A, Seror D, Vromen A, Pffeffermann R. (1991). Horner syndrome: A rare complication of internal jugular vein cannulation. *J Parent Enter Nutrition 15*:199.
Zito G, Gennaro P. (1982). Clinical evaluation of anisocoria. *Arch Neurol 39*:604.

♦ Index ♦

Page numbers in *italic* indicate figures. Page numbers followed by "t" indicate tables.